Nurse's
Quick
Check

Signs &
Symptoms

Nurse's
Quick
Check

Signs &
Symptoms

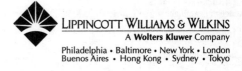

LIPPINCOTT WILLIAMS & WILKINS
A **Wolters Kluwer** Company

Philadelphia • Baltimore • New York • London
Buenos Aires • Hong Kong • Sydney • Tokyo

STAFF

Executive Publisher
Judith A. Schilling McCann, RN, MSN

Editorial Director
William J. Kelly

Clinical Director
Joan M. Robinson, RN, MSN

Senior Art Director
Arlene Putterman

Editorial Project Manager
Christiane L. Brownell

Clinical Project Manager
Mary Perrong, RN, CRNP, MSN, APRN,BC

Editor
Carol Koetke

Clinical Editors
Marcy Caplin, RN, MSN; Kathryn Henry, RN, BSN, CCRC; Carol A. Saunderson, RN, BA, BS

Designers
Will Boehm (book design),
Susan L. Sheridan (project manager)

Digital Composition Services
Diane Paluba (manager), Joyce Rossi Biletz,
Donna S. Morris

Manufacturing
Patricia K. Dorshaw (director), Beth J. Welsh

Editorial Assistants
Megan L. Aldinger, Karen J. Kirk, Linda K. Ruhf

Indexer
Barbara Hodgson

Library of Congress Cataloging-in-Publication Data

Nurse's quick check. Signs & symptoms.
   p. ; cm.
   Includes bibliographical references and index.
   1. Nursing assessment—Handbooks, manuals, etc. 2. Nursing diagnosis—Handbooks, manuals, etc. 3. Symptoms—Handbooks, manuals, etc. I. Title: Signs & symptoms. II. Lippincott Williams & Wilkins.
   [DNLM: 1. Nursing Assessment--Handbooks. 2. Signs and Symptoms—Handbooks. WY 49 N97425 2006]
   RT48.N853 2006
   616.07'5—dc22
   ISBN 1-58255-413-7 (alk. paper)   2004029627

Contents

Contributors
and consultants

Valerie J. Flattes, APRN,BC, ANP
Associate Instructor, Clinical
University of Utah College of Nursing
Salt Lake City

Stephen Gilliam, APRN,BC, PhD, FNP
Assistant Professor
Medical College of Georgia
School of Nursing
Athens

Janice D. Hausauer, RN, MS, FNP
Adjunct Assistant Professor
Montana State University College of Nursing
Bozeman

Nancy Banfield Johnson, RN, MSN
Nurse-Manager
Kendal at Ithaca (N.Y.)

Priscilla A. Lee, MN, FNP-C
Nurse Practitioner
Priscilla A. Lee, FNP Nursing, Inc.
Westlake Village, Calif.

Rosemary Macy, RN, PhD(c)
Assistant Professor
Boise (Idaho) State University

Donna Scemons, RN, MSN, CNS, CWOCN, FNP-C
Family Nurse Practitioner
Healthcare Systems, Inc.
Castaic, Cailf.

Sandra M. Waguespack, RN, MSN
Clinical Instructor
Louisiana State University Health Sciences Center
  School of Nursing
New Orleans

Marsha Wamsley, RN, MS
Associate Professor
Sinclair Community College
Dayton, Ohio

Foreword

Nursing in the 21st century is recognized as a highly rewarding profession that's distinguished for its unique knowledge and expertise. Nurses today acquire this knowledge and expertise through formal education and later through experience, seminars, and useful reference texts.

Nurse's Quick Check: Signs & Symptoms is a book that offers nurses an excellent reference on common signs and symptoms. As an assistant professor of nursing, I highly recommend this text, which is valuable for all areas of nursing. The text is geared toward registered nurses, licensed practical nurses, and nursing students; other health care providers will also find it useful. The easy-reading bullet points outline more than 200 common signs and symptoms in alphabetical order, each in its own two- or four- page entry.

The Overview section defines each sign or symptom and gives possible causes and other key specifications. The Assessment section tells you which specific history questions to ask and identifies the physical signs that may arise. The Physical Assessment section tells you which body systems to examine and which specific findings to look for. For the expert nurse, this book may be a review, but for the novice or student nurse, it gives information needed to become an expert.

The Medical Causes section provides an extensive list of common diagnoses for each sign or symptom with bullet points of findings for the specific diagnosis. The section also covers which symptoms can be expected as the illness progresses. Other Causes appear separately as possible origins of the sign or symptom that aren't related to illness and usually are a result of a diagnostic test or treatment.

Nursing Considerations offers a care plan for the nurse that can be personalized for the patient and include pointers for pediatric (children from birth to age 18) and geriatric (adults age 65 and older) care. The last section also includes Patient Teaching bullets offering techniques and advice that allow for optimal care.

To help readers find key information quickly, the book highlights two recurring themes: emergency actions and assessment tips. Emergency actions, appearing in italic type with a special symbol, identify emerging events and outline which actions the nurse should take. Throughout the book, you'll see boxes called "Assessment tip." These tips show, usually with a picture, drawing, or flowchart, exactly what to do to effectively assess your patient.

The profession of nursing is rapidly progressing; nurses are caring for patients with increasing medical complexities and multiple diagnoses. Nurses are being recognized for their knowledge, expertise, and dedication to study. The signs and symptoms in this book represent those that will be encountered in almost every nurse's professional practice. A nurse will be able to use this book, either at the nurse's station as a reference or at the bedside of a patient with a specific sign or symptom.

Joanne Haeffele, RN, MSN, FNP
Assistant Professor of Nursing
University of Utah College of Nursing
Salt Lake City

*Nurse's
Quick
Check*

Signs &
Symptoms

Abdominal distention

Overview

- Increased abdominal girth from increased intra-abdominal pressure
- Occurs when increased fluid and gas can't pass freely through the GI tract
- Can be mild or severe, localized or diffuse, and gradual or sudden
- May reflect acute bleeding, accumulation of ascitic fluid, or buildup of air from perforation of an abdominal organ

⭐ Emergency actions

Quickly check for signs of hypovolemia, difficulty breathing, or severe abdominal pain. Ask about recent accidents and observe for signs of trauma and peritoneal bleeding, such as Cullen's sign (ecchymosis around the umbilicus) or Turner's sign (ecchymosis over the flanks). Auscultate all abdominal quadrants, noting rapid and high-pitched, diminished, or absent bowel sounds. Gently palpate the abdomen for rigidity.

If you detect rigidity along with abnormal bowel sounds, and the patient complains of pain, begin emergency interventions. Place the patient in the supine position, administer oxygen, and insert an I.V. line for fluid replacement. Insert a nasogastric tube to relieve acute intraluminal distention and get the patient ready for surgery.

Assessment

History

- Ask about onset and duration.
- Localized distention may cause a sensation of pressure, fullness, or tenderness.
- Generalized distention may cause perceived bloating, heart pounding, and difficulty breathing when lying flat or breathing deeply.
- Other signs and symptoms may include abdominal pain, fever, nausea, vomiting, anorexia, altered bowel habits, and weight gain or loss.
- Obtain a medical history, noting GI or biliary disorders, chronic constipation, abdominal surgery, and recent accidents.

Physical assessment

- Observe the recumbent patient for abdominal asymmetry.
- Assess abdominal contour.
- Inspect for tense, glistening skin and bulging flanks, which may indicate ascites.
- Observe for everted or inverted umbilicus.
- Inspect the abdomen for signs of inguinal or femoral hernia and for incisions.
- Auscultate for bowel sounds, abdominal rubs, and bruits.
- Percuss and palpate the abdomen.
- Prepare the patient for pelvic or genital examination.
- Measure abdominal girth for a baseline value.

Medical causes

Abdominal cancer

- Generalized distention may occur when advanced cancer (ovarian, hepatic, or pancreatic) produces ascites.
- Other signs and symptoms may include severe abdominal pain, anorexia, jaundice, GI hemorrhage, dyspepsia, weight loss, abdominal mass, and muscle weakness and atrophy.

Abdominal trauma

- Acute and dramatic distention may occur with brisk internal bleeding.
- Other signs and symptoms include abdominal rigidity with guarding, decreased or absent bowel sounds, vomiting, tenderness, abdominal bruising, pain over the trauma site or scapula, and, if blood loss is significant, hypovolemic shock.

Bladder distention

- Distention occurs in the lower abdomen.
- In mild bladder distention, slight dullness on percussion above the symphysis pubis.
- In severe bladder distention, there's a palpable, smooth, rounded suprapubic mass.

Cirrhosis

- Ascites causes generalized distention.
- Umbilical eversion and *caput medusae* (dilated veins around the umbilicus) are common.
- The patient may report a feeling of fullness or weight gain.
- Other signs and symptoms include vague abdominal pain, hepatomegaly, fever, anorexia, nausea, vomiting, constipation or diarrhea, bleeding tendencies, severe pruritus, palmar erythema, spider angiomas, leg edema, and jaundice (a late sign).

Heart failure

- In severe cardiovascular impairment, ascites causes generalized abdominal distention.
- Hallmark signs and symptoms include peripheral edema, jugular vein distention, dyspnea, and tachycardia.
- Other signs and symptoms include hepatomegaly, nausea, vomiting, productive cough, crackles, cool extremities, cyanotic nail beds, nocturia, exercise intolerance, nocturnal wheezing, diastolic hypertension, and cardiomegaly.

Irritable bowel syndrome

○ Periodic intestinal spasms may cause intermittent, localized distention.
○ Lower abdominal pain or cramping typically accompanies intestinal spasms.
○ Pain is usually relieved by defecation or passage of intestinal gas and is aggravated by stress.
○ Other signs and symptoms include diarrhea that may alternate with constipation or normal bowel function; nausea; dyspepsia; straining or urgency at defecation; feeling of incomplete evacuation; and small, mucus-streaked stools.

Large-bowel obstruction

○ A life-threatening disorder — it's characterized by dramatic abdominal distention.
○ Constipation precedes distention.
○ Other findings include tympany, high-pitched bowel sounds, and the sudden onset of colicky lower abdominal pain.
○ Late signs include fecal vomiting and diminished peristaltic waves.

Mesenteric artery occlusion (acute)

○ A life-threatening disorder — abdominal distention usually occurs several hours after the sudden onset of severe, colicky periumbilical pain and rapid or forceful bowel evacuation.
○ Pain later becomes constant and diffuse.
○ Other signs and symptoms include severe abdominal tenderness with guarding and rigidity, absent bowel sounds, vomiting, anorexia, diarrhea, constipation, and, occasionally, a bruit in the right iliac fossa.
○ Late signs include fever; tachycardia; tachypnea; hypotension; and cool, clammy skin.

Nephrotic syndrome

○ Massive edema causes generalized distention with a fluid wave and shifting dullness.

Ovarian cysts

○ Lower abdominal distention is accompanied by umbilical eversion.
○ Lower abdominal pain and a palpable mass may be present.

Paralytic ileus

○ Generalized distention occurs with a tympanic percussion note.
○ Bowel sounds may be absent or hypoactive.
○ Other signs and symptoms include vomiting and severe constipation or flatus with small, frequent stools.

Peritonitis

○ Localized or generalized abdominal distention with sudden and severe abdominal pain that worsens with movement.
○ Rebound tenderness and abdominal rigidity may be present.

○ Other signs and symptoms include hypoactive or absent bowel sounds, fever, chills, nausea, vomiting, and signs of shock (with significant blood loss).

Small-bowel obstruction

○ A life-threatening disorder — abdominal distention is most pronounced during late obstruction, especially in the distal small bowel.
○ Bowel sounds may be hypoactive or hyperactive, with tympany.
○ Other signs and symptoms include colicky periumbilical pain, constipation, nausea, vomiting, drowsiness, malaise, dehydration, and signs of hypovolemic shock.

Toxic megacolon (acute)

○ A life-threatening disorder — dramatic abdominal distention usually develops gradually.
○ Bowel sounds may be diminished or absent.
○ Abdominal pain and rebound tenderness, fever, tachycardia, and dehydration are also present.

Nursing considerations

○ Position the patient comfortably, using pillows for support.
○ Place him on his left side to help flatus escape.
○ If the patient has ascites, elevate the head of the bed to ease breathing.
○ Give the patient drugs that relieve pain.
○ Offer emotional support.
○ Prepare the patient for diagnostic tests.

Pediatric pointers

○ Distention may be difficult to observe in children.
○ Ascites, congenital malformations of the GI tract, overeating, and constipation are likely causes in children.
○ In neonates, abdominal distention caused by ascites usually results from GI or urinary perforation; in older children, from heart failure, cirrhosis, or nephrosis.

Geriatric pointers

○ Don't confuse distention with a potbelly, a common effect of aging.

Patient teaching

○ Teach the patient to use slow breathing to help relieve abdominal discomfort.
○ If the patient has an obstruction or ascites, tell him which foods and fluids to avoid.
○ Emphasize the importance of oral hygiene to prevent dry mouth.

Abdominal mass

Overview

○ Manifests as localized swelling in one abdominal quadrant
○ May signify an enlarged organ, a neoplasm, an abscess, a vascular defect, or a fecal mass

⚡ Emergency actions

If the patient has a pulsating midabdominal mass and severe abdominal or back pain, suspect an abdominal aneurysm. Quickly take vital signs. Withhold food and fluids until the patient is examined. Administer oxygen and to start an I.V. infusion for fluid and blood replacement. Look for signs of shock, which occurs with significant blood loss.

Assessment

History

○ If mass is painful, ask if pain is constant or occurs only with palpation and is localized or generalized.
○ Ask if mass has changed size or location.
○ Obtain a medical history, noting GI disorders.
○ Other symptoms may include constipation, diarrhea, rectal bleeding, abnormally colored stools, vomiting, and changes in appetite.
○ Ask women to describe their menstrual cycles.

Physical assessment

○ Auscultate first, listening for bruits or rubs.
○ Percuss the mass, noting the sound.
○ Lightly palpate and then deeply palpate the abdomen, assessing painful or suspicious areas last.
○ Estimate the size of the mass and determine its shape and consistency.
○ Note whether mass is palpable in supine and side-lying positions.
○ Determine if the mass moves with your hand or in response to respiration.
○ Note contour and consistency of the mass.

Medical causes

Abdominal aortic aneurysm

○ A life-threatening disorder — it produces severe upper abdominal pain or, less often, lower back or dull abdominal pain if rupture occurs.
○ Condition may persist for years, producing only a pulsating periumbilical mass with a systolic bruit over the aorta.
○ Other signs and symptoms of rupture include mottled skin below the waist, absent femoral and pedal pulses, lower blood pressure in the legs than in the arms, mild to moderate tenderness with guarding, abdominal rigidity, and shock (with significant blood loss).

Bladder distention

○ A smooth, rounded, fluctuant suprapubic mass develops.
○ With extreme distention, the mass may extend to the umbilicus.
○ Severe suprapubic pain and urinary frequency may also develop.

Cholecystitis

○ Deep palpation below the liver border may reveal a smooth, firm, sausage-shaped mass.
○ With acute inflammation, the gallbladder may be too tender to be palpated.
○ May produce severe right-upper-quadrant pain that may radiate to the right shoulder, chest or back; abdominal rigidity and tenderness; fever; pallor; diaphoresis; anorexia; nausea; and vomiting.
○ Attacks typically occur 1 to 6 hours after meals.
○ Murphy's sign (inspiratory arrest brought about while palpating the right upper quadrant when the patient takes a deep breath) is common.

Cholelithiasis

○ A painless, smooth, and sausage-shaped mass develops in the right upper quadrant.
○ Other signs and symptoms include anorexia, nausea, vomiting, chills, diaphoresis, restlessness, low-grade fever, jaundice (if common bile duct is obstructed), intolerance to fatty foods, and indigestion.
○ Passage of a calculus through the bile duct or cystic duct may cause severe right-upper-quadrant pain that radiates to the epigastrium, back, or shoulder blades.

Colon cancer

○ If in the right colon, a right-lower-quadrant mass may occur with occult bleeding and anemia and abdominal aching, pressure, or dull cramps.
○ Other signs and symptoms of right colon cancer include weakness, fatigue, exertional dyspnea, vertigo, and, with intestinal obstruction, obstipation and vomiting.
○ If in the left colon, a palpable mass produces rectal bleeding and pressure, intermittent abdominal fullness or cramping, and pain relief with defecation.
○ Late signs of left colon cancer include obstipation; diarrhea; or pencil-shaped, grossly bloody, or mucus-streaked stools.

Crohn's disease

○ Tender, sausage-shaped masses are usually palpable in the right lower quadrant and, at times, in the left lower quadrant.
○ Colicky right-lower-quadrant pain and diarrhea are common.
○ Other signs and symptoms include fever; anorexia; weight loss; hyperactive bowel sounds; nausea; ab-

dominal tenderness with guarding; and perirectal, skin, or vaginal fistulas.

Diverticulitis

○ A left-lower-quadrant mass that's usually tender, firm, and fixed may develop.
○ Other signs and symptoms may include intermittent abdominal pain that's relieved by defecating or passing flatus, alternating diarrhea and constipation, nausea, low-grade fever, and a distended and tympanic abdomen.

Gallbladder cancer

○ A moderately tender, irregular mass may develop in the right upper quadrant.
○ Chronic, progressively severe epigastric or right-upper-quadrant pain that may radiate to the right shoulder occurs.
○ Other signs and symptoms include nausea, vomiting, anorexia, weight loss, jaundice and, at times, hepatomegaly.

Gastric cancer

○ An epigastric mass may develop.
○ Early findings include chronic dyspepsia and epigastric discomfort.
○ Late findings include weight loss, feeling of fullness, fatigue and, occasionally, coffee-ground vomitus or melena.

Hepatic cancer

○ A tender, nodular mass in the right upper quadrant or right epigastric area develops.
○ Pain is aggravated by jolting.
○ Other signs and symptoms may include weight loss, weakness, anorexia, nausea, fever, dependent edema, jaundice, ascites, and a bruit or hum (if the tumor is large).

Hepatomegaly

○ A firm, blunt, irregular mass in the epigastric region or below the right costal margin
○ Ascites, right-upper-quadrant pain and tenderness, anorexia, nausea, vomiting, leg edema, jaundice, palmar erythema, spider angiomas, gynecomastia, testicular atrophy, and splenomegaly

Hydronephrosis

○ A smooth, boggy mass in one or both flanks
○ Severe colicky renal pain or dull flank pain that radiates to the groin, vulva, or testes
○ Hematuria, pyuria, dysuria, alternating oliguria and polyuria, nocturia, accelerated hypertension, nausea, and vomiting

Ovarian cyst

○ A smooth, rounded, fluctuant mass may develop in the suprapubic region.
○ Mild pelvic discomfort, lower back pain, menstrual irregularities, and hirsutism may occur with large or multiple cysts.

○ Abdominal tenderness, distention, and rigidity may occur with twisted or ruptured cysts.

Pancreatic abscess

○ Occasionally, a palpable epigastric mass may develop.
○ Epigastric pain and tenderness occur.
○ Other signs and symptoms may include nausea, vomiting, diarrhea, tachycardia, hypotension, and an abrupt rise in temperature (although it may also rise steadily).

Renal cell cancer

○ A smooth, firm, nontender mass develops near the affected kidney.
○ Dull, constant abdominal or flank pain and hematuria occur.
○ Other signs and symptoms include elevated blood pressure, fever, and urine retention.
○ Weight loss, nausea, vomiting, and leg edema occur in late stages.

Splenomegaly

○ The spleen is palpable in the left upper quadrant.
○ Other signs and symptoms may include a feeling of abdominal fullness, left-upper-quadrant pain and tenderness, splenic rub, splenic bruits, and low-grade fever.

Uterine leiomyomas (fibroids)

○ A round, multinodular mass may develop in the suprapubic region.
○ Menorrhagia, a feeling of heaviness in the abdomen, back pain, constipation, urinary frequency and urgency, and edema and varicosities of the leg may occur.

Nursing considerations

○ Offer emotional support to the patient and his family.
○ Position the patient comfortably.
○ Give drugs for pain or anxiety as needed.
○ If bowel obstruction occurs, watch for indications of peritonitis and shock.

Pediatric pointers

○ In neonates, most abdominal masses result from renal disorders.
○ In older infants and children, abdominal masses are usually caused by enlarged organs.
○ Other common causes include Wilms' tumor, neuroblastoma, intussusception, volvulus, Hirschsprung's disease (congenital megacolon), pyloric stenosis, and abdominal abscess.

Geriatric pointers

○ Ultrasonography is used to evaluate a prominent midepigastric mass in thin, elderly patients.

Patient teaching

○ Explain any diagnostic tests that are needed.

Ababdominal pain

Overview

○ Abdominal pain arises from the abdominopelvic viscera, the parietal peritoneum, or the capsules of the liver, kidney, or spleen.
○ Pain may be acute or chronic, diffuse or localized.
○ Visceral pain develops slowly into a deep, dull, aching pain that's poorly localized in the epigastric, periumbilical, or lower midabdominal region.
○ Somatic (parietal, peritoneal) pain produces a sharp, more intense, and well-localized discomfort that rapidly follows the insult and is aggravated by coughing.
○ Sharp, well-localized, referred pain is felt in skin or deeper tissues.

⭐ Emergency actions

If the patient is experiencing sudden and severe abdominal pain, quickly take his vital signs and palpate pulses below the waist. Be alert for signs of hypovolemic shock. Start an I.V. line. If skin is mottled below the waist with a pulsating epigastric mass or rebound tenderness and rigidity, the patient may need emergency surgery.

Assessment

History

○ Obtain a medical history, noting previous abdominal pain; substance abuse; vascular, GI, genitourinary, or reproductive disorders; and menstrual patterns and changes.
○ Ask the patient to describe pain, including quality, quantity, frequency, duration, location, radiation, and what aggravates and alleviates pain.
○ Other signs and symptoms may include changes in appetite, increased flatulence, constipation, diarrhea, changes in bowel movements, and urinary frequency and urgency, and painful urination.
○ Constant, steady abdominal pain suggests organ perforation, ischemia, or inflammation or blood in the abdominal cavity.
○ Intermittent, cramping abdominal pain suggests an obstruction of a hollow organ.

Physical assessment

○ Take the patient's vital signs.
○ Assess skin turgor and mucous membranes.
○ Inspect the patient's abdomen for distention or visible peristaltic waves and measure his abdomen.
○ Auscultate for bowel sounds and characterize their motility.
○ Percuss all quadrants, noting the percussion sounds.
○ Palpate the entire abdomen for masses, rigidity, and tenderness.

○ Check for costovertebral angle tenderness, abdominal tenderness with guarding, and rebound tenderness.

Medical causes

Abdominal aortic aneurysm (dissecting)

○ A life-threatening disorder — it's characterized initially by dull lower abdominal, lower back, or severe chest pain.
○ Constant upper abdominal pain may worsen when the patient lies down and subside when the patient leans forward or sits up.
○ Pulsating epigastric mass may be palpated before rupture but not after it.
○ Other signs and symptoms include mottled skin and absent pulses below the waist, lower blood pressure in the legs than in the arms, abdominal tenderness with guarding, abdominal rigidity, and signs of shock.

Abdominal trauma

○ Generalized or localized abdominal pain occurs with abdominal tenderness, vomiting, and ecchymoses on the abdomen.
○ Hemorrhage into the peritoneal cavity, causes abdominal rigidity.
○ Bowel sounds are decreased or absent.
○ Hypovolemic shock may occur.

Adrenal crisis

○ Severe abdominal pain appears early.
○ Other signs and symptoms include nausea, vomiting, dehydration, profound weakness, anorexia, and fever.
○ Late signs include progressive loss of consciousness; hypotension; tachycardia; oliguria; cool, clammy skin; and increased motor activity, which may progress to delirium or seizures.

Anthrax, GI

○ Initial signs and symptoms include loss of appetite, nausea, vomiting, and fever.
○ Abdominal pain, severe bloody diarrhea, and hematemesis are late signs and symptoms.

Appendicitis

○ A life-threatening disorder — pain initially occurs in the epigastric or umbilical region then localizes at McBurney's point in the right lower quadrant.
○ Pain is accompanied by abdominal rigidity, tenderness, and rebound tenderness.
○ Other signs and symptoms include anorexia, nausea, and vomiting.
○ Late signs include malaise, constipation (or diarrhea), low-grade fever, and tachycardia.

Cholecystitis

○ Severe pain in the right upper quadrant may arise suddenly or increase gradually over several hours, usually after meals.
○ Pain may radiate to right shoulder, chest, or back.

- Other signs and symptoms are anorexia, nausea, vomiting, fever, abdominal rigidity, tenderness, pallor, and diaphoresis.
- Murphy's sign (inspiratory arrest brought about by palpating the right upper quadrant while the patient takes a deep breath) is common.

Cholelithiasis
- Sudden, severe, and paroxysmal pain in the right upper quadrant may radiate to the epigastrium, back, or shoulder blades.
- Other signs and symptoms include anorexia, nausea, vomiting (sometimes bilious), diaphoresis, restlessness, abdominal tenderness with guarding, fatty food intolerance, and indigestion.

Cirrhosis
- Dull abdominal aching early in the disorder's progression
- Abdominal aching with anorexia, indigestion, nausea, vomiting, constipation, or diarrhea
- Worse pain in the right upper quadrant when the patient sits up or leans forward
- Fever, ascites, leg edema, weight gain, hepatomegaly, jaundice, severe pruritus, bleeding tendencies, palmar erythema, and spider angiomas

Crohn's disease
- Acute attacks result in severe cramping pain in lower abdomen.
- Weeks or months of milder cramping pain typically precede an attack.
- Abdominal pain may be relieved by defecation.
- Chronic signs and symptoms include right-lower-quadrant pain with diarrhea, steatorrhea, and weight loss.
- Other signs include diarrhea, hyperactive bowel sounds, dehydration, weight loss, fever, abdominal tenderness with guarding, and a palpable mass in a lower quadrant.

Cystitis
- Abdominal pain and tenderness are usually suprapubic.
- Associates signs and symptoms include malaise, flank pain, low back pain, nausea, vomiting, urinary frequency and urgency, nocturia, dysuria, fever, and chills.

Diverticulitis
- Intermittent, diffuse left-lower-quadrant pain usually occurs in mild cases.
- Pain may be relieved by defecation or passage of flatus and worsened by eating.
- Rupture causes severe left-lower-quadrant pain, abdominal rigidity and, possibly, signs and symptoms of shock and sepsis.
- Other signs and symptoms include nausea, constipation or diarrhea, low-grade fever, and a palpable abdominal mass that's usually tender, firm, and fixed.

Duodenal ulcer
- Pain is localized and steady, gnawing, burning, aching, or hungerlike.
- Pain typically occurs 2 to 4 hours after a meal and may cause nocturnal awakening.
- Pain may be high in the midepigastrium, slightly off-center, usually on the right.
- Other symptoms include changes in bowel habits and heartburn or retrosternal burning.

Ectopic pregnancy
- Pain occurs in lower abdomen and may be sharp, dull, or cramping, and constant or intermittent.
- Rupture of the fallopian tube produces sharp lower abdominal pain, which may radiate to the shoulders and neck, and signs of shock may occur.
- Other signs and symptoms include vaginal bleeding, nausea, vomiting, urinary frequency, a tender adnexal mass, and a 1- to 2-month history of amenorrhea.

Endometriosis
- Constant, severe pain in the lower abdomen usually begins 5 to 7 days before the start of menses.
- Pain may be aggravated by defecation.
- Other symptoms include constipation, abdominal tenderness, dysmenorrhea, dyspareunia, and deep sacral pain.

Escherichia coli 0157:H7 infection
- Abdominal cramps, watery or bloody diarrhea, nausea, vomiting, and fever occur after eating contaminated foods.
- Hemolytic uremia may occur in children younger than age 5 and in elderly patients, possibly leading to acute renal failure.

Gastric ulcer
- Diffuse, gnawing, burning pain in the left upper quadrant or epigastric area occurs 1 to 2 hours after meals.
- Pain may be relieved by ingesting food or antacids.
- Vague bloating and nausea after meals, indigestion, weight change, anorexia, and GI bleeding may also occur.

Gastritis
- Onset of pain is rapid.
- Pain ranges from mild epigastric discomfort to burning in the left upper quadrant.
- Belching, fever, malaise, anorexia, nausea, bloody or coffee-ground vomitus, and melena may also occur.

Gastroenteritis
- Cramping or colicky pain originates in the left upper quadrant and then radiates or migrates to the other quadrants.
- Pain is accompanied by diarrhea, hyperactive bowel sounds, headache, myalgia, nausea, and vomiting.

Heart failure

○ Right-upper-quadrant pain is common.
○ Hallmark signs and symptoms include jugular vein distention, dyspnea, tachycardia, and peripheral edema.
○ Other findings include nausea, vomiting, ascites, productive cough, crackles, cool extremities, and cyanotic nail beds.

Hepatitis

○ Liver enlargement causes discomfort or dull pain and tenderness in the right upper quadrant.
○ Other signs and symptoms include dark urine, clay-colored stools, nausea, vomiting, anorexia, jaundice, malaise, and pruritus.

Herpes zoster

○ Abdominal and chest pain may occur in the areas served by the nerves affected by the infection.
○ Pain, tenderness, fever, and erythematous papules (which rapidly evolve into vesicles) also occur.

Intestinal obstruction

○ A life-threatening disorder — short episodes of intense, colicky, cramping pain alternate with pain-free intervals.
○ Accompanying signs and symptoms include abdominal distention, tenderness, and guarding; visible peristaltic waves; high-pitched, tinkling, or hyperactive sounds near the obstruction and hypoactive or absent sounds distally; obstipation; and pain-induced agitation.
○ A late sign is hypovolemic shock.
○ In jejunal and duodenal obstruction, nausea and bilious vomiting occur early.
○ In distal obstruction, nausea and vomiting are commonly feculent.
○ Bowel sounds are absent in complete obstruction.

Irritable bowel syndrome

○ Lower abdominal cramping or pain is aggravated by ingestion of coarse or raw foods.
○ Pain may be alleviated by defecation or passage of flatus.
○ Other findings include abdominal tenderness, diarrhea alternating with constipation or normal bowel function, small stools with visible mucus, dyspepsia, nausea, and abdominal distention with a feeling of incomplete evacuation.
○ Stress, anxiety, and emotional lability intensify the symptoms.

Listeriosis

○ Abdominal pain, fever, myalgia, nausea, vomiting, and diarrhea occur after eating contaminated food.
○ Meningitis may develop if the infection spreads to the nervous system.

Mesenteric artery ischemia

○ Sudden, severe abdominal pain develops after 2 or 3 days of colicky periumbilical pain and diarrhea.
○ Condition tends to occur in patients older than age 50 with chronic heart failure, cardiac arrhythmia, cardiovascular infarct, or hypotension.
○ Initially, abdomen is soft and tender with decreased bowel sounds.
○ Other findings include vomiting, anorexia, alternating periods of diarrhea and constipation and, in late stages, extreme abdominal tenderness with rigidity, tachycardia, tachypnea, absent bowel sounds, and cool, clammy, skin.

Ovarian cyst

○ Torsion or hemorrhage causes pain and tenderness in the right or left lower quadrant.
○ Pain is sharp and severe if the patient suddenly stands or stoops.
○ Pain becomes brief and intermittent if torsion self-corrects or dull and diffuse after several hours if it doesn't.
○ Other findings include slight fever, mild nausea and vomiting, abdominal tenderness, palpable abdominal mass, amenorrhea, and abdominal distention.

Pancreatitis

○ A life-threatening disorder — fulminating, continuous upper abdominal pain may radiate to both flanks and to the back in acute pancreatitis.
○ Early findings include abdominal tenderness, nausea, vomiting, fever, pallor, tachycardia, abdominal rigidity, rebound tenderness, and hypoactive bowel sounds.
○ Turner's sign (ecchymosis of the abdomen or flank) or Cullen's sign (a bluish tinge around the umbilicus) signals hemorrhagic pancreatitis.
○ Jaundice may occur as inflammation subsides.
○ In chronic pancreatitis, severe left-upper-quadrant or epigastric pain radiates to the back.

Pelvic inflammatory disease

○ Pain occurs in the right or left lower quadrant.
○ Extent of pain ranges from vague discomfort to deep, severe, and progressive pain.
○ Metrorrhagia may precede or accompany the onset of pain.
○ Other findings include abdominal tenderness, palpable abdominal or pelvic mass, fever, chills, nausea, vomiting, urinary discomfort, and abnormal vaginal bleeding or purulent vaginal discharge.

Perforated ulcer

○ A life-threatening disorder — sudden, severe, and prostrating epigastric pain may radiate through the abdomen to the back or to the right shoulder.
○ Other findings include abdominal rigidity, tenderness with guarding, generalized rebound tenderness, absent bowel sounds, grunting and shallow respirations, fever, tachycardia, hypotension, and syncope.

Peritonitis

○ A life-threatening disorder — sudden and severe pain can be diffuse or localized.

- Movement worsens the pain.
- Findings include fever; chills; nausea; vomiting; hypoactive or absent bowel sounds; abdominal tenderness, distention, and rigidity; rebound tenderness and guarding; hyperalgesia; tachycardia; hypotension; tachypnea; and psoas and obturator signs.

Prostatitis
- Vague abdominal pain or discomfort in the lower abdomen, groin, perineum, or rectum may develop.
- Other findings include dysuria, urinary frequency and urgency, fever, chills, low back pain, myalgia, arthralgia, and nocturia.
- Scrotal pain, penile pain, and pain on ejaculation may occur in chronic cases.

Pyelonephritis (acute)
- Progressive lower quadrant pain in one or both sides, flank pain, and costovertebral tenderness occur.
- Pain may radiate to the lower midabdomen or the groin.
- Additional signs and symptoms include abdominal and back tenderness, high fever, shaking chills, nausea, vomiting, and urinary frequency and urgency.

Renal calculi
- Depending on the location of calculi, severe abdominal or back pain may occur.
- The classic symptom is severe, colicky pain that travels from the costovertebral angle to the flank, suprapubic region, and external genitalia.
- Other findings include pain-induced agitation, nausea, vomiting, abdominal distention, fever, chills, hypertension, and urinary urgency.

Sickle cell crisis
- Sudden, severe abdominal pain may accompany chest, back, hand, or foot pain.
- Other signs and symptoms include weakness, aching joints, dyspnea, and scleral jaundice.

Smallpox (variola major)
- Abdominal pain, high fever, malaise, prostration, severe headache, and backache appear initially.
- A maculopapular rash develops at the same time on the mucosa of the mouth, pharynx, face, and forearms and spreads to the trunk and legs.
- Within 2 days, the rash becomes vesicular and later becomes round, firm pustules embedded in the skin.
- After 8 to 9 days, the pustules form a crust.

Splenic infarction
- Sudden, severe pain in the left upper quadrant occurs along with chest pain that may worsen during inspiration.
- Pain radiates to the left shoulder with splinting of the left diaphragm, abdominal guarding, and, occasionally, a splenic rub.

Ulcerative colitis
- Initially, vague abdominal discomfort leads to cramping lower abdominal pain.
- Pain may become steady and diffuse, increasing with movement and coughing.
- Recurrent and possibly severe diarrhea with blood, pus, and mucus may relieve pain.
- Other findings include a soft, squashy, and extremely tender abdomen; high-pitched, infrequent bowel sounds; nausea; vomiting; anorexia; weight loss; and mild, intermittent fever.

Other causes

Drugs
- Salicylates and nonsteroidal anti-inflammatory drugs commonly cause burning and gnawing pain in the left upper quadrant or epigastric area.

Nursing considerations

- Have the patient lie in a supine position with his knees slightly flexed.
- Monitor for findings — such as tachycardia, hypotension, clammy skin, abdominal rigidity, rebound tenderness, changes in the pain's location or intensity, or sudden relief from pain — that signal life-threatening developments.
- Withhold food and fluids.
- Prepare for I.V. infusion and insertion of a nasogastric or other intestinal tube.
- Peritoneal lavage or abdominal paracentesis may be required.

Pediatric pointers
- Abdominal pain can signal a disorder with different signs in children than in adults.
- Because children have difficulty describing abdominal pain, pay attention to nonverbal cues.
- A child's complaint of abdominal pain may reflect an emotional need such as a wish to avoid school or to gain adult attention.

Geriatric pointers
- Advanced age may decrease the manifestations of acute abdominal disease.

Patient teaching
- Explain the diagnostic tests the patient will need.
- Explain which foods and fluids the patient shouldn't have.
- Tell the patient to report any changes in bowel habits.
- Instruct the patient how to position himself to alleviate symptoms.

Abdominal rigidity

Overview

- Also known as *abdominal muscle spasm* or *involuntary guarding*
- Involves abnormal muscle tension or inflexibility of the abdomen
- May be *voluntary* (from fear or nervousness) or *involuntary* (reflecting potentially life-threatening peritoneal irritation or inflammation (see *Distinguishing voluntary from involuntary rigidity*)
- Involuntary rigidity most commonly from GI disorders but also from pulmonary or vascular disorders and from the effects of insect toxins.

Emergency actions

Quickly take the patient's vital signs. Give oxygen and insert an I.V. line for fluid and blood replacement. Anticipate the need for drugs to support blood pressure. Insert nasogastric tube to relieve abdominal distention. Prepare the patient for catheterization, and monitor intake and output of fluids. Because surgery may be necessary, prepare the patient for laboratory tests and X-rays.

Assessment

History

- Ask about the onset of abdominal rigidity.
- Ask if abdominal pain is present and when it began.
- Determine the location of rigidity (localized or generalized).

Assessment tip
Distinguishing voluntary from involuntary rigidity

Distinguishing voluntary from involuntary abdominal rigidity is a must for accurate assessment. Review this comparison so that you can quickly tell the two apart.

Voluntary rigidity
- Usually symmetrical
- More rigid on inspiration (expiration causes muscle relaxation)
- Eased by relaxation techniques, such as positioning the patient comfortably and talking to him in a calm, soothing manner
- Painless when the patient sits up using his abdominal muscles alone

Involuntary rigidity
- Usually asymmetrical
- Equally rigid on inspiration and expiration
- Unaffected by relaxation techniques
- Painful when the patient sits up using his abdominal muscles alone

- Ask about aggravating and alleviating factors, such as position changes, coughing, vomiting, elimination, and walking.

Physical assessment

- Inspect the abdomen for peristaltic waves.
- Check for a visibly distended bowel loop.
- Auscultate bowel sounds.
- Perform light palpation to locate the rigidity and to determine its severity.
- Check for signs of dehydration, such as poor skin turgor and dry mucous membranes.

Medical causes

Abdominal aortic aneurysm (dissecting)

- A life-threatening disorder — mild to moderate abdominal rigidity occurs.
- Constant upper abdominal pain may radiate to the lower back.
- A pulsating mass may be present in the epigastrium with a systolic bruit over the aorta before rupture.
- After rupture, the mass stops pulsating.
- Other findings include mottled skin and absent pulses below the waist, lower blood pressure in the legs than in the arms, and mild to moderate tenderness with guarding.
- Significant blood loss causes signs of shock (tachycardia, tachypnea, and cool and clammy skin).

Insect toxins

- Rigidity usually accompanies generalized, cramping abdominal pain.
- Other findings include low-grade fever, nausea, vomiting, tremors, burning sensations in the hands and feet, increased salivation, hypertension, paresis, and hyperactive reflexes.

Mesenteric artery ischemia

- Sudden, severe abdominal pain and rigidity occur in the central or periumbilical region after 2 or 3 days of persistent, low-grade abdominal pain and diarrhea.
- Rigidity is accompanied by severe abdominal tenderness, fever, vomiting, anorexia, diarrhea, constipation, and signs of shock.
- Suspect mesenteric artery ischemia in patients older than age 50 with a history of heart failure, arrhythmia, cardiovascular infarct, or hypotension.

Peritonitis

- Rigidity is localized or generalized depending on the cause of peritonitis.
- Other findings include abdominal tenderness and distention, rebound tenderness, guarding, hyperalgesia, hypoactive or absent bowel sounds, nausea, vomiting, fever, chills, tachycardia, tachypnea, and hypotension.

Nursing considerations

○ Monitor the patient closely for signs of shock.
○ Position the patient in a supine position with knees slightly flexed.
○ Withhold analgesics until a tentative diagnosis has been made.
○ Withhold food and fluids.
○ Administer an I.V. antibiotic because emergency surgery may be required.
○ Prepare for diagnostic tests which may include blood, urine, and stool studies; chest and abdominal X-rays, computed tomography, magnetic resonance imaging, gastroscopy, and colonoscopy.

Pediatric pointers

○ Voluntary rigidity may be difficult to distinguish from involuntary rigidity if associated pain makes the child restless, tense, or apprehensive.
○ It may stem from gastric perforation, hypertrophic pyloric stenosis, duodenal obstruction, meconium ileus, intussusception, cystic fibrosis, celiac disease, and appendicitis.
○ When involuntary rigidity is suspected, monitor for early signs of dehydration and shock, which can rapidly become life-threatening.

Geriatric pointers

○ Advanced age and impaired cognition decrease pain perception and intensity.
○ Weakening of abdominal muscles with aging means less muscle spasms and decreased rigidity.

Patient teaching

○ Explain diagnostic tests or surgery the patient will need.
○ Instruct the patient on measures to take to reduce anxiety.

Accessory muscle use

Overview

○ Stabilizes the thorax during respiration when breathing requires extra effort
○ May indicate acute respiratory distress, diaphragmatic weakness, fatigue, or chronic respiratory disease (see *Accessory muscles: Locations and functions*)

⭐ Emergency actions

Look for signs of acute respiratory distress. Quickly auscultate for abnormal, diminished, or absent breath sounds. Check for airway obstruction and attempt to restore airway patency. Begin suctioning and manual or mechanical ventilation. Assess oxygen saturation using pulse oximetry and administer oxygen. You may need to use a high flow rate initially, but be attentive to the patient's respiratory drive. (Too much oxygen may decrease respiratory drive.) If the patient has chronic obstructive pulmonary disease, use a low flow rate for mild exacerbations. Start an I.V. line.

Assessment

History

○ Ask about the onset, duration, and severity of signs and symptoms.
○ Obtain a medical and family history, including respiratory, cardiac, and infectious disorders.
○ Ask about recent trauma, pulmonary function testing, or respiratory therapy.
○ Determine smoking and occupational hazards.

Physical assessment

○ Perform a detailed chest assessment, noting abnormal respiratory rate, pattern, or depth.
○ Assess skin color, temperature, and turgor.
○ Check for clubbing of the fingers.

Medical causes

Acute respiratory distress syndrome

○ A life-threatening disorder — accessory muscle use increases in response to hypoxia.
○ Intercostal, supracostal, and sternal retractions occur on inspiration.
○ Grunting occurs on expiration.
○ Other findings include tachypnea, dyspnea, diaphoresis, diffuse crackles, anxiety, tachycardia, mental sluggishness, and a cough with pink, frothy sputum.

Airway obstruction

○ A life-threatening disorder — inspiratory stridor is a characteristic sign.

○ Accessory muscle use increases.
○ Other signs and symptoms include dyspnea, tachypnea, gasping, wheezing, coughing, intercostal retractions, cyanosis, and tachycardia.

Amyotrophic lateral sclerosis

○ Accessory muscle use increases as disorder affects the diaphragm.
○ Other signs and symptoms include fasciculations, muscle atrophy and weakness, spasticity, incoordination, and hyperactive deep tendon reflexes.
○ Other findings include impaired speech; difficulty chewing, swallowing, and breathing; choking; and excessive drooling.

Asthma

○ Accessory muscle use increases during acute attacks.
○ Severe dyspnea, tachypnea, wheezing, cough, nasal flaring, cyanosis, tachycardia, diaphoresis, and apprehension occur.
○ Auscultation reveals faint or absent breath sounds, inspiratory and expiratory wheezing, and coarse rhonchi.

Chronic bronchitis

○ Productive cough and exertional dyspnea precede accessory muscle use.
○ Accompanying findings include wheezing, barrel chest, clubbing of the fingers, cyanosis, and edema.

Emphysema

○ Increased accessory muscle use occurs with progressive exertional dyspnea and a minimally productive cough.
○ Other findings include pursed-lip breathing, tachypnea, peripheral cyanosis, anorexia, weight loss, malaise, barrel chest, and clubbing of the fingers.
○ Auscultation reveals decreased breath sounds and distant heart sounds.

Pneumonia

○ Increased accessory muscle use is accompanied by a sudden high fever with chills.
○ Other findings include chest pain, productive cough, dyspnea, tachypnea, and tachycardia.

Pulmonary edema

○ Increased accessory muscle use is accompanied by dyspnea, tachypnea, orthopnea, crepitant crackles, wheezing, and a cough with pink, frothy sputum.
○ Other findings include restlessness; tachycardia; ventricular gallop; and cool, clammy, cyanotic skin.

Pulmonary embolism

○ A life-threatening disorder — it may cause increased accessory muscle use.
○ Common findings include dyspnea, tachycardia, and pleuritic or substernal chest pain.
○ Other findings include restlessness, anxiety, tachycardia, productive cough, hemoptysis, and cyanosis.

Physical exertion and pulmonary disease usually increase the work of breathing, taxing the diaphragm and external intercostal muscles. When this happens, accessory muscles provide the extra effort needed to maintain respirations. The scalene, sternocleidomastoid, and trapezius muscles assist with inspiration, whereas the upper chest, sternum, internal intercostal, and abdominal muscles assist with expiration.

In inspiration, the scalene muscles elevate, fix, and expand the upper chest. The sternocleidomastoid muscles raise the sternum, expanding the chest's anteroposterior and longitudinal dimensions. The pectoralis major muscles elevate the chest, increasing its anteroposterior size, and the trapezius muscles raise the thoracic cage.

With expiration, the internal intercostals depress the ribs, decreasing the chest size. The abdominal muscles pull the lower chest down, depress the lower ribs, and compress the abdominal contents—all of which exert pressure on the chest.

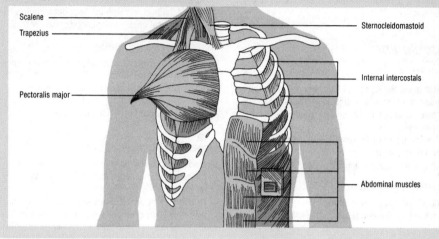

Spinal cord injury

○ Injury to cervical vertebrae C3 to C5 affects the upper respiratory muscles and diaphragm, causing increased accessory muscle use.
○ Other findings include unilateral or bilateral Babinski's reflex; hyperactive deep tendon reflexes; spasticity; and variable or total loss of pain and temperature sensation, proprioception, and motor function.

Thoracic injury

○ Increased accessory muscle use may occur depending on the type and extent of injury.
○ Other signs and symptoms include an obvious chest wound or bruising, chest pain, and dyspnea.
○ Signs of shock occur with significant blood loss.

Nursing considerations

○ If the patient is alert, elevate the head of the bed to make his breathing as easy as possible.
○ Encourage the patient to get plenty of rest.
○ Encourage the patient to drink plenty of fluids to liquefy secretions unless on fluid restriction.
○ Administer oxygen.
○ Prepare the patient for diagnostic tests, such as pulmonary function studies, chest X-ray, lung scans, arterial blood gas analysis, and sputum culture.

Pediatric pointers

○ Upper airway obstruction usually produces respiratory distress and increased accessory muscle use.
○ Disorders associated with airway obstruction include acute epiglottitis, croup, pertusis, cystic fibrosis, and asthma.
○ Suprasternal, intercostal, or abdominal retractions indicate accessory muscle use.
○ Respiratory distress can rapidly progress to respiratory failure because a child's accessory muscles tire sooner than those of an adult.

Geriatric pointers

○ Because of age-related loss of elasticity in the rib cage, accessory muscle use may be part of an older person's normal breathing pattern.

Patient teaching

○ Teach the patient relaxation techniques to reduce his apprehension.
○ Provide resources for quitting smoking.
○ Explain measures to prevent infection.
○ Explain prescribed drugs and how to take them.
○ Provide instruction on pursed-lip, diaphragmatic breathing to ease the work of breathing for patients with chronic lung disorders.
○ Teach the patient coughing and deep-breathing exercises to keep airways clear.

Agitation

Overview

- Refers to a state of hyperarousal, increased tension, and irritability
- Can lead to confusion, hyperactivity, and overt hostility
- Can arise gradually or suddenly and last for minutes or months

Assessment

History

- Determine the severity of agitation, including the number and quality of agitation-induced behaviors.
- Obtain a history, including the patient's diet and known allergies.
- Ask about past or present illnesses, trauma, stress, and sleep patterns.
- Question the patient about drug and alcohol use.

Physical assessment

- Check for signs of drug abuse.
- Obtain baseline vital signs and neurologic status.

Medical causes

Affective disturbance

- Agitation may occur in depressed and manic phases and in personality disorders.
- Psychomotor agitation may involve an inability to sit still, hand-wringing, pacing, and irritability.

Alcohol withdrawal syndrome

- Mild to severe agitation occurs along with hyperactivity, tremors, and anxiety.
- Severe agitation accompanies hallucinations, insomnia, diaphoresis, and depressed mood in alcohol withdrawal syndrome, the potentially life-threatening stage of alcohol withdrawal.

Anxiety

- Varying degrees of agitation result.
- Other findings include nausea, vomiting, diarrhea, cool and clammy skin, frontal headache, back pain, insomnia, and tremors.

Chronic renal failure

- Moderate to severe agitation occurs, marked especially by confusion and memory loss.
- Other findings include nausea, vomiting, anorexia, mouth ulcers, ammonia breath odor, GI bleeding, pallor, edema, dry skin, and uremic frost.

Dementia

- Mild to severe agitation can result from many common syndromes, such as Alzheimer's disease and Huntington's disease.
- Other findings include hypoactivity; wandering; hallucinations; aphasia; insomnia; and decreased memory, attention span, problem-solving ability, and alertness.

Drug withdrawal syndrome

- Mild to severe agitation occurs.
- Related findings vary with the drug but include anxiety, abdominal cramps, diaphoresis, and anorexia.

Hepatic encephalopathy

- Patients may experience agitation, drowsiness, stupor, fetor hepaticus (the peculiar breath odor characteristic of hepatic disease), asterixis, and hyperreflexia.
- Lethargy, aberrant behavior, and apraxia may also occur.

Hypersensitivity reaction

- Moderate to severe agitation may be the first sign.
- Urticaria, pruritus, and facial and dependent edema may occur.
- In anaphylactic shock, a potentially life-threatening hypersensitivity reaction, associated findings include the rapid onset of apprehension, urticaria or diffuse erythema, warm and moist skin, paresthesia, pruritus, edema, dyspnea, wheezing, stridor, hypotension, and tachycardia.

Hypoxemia

- Agitation starts as restlessness, then rapidly worsens.
- Other findings include confusion, impaired judgment and motor coordination, tachycardia, tachypnea, dyspnea, and cyanosis.

Increased intracranial pressure

- Agitation precedes other early signs and symptoms, such as headache, nausea, and vomiting.
- Other findings include respiratory changes; sluggish, nonreactive, or unequal pupils; widening pulse pressure; tachycardia; decreased level of consciousness; seizures; and motor changes.

Post-head-trauma syndrome

- Agitation is characterized by disorientation, loss of concentration, angry outbursts, and emotional lability.
- Other findings include fatigue, wandering, and poor judgment.

Vitamin B$_6$ deficiency

- Agitation ranges from mild to severe.
- Other effects include seizures, peripheral paresthesia, oculogyric crisis, and dermatitis.

Other causes

Drugs

○ Mild to moderate agitation may occur with central nervous system stimulants.

Radiographic contrast media

○ Agitation may occur as a hypersensitivity reaction to injected contrast medium.

Nursing considerations

○ Monitor the patient's vital signs and neurologic status.
○ Eliminate stressors, which can increase agitation.
○ Provide adequate lighting.
○ Maintain a calm environment.
○ Allow the patient time to sleep.
○ Ensure a balanced diet and provide vitamin supplements and hydration.
○ Remain calm, nonjudgmental, and nonargumentative.
○ Prepare the patient for diagnostic tests, such as computed tomography scanning, magnetic resonance imaging, and blood studies.

Pediatric pointers

○ In children, agitation accompanies the expected childhood diseases and more severe disorders — such as hyperbilirubinemia, phenylketonuria, vitamin A deficiency, hepatitis, frontal lobe syndrome, increased intracranial pressure, and lead poisoning — that can lead to brain damage.
○ In neonates, agitation can stem from alcohol or drug withdrawal.

Geriatric pointers

○ Environmental change or deviation from usual activities (or rituals) may provoke agitation.

Patient teaching

○ Provide the patient with an orientation to the unit and its procedures and routines.
○ Explain stress-reduction measures.
○ Provide a quiet environment.
○ Provide reassurance and emotional support.

Alopecia

Overview

- Hair loss that usually develops gradually; hair loss may be diffuse or patchy
- Can be scarring (permanent; follicles are destroyed) or nonscarring (temporary; follicles are damaged)

Assessment

History

- Ask about the onset of hair loss or thinning.
- Determine which areas of the body are affected.
- Question the patient about associated signs and symptoms, such as itching and rashes.
- Obtain a medical history
- Ask about menstrual irregularities in women and sexual dysfunction in men.
- Ask about hair care and habits.
- Check for a family history of alopecia.

Physical assessment

- Assess the extent and pattern of scalp hair loss.
- Inspect the underlying skin for follicular openings, erythema, loss of pigment, scaling, induration, broken hair shafts, and hair regrowth.
- Examine the rest of the skin for jaundice, edema, hyperpigmentation, pallor, or duskiness. Note the size, color, texture, and location of any lesions.
- Examine nails for vertical or horizontal pitting, thickening, brittleness, or whitening.
- Palpate for lymphadenopathy, enlarged thyroid or salivary glands, and masses in the abdomen or chest.

Medical causes

Alopecia areata

- Well-circumscribed patches of nonscarring scalp alopecia develop.
- Patches of alopecia are bordered by loose hairs with rough, brushlike tips on narrow, less-pigmented shafts.
- Horizontal or vertical nail pitting may occur.

Arterial insufficiency

- Patchy alopecia occurs, typically on the legs.
- Alopecia may be accompanied by thin, shiny, atrophic skin and thickened nails.
- Skin on the legs turns pale when the legs are elevated and dusky when they're dependent.
- Other findings include weak or absent peripheral pulses, cool extremities, paresthesia, leg ulcers, and intermittent claudication.

Burns

- Scarring or keloid formation from full-thickness or third-degree burns causes permanent alopecia.

Cutaneous T-cell lymphoma

- Alopecia mucinosa may occur in the premycotic stage and may persist through the plaque and tumor stages.
- Scattered papules or plaques may occur on clothed areas, or a zebralike pattern of scaly erythema may form on the trunk.

Exfoliative dermatitis

- Loss of scalp and body hair is preceded by several weeks of generalized scaling and erythema.
- Other findings include nail loss, pruritus, malaise, fever, weight loss, lymphadenopathy, and gynecomastia.

Fungal infections

- Tinea capitis produces irregular balding areas, scaling, and erythematous lesions.
- Broken scalp hairs surround the balding areas.
- Classic ring-shaped appearance occurs as lesions enlarge and the centers heal.
- Pruritus and thick, whitish nails may occur.

Hodgkin's disease

- Permanent alopecia may occur if lymphoma infiltrates the scalp.
- Alopecia may be accompanied by edema, pruritus, and hyperpigmentation.

Hypopituitarism

- In women, sparse or absent pubic and axillary hair, infertility, and breast atrophy occur.
- In men, decreased facial and body hair, infertility, decreased libido, impotence, and poor muscle development occur.

Hypothyroidism

- Hair on the face, scalp, and genitals thins and becomes dull, coarse, and brittle.
- Hair loss in the outer one-third of the eyebrows occurs.
- Other signs and symptoms include fatigue; constipation; cold intolerance; weight gain; dry, flaky, inelastic skin; puffy face, hands, and feet; thick, brittle nails; slow mental function; bradycardia; menorrhagia, and myalgia.

Lupus erythematosus

- Hair becomes brittle and falls out in patches in discoid and systemic lupus.
- Broken hairs commonly appear above the forehead.
- Characteristic findings in both types of lupus include raised, red, scaling plaques with follicular plugging, telangiectasia, central atrophy, and facial plaques in a butterfly-shaped pattern.

- Rash may vary in severity from malar erythema to discoid lesions in systemic lupus.
- Systemic lupus affects multiple body systems and may produce photosensitivity, weight loss, fatigue, lymphadenopathy, arthritis, and emotional lability.

Myotonic dystrophy

- Premature baldness occurs in the adult form.
- Myotonia, the inability to relax a muscle after its contraction, is a primary sign.
- Other signs include muscle wasting and cataracts.

Protein deficiency

- Hair becomes brittle, fine, dry, and thin, possibly with pigment changes.
- Characteristic muscle wasting may be accompanied by edema, hepatomegaly, apathy, irritability, anorexia, diarrhea, and dry and flaky skin.

Sarcoidosis

- If sarcoidosis infiltrates the scalp, scarring alopecia occurs.
- Accompanying findings include fever, weight loss, fatigue, lymphadenopathy, substernal pain, cough, shortness of breath, muscle weakness, arthralgia, myalgia, cranial nerve palsies, and various lesions of the face and the oral and nasal mucosa.

Seborrheic dermatitis

- Hair loss on the scalp may occur, beginning at the vertex and frontal areas.
- Pruritus occurs along with reddened, dry skin with branlike scales that flake off easily.

Skin cancer (metastasized)

- Scarring alopecia may develop slowly along with scalp induration and atrophy.
- Related findings include weight loss, fever, altered bowel habits, abdominal pain, and lymphadenopathy.

Thyrotoxicosis

- Diffuse hair loss occurs.
- Hair loss may be accentuated at the temples.
- Hair becomes fine, soft, and friable.
- Skin is uniformly flushed and thickened, marked by red, raised, pruritic patches.
- Characteristic findings include fine tremors, nervousness, an enlarged thyroid gland, sweating, heat intolerance, amenorrhea, palpitations, weight loss despite increased appetite, diarrhea, and exophthalmos.

Other causes

Drugs

- Chemotherapeutic drugs may cause patchy, reversible alopecia.

- Other drugs that may cause diffuse hair loss include allopurinol, antithyroid drugs, beta blockers, carbamazepine, colchicine, excessive doses of vitamin A, gentamicin, heparin, hormonal contraceptives, indomethacin, lithium, trimethadione, valproic acid, and warfarin.

Radiation therapy

- Radiation therapy produces reversible hair loss a few weeks after exposure.

Nursing considerations

- Explain to the patient that hair loss resulting from chemotherapy is reversible.
- A skin biopsy may be performed to determine the cause of alopecia.
- Microscopic examination of a plucked hair may aid diagnosis.
- For patients with partial baldness or alopecia areata, topical application of minoxidil for several months stimulates localized hair growth.

Pediatric pointers

- Alopecia normally occurs during the first 6 months of life.
- If the infant is always placed in same position, advise parents to change the infant's position regularly.
- Common causes include use of chemotherapy or radiation therapy, seborrheic dermatitis, alopecia mucinosa, tinea capitis, hypopituitarism, trichotillomania, progeria, and congenital hair shaft defects.

Patient teaching

- Teach the patient to use gentle hair care.
- Tell the patient about head wear and hairpieces.
- Explain the importance of head protection (sunblock, hat).

Amenorrhea

Overview

- Amenorrhea is the absence of menstrual flow.
- Menstruation fails to begin before age 16 in primary amenorrhea.
- Menstruation begins at appropriate age but later ceases for 3 or more months in the absence of physiologic causes in secondary amenorrhea.
- Anovulation or physical obstruction to menstrual outflow occurs in pathologic amenorrhea.
- Anovulation may result from hormonal imbalance, debilitating disease, stress or emotional disturbances, strenuous exercise, malnutrition, obesity, drug or hormonal treatments, or anatomic abnormalities.

Assessment

History

- Ask about frequency and duration of the patient's previous menses.
- Obtain the date of her last menses.
- Determine the onset and nature of menstrual pattern changes.
- Ask about related signs (breast swelling or weight changes).
- Obtain a medical history, including illnesses, use of hormonal contraceptives, exercise and eating habits, emotional state, weight changes, and stress levels.
- Obtain family medical and menstrual history.

Physical assessment

- Observe for secondary sex characteristics and signs of virilization.
- If performing a pelvic examination, check for anatomic aberrations of the outflow tract.

Medical causes

Adrenal tumor

- Amenorrhea may be accompanied by acne, thinning scalp hair, hirsutism, increased blood pressure, truncal obesity, and psychotic changes.
- Asymmetrical ovarian enlargement and rapid onset of signs of virilizing are key findings.

Adrenocortical hyperplasia

- Amenorrhea precedes characteristic cushingoid signs, such as truncal obesity, moon face, "buffalo hump," bruises, purple striae, hypertension, renal calculi, psychiatric disturbances, and widened pulse pressure.
- Thinning scalp hair and hirsutism typically appear.

Adrenocortical hypofunction

- Amenorrhea, fatigue, irritability, weight loss, increased pigmentation, nausea, vomiting, and orthostatic hypotension may result.

Anorexia nervosa

- Primary or secondary amenorrhea may occur.
- Related findings include weight loss, emaciated appearance, dry skin, compulsive behavior patterns, blotchy or sallow complexion, constipation, reduced libido, decreased pleasure in once-enjoyable activities, loss of scalp hair, lanugo (downy hair) on the face and arms, skeletal muscle atrophy, and sleep disturbances.

Congenital absence of ovaries and uterus

- Primary amenorrhea and absence of secondary sex characteristics occur.

Corpus luteum cysts

- Sudden amenorrhea
- Abdominal pain and breast swelling

Hypothyroidism

- Amenorrhea may be primary or secondary.
- Early findings include fatigue, forgetfulness, cold intolerance, weight gain, and constipation.
- Subsequent findings include dry, flaky, inelastic skin; puffy face, hands, and feet; hoarseness; dry, sparse hair; thick, brittle nails; slow mental function; bradycardia; and myalgia.
- Other common findings include anorexia, abdominal distention, decreased libido, ataxia, intention tremor, nystagmus, and delayed reflex relaxation time.

Pituitary infarction

- The postpartum patient fails to lactate and resume menses.
- Other signs and symptoms include headaches, visual field defects, oculomotor palsies, loss of pubic and axillary hair, and an altered level of consciousness.

Pituitary tumor

- Amenorrhea may be the first sign.
- Other findings include headache, vision disturbances, cushingoid signs, and acromegaly.

Polycystic ovary syndrome

- Irregular menstrual cycles, oligomenorrhea, and secondary amenorrhea or periods of profuse bleeding may alternate with periods of amenorrhea.
- Other findings include obesity; hirsutism; slight deepening of the voice; and enlarged ovaries.

Pseudoamenorrhea

- An anatomic anomaly obstructs menstrual flow, causing primary amenorrhea.
- Examination may reveal a bulging pink or blue hymen.

Testicular feminization
○ Primary amenorrhea may indicate this form of male pseudohermaphroditism.
○ The patient is outwardly female but genetically male, with breast and external genital development but scant or absent pubic hair.

Thyrotoxicosis
○ Overproduction of thyroid hormone may result in amenorrhea.
○ Classic findings include an enlarged thyroid gland, nervousness, heat intolerance, diaphoresis, tremors, palpitations, tachycardia, dyspnea, weakness, and weight loss despite increased appetite.

Turner's syndrome
○ Primary amenorrhea and failure to develop secondary sex characteristics may signal this syndrome.
○ Typical features include short stature, webbing of the neck, low nuchal hairline, a broad chest with widely spaced nipples, poor breast development, underdeveloped genitals, and edema of the legs and feet.

Other causes

Drugs
○ Busulfan, chlorambucil, injectable or implanted contraceptives, cyclophosphamide, and phenothiazines may cause amenorrhea.
○ Hormonal contraceptives may cause anovulation and amenorrhea when stopped.

Radiation therapy
○ Irradiation of the abdomen may damage the endometrium or ovaries, causing amenorrhea.

Surgery
○ Surgical removal of the ovaries or uterus produces amenorrhea.

Nursing considerations

○ In patients with secondary amenorrhea, rule out pregnancy before starting diagnostic testing.
○ Provide emotional support, since amenorrhea can cause severe emotional distress.

Pediatric pointers
○ Adolescent girls are prone to amenorrhea caused by emotional upsets stemming from school, social, or family problems.

Geriatric pointers
○ In women older than age 50, amenorrhea usually represents the onset of menopause.

Patient teaching
○ Explain treatment and expected outcomes.

○ Encourage the patient to discuss her fears.
○ Refer the patient for psychological counseling if needed.

Anhidrosis

Overview

- Anhidrosis is an abnormal deficiency of sweat.
- The disorder is classified as generalized (complete) or localized (partial).
- Generalized anhidrosis can lead to life-threatening impairment of thermoregulation.
- Anhidrosis results from neurologic and skin disorders; congenital abnormalities of sweat glands; atrophic or traumatic changes to sweat glands; and the use of certain drugs.
- The absence, obstruction, atrophy, or degeneration of sweat glands can produce anhidrosis at the skin surface, even if neurologic stimulation is normal.

✦ Emergency actions

If anhidrosis is suspected in a patient with hot, flushed skin, nausea, dizziness, palpitations, and substernal tightness, quickly take a rectal temperature and other vital signs and assess level of consciousness (LOC). If the rectal temperature is higher than 102.2° F (39° C) and is accompanied by tachycardia, tachypnea, altered blood pressure, and decreased LOC, suspect life-threatening anhidrotic asthenia (heatstroke). Start rapid cooling measures and give I.V. fluid replacement. Frequently check vital signs, hemodynamic status, and neurologic status until the patient's temperature drops below 102° F (38.9° C). Then place him in an air-conditioned room.

Assessment

History
- Obtain a description of previous sweating.
- Determine when onset of anhidrosis occurred.
- Question the patient about recent exposure to heat.
- Obtain a medical history, including neurologic, skin, and autoimmune disorders and systemic diseases.
- Obtain a drug history.

Physical assessment
- Perform a neurologic assessment to detect a disorder of the central or peripheral nervous system as a cause of anhidrosis.
- Inspect skin color, texture, and turgor.
- Document appearance of skin lesions.

Medical causes

Anhidrotic asthenia (heat stroke)
- A life-threatening condition — generalized anhidrosis occurs with hot, flushed skin; tachycardia; tachypnea; confusion; and seizure or loss of consciousness.
- In early stages, rectal temperature may exceed 102.2° F.
- Other findings include severe headache and muscle cramps, which later disappear; fatigue; nausea and vomiting; dizziness; palpitations; substernal tightness; and elevated blood pressure followed by hypotension.

Burns
- Burns destroy eccrine glands, causing permanent anhidrosis in affected areas.
- Blistering, edema, and pain or loss of sensation may also occur.

Miliaria crystallina
- Anhidrosis and clear, tiny, fragile blisters develop under the arms and breasts.
- Typically occurs in a neonate and can be widespread on the body.

Miliaria profunda
- Localized anhidrosis occurs with compensatory facial hyperhidrosis.
- Whitish papules appear mostly on the trunk.
- Other findings include inguinal and axillary lymphadenopathy, weakness, shortness of breath, palpitations, and fever.
- If severe and extensive, miliaria profunda can progress to life-threatening anhidrotic asthenia.

Miliaria rubra (prickly heat)
- Anhidrosis is localized.
- Small, erythematous papules with centrally placed blisters appear on trunk and neck.
- Related symptoms include paroxysmal itching and paresthesia.

Nervous system disorders
- Cerebral cortex and brain stem lesions may cause anhidrotic palms and soles.
- Peripheral neuropathy causes anhidrosis over the legs with compensatory hyperhidrosis over the head and neck.

Shy-Drager syndrome
- This degenerative neurologic syndrome causes ascending anhidrosis in the legs.
- Other findings include severe orthostatic hypotension, loss of leg hair, decreased salivation and tearing, mydriasis, and eventually focal neurologic signs, such as leg tremors, incoordination, and muscle wasting.

Spinal cord lesions
- Anhidrosis may occur symmetrically below the level of the lesion.
- Compensatory hyperhidrosis occurs in adjacent areas.

Other causes

Drugs

○ Anticholinergics such as atropine can cause generalized anhidrosis.

Nursing considerations

○ Perform tests to evaluate anhidrosis and observe sweat patterns.
○ Apply a topical agent to detect sweat on the skin, and give a systemic cholinergic to stimulate sweating.

Pediatric pointers

○ In infants, common causes of anhidrosis include miliaria rubra and congenital skin disorders.
○ Because slow development of the thermoregulatory center makes an infant, especially a premature one, anhidrotic for several weeks after birth, caution parents against overdressing their infant.

Patient teaching

○ Advise about ways to stay cool, such as maintaining a cool environment, moving slowly during warm weather, and avoiding strenuous exercise and hot foods.
○ Discuss with the patient the anhidrotic effects of drugs he's receiving.

Anorexia

Overview

- Lack of appetite in the presence of a physiologic need for food
- Appears as a common symptom of GI and endocrine disorders
- May indicate a severe psychological disturbance
- If chronic, leads to life-threatening malnutrition

Assessment

History

- Ask about weight history.
- Explore dietary and exercise habits.
- Obtain a dental history.
- Obtain a medical history, including stomach or bowel disorders and changes in bowel habits.
- Ask about alcohol and drug use.
- Explore situational or psychological causes of appetite loss.

Physical assessment

- Take the patient's vital signs and weigh the patient.
- Perform a complete physical examination.

Medical causes

Acquired immunodeficiency syndrome

- Infections and Kaposi's sarcoma in the GI and respiratory tracts may lead to anorexia.
- Other findings include fatigue, afternoon fevers, night sweats, diarrhea, cough, bleeding, lymphadenopathy, oral thrush, gingivitis, and skin disorders.

Adrenocortical hypofunction

- Anorexia may begin slowly and subtly; weight loss is gradual.
- Other common findings include nausea and vomiting, abdominal pain, diarrhea, weakness, fatigue, malaise, vitiligo, bronze-colored skin, and purple striae.

Alcoholism

- Chronic anorexia leads to malnutrition.
- Other findings include signs of liver damage, paresthesia, tremors, increased blood pressure, bruising, GI bleeding, and abdominal pain.

Anorexia nervosa

- Chronic anorexia begins insidiously, leading to life-threatening malnutrition.
- Skeletal muscle atrophy, loss of fatty tissue, constipation, amenorrhea, and dry and blotchy or sallow skin, anhedonia, decreased libido, alopecia, sleep disturbances, and distorted self-image may occur.
- Complicated food preparation and eating rituals and avid exercise are common.

Appendicitis

- Anorexia follows the abrupt onset of epigastric pain, nausea, and vomiting.
- Anorexia continues as pain localizes in the right lower quadrant (McBurney's point) and abdominal rigidity, rebound tenderness, constipation (or diarrhea), slight fever, and tachycardia appear.

Cancer

- Chronic anorexia occurs along with possible weight loss, weakness, apathy, and cachexia.
- Other findings include nausea, vomiting, oral lesions, and changes in bowel habits.

Chronic renal failure

- Chronic anorexia is common and insidious.
- Accompanying changes occur in all body systems, such as nausea, vomiting, mouth ulcers, ammonia breath odor, metallic taste, GI bleeding, constipation or diarrhea, drowsiness, confusion, tremors, pallor, dry and scaly skin, pruritus, alopecia, purpuric lesions, and edema.

Cirrhosis

- Anorexia occurs early and continues after other early signs and symptoms subside.
- Weakness, nausea, vomiting, constipation or diarrhea, and dull abdominal pain are early signs.
- Accompanying findings include lethargy, slurred speech, bleeding tendencies, ascites, severe pruritus, dry skin, hepatomegaly, fetor hepaticus (breath odor characteristic of hepatic disease), jaundice, edema, gynecomastia, and right-upper-quadrant pain.

Crohn's disease

- Anorexia causes marked weight loss.
- Other signs may include diarrhea, abdominal pain, fever, abdominal mass, weakness, and perianal or vaginal fistulas.
- Acute inflammatory signs and symptoms mimic those of appendicitis.

Depression

- Anorexia reflects anhedonia in depressive syndrome.
- Other findings include poor concentration, indecisiveness, delusions, menstrual irregularities, decreased libido, insomnia or hypersomnia, fatigue, mood swings, poor self-image, and gradual social withdrawal.

Gastritis

- Onset of anorexia may be sudden.
- Postprandial epigastric distress, with nausea, vomiting (commonly hematemesis), fever, belching, hiccups, and malaise, may occur.

Hepatitis

○ In viral hepatitis, anorexia begins in the preicteric phase, accompanied by fatigue, malaise, headache, arthralgia, myalgia, photophobia, nausea and vomiting, fever, hepatomegaly, and lymphadenopathy.
○ Anorexia may continue through the icteric phase, along with weight loss, dark urine, clay-colored stools, jaundice, right-upper-quadrant pain, irritability, and severe pruritus.

Hypopituitarism

○ Anorexia usually develops slowly.
○ Accompanying signs and symptoms include amenorrhea; decreased libido; lethargy; cold intolerance; pale, thin, and dry skin; dry, brittle hair; and decreased temperature, blood pressure, and pulse rate.

Hypothyroidism

○ Anorexia is usually insidious.
○ Vague early findings include fatigue, forgetfulness, cold intolerance, unexplained weight gain, and constipation.
○ Subsequent findings include decreased mental stability; dry, flaky, and inelastic skin; edema of the face, hands, and feet; ptosis; hoarseness; thick, brittle nails; coarse, broken hair; and bradycardia.

Pernicious anemia

○ Insidious anorexia may cause considerable weight loss.
○ Burning tongue, general weakness, and numbness and tingling in the extremities are the classic triad of this disorder.
○ Other findings include alternating constipation and diarrhea, abdominal pain, nausea and vomiting, bleeding gums, ataxia, positive Babinski's and Romberg's signs, diplopia and blurred vision, irritability, headache, malaise, and fatigue.

Other causes

Drugs

○ Anorexia may occur with digoxin toxicity.
○ Amphetamines, chemotherapeutic agents, sympathomimetics, and some antibiotics may cause anorexia.

Radiation therapy

○ Radiation treatments may cause anorexia.

Total parenteral nutrition

○ Maintenance of glucose levels by I.V. therapy may cause anorexia.

Nursing considerations

○ Promote protein and calorie intake by providing high-calorie snacks or frequent, small meals.
○ Take a 24-hour diet history daily.
○ Maintain strict calorie and nutrient counts for meals because the patient may exaggerate his intake.
○ In severe malnutrition, provide supplemental nutrition.
○ Encourage the family to provide favorite foods to stimulate appetite.
○ Monitor the patient for infection.

Pediatric pointers

○ Anorexia occurs in many illnesses but usually resolves promptly.
○ In preadolescent or adolescent girls, be alert for subtle signs of anorexia nervosa.

Patient teaching

○ Explain the condition.
○ Stress the importance of proper nutrition.
○ Instruct the patient in performing oral hygiene before meals.
○ Teach the patient useful techniques to help manage the disorder, including establishing a target weight, recording his weight daily, and maintaining a record of his progress by keeping a weight log.
○ Encourage the patient to seek psychological and nutritional counseling.

Anosmia

Overview

- Is the absence of a sense of smell
- Results from nasal mucosa irritation or swelling that obstructs the olfactory area (temporary)
- Occurs if the olfactory neuroepithelium or part of the olfactory nerve is destroyed (permanent)
- May be accompanied by ageusia, the loss of the sense of taste

Assessment

History

- Ask about the onset and duration of anosmia.
- Determine the presence or history of any other signs and symptoms, such as nasal congestion, discharge or bleeding, postnasal drip, sore throat, loss of sense of taste or appetite, and facial or eye pain.
- Obtain a history of nasal disease, allergies, or head trauma.
- Question the patient about heavy smoking, use of nose drops or nasal spray, and cocaine use.

Physical assessment

- Inspect and palpate the nasal area for obvious injury, inflammation, deformities, and septal deviation or perforation.
- Observe the contour and color of the nasal mucosa and the size and color of the turbinates.
- Assess for nasal obstruction and discharge.
- Palpate the sinus area for tenderness and contour.
- Test olfactory nerve function (cranial nerve I) by having the patient identify common odors.

Medical causes

Anterior cerebral artery occlusion

- Permanent anosmia may follow vascular damage involving the olfactory nerve.
- Other findings include contralateral weakness and numbness, confusion, and impaired motor and sensory functions.

Degenerative brain disease

- Anosmia may occur with Alzheimer's disease, Parkinson's disease, and other degenerative central nervous system disorders.
- Other findings include dementia, tremor, rigidity, and gait disturbance.

Head trauma

- Permanent anosmia may follow trauma that results in damage to the olfactory nerve.

- Other signs and symptoms include epistaxis, headache, nausea and vomiting, altered level of consciousness, blurred or double vision, "raccoon eyes", Battle's sign, and otorrhea.

Lead poisoning

- Anosmia may be permanent or temporary, depending on the extent of damage to the nasal mucosa.
- Other signs and symptoms include abdominal pain, weakness, headache, nausea, vomiting, constipation, wristdrop or footdrop, lead line on the gums, metallic taste, seizures, delirium, and coma.

Neoplasm (brain, nasal, or sinus)

- Anosmia may be permanent if a neoplasm destroys or displaces the olfactory nerve.
- Other findings include unilateral or bilateral epistaxis, swelling and tenderness in the affected area, vision disturbances, decreased tearing, and elevated intracranial pressure.

Pernicious anemia

- May be temporary or permanent.
- Accompanied by the classic triad: weakness; sore, pale tongue; and numbness and tingling in the extremities.
- Related findings include distortion of taste, pallor, headache, irritability, dizziness, nausea, vomiting, diarrhea, and shortness of breath.

Polyps (nasal)

- Temporary anosmia occurs when multiple polyps obstruct nasal cavities.
- Nasal obstruction may be accompanied by a sensation of fullness in the face, nasal discharge, headache, and shortness of breath.
- Examination reveals smooth, pale, grapelike polyp clusters.

Rhinitis

- Temporary anosmia occurs.
- In viral rhinitis, findings include nasal congestion, sneezing, watery or purulent nasal discharge, dryness or tickling sensation in the nasopharynx, headache, low-grade fever, chills, and red, swollen nasal mucosa.
- In allergic rhinitis, findings include nasal congestion, itching mucosa, thin nasal discharge, sneezing, tearing, and headache.
- In atrophic rhinitis, findings include purulent, yellow-green, foul-smelling crusts on sclerotic mucus membranes; paradoxical nasal congestion in an airway that's more open than usual; thin, atrophic turbinates; and dry nasopharynx.
- In vasomotor rhinitis, findings include chronic nasal congestion, watery nasal discharge, postnasal drip, sneezing, and pale nasal mucosa.

Septal fracture

○ Anosmia is usually temporary, caused by airflow obstruction.
○ Other findings include septal deviation, swelling, epistaxis, hematoma, nasal congestion, and ecchymoses.

Septal hematoma

○ Anosmia is temporary.
○ Related findings include epistaxis, headache, mouth breathing, and dusky red, inflamed nasal mucosa.

Sinusitis

○ Anosmia is temporary.
○ Anosmia may be associated with nasal congestion; sinus pain, tenderness, and swelling; severe headache; watery or purulent discharge; postnasal drip; inflamed throat and nasal mucosa; enlarged, purulent turbinates; malaise; low-grade fever; and chills.

Other causes

Drugs

○ Anosmia may result from prolonged use of nasal decongestants, which produces rebound nasal congestion.
○ Anosmia can also result from use of naphazoline, reserpine, amphetamines, phenothiazines, and estrogen.

Radiation therapy

○ May cause permanent anosmia.

Surgery

○ Temporary anosmia may result from damage to the olfactory nerve or nasal mucosa during nasal or sinus surgery.
○ Permanent anosmia accompanies a permanent tracheostomy, which disrupts nasal breathing.

Nursing considerations

For anosmia from nasal congestion:
○ Give a local decongestant or antihistamine.
○ Provide a vaporizer or humidifier.
○ Advise against excessive use of local decongestants.
For permanent anosmia:
○ Administer vitamin A orally or by injection, which may improve symptoms.

Pediatric pointers

○ Anosmia in children may result from nasal obstruction by a foreign body or enlarged adenoids.

Patient teaching

○ Explain proper use of nose drops and sprays.
○ If the patient is mouth breathing, give instruction on oral hygiene.

Anuria

Overview

○ Urine output of less than 100 ml in 24 hours
○ Indicates either urinary tract obstruction or acute renal failure (see *Major causes of acute renal failure*)
○ Without immediate treatment, may rapidly cause uremia and other complications of urine retention

⚡ Emergency actions

Determine if urine formation is occurring. Prepare to catheterize to relieve any lower urinary tract obstruction and to check for residual urine. If you collect more than 75 ml of urine, suspect lower urinary tract obstruction. If you collect less than 75 ml, suspect renal dysfunction or obstruction higher in the urinary tract.

Assessment

History

○ Ask about any changes in voiding pattern.
○ Determine the amount of fluid normally ingested and amount ingested in last 24 to 48 hours.
○ Note the time and amount of last urination.
○ Ask about drug use.
○ Review the medical history, noting previous renal or urinary tract disease, prostate problems, congenital abnormalities, and abdominal, renal, or urinary tract surgery.

Physical assessment

○ Inspect and palpate the abdomen for asymmetry, distention, or bulging.
○ Inspect the flank area for edema or erythema.

Major causes of acute renal failure

Prerenal causes
• Decreased cardiac output
• Hypovolemia
• Peripheral vasodilation
• Renovascular obstruction
• Severe vasoconstriction

Intrarenal causes
• Acute tubular necrosis
• Glomerulonephritis
• Renovascular occlusion
• Vasculitis

Postrenal causes
• Bladder obstruction
• Ureteral obstruction
• Urethral obstruction

○ Percuss and palpate the bladder.
○ Palpate the kidneys and percuss the costovertebral angle.
○ Auscultate over the renal arteries for bruits. (See *Assessing for renal bruits.*)

Medical causes

Acute tubular necrosis

○ Anuria occurs occasionally; oliguria (diminished urine output) is more common.
○ Oliguria precedes the onset of diuresis.
○ Other findings reflect the underlying cause and may include signs and symptoms of hyperkalemia, uremia, and heart failure.

Glomerulonephritis (acute)

○ Anuria or oliguria occurs.
○ Related findings include mild fever, malaise, flank pain, gross hematuria, edema, elevated blood pressure, headache, nausea, vomiting, abdominal pain, crackles, and dyspnea.

Hemolytic-uremic syndrome

○ Anuria occurs in the initial stages and lasts 1 to 10 days.
○ Other findings include vomiting, diarrhea, abdominal pain, hematemesis, melena, purpura, fever, elevated blood pressure, hepatomegaly, ecchymoses, edema, hematuria, pallor, and signs of upper respiratory tract infection.

Renal artery occlusion (bilateral)

○ Anuria or severe oliguria is accompanied by severe, continuous upper abdominal and flank pain; nausea and vomiting; decreased bowel sounds; fever; and diastolic hypertension.

Renal vein occlusion (bilateral)

○ Anuria sometimes develops with lower back pain, fever, flank tenderness, and hematuria.
○ Development of pulmonary emboli, a common complication, produces sudden dyspnea, pleuritic pain, tachypnea, tachycardia, crackles, and possibly hemoptysis.

Urinary tract obstruction

○ Acute or total anuria may alternate with or precede burning pain on urination, overflow incontinence or dribbling, urinary frequency and nocturia, voiding in small amounts, or altered urine stream.
○ Other findings include bladder distention, pain and a sensation of fullness in the lower abdomen and groin, upper abdominal and flank pain, nausea and vomiting, and signs of secondary infection.

Use the bell of your stethoscope to auscultate for bruits at the sites shown in the illustration.

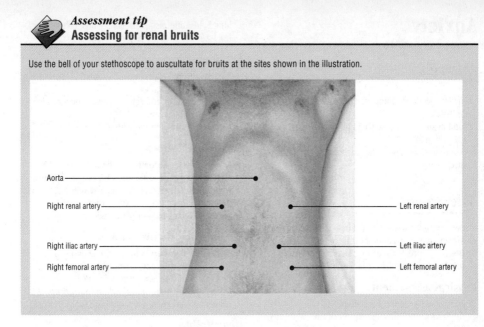

Aorta

Right renal artery — Left renal artery

Right iliac artery — Left iliac artery

Right femoral artery — Left femoral artery

Other causes

Diagnostic tests

○ Contrast media can cause nephrotoxicity, producing oliguria and, rarely, anuria.

Drugs

○ Nephrotoxic drugs that can cause anuria or oliguria include antibiotics (especially aminoglycosides), adrenergics, anesthetics, anticholinergics, ethyl alcohol, heavy metals, and organic solvents.

Nursing considerations

○ If catheterization fails to initiate urine flow, prepare the patient for diagnostic studies, such as ultrasonography, cystoscopy, retrograde pyelography, and renal scan to detect any obstruction higher in the urinary tract.
○ If an obstruction is present, prepare the patient for surgery and insert a nephrostomy tube or ureterostomy tube to drain the urine.
○ Monitor vital signs and measure intake and output, saving urine for inspection.
○ Restrict daily fluids to 600 ml more than the previous day's total urine output.
○ Restrict foods and juices high in potassium and sodium.
○ Have the patient maintain a balanced diet and control protein intake.
○ Record fluid intake and output and weigh the patient daily.

Pediatric pointers

○ In neonates, anuria is the absence of urine output for 24 hours.
○ Anuria in children commonly results from loss of renal function.

Geriatric pointers

○ Hospitalized or bedridden patients may be unable to generate pressure to void in a supine position.

Patient teaching

○ Discuss fluids and foods the patient should avoid.
○ Instruct the patient on nephrostomy tube or ureterostomy tube care, if needed.

Anxiety

Overview

- Anxiety produces a nonspecific feeling of uneasiness or dread.
- Mild anxiety can cause slight physical or psychological discomfort.
- Severe anxiety may be incapacitating or even life-threatening.

Assessment

- Determine the patient's chief complaint.
- Ask about the duration of the anxiety.
- Determine precipitating or exacerbating factors.
- Obtain a medical history, including drug use.

Physical assessment

- Perform a physical examination.
- Focus on complaints that trigger or are aggravated by anxiety.
- Assess level of consciousness (LOC) and observe behavior.

Medical causes

Acute respiratory distress syndrome

- Acute anxiety occurs along with tachycardia, mental sluggishness and, in severe cases, hypotension.
- Respiratory findings include dyspnea, tachypnea, intercostal and suprasternal retractions, crackles, and rhonchi.

Anaphylactic shock

- Acute anxiety signals the onset of anaphylactic shock.
- Anxiety is accompanied by urticaria, angioedema, pruritus, and shortness of breath.
- Others findings include light-headedness, hypotension, tachycardia, nasal congestion, sneezing, wheezing, dyspnea, barking cough, abdominal cramps, vomiting, diarrhea, and urinary urgency and incontinence.

Angina pectoris

- Acute anxiety may precede or follow an attack.
- Sharp and crushing substernal or anterior chest pain that may radiate to the back, neck, arms, or jaw occur during an attack.
- Nitroglycerin or rest may relieve the pain, easing anxiety.

Asthma

- Acute anxiety occurs with dyspnea, wheezing, productive cough, accessory muscle use, hyperresonant lung fields, diminished breath sounds, coarse crackles, cyanosis, tachycardia, and diaphoresis.

Autonomic hyperreflexia

- Anxiety, severe headache, and dramatic hypertension may be early signs.
- Pallor and motor and sensory deficits occur below the level of the lesion.
- Flushing occurs above the level of the lesion.

Cardiogenic shock

- Acute anxiety is accompanied by cool, pale, clammy skin; tachycardia; weak, thready pulse; tachypnea; ventricular gallop; crackles; jugular vein distention; decreased urine output; hypotension; narrowing pulse pressure; and peripheral edema.

Chronic obstructive pulmonary disease

- Acute anxiety occurs with exertional dyspnea, cough, wheezing, crackles, hyperresonant lung fields, tachypnea, and accessory muscle use.
- Other signs include "barrel" chest, pursed-lip breathing, and finger clubbing (late in the disease).

Heart failure

- Acute anxiety is a symptom of inadequate oxygenation.
- Other findings include restlessness, shortness of breath, tachypnea, decreased LOC, edema, crackles, ventricular gallop, hypotension, diaphoresis, and cyanosis.

Hyperthyroidism

- Acute anxiety may be an early sign.
- Classic findings include heat intolerance, weight loss despite increased appetite, nervousness, tremor, palpitations, sweating, an enlarged thyroid gland, exophthalmos, and diarrhea.

Hyperventilation syndrome

- Anxiety, pallor, and circumoral and peripheral paresthesia occur.
- Other findings include carpopedal spasms, chest pain, tachycardia, belching, flatus, and dizziness.

Hypochondriasis

- Mild to moderate chronic anxiety occurs.
- Patient is focused more on the belief that he has a specific serious disease than on the actual symptoms.
- Difficulty swallowing, back pain, light-headedness, and upset stomach are common complaints.

Hypoglycemia

- Anxiety is mild to moderate.
- Anxiety is associated with hunger, mild headache, palpitations, blurred vision, weakness, and diaphoresis.

Mitral valve prolapse

- Panic may occur.
- Hallmark sign of mitral valve prolapse is a midsystolic click, followed by an apical murmur.
- Paroxysmal palpitations with sharp, stabbing, or aching precordial pain may also occur.

Mood disorder

- Anxiety may be the chief complaint in the depressive or manic form.
- Other findings of the depressive form include dysphoria; anger; insomnia or hypersomnia; decreased libido, energy, and concentration; appetite disturbance; multiple somatic complaints; and suicidal thoughts.
- In the manic form, the patient may exhibit a reduced need for sleep, hyperactivity, increased energy, rapid or pressured speech and, in severe cases, paranoid ideas and other psychotic symptoms.

Myocardial infarction

- A life-threatening disorder — acute anxiety occurs with persistent, crushing substernal pain that may radiate.
- Anxiety may be accompanied by shortness of breath, nausea, vomiting, diaphoresis, and cool, pale skin.

Obsessive-compulsive disorder

- Chronic anxiety occurs along with thoughts or impulses to perform ritualistic acts.
- Anxiety builds if the patient can't perform rituals and diminishes if he can.
- The patient recognizes the acts as irrational, but he can't control them.

Pheochromocytoma

- Acute, severe anxiety accompanies the main sign of persistent or paroxysmal hypertension.
- Common signs and symptoms include tachycardia, diaphoresis, orthostatic hypotension, tachypnea, flushing, severe headache, palpitations, nausea, vomiting, epigastric pain, and paresthesia.

Phobias

- Chronic anxiety occurs along with persistent fear of an object, activity, or situation that results in a compelling desire to avoid it.
- The patient recognizes the fear as irrational, but he can't suppress it.

Postconcussion syndrome

- Chronic anxiety or periodic attacks of acute anxiety may occur, especially in situations demanding attention, judgment, or comprehension.
- Other findings include irritability, insomnia, dizziness, and mild headache.

Posttraumatic stress disorder

- Chronic anxiety occurs with thoughts of the extreme traumatic event.

- Intrusive, vivid memories and thoughts of the traumatic event also occur.
- The event is relived in dreams and nightmares.
- Insomnia, depression, and feelings of numbness and detachment are common.

Pulmonary edema

- Acute anxiety occurs along with dyspnea, orthopnea, cough with frothy sputum, tachycardia, tachypnea, crackles, ventricular gallop, hypotension, thready pulse, and cool, clammy skin.

Pulmonary embolism

- Hypoxia may result in acute anxiety and restlessness.
- The patient may also experience dyspnea, tachypnea, chest pain, tachycardia, blood-tinged sputum, and low-grade fever.

Somatoform disorder

- Anxiety and multiple somatic complaints that can't be explained are severe enough to impair functioning.

Other causes

Drugs

- Many drugs cause anxiety, especially sympathomimetics and central nervous system stimulants.
- Antidepressants may cause paradoxical anxiety.

Nursing considerations

- Provide a calm, quiet atmosphere.
- Encourage the patient to express his feelings and concerns freely.
- Encourage anxiety-reducing measures, such as distraction, relaxation techniques, or biofeedback.

Pediatric pointers

- Anxiety usually results from painful physical illness or inadequate oxygenation.
- The autonomic signs of anxiety tend to be more common and dramatic in children than in adults.

Geriatric pointers

- Distractions from ritualistic activity may provoke anxiety or agitation.

Patient teaching

- Instruct the patient in relaxation techniques.
- Encourage the patient's verbalization of anxiety.
- Help the patient to identify stressors.
- Help the patient understand more about coping mechanisms.

Aphasia (dysphasia)

Overview

- The impaired expression or comprehension of written or spoken language, caused by disease or injury to these centers of the brain (see *Where language originates*)
- May slightly impede communication or make it impossible
- May be classified as anomic, Broca's, global, or Wernicke's (see *Identifying types of aphasia*)
- Anomic aphasia: eventually resolves in more than half of patients; global aphasia: usually irreversible

★ *Emergency actions*

Look for signs and symptoms of increased intracranial pressure (ICP). If you detect increased ICP, administer mannitol I.V. to reduce cerebral edema. Make sure emergency resuscitation equipment is available, and anticipate preparing the patient for emergency surgery.

Assessment

History

- Perform a complete neurologic examination.
- Take a medical history including headaches, hypertension, seizure disorders, or drug use.
- Determine the patient's preaphasia ability to communicate and perform routine tasks.

Physical assessment

- Check for obvious signs of neurologic deficit.
- Take the patient's vital signs and assess his level of consciousness (LOC).
- Assess the patient's pupillary response, eye movements, and motor function.

Medical causes

Alzheimer's disease

- Anomic aphasia may begin insidiously and then progress to severe global aphasia.
- Other findings include behavioral changes, loss of memory, poor judgment, restlessness, myoclonus, and muscle rigidity.
- Incontinence is a late sign.

Brain abscess

- Any type of aphasia may occur.
- Aphasia may be accompanied by hemiparesis, ataxia, facial weakness, and signs of increased ICP.

Brain tumor

- Any type of aphasia
- As the tumor enlarges, behavioral changes, memory loss, motor weakness, seizures, auditory hallucinations, visual field deficits, and increased ICP

Creutzfeldt-Jakob disease

- Aphasia with a rapidly progressive dementia
- Aphasia possibly with myoclonic jerking, ataxia, vision disturbances, and paralysis

Encephalitis

- Transient aphasia

Where language originates

Aphasia reflects damage to one or more of the brain's primary language centers, which are usually located in the left hemisphere. Broca's area lies next to the region of the motor cortex that controls the muscles necessary for speech. Wernicke's area is the center of auditory, visual, and language comprehension. It lies between Heschl's gyrus, the primary receiver of auditory stimuli, and the angular gyrus, which is between the brain's auditory and visual regions. Connecting Wernicke's and Broca's areas is a large nerve bundle, the arcuate fasciculus, that enables repetition of speech.

Angular gyrus

Arcuate fasciculus

Broca's area

Wernicke's area

Heschl's gyrus

The location of the lesion as well as its signs and symptoms help to differentiate among types of aphasia.

Type	Location of lesion	Signs and symptoms
Anomic aphasia	Temporal-parietal area; may extend to angular gyrus, but sometimes is poorly localized	Patient's understanding of written and spoken language is relatively unimpaired. His speech, although fluent, lacks meaningful content. Word-finding difficulty and circumlocution are characteristic. Rarely, the patient also displays paraphasias.
Broca's aphasia (expressive aphasia)	Broca's area; usually in third frontal convolution of left hemisphere	Patient's understanding of written and spoken language is relatively unimpaired, but speech is nonfluent, with evidence of word-finding difficulty, jargon, paraphasias, limited vocabulary, and simple sentence construction. He can't repeat words and phrases that are spoken to him. If Wernicke's area is intact, he recognizes speech errors and shows frustration. He's commonly hemiparetic.
Global aphasia	Broca's area and Wernicke's area	Patient has profoundly impaired receptive and expressive ability. He can't repeat words or phrases that are spoken to him and can't follow directions. His occasional speech is marked by paraphasias or jargon.
Wernicke's aphasia (receptive aphasia)	Wernicke's area; usually in posterior or superior temporal lobe	Patient has difficulty understanding written and spoken language. He can't repeat words or phrases that are spoken to him and can't follow directions. His speech is fluent but may be rapid and rambling, with paraphasias. He has difficulty naming objects (anomia) and is unaware of speech errors.

○ Early on, fever, headache, and vomiting
○ Seizures, confusion, stupor or coma, hemiparesis, asymmetrical deep tendon reflexes, positive Babinski's reflex, ataxia, myoclonus, nystagmus, oculomotor palsies, and facial weakness

Head trauma
○ Sudden aphasia
○ Transient or permanent, depending on the extent of brain damage.
○ Blurred or double vision, headache, pallor, diaphoresis, numbness and paresis, discharge — containing cerebrospinal fluid — from the ear or nose, altered respirations, tachycardia, behavioral changes, and increased ICP.

Seizure disorder
○ Transient aphasia may occur if the seizures involve the language centers.

Stroke
○ Wernicke's, Broca's, or global aphasia
○ Decreased LOC, right-sided hemiparesis, homonymous hemianopsia, paresthesia, loss of sensation.

Transient ischemic attack
○ Sudden aphasia resolving within 24 hours

○ Transient hemiparesis, hemianopsia, paresthesia, dizziness, and confusion

Nursing considerations
○ Tell the patient frequently what has happened, where he is and why, and what the date is.
○ Expect periods of depression as the patient recognizes his disability.
○ Help the patient communicate by providing a relaxed environment with minimal distracting stimuli.

Pediatric pointers
○ Brain damage associated with aphasia most commonly follows anoxia — the result of near drowning or airway obstruction.

Geriatric pointers
○ Although a stroke can strike at any age, usually patients are men older than age 65.
○ When assessing speech in an elderly patient, make sure that his dentures and hearing aid are in place.

Patient teaching
○ Discuss alternate means of communication.
○ Discuss the risk reduction factors for stroke.

Apraxia

Overview

○ Inability to perform purposeful movements in the absence of significant weakness, sensory loss, poor coordination, or lack of comprehension or motivation
○ Classified as ideational, ideomotor, or kinetic, or by type of impairment (see *How apraxia interferes with purposeful movement*)
○ Indicative of a lesion in the cerebral hemisphere

⭐ Emergency actions

If signs and symptoms of increased intracranial pressure (ICP) are present, elevate the head of the bed 30 degrees and monitor for altered pupil size and reactivity, bradycardia, widened pulse pressure, and irregular respirations. Have emergency resuscitation equipment available and be prepared to give mannitol I.V. to decrease cerebral edema.

If the patient is having seizures, stay with the patient and have another nurse notify the physician immediately. Position the patient in a supine position, loosen tight clothing, and place a pillow or other soft object beneath his head. Avoid restraining the patient. If the patient's teeth are clenched, don't force anything into his mouth. Turn the patient's head to provide an open airway. After the seizure, reassure the patient that he's alright, and orient him to time and place.

Assessment

History

○ Ask about a history of headaches or dizziness.
○ Obtain a medical history, including previous neurologic, cerebrovascular, neoplastic, or hepatic disease; atherosclerosis; or infection.

Physical assessment

○ Perform a neurologic assessment.
○ Take vital signs and assess level of consciousness.
○ Test the patient's motor and sensory function.
○ Check deep tendon reflexes for quality and symmetry.
○ Test for visual field defects.

Medical causes

Alzheimer's disease

○ Gradual and irreversible ideomotor apraxia sometimes occurs.
○ Other findings may also include amnesia, anomia, decreased attention span, apathy, aphasia, restlessness, agitation, paranoid delusions, incontinence, social withdrawal, ataxia, and tremors.

Brain abscess

○ Apraxia occasionally results from a large brain abscess; it resolves spontaneously after the infection subsides.
○ Depending on the location of the abscess, other findings may include headache, fever, drowsiness, decreased metal acuity, aphasia, dysarthria, hemiparesis, hyperreflexia, incontinence, focal or generalized seizures, and ocular disturbances.

Brain tumor

○ May occur with or after early signs of increased ICP.
○ Apraxia may be preceded by decreased mental acuity, headache, dizziness, and seizures.

How apraxia interferes with purposeful movement

Type of apraxia	Description	Examination technique
Ideational apraxia	The patient can physically perform the steps required to complete a task but fails to remember the sequence in which they're performed.	Ask the patient to tie his shoelace. Typically, he'll be able to grasp the shoelace, loop it, and pull on it. However, he'll fail to remember the sequence of steps needed to tie a knot.
Ideomotor apraxia	The patient understands and can physically perform the steps required to complete the task but can't formulate a plan to carry them out.	Ask the patient to wave or cross his arms. Typically he won't respond, but he may be able to spontaneously perform the gesture.
Kinetic apraxia	The patient understands the task and formulates a plan but fails to set the proper muscles in motion.	Ask the patient to comb his hair. Typically, he'll fail to move his arm and hand correctly to do the task. However, he'll be able to state that he needs to pick up the comb and draw it through his hair.

- Localizing signs and symptoms of the tumor may include aphasia, dysarthria, visual field deficits, weakness, stiffness, and hyperreflexia in the extremities.

Hepatic encephalopathy

- Onset of constructional apraxia (the inability to copy simple drawings or patterns) is gradual and may be reversible with treatment.
- Early associated signs and symptoms include disorientation, amnesia, slurred speech, dysarthria, asterixis, and lethargy.
- Later signs include hyperreflexia, positive Babinski's reflex, agitation, seizures, *fetor hepaticus* (breath odor characteristic of liver disease), stupor, and coma.

Stroke

- Onset of apraxia is sudden and commonly resolves spontaneously.
- Other findings include headache, confusion, coma, hemiplegia, visual field deficits, aphasia, agnosia, dysarthria, and incontinence.

Nursing considerations

- Prepare the patient for diagnostic studies such as computed tomography scanning.
- Because weakness, sensory deficits, confusion, and seizures may accompany apraxia, take measures to ensure the patient's safety.

Pediatric pointers

- Sudden inability to perform a previously accomplished movement warrants prompt neurologic evaluation.
- Brain tumor is the most common cause of apraxia in children.
- Developmental apraxia may be caused by brain damage.

Patient teaching

- Provide an explanation of apraxia.
- Demonstrate routine tasks.
- Refer the patient to physical or occupational therapy.

Arm pain

Overview

○ Usually results from musculoskeletal disorders
○ May be referred from another area
○ Can be sharp or dull, burning or numbing, and shooting or penetrating

Assessment

History

○ Ask about history of injury.
○ Determine onset, duration, and description of pain.
○ Determine the location of referred pain.
○ Ask about factors that aggravate or alleviate pain.
○ Obtain a medical history including current drug therapy.
○ Determine whether a family history of gout or arthritis exists.

Physical assessment

○ Inspect the arm; compare it with the opposite arm for symmetry, movement, and muscle atrophy.
○ Palpate for swelling, nodules, and tender areas.
○ Assess circulation in both arms.
○ Compare active range of motion, muscle strength, and reflexes bilaterally.
○ Check responses to vibration, temperature, and pinprick.
○ Examine the neck for pain, point tenderness, or muscle spasms.
○ Check for arm pain when the neck is extended with the head toward the involved side.

Medical causes

Angina

○ Inner arm, chest, and jaw pain follows exertion.
○ Pain lasts for 2 to 10 minutes.
○ Dyspnea, diaphoresis, and apprehension accompany pain.
○ Rest or vasodilators relieve pain.

Cellulitis

○ Leg pain usually occurs, but arms may also be affected.
○ Redness, tenderness, and edema accompany the pain.
○ Fever, chills, tachycardia, headache, and hypotension may also occur.

Cervical nerve root compression

○ If nerves supplying upper arm are affected, chronic arm and neck pain occurs.

○ Pain may worsen with movement or prolonged sitting.
○ Muscle weakness, paresthesia, and decreased reflex response may also occur.

Compartment syndrome

○ Severe pain with passive muscle stretching is the main sign.
○ Other findings include muscle weakness, decreased reflex response, paresthesia, and edema.
○ Ominous signs include paralysis and absent pulse.

Fractures

○ Pain may occur at the site of injury and radiate throughout the arm.
○ Pain with a fresh fracture is intense and worsens with movement.
○ Other signs and symptoms include crepitus, deformity, ecchymosis, edema, impaired distal circulation and sensation, and paresthesia.

Muscle contusion or strain

○ Pain occurs in the area of injury.
○ Local swelling and ecchymosis may occur.
○ Mild to moderate pain occurs with movement, possibly leading to muscle weakness and atrophy.

Myocardial infarction

○ A life-threatening disorder — left arm pain may occur with deep, crushing chest pain.
○ Other findings include weakness, pallor, nausea, vomiting, diaphoresis, altered blood pressure, tachycardia, dyspnea, and feelings of apprehension or impending doom.

Neoplasms of the arm

○ Continuous, deep, and penetrating pain develops and worsens at night.
○ Redness and swelling accompany arm pain.
○ Late findings include skin breakdown, impaired circulation, and paresthesia.

Osteomyelitis

○ Vague and evanescent localized arm pain and fever occur.
○ Other findings include local tenderness, painful and restricted movement, malaise, tachycardia and, later, swelling.

Nursing considerations

○ Prepare the patient for diagnostic tests or X-rays.
○ Monitor for worsening pain, numbness, or decreased circulation distal to injury site.
○ Monitor vital signs and look for tachycardia, hypotension and diaphoresis. Take emergency actions for cardiovascular disorders (myocardial infarction).
○ Apply a sling or splint to immobilize the arm.

- Make the patient comfortable by elevating the arm and applying ice.
- Clean abrasions and lacerations and apply dry, sterile dressings.

Pediatric pointers

- Arm pain commonly results from fractures, muscle sprain, muscular dystrophy, or rheumatoid arthritis.
- If the child has a fracture or sprain, obtain a complete account of the injury; don't dismiss the possibility of child abuse.

Geriatric pointers

- Patients with osteoporosis are prone to degenerative joint disease and may experience fractures from simple trauma, heavy lifting, or unexpected movements.

Patient teaching

- Explain the signs and symptoms of circulatory impairment caused by a tight cast.
- Discuss the signs and symptoms of an ischemic event.

Ataxia

Overview

○ Incoordination and irregularity of voluntary, purposeful movements
○ Has acute (possibly life-threatening) and chronic forms
○ Can be classified as cerebellar (resulting from disease of the cerebellum) or sensory (resulting from proprioception)
○ Gait, trunk, limb and, possibly, speech disorders with the cerebellar form
○ Gait disorders with the sensory form

⚡ Emergency actions

If ataxic movements occur suddenly, examine for signs of increased intracranial pressure and impending herniation. Determine the level of consciousness (LOC) and be alert for pupillary changes, motor weakness or paralysis, neck stiffness or pain, and vomiting. Check vital signs, especially respirations. Elevate the head of the bed. Have emergency resuscitation equipment readily available. Prepare the patient for computed tomography scanning or surgery.

Assessment

History

○ Ask about a history of multiple sclerosis, diabetes, central nervous system infection, neoplastic disease, or stroke.
○ Inquire about a family history of ataxia.
○ Ask about chronic alcohol abuse or prolonged exposure to industrial toxins.
○ Find out if the ataxia developed suddenly or gradually.

Physical assessment

○ Perform Romberg's test to help distinguish between cerebellar and sensory ataxia.
○ Check motor strength.

Medical causes

Cerebellar abscess

○ Limb ataxia occurs on the same side as the lesion, with gait and truncal ataxia.
○ Initial symptom is headache localized behind the ear or in the occipital region.
○ Other findings include oculomotor palsy, fever, vomiting, altered LOC, and coma.

Cerebellar hemorrhage

○ A life-threatening disorder — ataxia is usually acute but transient; it may affect the trunk, gait, or limbs.
○ Initial signs include repeated vomiting, occipital headache, vertigo, oculomotor palsy, dysphagia, and dysarthria.
○ Late signs, such as decreased LOC or coma, signal impending herniation.

Creutzfeldt-Jakob disease

○ Ataxia accompanies other neurologic signs, such as myoclonic jerking, aphasia, and rapidly progressing dementia.

Diabetic neuropathy

○ Peripheral nerve damage may cause sensory ataxia.
○ Other findings include arm or leg pain, slight leg weakness, skin changes, bowel and bladder dysfunction, unsteady gait and, as neuropathy progresses, numbness in the feet.

Diphtheria

○ A life-threatening disorder — sensory ataxia may occur within 4 to 8 weeks of the onset of symptoms.
○ Other findings include fever, paresthesia, and paralysis of the limbs and, sometimes, the respiratory muscles.

Hepatocerebral degeneration

○ Residual neurologic defects, including mild cerebellar ataxia with a wide-based and unsteady gait, occur in those who survive hepatic coma.
○ Other symptoms include altered LOC, dysarthria, rhythmic arm tremors, and choreoathetosis of the face, neck, and shoulders.

Hyperthermia

○ If the patient survives the coma and seizures characteristic of the acute phase, cerebellar ataxia can occur.
○ Subsequent findings include spastic paralysis, dementia, and slowly resolving confusion.

Metastatic cancer

○ If cancer metastasizes to the cerebellum, gait ataxia may occur along with headache, dizziness, nystagmus, decreased LOC, nausea, and vomiting.
○ With a cerebellar tumor, gait ataxia may occur as well as dizziness, muscle incoordination, and nystagmus.
○ Falling toward the side of the lesion may occur.

Multiple sclerosis

○ Cerebellar ataxia may occur.
○ Spinal cord involvement may cause speech and sensory ataxia.
○ Ataxia may subside or disappear during remissions.
○ Other findings include optic neuritis, optic atrophy, numbness and weakness, diplopia, dizziness, and bladder dysfunction.

Poisoning

○ Chronic arsenic poisoning may cause sensory ataxia along with headache, seizures, altered LOC, motor deficits, and muscle aching.
○ Chronic mercury poisoning causes gait and limb ataxia, principally of the arms as well as dysarthria, mood changes, mental confusion, and tremors of the extremities, tongue, and lips.

Polyarteritis nodosa

○ Sensory ataxia, abdominal and limb pain, hematuria, and elevated blood pressure may occur.
○ Other findings include myalgia, headache, joint pain, and weakness.

Polyneuropathy

○ Ataxia, severe motor weakness, muscle atrophy, and sensory loss in the limbs occur.
○ Pain and skin changes may also occur.

Posterior fossa tumor

○ Gait, truncal, or limb ataxia is an early sign; ataxia may worsen as the tumor enlarges.
○ Other findings include vomiting, headache, papilledema, vertigo, oculomotor palsy, decreased LOC, and motor and sensory impairment on the same side as the lesion.

Spinocerebellar ataxia

○ Fatigue occurs initially, followed by stiff-legged gait ataxia.
○ Eventually, limb ataxia, dysarthria, static tremor, nystagmus, cramps, paresthesia, and sensory deficits occur.

Stroke

○ Infarction in medulla, pons, or cerebellum may lead to ataxia, which may remain as a residual symptom.
○ Worsening ataxia during acute phase may indicate extension of stroke or severe swelling of the brain.
○ Accompanying findings include motor weakness, sensory loss, vertigo, nausea, vomiting, oculomotor palsy, dysphagia and, possibly, altered LOC.

Wernicke's disease

○ Gait ataxia occurs.
○ With severe ataxia, the patient may not be able to stand or walk.
○ Other findings include nystagmus, diplopia, oculomotor palsies, confusion, tachycardia, exertional dyspnea, and orthostatic hypotension.

Other causes

Drugs

○ Aminoglutethimide may cause ataxia that disappears 4 to 6 weeks after the drug is stopped.
○ Toxic levels of anticonvulsants, anticholinergics, and tricyclic antidepressants may result in ataxia.

Nursing considerations

○ If toxic drug levels are the cause, stop the drug.
○ Encourage physical therapy to improve function following a stroke.
○ If the patient has a brain tumor, prepare him for surgery, chemotherapy, or radiation therapy.

Pediatric pointers

○ Acute ataxia may stem from febrile infection, brain tumors, mumps, and other disorders.
○ Chronic ataxia may stem from Gaucher's disease, Refsum's disease, and other inborn errors of metabolism.
○ If you suspect ataxia, refer the child for a neurologic evaluation to rule out a brain tumor.

Patient teaching

○ Help the patient to identify rehabilitation goals.
○ Stress safety measures.
○ Discuss use of assistive devices.
○ Refer the patient to counseling as needed.

Athetosis

Overview

○ Athetosis is an extrapyramidal sign characterized by slow, continuous, and twisting involuntary movements of the face, neck, and distal extremities.
○ Facial grimaces, jaw and tongue movements, and occasional phonation are associated with neck movements.
○ Worsened during stress and voluntary activity, movements may subside during relaxation and disappear during sleep.
○ Commonly a lifelong disorder, athetosis may be difficult to distinguish from chorea. Typically, athetoid movements are slower than choreiform movements. (See *Distinguishing athetosis from chorea.*)

Assessment

History

○ Obtain a medical history, including prenatal and postnatal complications, drug therapy, and family history.
○ Determine the onset and duration of symptoms.
○ Ask about the effects of rest, stress, and routine activity on symptoms.

Distinguishing athetosis from chorea

In *athetosis*, movements are typically slow, twisting, and writhing. They're associated with spasticity and most commonly involve the face, neck, and distal extremities.

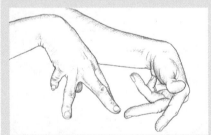

In *chorea*, movements are brief, rapid, jerky, and unpredictable. They can occur at rest or during normal movement. Typically, they involve the hands, lower arm, face, and head.

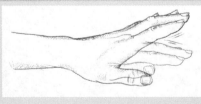

Physical assessment

○ Test muscle strength and tone, range of motion, fine-muscle movements, and ability to perform rapidly alternating movements.
○ Observe limb muscles during voluntary movements, noting the rhythm and duration of contraction and relaxation.

Medical causes

Brain tumor

○ Opposite-side choreoathetosis occurs.
○ Other signs vary with the type of tumor and degree of invasion.

Calcification of the basal ganglia

○ Characterized by choreoathetosis and rigidity
○ Usually arises in adolescence or early adult life

Cerebral infarction

○ Opposite-side athetosis is accompanied by altered level of consciousness.
○ Opposite-side paralysis of the face or limbs may also occur.

Hepatic encephalopathy

○ Episodic or persistent choreoathetosis occurs in the chronic stage.
○ Other findings include cerebellar ataxia, myoclonus of the face and limbs, asterixis, dysarthria, and dementia.

Huntington's disease

○ Athetosis and chorea progressively develop.
○ Other findings include dystonia, dysarthria, facial apraxia, rigidity, depression, and progressive mental deterioration leading to dementia.

Wilson's disease

○ Initially, choreoathetoid movements involve the fingers and hands and then spread to the arms, head, trunk, and legs.
○ Other findings include Kayser-Fleischer rings, arm and hand tremors, facial and muscular rigidity, dysarthria, dysphagia, drooling, and progressive dementia.
○ Hepatomegaly, splenomegaly, jaundice, hematemesis, and spider angiomas may also occur.

Other causes

Drugs

○ Athetoid or choreoathetoid movements may occur with toxic levels of levodopa and phenytoin.
○ Athetosis may occur with phenothiazine and other antipsychotics.

Nursing considerations

○ Stop the drug that is causing the athetosis.
○ Prepare the patient for diagnostic tests, such as computed tomography scanning, magnetic resonance imaging, lumbar puncture, EEG, and urine and blood studies.
○ Assist with rehabilitation.
○ Encourage exercise to maintain coordination, reduce the rate of deterioration, and minimize antisocial behavior.
○ Encourage verbalization of feelings.
○ Help the patient adapt to assistive devices to perform fine motor tasks.

Pediatric pointers

○ Athetosis may be acquired or inherited.
○ Refer parents or caregivers to special education services, rehabilitation centers, and support groups.
○ Promote the patient's self-esteem and positive self-image.

Geriatric pointers

○ Carefully question elderly patients about tremors; many older adults believe that tremors are a part of aging and may not report them.
○ Tremors may result from vascular or neoplastic lesions, degenerative disease, drug toxicity, or hypoxia.

Patient teaching

○ Provide information about self-help groups and appropriate support services such as physical therapy.
○ Give instruction in use of assistive devices.
○ Stress safety measures to prevent falls.

Babinski's reflex

Overview

- Also known as *extensor plantar reflex* or *toe sign*
- Refers to dorsiflexion of the great toe with extension and fanning of the other toes
- Elicited by firmly stroking the side of the sole of the foot with a moderately sharp object (see *How to test for Babinski's reflex*)
- A normal response in infants; in normal adults and infants, toes curl toward the sole
- May be on one side or both
- May be temporary or permanent
- Permanent: Indicates corticospinal damage
- Temporary: Occurs in the postictal state of a seizure

Assessment

History

- Ask about recent head trauma, spinal cord injury, or animal bite.
- Find out about a personal or family history of neurologic disorders.

Physical assessment

- Evaluate other neurologic signs.
- Evaluate muscle strength and tone in each extremity.
- Observe coordination.
- Test deep tendon reflexes (DTRs) in the elbow, antecubital area, wrist, knee, and ankle.
- Evaluate pain sensation and proprioception in the feet.

Medical causes

Amyotrophic lateral sclerosis

- One-sided Babinski's reflex may occur with hyperactive DTRs and spasticity.
- Fasciculations are accompanied by muscle atrophy and weakness.
- Other findings include incoordination; impaired speech; difficulty chewing, swallowing, and breathing; urinary frequency and urgency; and choking and excessive drooling.

Brain tumor

- Only if the tumor involves the corticospinal tract.
- Other findings include hHyperactive DTRs, spasticity, seizures, cranial nerve dysfunction, hemiparesis or hemiplegia, decreased pain sensation, unsteady gait, incoordination, headache, emotional lability, and decreased level of consciousness (LOC).

Head trauma

- From primary corticospinal damage or secondary injury associated with increased intracranial pressure
- Hyperactive DTRs, spasticity, weakness, and incoordination
- Depending on the type of head trauma, headache, vomiting, behavior changes, altered vital signs, and decreased LOC with abnormal pupillary size and response to light.

Meningitis

- Babinski's reflex of both feet follows fever, chills, and malaise.
- Nausea and vomiting occur.
- Decreased LOC, nuchal rigidity, positive Brudzinski's and Kernig's signs, hyperactive DTRs, and opisthotonos occur as meningitis progresses.
- Other findings include irritability, photophobia, diplopia, delirium, and deep stupor that may progress to coma.

Multiple sclerosis

- Babinski's reflex starts in one foot but eventually occurs in both.
- Initial signs and symptoms include paresthesia, nystagmus, and blurred or double vision.
- Other findings include scanning speech (syllables separated by pauses), dysphagia, intention tremor, weakness, incoordination, spasticity, gait ataxia, seizures, paraparesis or paraplegia, bladder incontinence, emotional lability, and loss of pain and temperature sensation and proprioception.

Pernicious anemia

- Babinski's reflex occurs in both feet late in the progression of the disorder.
- Burning tongue, general weakness, and numbness and tingling in the extremities are the classic triad of symptoms in pernicious anemia.
- Other findings include constipation, diarrhea, abdominal pain, nausea and vomiting, bleeding gums, ataxia, anorexia, diplopia and blurred vision, positive Romberg's sign, tachycardia, irritability, headache, malaise, and fatigue.

Rabies

- Babinski's reflex in both feet occurs during the excitation phase, 2 to 10 days after the onset of symptoms.
- Occurring 30 to 40 days after a bite from an infected animal, prodromal findings include fever, malaise, and irritability.
- Characterized by restlessness and extremely painful pharyngeal muscle spasms.
- Difficulty swallowing, excessive drooling, hydrophobia, seizures, and hyperactive DTRs may also occur.

Spinal cord injury

- Babinski's reflex can be elicited as spinal shock resolves.

Firmly stroke the side of the sole of the patient's foot with your thumbnail or another moderately sharp object. Normally, this elicits flexion of all toes (a negative Babinski's reflex), as shown below left. With a positive Babinski's reflex, the great toe dorsiflexes and the other toes fan out, as shown below right.

NORMAL TOE FLEXION

POSITIVE BABINSKI'S REFLEX

○ Babinski's reflex occurs on one side if injury affects only one side of the spinal cord (Brown-Séquard's syndrome), both sides if injury affects both sides.
○ Other findings include hyperactive DTRs, spasticity, and variable or total loss of pain and temperature sensation, proprioception, and motor function.
○ Horner's syndrome — marked by one-sided ptosis, pupillary constriction, and facial anhidrosis — may occur with lower cervical cord injury.

Spinal cord tumor

○ Babinski's reflex in both feet occurs with paresis and paralysis below the level of the tumor.
○ Other findings include spasticity, hyperactive DTRs, absent abdominal reflexes, incontinence, and diffuse pain at the level of the tumor.

Stroke

○ Cerebral involvement produces Babinski's reflex in one foot with hemiplegia or hemiparesis, one-sided hyperactive DTRs, hemianopsia, and aphasia.
○ Brain stem involvement produces Babinski's reflex in both feet with weakness or paralysis, bilateral hyperactive DTRs, cranial nerve dysfunction, incoordination, and unsteady gait.
○ Generalized findings include headache, vomiting, fever, disorientation, nuchal rigidity, seizures, and coma.

Nursing considerations

○ Assist the patient with activity.
○ Keep his environment free from obstructions.

Pediatric pointers

○ Babinski's reflex occurs normally in infants up to age 2, reflecting immaturity of the corticospinal tract.
○ After age 2, Babinski's reflex is pathologic and may result from hydrocephalus or any of the causes more commonly seen in adults.

Patient teaching

○ Caution the patient about the need to call for assistance when getting out of bed.
○ Discuss ways to maintain a safe environment.
○ Instruct the patient in the use of adaptive devices

Back pain

Overview

- Affects about 80% of the U.S. population
- May be acute or chronic, constant or intermittent
- May be localized or radiate along the spine or legs
- May be referred from abdomen or flank, possibly signaling a life-threatening disorder (see *Managing acute, severe back pain*)

Assessment

History

- Obtain a medical, family, and drug history.
- Ask about unusual sensations in the legs.
- Ask about diet and alcohol use.

Physical assessment

- Observe skin color, especially in the legs.
- Observe posture and body alignment.
- Palpate skin temperature and femoral, popliteal, posterior tibial, and pedal pulses.
- Ask the patient to bend forward, backward, and side to side while you palpate for paravertebral muscle spasms.
- Palpate the dorsolumbar spine for point tenderness.
- Ask the patient to walk—first on heels, then on toes.
- Evaluate patellar tendon (knee), Achilles tendon, and Babinski's reflexes.
- Evaluate the strength of the extensor hallucis longus by asking the patient to hold up his big toe against resistance.
- Measure leg length and hamstring and quadriceps muscles.

- Position the patient supine. Grasp his heel and slowly lift his leg. Note the pain's exact location and the angle between the table and his leg when it occurs. Repeat this maneuver with the opposite leg.
- Note the range of motion of the hip and knee.
- Palpate and percuss the flanks to elicit costovertebral angle tenderness.

Medical causes

Abdominal aortic aneurysm (dissecting)

- A life-threatening disorder—initially lower back pain or dull abdominal pain may occur.
- Upper abdominal pain is more common.
- A pulsating epigastrium mass may be palpated; pulsating stops after rupture.
- Other findings include mottled skin below the waist, absent femoral and pedal pulses, lower blood pressure in the legs than in the arms, abdominal rigidity, mild to moderate tenderness with guarding, and shock (if blood loss is significant).

Ankylosing spondylitis

- Sacroiliac pain radiates up the spine and is aggravated by pressure on the side of the pelvis.
- Pain is usually most severe in the morning or after a period of inactivity and isn't relieved by rest.
- Abnormal rigidity of the lumbar spine with forward flexion is characteristic.
- Other findings include local tenderness, fatigue, fever, anorexia, weight loss, and occasional iritis.

Intervertebral disk rupture

- Gradual or sudden lower back pain occurs with or without sciatica.
- Pain begins in the back and radiates to the buttocks and legs.

Emergency actions
Managing acute, severe back pain

If the patient reports acute, severe back pain, quickly take his vital signs; then perform a rapid assessment to rule out life-threatening causes:

- Ask him when the pain began. Can he relate it to any causes? For example, did the pain occur after eating? After falling on ice?
- Ask the patient to describe the pain. Is it burning, stabbing, throbbing, or aching? Is it constant or intermittent? Does it radiate to the buttocks or legs? Does he have leg weakness? Does the pain seem to originate in the abdomen and radiate to the back? Has he had a pain like this before? What makes it better or worse? Is it affected by activity or rest? Is it worse in the morning or evening? Does it wake him up? Typically, visceral-referred back pain is unaffected by activity and rest. In contrast, spondylogenic-referred back pain worsens

with activity and improves with rest. Pain of neoplastic origin is usually relieved by walking and worsens at night.

If the patient describes deep lumbar pain unaffected by activity, palpate for a pulsating epigastric mass. If this sign is present, suspect dissecting abdominal aortic aneurysm. Withhold food and fluid in anticipation of emergency surgery. Prepare for I.V. fluid replacement and for oxygen administration.

If the patient describes severe epigastric pain that radiates through the abdomen to the back, assess him for absent bowel sounds and for abdominal rigidity and tenderness. If these occur are present, suspect perforated ulcer or acute pancreatitis. Start an I.V. line for fluids and drugs, administer oxygen, and insert a nasogastric tube while withholding food.

- Pain is exacerbated by activity, coughing, and sneezing and is eased by rest.
- The patient walks slowly and rises from sitting to standing with extreme difficulty.
- Other findings include paresthesia, paravertebral muscle spasm, and decreased reflexes on the affected side.

Lumbosacral sprain

- Aching, localized pain and tenderness is associated with muscle spasm upon sideways motion.
- Flexion of the spine and movement intensify the pain; rest and lying recumbent with knees and hips flexed relieves it.

Pancreatitis (acute)

- A life-threatening disorder — upper abdominal pain may radiate to the flanks and back.
- Bending forward, drawing the knees to the chest, or moving around may relieve pain.
- Early findings include abdominal tenderness, nausea, vomiting, fever, pallor, tachycardia, hypoactive bowel sounds, rebound tenderness, and abdominal guarding and rigidity.
- Turner's sign (ecchymosis of the abdomen or flank) or Cullen's sign (bluish discoloration of skin around the umbilicus and in both flanks) signals hemorrhagic pancreatitis.

Perforated ulcer

- A life-threatening disorder — sudden, prostrating epigastric pain may radiate throughout the abdomen and to the back.
- Other findings include boardlike abdominal rigidity, tenderness with guarding, generalized rebound tenderness, absent bowel sounds, fever, tachycardia, hypotension, and grunting, shallow respirations.

Prostate cancer

- Chronic aching back pain may be the only symptom, appearing in the advanced stages.
- Other late findings include hematuria, difficulty initiating a urine stream, dribbling, urine retention, unexplained cystitis, and a decrease in the urine stream.

Pyelonephritis (acute)

- Progressive flank and lower abdominal pain accompanies back pain or tenderness (especially over the costovertebral angle).
- Other findings include high fever and chills, nausea, vomiting, flank and abdominal tenderness, and urinary frequency and urgency.

Renal calculi

- Colicky pain travels from the costovertebral angle to the flank, suprapubic region, and external genitalia.
- If calculi travel down a ureter, the patient may feel excruciating pain.
- If calculi are in the renal pelvis and calyces, the patient may feel dull and constant flank pain.

- Other findings include nausea, vomiting, urinary urgency, hematuria, and agitation.

Sacroiliac strain

- Sacroiliac pain may radiate to the buttock, hip, and lateral aspect of the thigh.
- Weight bearing on the affected side and abduction with resistance of the leg aggravates the pain.

Spinal stenosis

- Back pain occurs with or without sciatica.
- Pain may radiate to the toes and, if the patient doesn't rest, may progress to numbness or weakness.

Transverse process fractures and vertebral compression fractures

- Severe localized back pain occurs with muscle spasm and hematoma in a transverse process fracture.
- Pain may not occur for several weeks in a vertebral compression fracture, then back pain aggravated by weight bearing and local tenderness occurs.

Vertebral osteoporosis

- Chronic, aching back pain is aggravated by activity and relieved somewhat by rest.
- Vertebral collapse, causing a backache with pain that radiates around the trunk, is the most common characteristic.

Nursing considerations

- If the cause is life-threatening, monitor the patient closely.
- Look for increasing pain, altered neurovascular condition of the legs, loss of bowel or bladder control, altered vital signs, sweating, and cyanosis.
- Withhold food and fluids in case surgery is needed.
- Elevate the head of the bed and place a pillow under the knees.
- Fit the patient for a corset or lumbosacral support.
- Apply heat or cold therapy, backboard, foam mattress, or pelvic traction.

Pediatric pointers

- Back pain may stem from diskitis, neoplasms, idiopathic juvenile osteoporosis, and spondylolisthesis.

Patient teaching

- Provide information about use of anti-inflammatory drugs and analgesics.
- Discuss lifestyle changes, such as losing weight or correcting posture.
- Teach relaxation techniques such as deep breathing.
- Instruct the patient on correct use of corset or lumbosacral support.
- Provide information about alternatives to drug therapy, such as biofeedback and transcutaneous electrical nerve stimulation.

Barrel chest

Overview

○ A rounded chest in which the anteroposterior diameter enlarges to approximate the transverse diameter
○ A late sign of chronic obstructive pulmonary disease (COPD) — results from increased lung volumes from chronic airflow obstruction (see *Recognizing barrel chest*)

Assessment

History

○ Ask about a history of pulmonary disease.
○ Note chronic exposure to environmental irritants such as asbestos.
○ Ask about smoking habits.
○ Inquire about a cough and, if it's productive, about the color and consistency of the sputum.
○ Ask if dyspnea or shortness of breath is present at rest or with activity.

Recognizing barrel chest

In the normal adult chest, the ratio of anteroposterior to transverse (or lateral) diameter is 1:2. In patients with barrel chest, this ratio approaches 1:1 as the anteroposterior diameter enlarges.

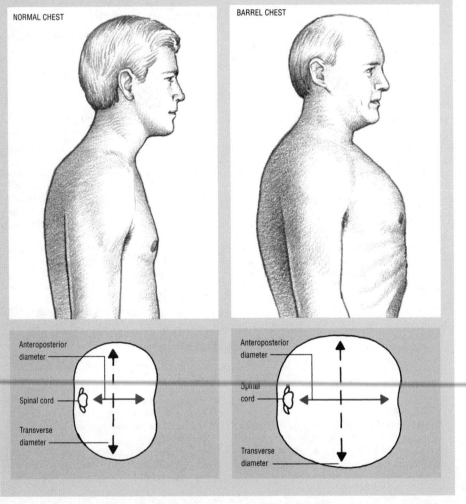

NORMAL CHEST

BARREL CHEST

Anteroposterior diameter

Spinal cord

Transverse diameter

Anteroposterior diameter

Spinal cord

Transverse diameter

Physical assessment

○ Auscultate for abnormal breath sounds.
○ Percuss the chest for hyperresonant sounds (indicating trapped air) and dull or flat sounds (indicating consolidation).
○ Observe for accessory muscle use, intercostal retractions, and tachypnea.
○ Note if central cyanosis of the cheeks, nose, and oral mucosa is present.
○ Check for peripheral cyanosis of the nail beds.
○ Observe for finger clubbing, a late sign of COPD.

Medical causes

Asthma

○ Barrel chest develops with chronic asthma.
○ Severe dyspnea, wheezing, and a productive cough occur with an acute asthma attack.
○ Prolonged expiratory time, accessory muscle use, tachycardia, perspiration, and flushing may also occur.

Chronic bronchitis

○ Barrel chest, a late sign, is preceded by dyspnea and a productive cough.
○ Other findings include cyanosis, tachypnea, wheezing, prolonged expiratory time, and accessory muscle use.

Emphysema

○ Barrel chest is a late sign.
○ Dyspnea is the initial symptom.
○ Eventually, anorexia, weight loss, malaise, accessory muscle use, pursed-lip breathing, tachypnea, peripheral cyanosis, clubbing of fingers, and a chronic cough occur.

Nursing considerations

○ Have the patient sit forward with his hands on his knees to support the upper torso and ease breathing.

Pediatric pointers

○ In infants, the ratio of anteroposterior to transverse diameter is normally 1:1.
○ By age 5 or 6, this ratio gradually changes to 1:2.
○ Cystic fibrosis and chronic asthma may cause barrel chest in the child.

Geriatric pointers

○ Senile kyphosis of the thoracic spine may be mistaken for barrel chest in an elderly patient, but signs of pulmonary disease are absent.

Patient teaching

○ Explain how to avoid bronchial irritants that may exacerbate COPD.

○ Emphasize the importance of quitting smoking, and provide information about resources to assist this goal.
○ Tell the patient the signs and symptoms of upper respiratory infection he should report.
○ Discuss the pacing of activities to minimize exertional dyspnea.

Battle's sign

Overview

- Ecchymosis over the temporal bone's mastoid process
- Develops 24 to 36 hours after a basilar skull fracture and is commonly the only outward sign of basilar skull fracture

⚡ Emergency actions

Basilar skull fracture, if untreated, can be fatal. Place the patient flat on his back in bed and monitor his neurologic status. If the patient has a large dural tear, prepare him for a craniotomy.

Assessment

History

- Ask about recent head trauma or accidents, such as severe head blow or motor vehicle accident.

Reviewing cranial nerves

The cranial nerves have either sensory or motor function or both. They're assigned Roman numerals and are written: CN I, CN II, CN III, and so forth. The function of each cranial nerve is listed below.
- CN I: Olfactory
Smell
- CN II: Optic
Vision
- CN III: Oculomotor
Most eye movement, pupillary constriction, upper eyelid elevation
- CN IV: Trochlear
Downward and inward eye movement
- CN V: Trigeminal
Chewing, corneal reflex, face and scalp sensations
- CN VI: Abducens
Lateral eye movement
- CN VII: Facial
Expressions in forehead, eye, and mouth; taste
- CN VIII: Acoustic
Hearing and balance
- CN IX: Glossopharyngeal
Swallowing, salivating, and tasting
- CN X: Vagus
Swallowing, gag reflex, talking; sensations of throat, larynx, and abdominal viscera; activities of thoracic and abdominal viscera, such as heart rate and peristalsis
- CN XI: Spinal accessory
Shoulder movement and head rotation
- CN XII: Hypoglossal
Tongue movement

Physical assessment

- Perform a complete neurologic examination, including mental status and speech, cranial nerve function, sensory and motor function, and reflexes. (See *Reviewing cranial nerves*.)
- Assess level of consciousness (LOC).
- Check vital signs; look for signs of increased intracranial pressure (ICP). (See *Signs of increased ICP*.)
- Evaluate pupillary size, response to light, and motor and verbal responses; relate data to the Glasgow Coma Scale.
- Note cerebrospinal fluid (CSF) leakage from the nose or ears.
- Look for the "halo" sign on bed linens or dressings.
- Test drainage with a glucose reagent strip to confirm that it's CSF. (If it's CSF, the strip will indicate presence of glucose.)
- Perform a complete physical examination of all body systems.

Medical causes

Basilar skull fracture

- Battle's sign may be the only outward sign.
- Other signs include periorbital ecchymosis ("raccoon" eyes), conjunctival hemorrhage, nystagmus, ocular deviation, epistaxis, anosmia, visible fracture lines on the external auditory canal, tinnitus, difficulty hearing, facial paralysis, vertigo, and a bulging tympanic membrane (from accumulation of CSF or blood).

Nursing considerations

- Keep the patient flat to decrease pressure on dural tears and to minimize CSF leakage.
- Monitor neurologic status.
- Avoid nasogastric intubation and nasopharyngeal suction, either of which may cause cerebral infection.
- Caution the patient against blowing his nose, which may worsen a dural tear.
- Prepare the patient for diagnostic tests, such as skull X-rays and computed tomography scan.
- Typically, basilar skull fracture and associated dural tears heal spontaneously within several days to weeks.
- A large dural tear may require a craniotomy to repair the tear with a graft patch.

Pediatric pointers

- Victims of abuse frequently sustain basilar skull fractures.
- If you suspect abuse, follow protocol for reporting the incident.

The earlier you can spot signs of increased intracranial pressure (ICP), the quicker you can intervene and the better your patient's chance of recovery. By the time late signs appear, interventions may be useless.

Assessment area	Early signs	Late signs
Level of consciousness	• Need for increased stimulation • Subtle orientation loss • Restlessness and anxiety • Sudden quietness	• Unable to be roused
Pupils	• Changes in pupil on side of lesion • Abnormal and exaggerated rhythmic contraction and dilation of one pupil (unilateral hippus) • Sluggish reaction of both pupils • Unequal pupils	• Pupils fixed and dilated or "blown"
Motor response	• Sudden weakness • Motor changes on side opposite the lesion • Positive pronator drift: With palms up, one hand pronates	• Profound weakness
Vital signs	• Intermittent increases in blood pressure	• Increased systolic pressure with widening pulse pressure, bradycardia, and abnormal respirations (Cushing's triad)

Patient teaching

○ Explain what activities the patient should avoid, and emphasize the importance of bed rest.
○ Explain to the patient (or caregiver) the signs and symptoms to look for and report, such as changes in mental status, LOC, or breathing.
○ Tell the patient to take acetaminophen for headaches.
○ Explain what diagnostic tests the patient may need.
○ Discuss the prospect of surgery with the patient, and answer his questions and concerns.

Bladder distention

Overview

- Abnormal enlargement of the bladder
- Results from an inability to urinate
- Caused by a mechanical or anatomic obstruction, neuromuscular disorder, or the use of certain drugs
- If severe distention isn't corrected promptly, renal impairment
- Gradual distention: no symptoms until the stretched bladder produces discomfort
- Acute distention: suprapubic fullness, pressure, and pain

> ### ★ Emergency actions
>
> *With severe distention, insert an indwelling urinary catheter to relieve discomfort and prevent bladder rupture. If more than 700 ml is emptied when the catheter is inserted, compressed blood vessels dilate and may make the patient feel faint.*

Assessment

History

- Ask about voiding patterns and characteristics.
- Find out the time and amount of last voiding.
- Determine the amount of fluid consumed since last voiding.
- Obtain a medical history, including urinary tract obstruction or infections; sexually transmitted disease; neurologic, intestinal, or pelvic surgery; lower abdominal or urinary tract trauma; and systemic or neurologic disorders.
- Note drug history, including use of over-the-counter drugs.

Physical assessment

- Take vital signs.
- Percuss and palpate the bladder.
- Inspect the urethral meatus and measure its diameter.
- Describe the appearance and amount of discharge.
- Test for perineal sensation and anal sphincter tone.
- Digitally examine the prostate gland (in men).

Medical causes

Benign prostatic hyperplasia

- Bladder distention develops gradually as the prostate enlarges.
- Initial findings include urinary hesitancy, straining, and frequency; reduced force of the urine stream and the inability to stop the stream; nocturia; and postvoiding dribbling.

- Later findings include prostate enlargement, perineal pain, constipation, hematuria, and sensations of suprapubic fullness and incomplete bladder emptying.

Bladder cancer

- Neoplasms can cause bladder distention by blocking the urethra.
- Other findings include hematuria (the most common sign); urinary frequency and urgency; nocturia; dysuria; pyuria; pain in the bladder, rectum, pelvis, flank, back, or legs; vomiting; diarrhea; and sleeplessness.
- A mass may be palpable on manual examination.

Multiple sclerosis

- Urine retention and bladder distention result from interrupted upper-motor-neuron control of the bladder.
- Other findings include optic neuritis, paresthesia, impaired senses of position and vibration, diplopia, nystagmus, dizziness, abnormal reflexes, dysarthria, muscle weakness, emotional lability, Lhermitte's sign (transient, electric-like shocks that spread down the body when the head is dropped forward), Babinski's sign, and ataxia.

Prostatitis

- Bladder distention occurs rapidly along with perineal discomfort and suprapubic fullness.
- Other findings include perineal pain; tense, boggy, tender, and warm enlarged prostate; decreased libido; impotence; decreased force of the urine stream; dysuria; hematuria; urinary frequency and urgency; fatigue; malaise; myalgia; fever; chills; nausea; and vomiting.

Spinal neoplasms

- Upper-neuron control of the bladder is disrupted, causing neurogenic bladder and distention.
- Other findings include a sense of pelvic fullness, continuous overflow dribbling, back pain that typically mimics sciatic pain, constipation, tender vertebral processes, sensory deficits, and muscle weakness, flaccidity, and atrophy.

Urethral calculi

- Urethral obstruction causes bladder distention and interrupted urine flow.
- Pain from the obstruction radiates to the penis or vulva and then to the perineum or rectum.
- A palpable calculus and urethral discharge may also be present.

Urethral stricture

- Urine retention and bladder distention result.
- Urethral discharge and urinary frequency are common signs.

Other causes

Catheterization
○ Urine retention and bladder distention may occur from a kinked tube or an occluded lumen.

Drugs
○ Anesthetics, anticholinergics, ganglionic blockers, opiates, parasympatholytics, and sedatives may cause urine retention and bladder distention.

Nursing considerations

○ Monitor vital signs and the extent of bladder distention.
○ Encourage the patient to change positions to alleviate discomfort.
○ Give analgesics, if needed.
○ Prepare the patient for surgery as needed.
○ Provide privacy for voiding and encourage a normal voiding position.

Pediatric pointers
○ Look for urine retention and bladder distention in any infant who fails to void normal amounts of urine.
○ In boys, posterior urethral valves, meatal stenosis, phimosis, spinal cord anomalies, bladder diverticula, and other congenital defects may cause urinary obstruction and resultant bladder distention.

Geriatric pointers
○ Bladder distention is most common in elderly men with prostate disorders that cause urine retention.

Patient teaching
○ Teach the patient to use Valsalva's maneuver or Credé's method to empty the bladder.
○ Explain how to stimulate voiding.

Blood pressure decrease

Overview

- Inadequate intravascular pressure to maintain oxygen requirements
- Also called *hypotension*
- Typically defined as a reading below 90/60 mm Hg or a drop of 30 mm Hg from the baseline
- May affect the kidneys, brain, and heart, and may lead to a change in level of consciousness (LOC) or to myocardial ischemia
- May reflect an expanded intravascular space or reduced intravascular volume and cardiac output

⭐ *Emergency actions*

If the patient's systolic blood pressure is less than 80 mm Hg, or 30 mm Hg below baseline, suspect shock. Quickly evaluate the patient for decreased LOC. Check the apical pulse for tachycardia; check respirations for tachypnea. Inspect for cool, clammy skin. Elevate the patient's legs above the level of his heart, or place him in Trendelenburg's position. Start an I.V. line using a large-bore needle to replace fluids and blood or to give drugs. Administer oxygen with mechanical ventilation. Monitor intake of fluids and output of urine. Prepare for cardiac or hemodynamic monitoring. Insert a nasogastric tube to prevent aspiration in the comatose patient.

Assessment

History

- Ask about other symptoms, such as weakness, nausea, dizziness, and chest pain.

Physical assessment

- Obtain vital signs.
- Inspect skin for pallor, sweating, and clamminess.
- Palpate peripheral pulses.
- Auscultate for abnormal heart, breath, and bowel sounds and abnormal heart and breath rates, and rhythms.
- Look for signs of hemorrhage.
- Assess for abdominal rigidity and rebound tenderness and possible sources of infection.

Medical causes

Acute adrenal insufficiency

- Characteristic sign: orthostatic hypotension

- Other signs: fatigue; weakness; nausea; vomiting; abdominal discomfort; weight loss; fever; and tachycardia; pale, cool, clammy skin; restlessness; decreased urine output; tachypnea; hyperpigmentation of fingers, nails, scars, nipples, and body folds; and coma

Anaphylactic shock

- Blood pressure falls dramatically and pulse pressure narrows
- Initially, anxiety, restlessness, intense itching, pounding headache, and a feeling of doom occur.
- Later findings include weakness, sweating, nasal congestion, coughing, difficulty breathing, nausea, abdominal cramps, involuntary defecation, seizures, flushing, change or loss of voice, urinary incontinence, and tachycardia.

Anthrax (inhalation)

- Initial signs and symptoms are flulike and include fever, chills, weakness, cough, and chest pain.
- The second stage develops abruptly with rapid deterioration marked by fever, dyspnea, stridor, and hypotension.

Cardiac arrhythmia

- Blood pressure fluctuates between normal and low.
- Dizziness, chest pain, difficulty breathing, light-headedness, weakness, fatigue, and palpitations occur.
- Pulse rhythm is irregular, and heart rate is greater than 100 beats/minute or less than 60 beats/minute.

Cardiac tamponade

- Systolic pressure falls more than 10 mm Hg during inspiration (paradoxical pulse).
- Other findings include restlessness, cyanosis, tachycardia, jugular vein distention, muffled heart sounds, dyspnea, and Kussmaul's sign.

Cardiogenic shock

- Systolic pressure falls to less than 80 mm Hg or to 30 mm Hg less than baseline.
- Tachycardia; narrowed pulse pressure; diminished Korotkoff sounds; peripheral cyanosis; restlessness and anxiety, which may progress to disorientation and confusion; and pale, cool, clammy skin occur.
- Other findings include angina, dyspnea, jugular vein distention, oliguria, ventricular gallop, tachypnea, and weak, rapid pulse.

Cholera

- A life-threatening disorder — watery diarrhea and vomiting occur.
- Water and electrolyte losses cause thirst, weakness, muscle cramps, decreased skin turgor, oliguria, tachycardia, and hypotension.
- Without treatment, death occurs within hours.

Diabetic ketoacidosis

- Hypovolemia — triggered by osmotic diuresis in hyperglycemia — causes low blood pressure.

○ Other findings include polydipsia, polyuria, polyphagia, dehydration, weight loss, abdominal pain, nausea, vomiting, breath with fruity odor, Kussmaul's respirations, tachycardia, seizures, confusion, and stupor that may progress to coma.

Heart failure

○ Blood pressure fluctuates between normal and low.
○ Other findings include dyspnea of abrupt or gradual onset, exertional dyspnea, orthopnea, paroxysmal nocturnal dyspnea, fatigue, weight gain, pallor or cyanosis, sweating, and anxiety.
○ Auscultation reveals ventricular gallop, tachycardia, crackles, and tachypnea.
○ Dependent edema, jugular vein distention, and hepatomegaly may also occur.

Hypovolemic shock

○ Systolic pressure falls to less than 80 mm Hg or 30 mm Hg less than the patient's baseline because of acute blood loss or dehydration.
○ Other signs include diminished Korotkoff sounds; narrowed pulse pressure; cyanosis of the extremities; pale, cool, clammy skin; and rapid, weak, and irregular pulse; oliguria; confusion; disorientation; restlessness; and anxiety.

Hypoxemia

○ Initially, blood pressure may be normal or slightly elevated.
○ Blood pressure drops as hypoxemia becomes pronounced.
○ Tachycardia, tachypnea, dyspnea, confusion, and stupor that may progress to coma may occur.

Myocardial infarction

○ A life-threatening disorder — blood pressure may be low or high.
○ A precipitous drop in blood pressure may signal cardiogenic shock.
○ Other findings include chest pain that may radiate to the jaw, shoulder, arm, or epigastrium; dyspnea; anxiety; nausea or vomiting; sweating; and cool, pale, or cyanotic skin.

Neurogenic shock

○ Low blood pressure and bradycardia occur.
○ Other findings include warm, dry skin and, possibly, motor weakness of the limbs or diaphragm, depending on the cause of shock.

Pulmonary embolism

○ Low blood pressure with narrowed pulse pressure and diminished Korotkoff sounds
○ Initially, sharp chest pain, dyspnea, and cough
○ Tachycardia, tachypnea, paradoxical pulse, jugular vein distention, and hemoptysis.

Septic shock

○ Initially, fever and chills occur.

○ Low blood pressure, tachycardia, and tachypnea may develop early, but the skin remains warm.
○ Blood pressure continues to decrease, accompanied by a narrowed pulse pressure.
○ Other late findings include pale skin, cyanotic extremities, apprehension, thirst, oliguria, and coma.

Vasovagal syncope

○ Low blood pressure, pallor, cold sweats, nausea, palpitations or slowed heart rate, and weakness follow stressful, painful, or claustrophobic experiences.

Other causes

Diagnostic tests

○ Gastric acid stimulation test using histamine and X-ray studies using contrast media may cause low blood pressure.

Drugs

○ Alpha and beta blockers, anxiolytics, calcium channel blockers, diuretics, general anesthetics, most I.V. antiarrhythmics, monoamine oxidase inhibitors, opioid analgesics, tranquilizers, and vasodilators can cause low blood pressure.

Nursing considerations

○ Check vital signs frequently to determine if low blood pressure is constant or intermittent.
○ If blood pressure remains extremely low, place an arterial catheter to allow close monitoring.
○ Ensure bed rest.
○ Assist ambulatory patients as needed.
○ Don't leave a dizzy patient unattended when he's sitting or walking.

Pediatric pointers

○ Normal blood pressure is lower than that in adults.
○ Suspect trauma or shock as a possible cause of low blood pressure.
○ Dehydration may cause low blood pressure.

Geriatric pointers

○ Low blood pressure commonly results from taking several drugs that have this adverse effect.
○ Orthostatic hypotension may occur because of autonomic dysfunction.

Patient teaching

○ Advise the patient with orthostatic hypotension to stand up slowly from a sitting or lying position.
○ For patients with vasovagal syncope, discuss how to avoid triggers.
○ Discuss the need for cane or walker.
○ Emphasize the importance of dangling the feet and rising slowly when getting out of bed.

Blood pressure increase

Overview

○ Intermittent or sustained increase in blood pressure exceeding 140/90 mm Hg
○ Affects men more than women
○ May develop gradually or suddenly
○ A sudden, severe rise in blood pressure may indicate a life-threatening condition

⚡ Emergency actions

If blood pressure rises above 180/110 mm Hg, suspect hypertensive crisis and treat immediately. Maintain a patent airway in case the patient vomits, and use seizure precautions. Give an I.V. antihypertensive and a diuretic. Insert an indwelling urinary catheter to monitor urine output.

Assessment

History

○ Ask about a history of diabetes or cardiovascular, cerebrovascular, or renal disease.
○ Note a family history of high blood pressure.
○ Ask the patient about the onset of high blood pressure.
○ Note associated signs and symptoms, including headache, palpitations, blurred vision, sweating, wine-colored urine, and decreased urine output.
○ Take a drug history, including past and present prescriptions, herbal preparations, and over-the-counter (OTC) drugs.
○ If the patient is taking antihypertensives, determine compliance to the drug regimen.
○ Explore psychosocial or environmental factors that affect blood pressure control.

Physical assessment

○ Perform a funduscopic (ophthalmoscopic) examination.
○ Perform a cardiovascular assessment; check for carotid bruits and jugular vein distention.
○ Assess skin color, temperature, and turgor.
○ Palpate peripheral pulses.
○ Auscultate for abnormal heart sounds, rate, or rhythm.
○ Auscultate for abnormal breath sounds, rate, or rhythm.
○ Auscultate for abdominal bruits.
○ Palpate the abdomen for tenderness, masses, and liver or kidney enlargement.

Medical causes

Anemia

○ Elevated systolic pressure
○ Other findings: pulsations in the capillary beds, bounding pulse, tachycardia, systolic ejection murmur, and pale mucous membranes

Aortic aneurysm (dissecting)

○ Initially, a sudden rise in systolic pressure occurs, but diastolic pressure is stable.
○ Hypotension occurs as the body's ability to compensate fails.
○ Abdominal and back pain, weakness, sweating, tachycardia, dyspnea, a pulsating abdominal mass, restlessness, confusion, and cool, clammy skin may occur with abdominal aneurysm.
○ A ripping or tearing sensation in the chest, which may radiate to the neck, shoulders, lower back, or abdomen; pallor; syncope; blindness; loss of consciousness; sweating; dyspnea; tachycardia; cyanosis; leg weakness; murmur; and absent radial and femoral pulses may occur with a thoracic aneurysm.

Atherosclerosis

○ Systolic pressure rises.
○ Diastolic pressure remains normal or slightly elevated.
○ The patient may be asymptomatic.
○ Other findings may include a weak pulse, flushed skin, tachycardia, angina, and claudication.

Cushing's syndrome

○ Blood pressure elevates and pulse pressure widens.
○ Other findings include truncal obesity, "moon" face, and other cushingoid signs.

Hypertension

○ Essential hypertension develops insidiously; blood pressure increases gradually.
○ The patient may be without symptoms.
○ Malignant hypertension results when diastolic pressure abruptly rises above 120 mm Hg; systolic pressure may exceed 200 mm Hg.
○ Pulmonary edema is common.
○ Other findings include severe headache, confusion, blurred vision, tinnitus, epistaxis, muscle twitching, chest pain, nausea, and vomiting.

Increased intracranial pressure

○ Respiratory rate increases initially, followed by increased systolic pressure and widened pulse pressure.
○ Bradycardia is a late sign.
○ Other findings include headache, projectile vomiting, decreased level of consciousness, and fixed or dilated pupils.

Myocardial infarction

- Blood pressure may be high or low.
- Crushing chest pain may radiate to the jaw, shoulder, arm, or epigastrium.
- Other findings include dyspnea, anxiety, nausea, vomiting, weakness, diaphoresis, atrial gallop, and murmurs.

Pheochromocytoma

- Paroxysmal or sustained elevated blood pressure occurs with possible orthostatic hypotension.
- Other findings include anxiety, diaphoresis, palpitations, tremors, pallor, nausea, weight loss, and headache.
- Hematuria, life-threatening retroperitoneal bleeding, proteinuria, and colicky abdominal pain may occur in advanced stages.

Preeclampsia and eclampsia

- Blood pressure increases to 140/90 mm Hg or more in the first trimester of pregnancy, to 130/80 mm Hg or more in the second or third trimester, to 30 mm Hg above baseline systolic pressure, or to 15 mm Hg above baseline diastolic pressure.
- Other findings include generalized edema, sudden weight gain of 3 lb (1.4 kg) or more per week during the second or third trimester, severe frontal headache, blurred or double vision, decreased urine output, proteinuria, midabdominal pain, neuromuscular irritability, nausea, and seizures.

Renovascular stenosis

- Systolic and diastolic pressure rise abruptly.
- Other characteristic findings include bruits over the upper abdomen or in the costovertebral angles, hematuria, and acute flank pain.

Thyrotoxicosis

- A life-threatening disorder — elevated systolic pressure occurs.
- Other findings include widened pulse pressure, tachycardia, bounding pulse, pulsations in the capillary nail beds, palpitations, weight loss, exophthalmos, enlarged thyroid gland, weakness, diarrhea, fever, nervousness, emotional instability, heat intolerance, exertional dyspnea, decreased or absent menses, and warm, moist skin.

Other causes

Drugs

- Central nervous system stimulants, corticosteroids, hormonal contraceptives, monoamine oxidase inhibitors, nonsteroidal anti-inflammatory drugs, sympathomimetics, and OTC cold remedies can increase blood pressure.
- Cocaine use may increase blood pressure.

Treatments

- Kidney dialysis or transplant may cause temporary elevation of blood pressure.

Nursing considerations

- Stress the need for follow-up diagnostic tests.

Pediatric pointers

- Elevated blood pressure may result from such conditions as lead or mercury poisoning, chronic pyelonephritis, coarctation of the aorta, patent ductus arteriosus, glomerulonephritis, adrenogenital syndrome, or neuroblastoma.

Geriatric pointers

- Atherosclerosis produces isolated systolic hypertension.

Patient teaching

- Emphasize the importance of weight loss and exercise.
- Explain the need for sodium restriction.
- Discuss stress management.
- Discuss ways of reducing other risk factors for coronary artery disease.
- Discuss the importance of regular blood pressure monitoring.
- Explain how to take prescribed antihypertensives correctly.
- Explain what adverse drug reactions the patient should report.
- Emphasize the importance of long-term followup care.

Bowel sounds, absent (silent)

Overview

- Characterized by an inability to hear bowel sounds in any quadrant with a stethoscope after listening for at least 5 minutes (see *Are bowel sounds really absent?*)
- When mechanical or vascular obstruction or neurogenic inhibition halts peristalsis, bowel sounds are absent.
- Life-threatening complications include bowel perforation, peritonitis, sepsis, and hypovolemic shock.
- Abrupt stopping of bowel sounds with abdominal pain, rigidity, and distention signal a life-threatening crisis.
- Absent bowel sounds following a period of hyperactive sounds may indicate bowel strangulation or a mechanically obstructed bowel.

Emergency actions

If accompanied by sudden, severe abdominal pain and cramping or severe abdominal distention, insert a nasogastric (NG) or intestinal tube to suction lumen contents and decompress the bowel. Give I.V. fluids and electrolytes. Withhold oral intake in case surgery is needed. Take the patient's vital signs, and watch for signs of shock, such as hypotension, tachycardia, and cool, clammy skin. Measure abdominal girth to establish a baseline.

Assessment

History

- Ask about the onset and description of abdominal pain.

Assessment tip
Are bowel sounds really absent?

Before concluding that your patient has absent bowel sounds, ask yourself these three questions:

- *Did I use the diaphragm of your stethoscope to auscultate for the bowel sounds?* The diaphragm detects high-frequency sounds, such as bowel sounds, whereas the bell detects low-frequency sounds, such as a vascular bruit or a venous hum.
- *Did I listen for at least 5 minutes for the presence of bowel sounds?* Normally, bowel sounds occur every 5 to 15 seconds, but the duration of a single sound may be less than 1 second.
- *Did I listen for bowel sounds in all quadrants?* Bowel sounds may be absent in one quadrant but present in another.

- Obtain a description of bowel movements and ask the patient if he has had diarrhea or has passed pencil-thin stools (a possible sign of a developing luminal obstruction).
- Obtain a medical and surgical history, including recent accidents, abdominal tumors, hernias, adhesions from past surgery, acute pancreatitis, diverticulitis, gynecologic infection, uremia, or spinal cord injury.

Physical assessment

- Inspect abdominal contour.
- Observe for distention.
- Gently percuss and palpate the abdomen.
- Listen for dullness over fluid-filled areas and for tympany over pockets of gas.
- Palpate for abdominal rigidity and guarding.

Medical causes

Complete mechanical intestinal obstruction

- A potentially life-threatening condition — absent bowel sounds follow hyperactive sounds.
- Colicky abdominal pain, which may radiate, arises in the quadrant with the obstruction.
- Other findings include abdominal distention, bloating, constipation, nausea, and vomiting.
- Signs of shock, fever, rebound tenderness, and abdominal rigidity may occur in later stages.

Mesenteric artery occlusion

- Bowel sounds disappear after a brief period of hyperactive sounds.
- Midepigastric or periumbilical pain occurs next, followed by abdominal distention, bruits, vomiting, constipation, and signs of shock.
- Abdominal rigidity may appear later.

Paralytic ileus

- Absent bowel sounds are a main sign.
- Other signs include abdominal distention, generalized discomfort, and constipation or passage of small, liquid stools.
- If paralytic ileus follows acute abdominal infection, fever and abdominal pain may occur.

Other causes

Abdominal surgery

- Bowel sounds are normally temporarily absent after abdominal surgery.

Nursing considerations

○ After NG or intestinal tube insertion, elevate the head of the bed at least 30 degrees.
○ Turn the patient to facilitate passage of the tube through the GI tract.
○ Ensure tube patency.
○ Continue to give I.V. fluids and electrolytes.
○ Once mechanical obstruction and intra-abdominal sepsis have been ruled out, give drugs to control pain and stimulate peristalsis.

Pediatric pointers

○ Absent bowel sounds in children may result from Hirschsprung's disease or intussusception.
○ These conditions can lead to life-threatening obstruction.

Geriatric pointers

○ If a bowel obstruction doesn't respond to decompression, early surgical intervention should be considered to avoid the risk of bowel infarct.

Patient teaching

○ Explain diagnostic tests and therapeutic procedures that are needed.
○ Explain which foods and fluids the patient should avoid.
○ Explain the need for postoperative ambulation.

Bowel sounds, hyperactive

Overview

○ Reflect increased intestinal motility
○ Characterized as rapid, rushing, gurgling waves of sounds (see *Characterizing bowel sounds*)

Emergency actions

Take the patient's vital signs, and ask him about other symptoms, such as abdominal pain, vomiting, and diarrhea. If he has cramping abdominal pain or is vomiting, continue to auscultate for bowel sounds. If bowel sounds stop abruptly, suspect complete bowel obstruction. Assist with GI suction and decompression, give I.V. fluids and electrolytes, and get the patient ready for surgery.

If the patient has diarrhea, record its frequency, amount, color, and consistency. If you detect excessive watery diarrhea or bleeding, give an antidiarrheal, I.V. fluids and electrolytes and, possibly, blood transfusions.

Assessment

History

○ Obtain a medical and surgical history, including abdominal surgeries or previous inflammatory bowel disease.
○ Ask the patient about recent exposure to gastroenteritis.
○ Determine whether the patient has traveled recently.

Assessment tip
Characterizing bowel sounds

The sounds of swallowed air and fluid moving through the GI tract are known as bowel sounds. These sounds usually occur every 5 to 15 seconds, but their frequency may be irregular. For example, bowel sounds are normally more active just before and after a meal. Bowel sounds may last less than 1 second or up to several seconds.

To accurately assess bowel sounds, you need to be aware of the various types:
• *Normal bowel sounds* can be characterized as murmuring, gurgling, or tinkling.
• *Hyperactive bowel sounds* can be characterized as loud, gurgling, splashing, and rushing; they're higher pitched and occur more frequently than normal sounds.
• *Hypoactive bowel sounds* can be characterized as softer or lower in tone and less frequent than normal sounds.

○ Inquire about possible stress factors.
○ Ask about allergies and recent food and fluid consumption.

Physical assessment

○ Take vital signs.
○ Check for fever.
○ After auscultation, gently inspect, percuss, and palpate the abdomen.

Medical causes

Crohn's disease

○ Hyperactive bowel sounds arise insidiously.
○ Other findings include diarrhea, anorexia, low-grade fever, abdominal distention and tenderness, cramping abdominal pain that may be relieved by defecation, and a fixed mass in the right lower quadrant of the abdomen.
○ Muscle wasting, weight loss, and signs of dehydration may occur as the disease progresses.

Gastroenteritis

○ Hyperactive bowel sounds follow sudden nausea and vomiting.
○ The patient has explosive diarrhea.
○ Abdominal cramping or pain is common.
○ Fever may occur, depending on the causative organism.

GI hemorrhage

○ Hyperactive bowel sounds indicate upper GI bleeding.
○ Other findings include hematemesis, coffee-ground vomitus, abdominal distention, bloody diarrhea, rectal passage of bright red clots and jellylike material or melena, and pain.
○ Decreased urine output, tachycardia, and hypotension accompany blood loss.

Malabsorption

○ Lactose intolerance typically results in hyperactive bowel sounds.
○ Other findings include diarrhea and, possibly, nausea and vomiting, angioedema, and urticaria.

Mechanical intestinal obstruction

○ A potentially life-threatening disorder — hyperactive bowel sounds occur with cramping abdominal pain every few minutes.
○ Bowel sounds may later become hypoactive and then disappear.
○ Nausea and vomiting occur earlier and with greater severity in small-bowel obstruction than in large-bowel obstruction.
○ Abdominal distention and constipation accompany hyperactive bowel sounds in complete obstruction, although the bowel furthest from the obstruction may continue to empty for up to 3 days.

Ulcerative colitis (acute)

○ Hyperactive bowel sounds arise abruptly.
○ Bloody diarrhea with anorexia, abdominal pain, nausea and vomiting, fever, and tenesmus is a characteristic sign.
○ Weight loss, arthralgia, and arthritis may occur.

Nursing considerations

If the patient has GI bleeding:
○ Insert an I.V. line for giving fluids and blood.
○ Restrict food and oral fluids.
○ Give drugs such as vasopressin to manage bleeding.
○ Insert an NG tube to suction and monitor drainage.

Pediatric pointers

○ Hyperactive bowel sounds in children usually result from gastroenteritis, erratic eating habits, excessive ingestion of certain foods, or food allergy.

Patient teaching

○ Explain dietary changes that are necessary or beneficial.
○ Explain what physical activity the patient should avoid.
○ Discuss stress reduction techniques.

Bowel sounds, hypoactive

Overview

○ Bowel sounds diminished in regularity, tone, and loudness
○ Result if peristalsis is decreased, a situation that may occur as a result of bowel obstruction
○ May precede absent bowel sounds, a possible sign of a life-threatening condition

Assessment

History

○ Ask about the location, onset, frequency, and severity of pain — cramping or colicky abdominal pain usually indicates mechanical bowel obstruction, while diffuse abdominal pain usually indicates intestinal distention from paralytic ileus.
○ Obtain a description of any recent vomiting or constipation.
○ Obtain a medical and surgical history, including conditions that may cause mechanical bowel obstruction.
○ Note the patient's treatment history, including radiation and drug therapy.

Physical assessment

○ Inspect the abdomen for distention, noting surgical incisions and obvious masses.
○ Gently percuss and palpate the abdomen for masses, gas, fluid, tenderness, and rigidity.
○ Measure abdominal girth.
○ Check for signs of dehydration and electrolyte imbalance.

Medical causes

Mechanical intestinal obstruction

○ Bowel sounds may become hypoactive after a period of hyperactive bowel sounds.
○ Other findings include acute colicky abdominal pain in the quadrant with obstruction, possibly radiating to the flank or lumbar region; nausea and vomiting; and abdominal distention and bloating.
○ If obstruction becomes complete, signs of shock may occur.

Mesenteric artery occlusion

○ Bowel sounds become hypoactive after a brief period of hyperactivity and then quickly disappear, signifying a life-threatening crisis.

○ Other findings include fever; a history of colicky abdominal pain leading to sudden and severe mid-epigastric or periumbilical pain, followed by abdominal distention and possible bruits; vomiting; constipation; and signs of shock.
○ Abdominal rigidity is a late sign.

Paralytic ileus

○ Bowel sounds are hypoactive and may become absent.
○ Other signs and symptoms include abdominal distention and constipation or passage of small, liquid stools and flatus.
○ If the disorder follows acute abdominal infection, fever and abdominal pain may occur.

Other causes

Drugs

○ Anticholinergics, general or spinal anesthetics, opiates, phenothiazine, and vinca alkaloids

Surgery

○ Surgery involving the bowel may produce hypoactive bowel sounds from manipulation of the bowel. Motility and bowel sounds in the small intestine usually resume within 24 hours; colonic bowel sounds, in 3 to 5 days.

Nursing considerations

○ Frequently evaluate for signs and symptoms of shock.
○ Be alert for sudden absence of bowel sounds; monitor vital signs, and auscultate for bowel sounds every 2 to 4 hours.
○ If GI suction and decompression are needed, maintain tube patentcy and provide oral and nasal hygiene.
○ Withhold food and oral fluids.
○ If severe pain, abdominal rigidity, guarding, and fever accompany hypoactive bowel sounds, perform emergency interventions to treat paralytic ileus from peritonitis.
○ Give I.V. fluids and electrolytes.
○ Prepare the patient for diagnostic studies, such as X-rays and endoscopic procedures.

Pediatric pointers

○ Hypoactive bowel sounds in a child may be caused by bowel distention from excessive swallowing of air while eating or crying.
○ Observe the child for further signs of illness.

Patient teaching

○ Tell the caregiver that ambulation or frequent turning are important.
○ Teach the patient or caregiver about the need for diagnostic tests and procedures.
○ Tell the patient or caregiver to maintain food and fluid restrictions.

Bradycardia

Overview

○ Refers to a heart rate of fewer than 60 beats/minute
○ Occurs normally but can also result from pathologic causes (see *Managing life-threatening bradycardia*)

Assessment

History

○ Ask about a family history of slow pulse rate.
○ Obtain a medical history, including underlying metabolic disorders.
○ Ask about current drugs and the patient's compliance.
○ Find out if the patient is an athlete and his degree of physical activity.

Physical assessment

○ Monitor vital signs and oxygen saturation.
○ Perform a complete cardiac assessment.

Medical causes

Cardiac arrhythmia

○ Bradycardia may be transient or sustained, benign, or life-threatening.
○ Hypotension, palpitations, dizziness, weakness, dyspnea, chest pain, decreased urine output, altered level of consciousness (LOC), syncope, and fatigue may occur.

Cardiomyopathy

○ A life-threatening disorder—transient or sustained bradycardia may occur.
○ Other findings include dizziness, syncope, edema, fatigue, jugular vein distention, orthopnea, dyspnea, and peripheral cyanosis.

Cervical spinal injury

○ Bradycardia may be transient or sustained, depending on the severity of the injury.
○ Other findings include hypotension, decreased body temperature, slowed peristalsis, leg paralysis, and partial arm and respiratory muscle paralysis.

Hypothermia

○ Other symptoms include shivering, peripheral cyanosis, muscle rigidity, bradypnea, and confusion leading to stupor.
○ If the patient's core temperature drops below 86° F (30° C), he may not have a palpable pulse or audible heart sounds.

Hypothyroidism

○ Severe bradycardia is accompanied by fatigue, constipation, unexplained weight gain, and sensitivity to cold.
○ Related signs include cool, dry, thick skin; sparse, dry hair; facial swelling; periorbital edema; thick, brittle nails; and confusion leading to stupor.

Myocardial infarction

○ Sinus bradycardia is common.
○ Other findings include an aching, burning, or viselike pressure in the chest, which may radiate to the jaw, shoulder, arm, back, or epigastric area; nausea and vomiting; cool, clammy, and pale or cyanotic skin; anxiety; and dyspnea.
○ Abnormal heart sounds may be heard on auscultation.

Emergency actions
Managing life-threatening bradycardia

Bradycardia can signal a life-threatening disorder when accompanied by pain, shortness of breath, dizziness, syncope, or other symptoms; prolonged exposure to cold; or head or neck trauma. In such patients, quickly take vital signs. Connect the patient to a cardiac monitor, and insert an I.V. line. Depending on the cause of bradycardia, you'll need to administer fluids, atropine, steroids, or thyroid medication. If indicated, insert an indwelling urinary catheter. Intubation and mechanical ventilation may be necessary if the patient's respiratory rate falls. Assist with the placement of a pacemaker if medications don't increase the heart rate.

Perform a focused assessment to help locate the cause of bradycardia. For example, ask about pain. Viselike pressure or crushing or burning chest pain that radiates to the arms, back, or jaw may indicate an acute myocardial infarction (MI); a severe headache, increased intracranial pressure. Also, ask about nausea, vomiting, or shortness of breath—signs and symptoms associated with an acute MI and cardiomyopathy. Observe the patient for peripheral cyanosis, edema, or jugular vein distention, any of which may indicate cardiomyopathy. Look for a thyroidectomy scar because severe bradycardia may result from hypothyroidism caused by failure to take thyroid hormone replacements.

If the cause of bradycardia is evident, provide supportive care. For example, keep the hypothermic patient warm by applying blankets, and monitor his core temperature until it reaches 99° F (37.2° C); stabilize the head and neck of a trauma patient until cervical spinal injury is ruled out.

Other causes

Diagnostic tests

○ Cardiac catheterization and electrophysiologic studies can induce temporary bradycardia.

Drugs

○ Protamine and some antiarrhythmics, beta blockers, cardiac glycosides, calcium channel blockers, sympatholytics, and topical miotics may cause transient bradycardia.
○ Not taking a thyroid replacement may cause bradycardia.

Invasive treatments

○ Cardiac surgery can result in edema or damage to the conduction tissue, causing bradycardia.
○ Suctioning can induce hypoxia and vagal stimulation, causing bradycardia.

Nursing considerations

○ Look for changes in cardiac rhythm, respiratory rate, and LOC.
○ Prepare the patient for 24-hour Holter monitoring.

Pediatric pointers

○ Fetal bradycardia, characterized by heart rate less than 120 beats/minute, may occur during prolonged labor or complications of delivery.
○ Intermittent bradycardia commonly occurs in premature infants.
○ Congenital heart defects, acute glomerulonephritis, and transient or complete heart block associated with cardiac catheterization or cardiac surgery can cause bradycardia in full-term infants and in children.

Geriatric pointers

○ Sinus node dysfunction is the most common bradyarrhythmia in elderly patients.
○ Carefully scrutinize the patient's drug regimen.

Patient teaching

○ Inform the patient about signs and symptoms he should report.
○ Give instructions for pulse measurement, and explain the parameters for calling the physician and seeking emergency care.
○ If a patient is getting a pacemaker, explain its use.

Bradypnea

Overview

○ Involves a pattern of regular respirations with a rate of less than 10 breaths/minute
○ May precede life-threatening apnea or respiratory arrest
○ Results from neurologic and metabolic disorders and drug overdose, which depress the brain's respiratory control centers (see *Understanding how the nervous system controls breathing*)

Understanding how the nervous system controls breathing

Stimulation from the external sources and from higher brain centers acts on respiratory centers in the pons and medulla. These centers, in turn, send impulses to the various parts of the respiratory system to alter respiration patterns.

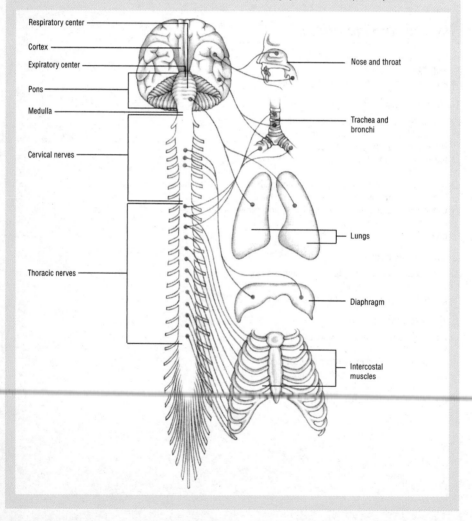

Respiratory center
Cortex
Expiratory center
Pons
Medulla
Cervical nerves
Thoracic nerves

Nose and throat
Trachea and bronchi
Lungs
Diaphragm
Intercostal muscles

Assessment

History

○ Ask about whether a drug overdose is possible; find out the names, doses, time frames, and routes of the drugs taken.
○ Obtain a medical history.

Physical assessment

○ Assess vital signs.
○ Perform a complete physical assessment, paying particular attention to the cardiopulmonary assessment.

Medical causes

Diabetic ketoacidosis

○ In patients with severe, uncontrolled diabetes, bradypnea occurs late.
○ Other signs and symptoms include decreased LOC, fatigue, weakness, fruity breath odor, and oliguria.

Increased intracranial pressure

○ Bradypnea is a late sign.
○ Bradypnea is preceded by decreased LOC, deteriorating motor function, and fixed, dilated pupils.
○ The triad of bradypnea, bradycardia, and hypertension is a classic sign of late medullary strangulation.

Respiratory failure

○ Bradypnea occurs during end-stage respiratory failure.
○ Other findings include cyanosis, diminished breath sounds, tachycardia, and mildly increased blood pressure.
○ Restlessness, confusion, irritability, and a decreased LOC may also occur.

Other causes

Drugs

○ Overdose with an opioid analgesic, sedative, barbiturate, phenothiazine, or another central nervous system (CNS) depressant can cause bradypnea.
○ Use of alcohol with these drugs can also cause bradypnea.

Nursing considerations

○ Check respiratory status frequently, and give ventilatory support if needed.
○ Draw blood for arterial blood gas analysis, electrolyte studies, and drug screening.
○ Give oxygen and prescribed drugs, avoiding CNS depressants, which can exacerbate bradypnea.
○ Review all drugs and dosages taken during the last 24 hours.

Respiratory rates in children

This graph shows normal respiratory rates in children, which are higher than normal rates in adults. Accordingly, bradypnea in a child is defined by the child's age.

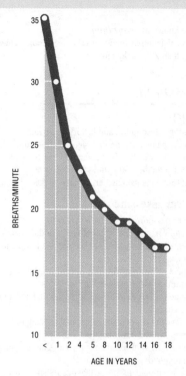

Pediatric pointers

○ Because respiratory rates are higher in children than in adults, bradypnea in children is defined according to age. (See *Respiratory rates in children*.)

Geriatric pointers

○ Older patients have a higher risk of developing bradypnea from drug toxicity.

Patient teaching

○ Explain the complications of opioid therapy—such as bradypnea.
○ Discuss the signs and symptoms of opioid toxicity.

Breast nodule

Overview

- Also known as *breast lumps*
- Two chief causes: benign breast disease and cancer
- Less than 20% malignant

Assessment

History

- Ask for a description and history of the lump.
- Ask the patient about other signs and symptoms.
- Determine whether the patient has ever breast-fed.
- Obtain a medical and family history.
- Determine the patient's breast cancer risk factors.

Physical assessment

- Perform a thorough breast examination.
- Carefully palpate a suspected breast nodule, noting its location, shape, size, consistency, mobility, and delineation.
- Inspect and palpate the skin over the nodule for warmth, redness, and edema.
- Palpate the lymph nodes of the breast and axilla for enlargement.
- Observe the contour of the breasts, looking for asymmetry and irregularities.
- Look for signs of retraction, such as skin dimpling and nipple deviation or flattening.
- Note any nipple discharge that occurs spontaneously, comes from only one breast, and isn't milky.

Medical causes

Adenofibroma

- The nodule usually occurs singly and feels firm, slippery, elastic, and round or lobular, with well-defined margins.
- The nodule is painless, grows rapidly, and usually lies around the nipple or upper outer quadrant.

Areolar gland abscess

- A tender, palpable abscess on the border of the areola develops following an inflammation of Montgomery's glands.
- Fever, local swelling, drainage, and malaise may also occur.

Breast abscess

- The nodule is localized, hot, tender, and fluctuant, with erythema and peau d'orange.
- Other findings include fever, chills, malaise, and generalized discomfort.

- With a chronic abscess, the nodule is nontender, irregular, firm, and may feel like a thick wall of fibrous tissue.
- With a chronic abscess, other findings include skin dimpling, peau d'orange, nipple retraction, and axillary lymphadenopathy.

Breast cancer

- The nodule is hard, poorly delineated, and fixed to the skin or underlying tissue.
- Nodules usually occur singly, developing in the upper outer quadrant 40% to 50% of the time.
- Satellite nodules may surround the main one.
- Other findings include serous or bloody nipple discharge (common); breast dimpling; nipple deviation or retraction; flattening of the nipple or breast contour; peau d'orange; erythema; tenderness; and axillary lymphadenopathy.
- Breast ulcer is a late sign.

Fibrocystic breast disease

- Smooth, round, slightly elastic, nodules, increase in size and tenderness just before menstruation.
- Nodules are mobile, which differentiates them from malignant nodules.
- May occur in fine, granular clusters in both breasts or as widespread, well-defined lumps in varying sizes.
- Other findings include thickening of adjacent tissue and premenstrual syndrome.

Intraductal papilloma

- Nodules are tiny, benign, soft, poorly delineated, and usually resist palpation.
- Serous or bloody nipple discharge is the primary sign.
- Breast pain and tenderness may occur.

Mammary duct ectasia

- A rubbery breast nodule lies under the areola.
- Other findings include transient pain, itching, tenderness, and erythema of the areola; thick, sticky, multicolored nipple discharge from multiple ducts; nipple retraction; bluish green or peau d'orange skin over the mass; and lymphadenopathy.

Mastitis

- Nodules feel firm and hard or tender, flocculent, and discrete.
- Skin dimpling; nipple deviation, retraction, or flattening; and nipple crack or abrasion may occur.
- Other findings include breast warmth, erythema, tenderness, peau d'orange, high fever, chills, malaise, and fatigue.

Paget's disease

- Paget's disease is characterized by a scaling, eczematoid, single nipple lesion that progresses to a deep mass.

○ Later, the nipple becomes reddened and excoriated and may eventually be completely destroyed.

Nursing considerations

○ Provide a simple explanation of your examination.
○ Encourage the patient to express feelings about nodules.
○ Although most nodules in breast-feeding women are from mastitis, the possibility of cancer demands careful evaluation.

Pediatric pointers

○ Most nodules in children and adolescents reflect the normal response of breast tissue to hormonal fluctuations.

Geriatric pointers

○ In women age 70 and older, 75% of all breast lumps are malignant.

Patient teaching

○ Teach the patient the techniques of breast self-examination.
○ Explain how to treat mastitis.

Breast pain

Overview

- Also called *mastalgia*
- Commonly results from benign breast disease
- May occur during rest or movement
- May be aggravated by manipulation or palpation
- May be in one or both breasts
- May be cyclic, intermittent or constant, dull or sharp
- May occur before menstruation as a result of increased mammary blood flow caused by hormonal changes
- May occur during pregnancy, a result of hormonal changes

Assessment

History

- Determine the onset and description of the pain.
- Ask about duration of pain (constant or intermittent).
- Find out if the patient is nursing, pregnant, menopausal, or postmenopausal.
- Question the patient about injury or changes to breast.

Physical assessment

- With the patient standing or sitting with arms at the sides, note breast size, symmetry, and contour, and the appearance of the skin.
- Note the size, shape, and symmetry of the nipples and areolae.
- Repeat your inspection with the patient's arms raised over the head and then with the hands pressed against the hips.
- Palpate the breasts with the patient seated and then lying down with a pillow placed under the shoulder on the side being examined.
- Palpate the nipple, noting tenderness and nodules; check for discharge.
- Palpate axillary lymph nodes, noting any enlargement.

Medical causes

Areolar gland abscess

- Montgomery's glands become inflamed.
- Abscess is tender and palpable and is located on the periphery of the areola.
- Other findings include fever, local swelling, drainage, and malaise.

Breast abscess (acute)

- Local pain, tenderness, erythema, *peau d'orange*, and warmth are associated with a nodule.
- Other findings include malaise, fever, chills, and enlarged axillary nodes.

Fat necrosis

- Local pain and tenderness may develop.
- Other findings include ecchymosis; erythema; a firm, irregular, fixed mass; skin dimpling; and nipple retraction.

Fibrocystic breast disease

- Cysts may cause pain before menstruation and produce no symptoms afterward.
- Later, pain may persist throughout the cycle.
- Cysts feel firm, mobile, and well-defined.
- A clear, serous nipple discharge may come from one or both breasts.
- The patient may experience signs and symptoms of premenstrual syndrome.

Intraductal papilloma

- Breast pain or tenderness may occur in one breast.
- Serous or bloody nipple discharge is the primary sign.
- Other signs include a small, soft, poorly delineated mass in the ducts beneath the areola.

Mammary duct ectasia

- Burning pain and itching around the areola may occur.
- Inflammation with pain, tenderness, erythema, and acute fever, or with pain and tenderness alone, may develop and subside in 7 to 10 days.
- Other findings include a rubbery, subareolar breast nodule; swelling and erythema around the nipple; nipple retraction; a bluish green discoloration or *peau d'orange* of the skin overlying the nodule; a thick, sticky, multicolored nipple discharge from multiple ducts; and axillary lymphadenopathy
- Breast ulcer is a late sign.

Mastitis

- Pain in one breast may be severe.
- Skin is typically red and warm at the inflammation site.
- Other findings include *peau d'orange*, breast dimpling, a firm area of induration, and nipple deviation, inversion, or flattening.
- High fever, chills, malaise, and fatigue are systemic findings.

Sebaceous cyst (infected)

- Pain may be reported with this cutaneous cyst.
- Other findings include a small, well-delineated nodule, localized erythema, and induration.

Nursing considerations

○ Provide emotional support for the patient.
○ Emphasize the importance of monthly breast self-examination.

Pediatric pointers

○ Transient gynecomastia can cause breast pain in boys during puberty.

Geriatric pointers

○ Breast pain from benign breast disease is rare in postmenopausal women.
○ Breast pain can be due to trauma from falls or physical abuse.
○ Because of decreased pain perception and decreased cognitive function, elderly patients may not report breast pain.

Patient teaching

○ Instruct the patient on correct type of brassiere.
○ Explain the use of warm or cold compresses.
○ Teach the techniques of breast self-examination, and stress the importance of monthly self-examination.

Breath with fecal odor

Overview

○ Typically occurs with fecal vomiting associated with a long-standing intestinal obstruction or gastrojejunocolic fistula
○ May indicate a late diagnostic clue to a life-threatening GI disorder (see *Managing fecal breath odor*)

Assessment

History

○ Ask about previous abdominal surgeries.
○ Note the onset, duration, and location of abdominal pain.
○ Find out about normal bowel habits, including time and description of last bowel movement.
○ Ask about loss of appetite.

Physical assessment

○ Auscultate for bowel sounds.
○ Inspect the abdomen, noting its contour and surgical scars.
○ Measure abdominal girth to provide a baseline.
○ Percuss for tympany or dullness.
○ Palpate for tenderness, distention, and rigidity.
○ Rectal and pelvic examinations should be performed.

Medical causes

Distal small-bowel obstruction

○ Fecal breath odor results from vomiting of fecal contents after vomiting of gastric contents and bilious contents.
○ Other symptoms include achiness, malaise, drowsiness, and polydipsia.

○ Bowel changes (ranging from diarrhea to constipation) are accompanied by abdominal distention, persistent epigastric or periumbilical colicky pain, and hyperactive bowel sounds and borborygmi.
○ Bowel sounds become hypoactive or absent as obstruction becomes complete.
○ Fever, hypotension, tachycardia, and rebound tenderness may indicate strangulation or perforation.

Gastrojejunocolic fistula

○ Fecal vomiting with resulting fecal breath odor may occur.
○ Diarrhea with abdominal pain is the most common chief complaint.
○ Other GI findings include anorexia, weight loss, abdominal distention, and marked malabsorption.

Large-bowel obstruction

○ Fecal vomiting with fecal breath odor occurs as a late sign.
○ Colicky abdominal pain appears suddenly, followed by continuous hypogastric pain.
○ Marked abdominal distention and tenderness occur.
○ Constipation develops, but defecation may continue for up to 3 days.
○ Leakage of stool is common with partial obstruction.

Nursing considerations

After a nasogastric or intestinal tube has been inserted:
○ Keep the head of the bed elevated at least 30 degrees.
○ Turn the patient to facilitate passage of the intestinal tube through the GI tract.
○ Don't tape the intestinal tube to the patient's face.
○ Ensure tube patency by monitoring drainage and checking that suction devices function properly.
○ Irrigate tube as needed.
○ Monitor GI drainage.
○ At least once per day, send serum specimens to the laboratory for electrolyte analysis.

⭐ Emergency actions
Managing fecal breath odor

Because fecal breath odor can signal a life-threatening intestinal obstruction, you'll need to quickly assess your patient's condition. Monitor his vital signs, and look for signs of shock, such as hypotension, tachycardia, narrowed pulse pressure, and cool, clammy skin. Ask the patient if he's nauseated or has vomited. Find out the frequency of vomiting as well as the color, odor, amount, and consistency of the vomitus. Have an emesis basin nearby to collect and accurately measure the vomitus.

Withhold all food and fluids because surgery may be necessary to relieve an obstruction or repair a fistula. Insert a nasogastric or intestinal tube for GI tract decompres-

sion. Insert a peripheral I.V. line for vascular access, or assist with central line insertion for large-bore access and central venous pressure monitoring. Obtain a blood sample and send it to the laboratory for complete blood count and electrolyte analysis, because large fluid losses and shifts can produce electrolyte imbalances. Maintain adequate hydration and support circulatory status with additional fluids. Give a physiologic solution — such as lactated Ringer's solution, normal saline solution, or human plasma protein fraction (Plasmanate) — to prevent metabolic acidosis from gastric losses and metabolic alkalosis from intestinal fluid losses.

Pediatric pointers

○ Carefully monitor the child's fluid and electrolyte status, because dehydration can develop rapidly from persistent vomiting.
○ Signs of dehydration include the absence of tears and dry or parched mucous membranes.

Geriatric pointers

○ Early surgical intervention may be necessary for a bowel obstruction that doesn't respond to decompression, because of the high risk of bowel infarct.

Patient teaching

○ Explain to the patient the procedures and treatments he needs.
○ Teach the patient the techniques of good oral hygiene.
○ Explain to the patient the food and fluid restrictions that are needed.

Breath with fruity odor

Overview

- Results from respiratory elimination of excess acetone
- Characteristically occurs with ketoacidosis, a potentially life-threatening condition (see *Managing fruity breath odor*)

Assessment

History

- Ask about the onset and duration of odor.
- Find out about changes in breathing patterns.
- Review other signs and symptoms, including increased thirst, frequent urination, weight loss, fatigue, and abdominal pain.
- Ask a woman if she has had candidal vaginitis or vaginal secretions with itching.
- If the patient has a history of diabetes mellitus, ask about stress, infections, and noncompliance to the managing regimen.
- If anorexia nervosa is suspected, obtain a dietary and weight history.

Physical assessment

- Take vital signs.
- Perform a physical examination.

Medical causes

Anorexia nervosa

- Severe weight loss may produce fruity breath odor.
- Nausea, constipation, and cold intolerance may be present.
- Dental enamel erosion and scars or calluses in the dorsum of the hand may indicate induced vomiting.

Ketoacidosis

- With alcoholic ketoacidosis, fruity breath odor occurs with vomiting, abdominal pain, abrupt onset of Kussmaul's respirations, signs of dehydration, minimal food intake over several days, and normal or slightly decreased blood glucose levels.
- With diabetic ketoacidosis (DKA), fruity breath odor occurs as DKA develops over 1 or 2 days.
- Other findings of DKA include polydipsia, polyuria, nocturia, weak and rapid pulse, hunger, weight loss, weakness, fatigue, nausea, vomiting, abdominal pain, and, eventually, Kussmaul's respirations, orthostatic hypotension, dehydration, tachycardia, confusion, stupor, and coma.
- With starvation ketoacidosis, fruity breath odor occurs with signs of cachexia and dehydration, decreased level of consciousness, bradycardia, and a history of severely limited food intake.

Other causes

Drugs

- Drugs that cause metabolic acidosis, such as nitroprusside and salicylates, can result in fruity breath odor.
- Low-carbohydrate diets may cause ketoacidosis and a fruity breath odor.

Nursing considerations

- When the patient is more alert and his condition stabilizes, remove the nasogastric tube and start him on an appropriate diet.
- Switch his insulin from I.V. to subcutaneous.

Pediatric pointers

- Fruity breath odor in an infant or a child usually stems from uncontrolled diabetes mellitus.
- Ketoacidosis develops rapidly because of low glycogen stores in this age-group.

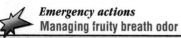

Emergency actions
Managing fruity breath odor

Check for Kussmaul's respirations, and examine the patient's level of consciousness. Take vital signs and check skin turgor. Check for rapid, deep respirations; stupor; and poor skin turgor. Obtain a brief history, noting especially diabetes mellitus, nutritional problems such as anorexia nervosa, and fad diets with scant or no carbohydrates. Obtain venous and arterial blood samples for complete blood count and glucose, electrolyte, acetone, and arterial blood gas (ABG) levels. Also obtain a urine specimen to test for glucose and acetone. Administer I.V. fluids and electrolytes to maintain hydration and electrolyte balance and, in patients with diabetic ketoacidosis, give regular insulin to reduce glucose levels.

If the patient is obtunded, insert endotracheal and nasogastric tubes. Suction as needed. Insert an indwelling urinary catheter, and monitor fluid intake and urine output. Insert central venous pressure and arterial lines to monitor the patient's fluid status and blood pressure. Place the patient on a cardiac monitor, monitor vital signs and neurologic status, and draw blood hourly to check glucose, electrolyte, acetone, and ABG levels.

Geriatric pointers

○ Consider factors, such as poor oral hygiene, increased dental caries, decreased salivary function, poor dietary intake, and use of multiple drugs when evaluating the condition of an elderly patient with mouth odor.

Patient teaching

○ Explain the signs of hyperglycemia.
○ Emphasize the importance of wearing medical identification.
○ Refer the patient to psychologist or support group, as needed.

Brudzinski's sign

Overview

○ Causes hips and knees to go into flexion in response to passive flexion of the neck
○ Signals meningeal irritation

○ An early indicator of life-threatening meningitis and subarachnoid hemorrhage (see *Testing for Brudzinski's sign*)

Emergency actions

Ask the patient about signs of increased intracranial pressure (ICP), such as *headache, neck pain, nausea,* and *vision disturbances. Observe for altered level of consciousness (LOC), pupillary changes, bradycardia, widened pulse pressure, Cheyne-Stokes*

Assessment tip
Testing for Brudzinski's sign

Here's how to test for Brudzinski's sign when you suspect meningeal irritation:

With the patient in a supine position, place your hands behind her neck and lift her head toward her chest.

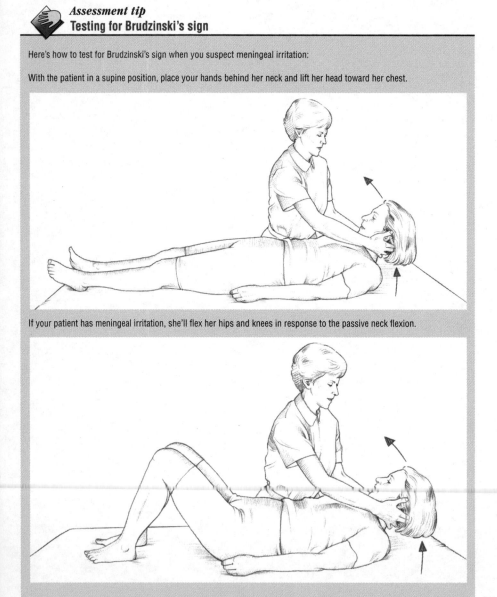

If your patient has meningeal irritation, she'll flex her hips and knees in response to the passive neck flexion.

or Kussmaul's respirations, vomiting, and moderate fever.

Keep artificial airways, intubation equipment, a handheld resuscitation bag, and suction equipment on hand. Elevate the head of the patient's bed 30 to 60 degrees to promote venous return. Give an osmotic diuretic to reduce cerebral edema. Monitor and look for ICP that continues to rise. You may have to provide mechanical ventilation and give a barbiturate and additional doses of a diuretic. Also, cerebrospinal fluid may have to be drained.

Assessment

History

○ Ask about a history of hypertension, spinal arthritis, recent head trauma, open-head injury, dental work or abscessed teeth, endocarditis, or I.V. drug abuse.
○ Ask about the sudden onset of headaches.

Physical assessment

○ Evaluate cranial nerve function, noting any motor or sensory deficits.
○ Look for Kernig's sign (resistance to knee extension after flexion of the hip), which is a further indication of meningeal irritation.
○ Look for signs of central nervous system infection, such as fever and nuchal rigidity.

Medical causes

Meningitis

○ A life-threatening disorder — a positive Brudzinski's sign can usually be elicited 24 hours after onset.
○ Other findings include headache, a positive Kernig's sign, nuchal rigidity, irritability or restlessness, deep stupor or coma, vertigo, fever, chills, malaise, hyperalgesia, muscular hypotonia, opisthotonos, symmetrical deep tendon reflexes, papilledema, ocular and facial palsies, nausea, vomiting, photophobia, diplopia, and unequal, sluggish pupils.
○ As ICP rises, arterial hypertension, bradycardia, widened pulse pressure, Cheyne-Stokes or Kussmaul's respirations, and coma may develop.

Subarachnoid hemorrhage

○ A life-threatening disorder — Brudzinski's sign may be elicited within minutes after initial bleeding.
○ Other findings include sudden onset of severe headache, nuchal rigidity, altered LOC, dizziness, photophobia, cranial nerve palsies, nausea, vomiting, fever, and a positive Kernig's sign.
○ Focal signs — such as hemiparesis, vision disturbances, or aphasia — may also occur.
○ As ICP rises, arterial hypertension, bradycardia, widened pulse pressure, Cheyne-Stokes or Kussmaul's respirations, and coma may develop.

Nursing considerations

○ Provide constant ICP monitoring and perform frequent neurologic checks.
○ Monitor vital signs, fluid intake and urine output, and cardiorespiratory status.
○ Maintain low lights and minimal noise and elevate the head of the bed to make the patient more comfortable.

Pediatric pointers

○ Bulging fontanels, a weak cry, fretfulness, vomiting, and poor feeding appear earlier in infants with meningeal irritation than Brudzinski's sign does.

Patient teaching

○ Discuss the signs and symptoms of meningitis and subdural hematoma.
○ Tell the patient when to seek immediate medical attention.

Bruit

Overview

- Bruits are swishing sounds caused by turbulent blood flow.
- Bruits are characterized by location, duration, intensity, pitch, and time of onset in the cardiac cycle.
- Bruits can indicate life- or limb-threatening vascular disease.
- Loud bruits produce a strong thrill.

Assessment tip
Preventing false bruits

Auscultating bruits accurately requires practice and skill. These sounds typically stem from arterial luminal narrowing or arterial dilation, but they can also result from excessive pressure applied to the stethoscope's bell during auscultation. This pressure compresses the artery, creating turbulent blood flow and a false bruit.

To prevent false bruits, place the bell lightly on the patient's skin. Also, if you're auscultating for a popliteal bruit, help the patient to a supine position, place your hand behind his ankle, and lift his leg slightly before placing the bell behind the knee.

NORMAL BLOOD FLOW, NO BRUIT

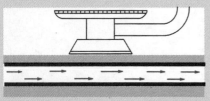

TURBULENT BLOOD FLOW AND RESULTANT BRUIT CAUSED BY ANEURYSM

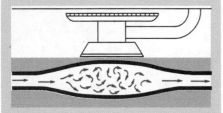

TURBULENT BLOOD FLOW AND FALSE BRUIT CAUSED BY COMPRESSION OF ARTERY

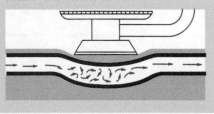

- When heard over the abdominal aorta; the renal, carotid, femoral, popliteal, or subclavian artery; or the thyroid gland, bruits are most significant. (See *Preventing false bruits.*)
- When heard consistently despite changes in the patient's position and when heard during diastole, bruits are also significant.

Assessment

History

- Obtain a medical history, including past injuries, illnesses, surgeries, and family medical history.
- Ask about alcohol use and diet.
- Take a drug and social history.

Physical assessment

- Perform cardiac assessment.
  If bruits are present over abdominal aorta:
- Check for a pulsating mass, Cullen's sign, or severe, tearing pain in the abdomen, flank, or lower back.
- Check peripheral pulses, comparing intensity in the upper versus lower extremities.
- Look for signs and symptoms of hypovolemic shock and dissection.
  If bruits occur over thyroid gland:
- Ask the patient about history of hyperthyroidism.
- Watch for signs and symptoms of life-threatening thyroid storm.
  If carotid artery bruits occur:
- Be alert for signs and symptoms of a transient ischemic attack (TIA).
- Evaluate frequently for changes in level of consciousness and muscle function.
  If bruits occur over femoral, popliteal, or subclavian artery:
- Watch for signs and symptoms of decreased or absent peripheral circulation.
- Ask if the patient has a history of intermittent claudication.
- Frequently check distal pulses and skin color and temperature.
- Watch for pallor, coolness, or the sudden absence of pulse.

Medical causes

Abdominal aortic aneurysm

- A systolic bruit over the aorta accompanies a pulsating periumbilical mass.
- Other findings include a rigid, tender abdomen; mottled skin; diminished peripheral pulses; and claudication.
- Sharp, tearing pain in the abdomen, flank, or lower back signals imminent dissection.

Abdominal aortic atherosclerosis

○ Loud systolic bruits in the epigastric and midabdominal areas are common.
○ Other findings may include leg weakness, numbness, paresthesia, or paralysis; leg pain; or decreased or absent femoral, popliteal, or pedal pulses.

Carotid artery stenosis

○ Systolic bruits can be heard over one or both carotid arteries.
○ Other signs and symptoms may be absent.
○ Dizziness, vertigo, headache, syncope, aphasia, dysarthria, sudden vision loss, hemiparesis, or hemiparalysis signals TIA and may signal a future stroke.

Peripheral arteriovenous fistula

○ A rough, continuous bruit with systolic accentuation may be heard over the fistula.
○ A palpable thrill is also common.
○ Other findings depend on the location of the fistula, but may include claudication, absent pulses, and cool skin.

Peripheral vascular disease

○ Bruits may be heard over the femoral artery and other arteries in the legs.
○ Other findings include diminished or absent femoral, popliteal, or pedal pulses; intermittent claudication; numbness, weakness, pain, and cramping in the legs, feet, and hips; and cool, shiny skin and hair loss on the affected extremity.
○ Lower-leg ulcers that are difficult to heal may also occur.

Renal artery stenosis

○ Systolic bruits are heard over abdominal midline and flank on affected side.
○ Hypertension commonly accompanies stenosis.
○ Headache, palpitations, tachycardia, anxiety, dizziness, retinopathy, hematuria, and mental sluggishness may also appear.

Subclavian steal syndrome

○ Systolic bruits may be heard over subclavian artery.
○ Other findings include decreased blood pressure and claudication in the affected arm, hemiparesis, vision disturbances, vertigo, and dysarthria.

Thyrotoxicosis

○ Systolic bruit is heard over the thyroid gland.
○ Characteristic findings include thyroid enlargement, fatigue, nervousness, tachycardia, heat intolerance, sweating, tremor, diarrhea, exophthalmos, and weight loss despite increased appetite.

Nursing considerations

○ Frequently check vital signs, and auscultate over affected arteries.

○ Check for bruits that become louder or develop a diastolic component.
○ Administer drugs, such as a vasodilator, anticoagulant, antihypertensive, or antiplatelet drug.

Pediatric pointers

○ Bruits are usually of little significance.
○ Auscultate for bruits in a child with port-wine spots or cavernous or diffuse hemangiomas.

Geriatric pointers

○ Elderly patients with atherosclerosis may experience bruits over several arteries.
○ Bruits from carotid artery stenosis are associated with stroke; close follow-up prompt surgical referral are mandatory.

Patient teaching

○ Tell the patient what symptoms of stroke are and that he should report them immediately.
○ Discuss lifestyle changes, such as quitting smoking, exercising regularly, and eating a balanced diet.

Butterfly rash

Overview

- Signals systemic lupus erythematosus (SLE) or dermatologic disorders
- Appears in a malar distribution across the nose and cheeks (see *Recognizing butterfly rash*)

Assessment

History

- Ask about the onset and extent of rash.
- Ask the patient about recent exposure to the sun.
- Determine whether the patient has had recent weight loss or hair loss.
- Ask about a family history of SLE.
- Note whether the patient is taking hydralazine or procainamide.

Physical assessment

- Inspect the rash, noting macules, papules, pustules, scaling, hypopigmentation, or hyperpigmentation.
- Look for blisters or ulcers in the mouth.
- Note inflamed lesions.
- Check for rashes elsewhere on the body.

Medical causes

Discoid lupus erythematosus

- One-sided or butterfly rash with erythematous, raised, sharply demarcated plaques, follicular plugging, and central atrophy of the plaque
- On the scalp, ears, chest, or other areas exposed to the sun
- At a late stage, telangiectasia, scarring, alopecia, and hypopigmentation or hyperpigmentation
- Conjunctival redness, dilated capillaries of the nail fold, parotid gland enlargement, oral lesions, and mottled, reddish blue skin on the legs

Erysipelas

- Rosy or crimson swollen lesions develop on the neck and head and along the nasolabial fold.
- The condition occurs primarily in infants and in adults older than age 30, after streptococcal infection.
- Other findings include fever, chills, cervical lymphadenopathy, and malaise.

Rosacea

- Initially, the rash may appear as a prominent, nonscaling, intermittent erythema limited to the lower half of the nose or including the chin, cheeks, and central forehead.
- As the rash develops, it remains longer and instead of disappearing after each episode, it subsides then rises again and is seen with telangiectasia.

Recognizing butterfly rash

With classic butterfly rash, lesions appear on the cheeks and the bridge of the nose, creating a characteristic butterfly pattern. The rash may vary in severity from malar erythema to discoid lesions (plaques).

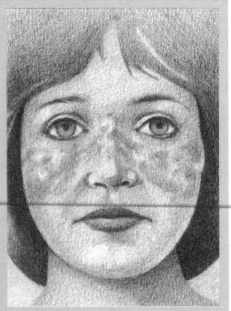

○ In advanced stages, skin is oily, with papules, pustules, nodules, and telangiectasis only on the central oval of the face.

Seborrheic dermatitis

○ Rash appears as greasy, scaling, slightly yellow macules and papules of varying size on the cheeks and the bridge of the nose.
○ The scalp, beard, eyebrows, portions of the forehead above the bridge of the nose, the nasolabial fold, or the trunk may be involved.
○ Other findings include crusts and fissures, pruritus, redness, blepharitis, styes, severe acne, and oily skin.

Systemic lupus erythematosus

○ Rash appears as a red, scaly, sharply demarcated macular eruption.
○ Rash may progress slowly to include the forehead, chin, the area around the ears, and other exposed areas.
○ Other findings include scaling, patchy alopecia, mucous membrane lesions, mottled erythema of the palms and fingers, periungual erythema with edema, reddish purple macular lesions on the palm side of the fingers, telangiectasis of the base of the nails or of the eyelids, purpura, petechiae, and ecchymoses.
○ Joint pain, stiffness, and deformities, particularly an ulnar deviation of the fingers and subluxation of the proximal interphalangeal joints, may accompany the rash.
○ Other findings include periorbital and facial edema, dyspnea, low-grade fever, malaise, weakness, fatigue, weight loss, anorexia, nausea, vomiting, lymphadenopathy, photosensitivity, and hepatosplenomegaly.

Other causes

Drugs

○ Hydralazine and procainamide can cause a lupuslike syndrome.

Nursing considerations

○ Withhold photosensitizing drugs.
○ Give local and systemic drugs.

Pediatric pointers

○ Rarely, butterfly rash may occur as part of an infectious disease such as erythema infectiosum.

Patient teaching

○ Urge the use of sunscreen.
○ Stress the avoidance of sun exposure.
○ Encourage the use of hypoallergenic makeup to conceal facial lesions.
○ Inform the patient about sources of support such as Lupus Foundation of America.

Capillary refill time, increased

Overview

- Increased time required for color to return to the nail bed after application of slight pressure
- Reflects the quality of peripheral vasomotor function
- Signals obstructive peripheral arterial disease or decreased cardiac output
- Normal capillary refill: Less than 3 seconds

Assessment

History

- Take a medical history, including previous peripheral vascular disease.
- Obtain a drug history, including tobacco.
- Ask about pain or other sensations in fingers or toes.

Physical assessment

- Perform a complete cardiovascular examination. (See *Assessing capillary refill.*)
- Observe skin color and check for edema.
- Check pulses in the affected limb.

Medical causes

Aortic aneurysm (dissecting)

- If aneurysm is in the thoracic aorta, capillary refill increases in the fingers and toes.
- If aneurysm is in abdominal aorta, capillary refill increases in the toes.
- Other findings include a pulsating abdominal mass, systolic bruit, and substernal, back, or abdominal pain.

Aortic arch syndrome

- Increased capillary refill in the fingers occurs early.
- Carotid pulses are absent, and radial pulses may be uneven.
- Other findings usually precede loss of pulses and include fever, night sweats, arthralgia, weight loss, anorexia, nausea, malaise, skin rash, splenomegaly, and pallor.

Arterial occlusion (acute)

- Increased capillary refill occurs early in the affected limb.
- Arterial pulses are usually absent far from the obstruction.
- The affected limb appears cool and pale or cyanotic.
- Intermittent claudication, moderate to severe pain, numbness, and paresthesia or paralysis of the affected limb may occur.

Buerger's disease

- Capillary refill is increased in the toes.
- Feet turn cold, cyanotic, and numb with exposure to low temperatures; later, feet redden, become hot, and tingle.
- Other findings include intermittent claudication of the instep and weak peripheral pulses.
- Ulceration, muscle atrophy, and gangrene may occur in later stages.
- Painful fingertip ulcerations may occur if the hands are affected.

Cardiac tamponade

- Increased capillary refill represents a late sign of decreased cardiac output.
- Other signs include paradoxical pulse, tachycardia, cyanosis, dyspnea, jugular vein distention, and hypotension.

Hypothermia

- Increased capillary refill may appear early as a response.
- Other findings include shivering, fatigue, weakness, decreased level of consciousness (LOC), slurred speech, ataxia, muscle stiffness or rigidity, tachycardia or bradycardia, hyporeflexia or areflexia, diuresis, oliguria, bradypnea, decreased blood pressure, and cold, pale skin.

Peripheral arterial trauma

- Trauma to a peripheral artery that reduces blood flow also increases capillary refill in the affected extremity.
- Other findings in the affected extremity include bruising, pulsating bleeding, weakened pulse, cyanosis, sensory loss, and cool, pale skin.

Raynaud's disease

- Capillary refill is prolonged in the fingers.
- Exposure to cold or stress produces blanching in the fingers, then cyanosis, and then erythema before the fingers return to normal temperature.
- Skin and other changes from poor circulation may occur with chronic disease.

Shock

- Increased capillary refill appears late in almost all types of shock.
- Other findings include hypotension, tachycardia, tachypnea, and cool, clammy skin.

Other causes

Diagnostic tests

- Cardiac catheterization can cause arterial hematoma or clot formation and increased capillary refill.

Fingernails normally appear pinkish with no markings. To estimate the rate of peripheral blood flow, assess the capillary refill in the fingernails (or toenails) by applying pressure to the nail for about 5 seconds, then assess the time it takes for color to return. In a patient with good arterial blood supply, the color should return in less than 3 seconds.

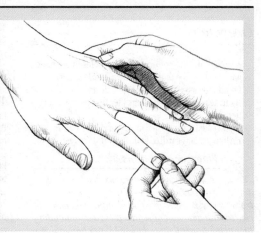

Drugs

○ Drugs that cause vasoconstriction (particularly alpha blockers) increase capillary refill.

Treatments

○ Arterial or umbilical lines can cause arterial hematoma and obstructed blood flow, leading to increased capillary refill time.
○ Improperly fitting casts can constrict circulation.

Nursing considerations

○ Frequently assess vital signs, LOC, and affected extremity; report any changes.
○ Prepare the patient for tests, which may include arteriography or Doppler ultrasonography.

Pediatric pointers

○ Increased capillary refill is normal in neonates with acrocyanosis.
○ Cardiac surgery is a common cause.

Patient teaching

○ Explain the signs and symptoms the patient needs to report.
○ Discuss with the patient ways to reduce risk of aggravating or reintroducing the underlying disorder.
○ Instruct the patient in ways to promote circulation.
○ Stress to the patient the importance of quitting smoking.

Carpopedal spasm

Overview

- A violent, painful contraction of muscles in the hands and feet (see *Recognizing carpopedal spasm*)
- Commonly associated with hypocalcemia
- Indicates tetany, a potentially life-threatening disorder
- If untreated: laryngospasm, seizures, cardiac arrhythmias, and cardiac and respiratory arrest

Emergency actions

Look for signs of respiratory distress or cardiac arrhythmias. Obtain blood samples for electrolyte analysis, especially for calcium, and obtain an electrocardiogram. Connect the patient to a monitor to watch for arrhythmias. Infuse I.V. calcium and provide emergency respiratory and cardiac support. If the calcium infusion doesn't control seizures, give a sedative.

Assessment

History

- Ask about the onset and duration of spasms.
- Explore the extent of pain.
- Note related signs and symptoms of hypocalcemia.
- Obtain the patient's immunization history.
- Ask about previous neck surgery, calcium or magnesium deficiency, tetanus exposure, hypoparathyroidism, or recent puncture wounds.

Physical assessment

- Take vital signs.
- Check for Chvostek's sign.
- Inspect the patient's skin and fingernails, noting any dryness or scaling or ridged, brittle nails caused by hypocalcemia.
- Assess his mental status and behavior.
- Complete the physical examination.

Medical causes

Hypocalcemia

- Carpopedal spasm is an early sign.
- Paresthesia of the fingers, toes, and perioral area; muscle weakness, twitching, and cramping; hyperreflexia; chorea; fatigue; and palpitations occur.
- Positive Chvostek's and Trousseau's signs can be elicited.
- Laryngospasm, stridor, and seizures may appear in severe hypocalcemia.
- In chronic hypocalcemia, mental status changes; cramps; dry, scaly skin; brittle nails; and thin, patchy hair and eyebrows occur.

Tetanus

- Muscle spasms and seizures develop.
- The patient has difficulty swallowing and low-grade fever.

Other causes

Treatments

- Multiple blood transfusions and parathyroidectomy may cause hypocalcemia.

Surgeries

- Surgeries that impair calcium absorption may cause hypocalcemia.

Assessment tip
Recognizing carpopedal spasm

In the hand, carpopedal spasm involves adduction of the thumb over the palm, followed by flexion of the metacarpophalangeal joints, extension of the interphalangeal joints (fingers together), adduction of the hyperextended fingers, and flexion of the wrist and elbow joints. Similar effects occur in the joints of the feet.

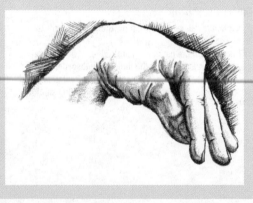

Nursing considerations

○ If hyperventilation occurs, help the patient slow his breathing.
○ To reduce the patient's anxiety, provide a quiet, dark environment.

Pediatric pointers

○ Monitor children with hypocalcemia caused by idiopathic hypoparathyroidism; carpopedal spasm may precede the onset of epileptiform seizures or generalized tetany.

Geriatric pointers

○ Suspect tetanus in anyone with carpopedal spasm, difficulty swallowing, and seizures.
○ Ask the elderly patient about his immunization record and recent wounds.

Patient teaching

○ Explain the importance of tetanus immunization and keeping an immunization record and schedule.

Chest expansion, asymmetrical

Overview

- Uneven extension of portions of the chest wall during inspiration
- May develop suddenly or gradually and may affect one or both sides of the chest wall
- May be a sign of a potentially life-threatening disorder (see *Recognizing life-threatening causes of asymmetrical chest expansion*)

![star icon] **Emergency actions**

First, suspect flail chest, a life-threatening emergency. Take the patient's vital signs, and look for signs of acute respiratory distress. Use tape or sandbags to temporarily splint the unstable flail segment. Administer oxygen by nasal cannula, mask, or mechanical ventilation, depending on the severity of respiratory distress. Insert an I.V. line to allow fluid replacement and administration of drugs for pain. Draw a blood sample for arterial blood gas analysis, and connect the patient to a cardiac monitor. Look for signs of respiratory distress.

Assessment

History

- Ask about the onset, duration, aggravating and alleviating factors, and extent of dyspnea or pain during breathing.
- Obtain a history of pulmonary or systemic illness, thoracic surgery, or blunt or penetrating chest trauma.
- Ask about job-related history.

Physical assessment

- Palpate the trachea for midline positioning.
- Examine the posterior chest wall for tenderness or deformity.
- Evaluate the extent of asymmetrical chest expansion.
- Palpate for vocal or tactile fremitus on both sides of the chest. Note asymmetrical vibrations and areas of enhanced, diminished, or absent fremitus.
- Percuss and auscultate to detect air and fluid in the lungs and pleural spaces.
- Auscultate all lung fields for abnormal breath sounds.
- Examine the patient's anterior chest wall.

Medical causes

Bronchial obstruction

- A life-threatening disorder — lack of chest movement indicates complete obstruction; lagging chest signals partial obstruction.
- Intercostal bulging during expiration and hyperresonance on percussion suggests air trapped in the chest.
- Dyspnea, accessory muscle use, decreased or absent breath sounds, and suprasternal, substernal, or intercostal retractions may occur.

Flail chest

- A life-threatening injury — the unstable portion of the chest wall collapses inward during inspiration and balloons outward during expiration. (See *Recognizing life-threatening causes of asymmetrical chest expansion*.)
- Ecchymoses and severe localized pain occur with traumatic injury to the chest wall.
- Rapid and shallow respirations, tachycardia, and cyanosis may also occur.

Hemothorax

- Life-threatening bleeding into the pleural space causes the chest to lag during inspiration.
- Other findings include signs of traumatic chest injury, stabbing pain at the injury site, anxiety, dullness on percussion, tachypnea, tachycardia, hypoxemia, and signs of shock.

Kyphoscoliosis

- Chest wall movement is decreased on the compressed-lung side.
- Intercostal muscles expand during inspiration on the opposite side.

Myasthenia gravis

- Progressive loss of ventilatory muscle function produces asynchrony of the chest and abdomen during inspiration.
- Shallow respirations and increased muscle weakness cause severe dyspnea, tachypnea, and possible apnea.

Phrenic nerve dysfunction

- The paralyzed hemidiaphragm fails to contract downward.
- Asynchrony of thorax and upper abdomen during inspiration develops on the affected side.
- Onset of phrenic nerve dysfunction may be gradual or sudden.

Pneumonia

- Asymmetrical chest expansion as inspiratory lagging chest or as chest-abdomen asynchrony.
- Fever, chills, tachycardia, fatigue, productive cough with rust-colored sputum, tachypnea, dyspnea, crackles, rhonchi, and chest pain that worsens with deep breathing.

Recognizing life-threatening causes of asymmetrical chest expansion

Asymmetrical chest expansion can result from several life-threatening disorders. Two common causes — bronchial obstruction and flail chest — produce distinctive chest wall movements that provide important clues about the underlying disorder.

With *bronchial obstruction,* only the unaffected portion of the chest wall expands during inspiration. Intercostal bulging during expiration may indicate that the air is trapped in the chest.

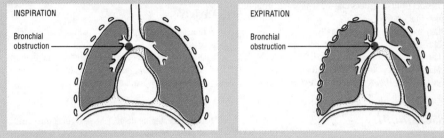

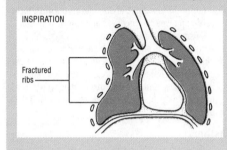

With *flail chest* — a disruption of the thorax due to multiple rib fractures — the unstable portion of the chest wall collapses inward at inspiration and balloons outward at expiration.

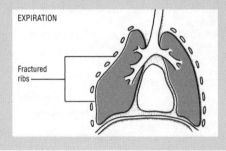

Pneumothorax

○ Lagging chest at end-inspiration can occur with this life-threatening condition.
○ The patient has sudden, stabbing chest pain that may radiate to the arms, face, back, or abdomen.
○ Other findings include tachypnea, decreased tactile fremitus, tympany on percussion, decreased or absent breath sounds over the trapped air, tachycardia, restlessness, and anxiety.
○ In tension pneumothorax, the same findings occur as in pneumothorax but more severe.
○ Other findings of tension pneumothorax include cyanosis; hypotension; subcutaneous crepitation of the upper trunk, neck, and face; mediastinal and tracheal deviation from the affected side; and a crunching sound on auscultation over the precordium with each heartbeat.

Other causes

Treatments

○ Treatments, such as pneumonectomy and surgical removal of several ribs, can cause asymmetrical chest expansion.
○ Mainstem bronchi intubation may also cause chest lag or the absence of chest movement.

Nursing considerations

○ Prepare patient for pulmonary studies.
○ Auscultate breath sounds in the lung peripheries.
○ Give supplemental oxygen during acute events.
 If the patient has a chest tube:
○ Maintain the water seal.
○ Check the system for air leaks.
○ Monitor drainage.

Pediatric pointers

○ Asymmetrical chest expansion may develop with acute respiratory illnesses, congenital abnormalities, cerebral palsy, and life-threatening diaphragmatic hernia.

Geriatric pointers

○ Asymmetrical chest expansion may be more difficult to determine because of the structural deformities associated with aging.

Patient teaching

○ Explain to the patient or caregiver how to recognize early signs and symptoms of respiratory distress and what to do if they occur.
○ Teach the patient coughing and deep-breathing exercises.
○ Teach the patient techniques that can help reduce his anxiety.

Chest pain

Overview

- Results from disorders that affect thoracic or abdominal organs
- Can arise suddenly or gradually
- May radiate to the arms, neck, jaw, or back
- Can be steady or intermittent, mild or acute
- May be an indicator of acute and life-threatening disorders (see *Managing severe chest pain*)

Assessment

History

- Ask about the onset and radiation of pain and its duration, quality, quantity, and what aggravates or alleviates it.
- Obtain a history of cardiac or pulmonary disease, chest trauma, GI disease, or sickle cell anemia.
- Obtain a drug history, including tobacco.

Physical assessment

- Take vital signs; note tachypnea, fever, tachycardia, oxygen saturation, paradoxical pulse, and hypertension or hypotension.
- Look for jugular vein distention and peripheral edema.
- Observe breathing pattern; inspect the chest for asymmetrical expansion.
- Auscultate for pleural rub, crackles, rhonchi, wheezing, and diminished or absent breath sounds.
- Auscultate for murmurs, clicks, gallops, and pericardial rub.
- Palpate for lifts, heaves, thrills, gallops, tactile fremitus, and abdominal masses or tenderness.

Medical causes

Angina pectoris

- Chest discomfort may be described as pain or a sensation of indigestion or expansion.
- Pain usually occurs in the retrosternal region behind the sternum and typically lasts 2 to 10 minutes.
- Pain may radiate to the neck, jaw, and arms.
- Emotional stress, exertion, or a heavy meal provoke anginal pain.
- Other signs and symptoms include dyspnea, nausea, vomiting, tachycardia, dizziness, diaphoresis, belching, and palpitations.
- With Prinzmetal's angina, pain occurs at rest and with shortness of breath, nausea, vomiting, dizziness, and palpitations.

Anthrax (inhalation)

- Initial stage: fever, chills, cough, and chest pain
- Second stage: develops abruptly with rapid deterioration marked by fever, dyspnea, stridor, and hypotension, generally leading to death within 24 hours

Anxiety

- Intermittent, sharp, stabbing pain behind the left breast
- Other findings: precordial tenderness, palpitations, fatigue, headache, insomnia, breathlessness, nausea, vomiting, diarrhea, and tremors

Aortic aneurysm (dissecting)

- A life-threatening disorder — excruciating tearing, ripping, stabbing chest and neck pain begins suddenly and radiates to the upper and lower back and abdomen.
- Other findings include abdominal tenderness; tachycardia; murmurs; syncope; blindness; loss of consciousness; weakness or transient paralysis of the arms or legs; hypotension; asymmetrical brachial pulses; lower blood pressure in the legs than in the arms; pale, cool, diaphoretic, and mottled skin below the waist; and weak or absent femoral or pedal pulses; a palpable abdominal mass; and systolic bruit.

Asthma

- Diffuse and painful chest tightness, dry cough, and mild wheezing arise suddenly.
- Signs may progress to a productive cough, audible wheezing, and severe dyspnea.
- Other respiratory findings include rhonchi, crackles, prolonged expirations, intercostal and supraclavicular retractions on inspiration, accessory muscle use, flaring nostrils, and tachypnea.
- Other signs and symptoms include anxiety, tachycardia, diaphoresis, flushing, and cyanosis.

Bronchitis

- The acute form produces a burning chest pain or a sensation of substernal tightness.
- Cough is initially dry but later productive.
- Other signs and symptoms include a low-grade fever, chills, sore throat, tachycardia, muscle and back pain, rhonchi, crackles, and wheezing.

Cardiomyopathy

- Hypertrophic cardiomyopathy may cause angina-like chest pain, dyspnea, a cough, dizziness, syncope, gallops, murmurs, and bradycardia associated with tachycardia.
- A medium-pitched systolic ejection murmur may be heard along the left sternal border and top of the heart.
- Palpation of peripheral pulses reveals a characteristic double impulse *(pulsus biferiens)*.

If the patient reports a sudden onset of pleuritic chest pain, described as crushing, shooting, and deep, assess him for diaphoresis, dyspnea, hemoptysis, and tachycardia. If you detect these signs and symptoms, suspect pulmonary embolism.

If the patient tells you his pain started suddenly and describes it as tearing, ripping, or stabbing chest pain, question him about syncope and hemiplegia. Check for differences in blood pressure between legs and arms as well as weak or absent femoral or pedal pulses. Begin interventions for *aortic aneurysm* if you assess these signs.

If the patient reports the sudden onset of severe substernal pain that radiates to his left arm, jaw, neck, or shoulder blades that he describes as squeezing, viselike, or burning, have him lie down. Assess for pallor, diaphoresis, nausea, vomiting, apprehension, weakness, fatigue, and dyspnea. If you detect these signs and symptoms, suspect *myocardial*

infarction.

If you suspect any of these life-threatening disorders, quickly take the patient's vital signs. Obtain a 12-lead electrocardiogram. Insert an I.V. line to administer fluids and drugs, and give oxygen. Check the patient's vital signs frequently to detect changes from baseline. Begin cardiac monitoring to detect arrhythmias. As appropriate, prepare the patient for emergency surgery.

If the patient reports a sudden onset of chest tightness, assess for wheezing, dry cough, dyspnea, tachycardia, and hyperventilation. The presence of these signs and symptoms suggests an acute *asthmatic attack.* Try to calm the patient to slow his respiratory rate. Ask him if he has ever had this pain before and, if so, what eased it. Give oxygen and insert an I.V. line to administer fluids and drugs. Expect to give epinephrine and a bronchodilator and to begin respiratory therapy.

Cholecystitis

○ Epigastric or right-upper-quadrant pain occurs abruptly.
○ Pain may be sharp or intensely aching, steady or intermittent.
○ Pain may radiate to the back or right shoulder.
○ Other findings include Murphy's sign, nausea, vomiting, fever, diaphoresis, and chills.
○ An abdominal mass, rigidity, distention, or tenderness may be palpable in the right upper abdomen.

Costochondritis

○ Pain and tenderness occur at the costochondral junctions, especially at the second costicartilage.
○ Pain is elicited by palpating the inflamed joint and worsens with movement.

Esophageal spasm

○ Substernal chest pain mimics angina.
○ Pain may last up to an hour and can radiate to the neck, jaw, arms, or back.
○ Other findings include dysphagia for solid foods, bradycardia, and nodal rhythm.

Herpes zoster (shingles)

○ Initially, pain is sharp, shooting, and one-sided; it may mimic myocardial infarction (MI).
○ About 4 to 5 days after onset, chest pain becomes burning, and small, red, nodular lesions erupt on the painful areas.
○ Associated signs and symptoms include fever, malaise, pruritus, and paresthesia or hyperesthesia of the affected areas.

Hiatal hernia

○ Heartburn and sternal ache or pressure occur and may radiate to left shoulder and arm.

○ Pain occurs after a meal and with bending or lying down.
○ Other findings include a bitter taste and pain while eating or drinking.

Interstitial lung disease

○ Pleuritic chest pain, progressive dyspnea, "cellophane" crackles, nonproductive cough, fatigue, weight loss, decreased exercise tolerance, clubbing and cyanosis occur.

Legionnaires' disease

○ Pleuritic chest pain, malaise, and headache develop.
○ Diarrhea, anorexia, diffuse myalgia, and general weakness may occur.
○ Within 12 to 24 hours, a sudden high fever, chills, and a nonproductive cough that progresses to yield mucoid and then mucopurulent sputum, and possibly hemoptysis, occurs.
○ Other findings include flushed skin, diaphoresis, prostration, nausea, vomiting, mild temporary amnesia, confusion, dyspnea, crackles, tachypnea, and tachycardia.

Mediastinitis

○ Severe retrosternal chest pain radiates to the epigastrium, back, or shoulder.
○ Pain may worsen with breathing, coughing, or sneezing.
○ Chills, fever, and dysphagia may also occur.

Mitral valve prolapse

○ Sharp, stabbing precordial chest pain or precordial ache may occur.
○ A midsystolic click is followed by a systolic murmur at the apex.

- Other signs and symptoms include cardiac awareness, migraine headache, dizziness, weakness, episodic severe fatigue, dyspnea, tachycardia, mood swings, and palpitations.

Muscle strain

- A superficial and continuous ache or pulling sensation in the chest may result from strain.
- Lifting, pulling, or pushing heavy objects may aggravate this discomfort.
- Fatigue, weakness, and rapid swelling of the affected area occur with acute strain.

Myocardial infarction

- Crushing substernal pain isn't relieved by nitroglycerin.
- Pain lasts 15 minutes to hours and may radiate to the left arm, jaw, neck, or shoulder blades.
- Other signs and symptoms include pallor, clammy skin, dyspnea, diaphoresis, nausea, vomiting, anxiety, restlessness, murmurs, crackles, hypotension or hypertension, a feeling of impending doom, and an atrial gallop.

Pancreatitis

- Acute form causes intense pain in the epigastric area.
- Pain radiates to the back and worsens in a supine position.
- Other findings include nausea, vomiting, fever, abdominal tenderness and rigidity, diminished bowel sounds, and crackles at the lung bases.
- Extreme restlessness, mottled skin, tachycardia, and cold, sweaty extremities may occur with severe pancreatitis.
- Massive hemorrhage, with resultant shock and coma, occurs with sudden, severe pancreatitis.

Peptic ulcer

- Sharp and burning pain arises in the epigastric region hours after food intake, commonly during the night.
- Pain is relieved by food or antacids.
- Other signs and symptoms include nausea, vomiting, melena, and epigastric tenderness.

Pericarditis

- Sharp or cutting precordial or retrosternal pain is aggravated by deep breathing, coughing, and position changes.
- Pain radiates to the shoulder and neck.
- Associated findings include pericardial rub, fever, tachycardia, and dyspnea.

Plague

- Signs and symptoms include productive cough, chest pain, tachypnea, dyspnea, hemoptysis, increasing respiratory distress, and cardiopulmonary insufficiency.

Pleurisy

- Sharp, usually one-sided, pain in the lower aspects of the chest arises abruptly, reaching maximum intensity within a few hours.
- Deep breathing, coughing, or thoracic movement aggravates pain.
- Decreased breath sounds, inspiratory crackles, and a pleural rub may be heard on auscultation.
- Other findings include dyspnea, shallow breathing, cyanosis, fever, and fatigue.

Pneumonia

- Pleuritic chest pain increases with deep inspiration.
- Shaking chills and fever occur.
- A dry, hacking cough occurs that later becomes productive.
- Other signs and symptoms include crackles, rhonchi, tachycardia, tachypnea, myalgia, fatigue, headache, dyspnea, abdominal pain, anorexia, cyanosis, decreased breath sounds, and diaphoresis.

Pneumothorax

- A life-threatening disorder — sudden, severe, sharp chest pain that's typically on one side and increases with chest movement.
- Dyspnea and cyanosis progressively worsen.
- Breath sounds are decreased or absent on the affected side, with hyperresonance or tympany, subcutaneous crepitation, and decreased vocal fremitus.
- Other findings include asymmetrical chest expansion, accessory muscle use, a nonproductive cough, tachypnea, tachycardia, anxiety, and restlessness.

Pulmonary embolism

- The patient first experiences sudden dyspnea with intense angina-like or pleuritic pain aggravated by deep breathing and thoracic movement.
- Other signs and symptoms include a choking sensation, tachycardia, tachypnea, cough, low-grade fever, restlessness, diaphoresis, crackles, pleural rub, diffuse wheezing, dullness on percussion, signs of respiratory collapse, paradoxical pulse, signs of cerebral ischemia, and signs of hypoxia.
- Cyanosis and distended neck veins occur with a large embolus.

Pulmonary hypertension (primary)

- Angina-like pain develops late.
- Pain typically occurs on exertion.
- Pain may radiate to the neck.
- Other signs and symptoms include exertional dyspnea, fatigue, syncope, weakness, cough, and hemoptysis.

Q fever

- Fever, chills, severe headache, malaise, chest pain, nausea, vomiting, and diarrhea occur.
- Hepatitis or pneumonia may develop in severe cases.

Rib fracture

○ Chest pain is usually sharp, severe, and aggravated by inspiration, coughing, or pressure on the affected area.
○ Other findings include dyspnea, cough, tenderness and slight edema at the fracture site, and shallow, splinted breathing.

Sickle cell crisis

○ Pain may be vague at first and located in the back, hands, or feet.
○ As pain worsens, it becomes generalized or localized to the abdomen or chest, causing severe pleuritic pain.
○ Abdominal distention and rigidity, dyspnea, fever, and jaundice may also occur.

Tuberculosis

○ Pleuritic chest pain and fine crackles occur after coughing.
○ Other findings include night sweats, anorexia, weight loss, fever, malaise, dyspnea, fatigue, mild to severe productive cough, hemoptysis, dullness on percussion, increased tactile fremitus, and amphoric breath sounds.

Tularemia

○ Pneumonia can develop, causing chest pain and hemoptysis.
○ Other signs and symptoms include the abrupt onset of fever, chills, headache, myalgia, nonproductive cough, dyspnea, and empyema.

Other causes

Chinese restaurant syndrome

○ A reaction to excessive ingestion of monosodium glutamate mimics the signs of an acute MI.

Drugs

○ Abrupt withdrawal from a beta blocker can cause rebound angina in the patient with coronary heart disease.

Nursing considerations

○ Prepare the patient for cardiopulmonary studies.
○ Perform a venipuncture to collect a serum specimen for cardiac enzyme and other studies.

Pediatric pointers

○ A child may complain of chest pain in an attempt to get attention or to avoid attending school.

Geriatric pointers

○ Because older patients have a higher risk of developing life-threatening conditions, carefully evaluate chest pain.

Patient teaching

○ Alert the patient or caregiver to signs and symptoms that require medical attention.
○ Explain the diagnostic tests the patient needs.
○ Provide details to the patient about his prescribed drugs and how to take them.

Cheyne-Stokes respirations

Overview

○ A waxing and waning period of hyperpnea that alternates with a shorter period of apnea (see *Respiratory pattern of Cheyne-Stokes*)
○ May occur normally in patients with heart or lung disease or those who live at high altitudes
○ Usually indicate increased intracranial pressure (ICP) from a deep cerebral or brain stem lesion or a metabolic disturbance in the brain

> ⭐ **Emergency actions**
>
> *In a patient with a history of head trauma, recent brain surgery, or another brain insult, quickly take his vital signs. Elevate the head of the bed 30 degrees, and perform a rapid neurological examination. Watch for signs of rising ICP, and anticipate ICP monitoring.*
>
> *Time the periods of hyperpnea and apnea, being alert for prolonged periods of apnea. Assess vital signs and neurological status frequently to detect changes. Maintain airway patency, and administer oxygen as needed. Mechanical ventilation may be necessary if the patient's condition worsens.*

Assessment

History
○ Obtain a medical and surgical history.
○ Ask about drug use.

Respiratory pattern of Cheyne-Stokes

When assessing a patient's respirations, you should determine the rate, rhythm, and depth. This schematic diagram shows respiratory pattern of Cheyne-Stokes. Respirations that gradually become faster and deeper than normal, then slower; alternates with periods of apnea.

Physical assessment
○ Perform a complete physical examination, focusing on the neurologic and cardiorespiratory systems.

Medical causes

Adams-Stokes syndrome
○ Adams-Stokes attacks may precede Cheyne-Stokes respirations.
○ A syncopal episode associated with atrioventricular block occurs.
○ Other findings include hypotension, a heart rate between 20 and 50 beats/minute, confusion, shaking, and paleness.

Heart failure
○ Cheyne-Stokes respirations may occur with exertional dyspnea and orthopnea in left-sided heart failure
○ Related signs and symptoms include fatigue, weakness, tachycardia, tachypnea, and crackles.

Hypertensive encephalopathy
○ A life-threatening disorder — severe hypertension precedes Cheyne-Stokes respirations.
○ Accompanying signs and symptoms include decreased level of consciousness (LOC), vomiting, seizures, severe headaches, vision disturbances, and transient paralysis.

Increased ICP
○ Cheyne-Stokes respirations are the first irregular respiratory pattern to occur as ICP rises.
○ Decreased LOC precedes respiratory changes.
○ Accompanying signs and symptoms include hypertension, headache, vomiting, impaired motor movement, and vision disturbances.
○ Bradycardia and widened pulse pressure are late signs of increased ICP.

Renal failure
○ Cheyne-Stokes respirations occur with end-stage chronic renal failure.
○ Other findings include bleeding gums, oral lesions, ammonia breath odor, and marked changes in every body system.

Other causes

Drugs
○ Large doses of an opioid, hypnotic, or barbiturate can precipitate Cheyne-Stokes respiratory pattern.

Nursing considerations

○ Don't mistake periods of hypoventilation or decreased tidal volume for complete apnea.

Pediatric pointers

○ Cheyne-Stokes respirations rarely occur in children except during late heart failure.

Geriatric pointers

○ Cheyne-Stokes respirations may occur normally in elderly people during sleep.

Patient teaching

○ Teach the patient and a responsible person to recognize the difference between sleep apnea and Cheyne-Stokes respirations.
○ Explain the causes and treatments of Cheyne-Stokes respirations.

Chills

Overview

- Extreme, involuntary muscle contractions with paroxysms of violent shivering and teeth chattering
- Signal onset of infection
- Commonly accompanied by fever

Assessment

History

- Ask about the onset and duration of chills (continuous or intermittent).
- Inquire about related signs and symptoms.
- Obtain a history of allergies or infectious disorders.
- Take a drug history.
- Ask about recent treatments (such as chemotherapy), travel, and exposure to animals or infection.

Physical assessment

- Take other vital signs.
- Note the pattern of temperature changes.
- Assess the skin, mucous membranes, liver, spleen, and lymph nodes.
- Check for drainage from skin lesions.
- Note skin color, temperature, and turgor.
- Percuss for costovertebral angle tenderness to determine if cystitis is present.
- Assess level of consciousness (LOC).

Medical causes

Acquired immunodeficiency syndrome

- Fatigue, fever, chills, anorexia, weight loss, diarrhea, diaphoresis, skin disorders, lymphadenopathy, and upper respiratory tract infection

Anthrax (inhalation)

- Initially fever, chills, weakness, cough, and chest pain
- Abrupt fever, dyspnea, stridor, and hypotension, leading to death within 24 hours

Cholangitis

- Charcot's triad: chills with spiking fever, abdominal pain, and jaundice
- Pruritus, weakness, fatigue, dark urine, and light-colored stools

Gram-negative bacteremia

- Infection causes sudden chills and fever, nausea, vomiting, diarrhea, and prostration.
- Other findings include tachypnea, hypotension, decreased urine output, and an altered LOC.

Hemolytic anemia

- Fulminating chills with fever and abdominal pain
- Rapidly developing jaundice and hepatomegaly
- Possible splenomegaly and brown or red urine

Hepatic abscess

- Chills, fever, nausea, vomiting, diarrhea, anorexia, and severe upper abdominal tenderness and pain
- Pain radiating to the right shoulder

Hodgkin's disease

- Several days or weeks of fever and chills alternate with periods of no fever and no chills.
- Regional lymphadenopathy may progress to hepatosplenomegaly.
- Other signs and symptoms include diaphoresis, fatigue, and pruritus.

Infective endocarditis

- Intermittent, shaking chills with fever occur abruptly.
- Accompanying findings include petechiae, Janeway lesions on the hands and feet, Osler's nodes on the palms and soles, murmur, hematuria, eye hemorrhage, Roth's spots, and signs of heart failure.

Influenza

- Onset of chills, high fever, malaise, headache, myalgia, and nonproductive cough is abrupt.
- Rhinitis, rhinorrhea, laryngitis, conjunctivitis, hoarseness, and sore throat may occur.
- Chills generally subside after the first few days.
- Intermittent fever, weakness, and cough may persist for up to 1 week.

Legionnaires' disease

- Sudden chills and high fever within 48 hours of disease onset
- Early sign and symptoms: malaise, headache, diarrhea, anorexia, myalgia, and weakness
- First, a nonproductive cough then a productive cough with mucoid or mucopurulent sputum
- Nausea, vomiting, confusion, pleuritic chest pain, dyspnea, tachypnea, crackles, tachycardia, and flushed and mildly diaphoretic skin

Lymphangitis

- Chills and other systemic signs and symptoms (such as fever, malaise, and headache) develop.
- Red streaks radiating from a wound and cellulitis draining toward tender, regional lymph nodes are characteristic.
- Lymph nodes along the course of drainage may be enlarged, red, and tender.

Malaria

- The paroxysmal cycle begins with a period of chills lasting 1 to 2 hours.
- Chills are followed by a high fever lasting 3 to 4 hours and then 2 to 4 hours of profuse diaphoresis.

- Headache, muscle pain, and hepatosplenomegaly may occur.

Miliary tuberculosis

- Intermittent chills, high fever, and night sweats
- Epididymal or testicular nodules and splenomegaly
- Fatigue, malaise, joint pain, and swollen lymph nodes

Otitis media

- Acute suppurative otitis media produces chills with fever and severe deep, throbbing ear pain.
- A mild conductive hearing loss and a bulging, hyperemic tympanic membrane may also occur.
- Other signs and symptoms include dizziness, nausea, and vomiting.

Plague

- Fever, chills, and swollen, inflamed, and tender lymph nodes near the site of a flea bite develop.
- The onset of the pneumonic form is usually sudden with chills, fever, headache, and myalgia.
- Pulmonary findings include productive cough, chest pain, tachypnea, dyspnea, hemoptysis, and increasing respiratory distress.

Pneumonia

- A single shaking chill signals the sudden onset of pneumococcal pneumonia.
- Other types of pneumonia cause intermittent chills.
- Related signs and symptoms include fever, productive cough, pleuritic chest pain, dyspnea, tachypnea, tachycardia, diaphoresis, crackles, rhonchi, and increased tactile fremitus.

Pyelonephritis

- Chills, high fever and possible nausea and vomiting over several hours to days
- Anorexia, fatigue, myalgia, flank pain, costovertebral angle tenderness, hematuria or cloudy urine, and urinary frequency, urgency, and burning

Q fever

- Fever, chills, severe headache, malaise, chest pain, nausea, vomiting, and diarrhea develop.
- In severe cases, hepatitis and pneumonia develop.

Rocky Mountain spotted fever

- Sudden onset of chills, fever, malaise, excruciating headache, and muscle, bone, and joint pain
- A thick white coating gradually turning brown on tongue
- After 2 to 6 days of fever and occasional chills, a macular or maculopapular rash on the hands and feet and then becomes generalized
- Petechial rash after a few days

Septic shock

- Initially, chills, fever and possible nausea, vomiting, and diarrhea

- Normal or slightly low blood pressure, tachycardia, tachypnea, and warm, flushed, dry skin
- Oliguria, thirst, anxiety, restlessness, confusion, hypotension, and cool, cyanotic limbs as shock progresses
- Late signs: cold, clammy skin; rapid, thready pulse; severe hypotension; oliguria or anuria; signs of respiratory failure; and coma

Tularemia

- Abrupt onset of fever, chills, headache, generalized myalgia, nonproductive cough, dyspnea, pleuritic chest pain, and empyema
- A red spot on the skin that enlarges to an ulcer, enlarged lymph nodes, conjunctivitis, diaphoresis, and joint stiffness

Other causes

Drugs

- Amphotericin B, I.V. bleomycin, oral antipyretics, and phenytoin may cause chills.

I.V. therapy

- Infection at the I.V. insertion site can cause chills, high fever, and local redness, warmth, induration, and tenderness.

Transfusion reaction

- A hemolytic reaction may cause chills during or immediately after the transfusion.

Nursing considerations

- Check vital signs often.
- Be alert for signs of progressive septic shock.
- Obtain samples of blood, sputum, or wound drainage for culture to determine the cause.
- Give the appropriate antibiotic.
- Keep room temperature even.
- Provide adequate hydration and nutrients.
- Administer an antipyretic.

Pediatric pointers

- Infants don't get chills because they have poorly developed shivering mechanisms.

Geriatric pointers

- Chill usually indicate an underlying infection.

Patient teaching

- Explain the importance of documenting temperature to reveal patterns.
- Explain treatment and antibiotics the patient needs.
- Explain the signs and symptoms of a worsening condition and when to seek medical attention.

Chorea

Overview

- Brief, unpredictable bursts of rapid, jerky motion that interrupt normal coordinated movement
- Indicates dysfunction of the extrapyramidal system
- Usually involves the face, head, lower arms, and hands
- Aggravated by excitement or fatigue; may disappear during sleep
- May be difficult to distinguish from athetosis (snakelike, writhing movements), although choreiform movements are generally more rapid than athetoid ones

Assessment

History

- Ask about the onset and description of choreiform movements.
- Note a family history of choreiform movements or Huntington's disease.
- Obtain a drug history.
- Obtain an occupational history, noting prolonged exposure to manganese or other metals.

Physical assessment

- Ask the patient to stick out his tongue and keep it out. Typically, he'll be unable to do this; instead, his tongue will dart in and out of his mouth.
- Observe arms and legs for involuntary jerky movements.
- Ask the patient to extend and flex his hand as if halting traffic, and note the choreiform movements — they'll be extremely evident in this position.
- Check for athetosis, rigidity, or tremor.
- Assess for choreoathetotic gait by asking the patient to walk (he may change the positions of his trunk and upper body parts with each step and jerk and tilt his head to one side. His legs may move slowly and awkwardly and his gait will have a dancing quality).

Medical causes

Cerebral infarction

- If thalamic area is involved, unilateral or bilateral chorea occurs.
- Other findings include dysarthria, tremors, rigidity, weakness, and sensory disturbances.

Encephalitis

- Chorea may occur in the recovery phase with low-grade fever, athetosis, hemiparesis, hemiplegia, and facial droop.

- Other signs and symptoms include headache, vomiting, photophobia, stiff neck, confusion, and drowsiness.

Huntington's disease

- Chorea may be the first sign or may occur with intellectual decline.
- Emotional disturbances and dementia occur.
- Choreoathetotic movements may occur, accompanied by dysarthria, dystonia, prancing gait, dysphagia, and facial grimacing.

Wilson's disease

- Chorea is an early indication of this disorder — in addition to dystonia that affects the arms and legs.
- The patient typically experiences dysarthria, tremors, hoarseness, dysphagia, and slowed body movements.
- Other findings include emotional and behavioral disturbances, drooling, rigidity and mental deterioration.
- The pathognomonic Kayser-Fleischer ring in the cornea appears as the disease progresses.

Other causes

Carbon monoxide poisoning

- The patient may experience chorea, rigidity, dementia, impaired sensory function, masklike facies, generalized seizures, and myoclonus.

Lead poisoning

- Chorea, seizures, headache, memory lapses, and severe mental impairment occur in later stages.
- Accompanying signs and symptoms include masklike facies, footdrop, wristdrop, dizziness, ataxia, weakness, lethargy, abdominal pain, anorexia, nausea, vomiting, constipation, lead line on the gums, and a metallic taste.

Manganese poisoning

- Chorea occurs with propulsive gait, dystonia, and rigidity.
- Masklike facies, a resting tremor, and personality changes develop initially.
- Extreme muscle weakness and lethargy occur later.

Drugs

- Phenothiazines, haloperidol, thiothixene, and loxapine commonly produce chorea.
- Metoclopramide, metyrosine, hormonal contraceptives, levodopa, and phenytoin may cause chorea.

Nursing considerations

- Pad the side rails of the patient's bed.
- Keep sharp objects out of the patient's environment.

- ○ Help minimize physical activity and emotional upset.
- ○ Provide adequate periods of rest and sleep.

Pediatric pointers

- ○ Sydenham's chorea occurs in childhood as a delayed manifestation of rheumatic fever.
- ○ Chorea can occur in children with athetoid cerebral palsy.

Patient teaching

- ○ Explain safety measures to reduce risk of falls and poisoning.
- ○ Discuss genetic counseling (for those with Huntington's disease).

Chvostek's sign

Overview

○ Chvostek's sign is a spasm of the facial muscles, elicited by lightly tapping the patient's facial nerve near his lower jaw. (See *Eliciting Chvostek's sign*.)
○ Positive sign suggests hypocalcemia.
○ Positive sign occurs normally in about 25% of patients.

> **Emergency actions**
>
> *Test for Trousseau's sign, a reliable indicator of hypocalcemia. Monitor for signs of tetany. The patient may have a seizure. Obtain an electrocardiogram to check for changes associated with hypocalcemia, which can predispose the patient to arrhythmias. Place the patient on a cardiac monitor.*

Assessment

History

○ Obtain a medical history, including hypoparathyroidism, hypomagnesemia, or a malabsorption disorder.
○ Ask about previous surgical removal of parathyroid glands.
○ Determine whether mental changes have occurred.
○ Question the patient about other symptoms, including tingling sensations around the mouth and in the fingertips and feet.

Physical assessment

○ Observe the patient's behavior.
○ Observe for seizures, tetany, and facial spasms.
○ Check for dry and scaling skin, brittle nails, and dry hair.
○ Take vital signs because an irregular pulse and hypotension suggest hypocalcemia.
○ Auscultate the lungs.
○ Note signs of bronchospasm, laryngospasm, and airway obstruction.

Medical causes

Hypocalcemia

○ The degree of muscle spasm elicited reflects the patient's calcium level.
○ Paresthesia in the fingers, toes, and circumoral area that progresses to muscle tension and carpopedal spasms occur initially.
○ Muscle weakness, muscle twitching, hyperactive deep tendon reflexes, choreiform movements, muscle cramps, fatigue, and palpitations may be present.
○ Mental status changes; diplopia; difficulty swallowing; abdominal cramps; dry, scaly skin; brittle nails; and thin, patchy scalp hair and eyebrows occur with chronic hypocalcemia.

Other causes

Treatments

○ Massive blood transfusion can lower calcium levels.

Assessment tip
Eliciting Chvostek's sign

Begin by telling the patient to relax his facial muscles. Then stand directly in front of him and tap the facial nerve either just anterior to the earlobe and below the zygomatic arch or between the zygomatic arch and the corner of his mouth. A positive response varies from twitching of the lip at the corner of the mouth to spasm of all facial muscles, depending on the severity of hypocalcemia.

Nursing considerations

○ Collect blood samples for ongoing calcium studies.
○ Administer oral or I.V. calcium supplements.
○ Look for Chvostek's sign postoperatively.

Pediatric pointers

○ This sign may be observed in healthy infants so it isn't used to detect neonatal tetany.

Geriatric pointers

○ Consider malabsorption and poor nutritional status in the elderly patient with Chvostek's sign and hypocalcemia.

Patient teaching

○ Explain which early signs and symptoms of hypocalcemia a patient should report.
○ Stress the important of seeking immediate medical attention if early signs and symptoms occur.

Clubbing

Overview

○ A painless increase in soft tissue around the tips of the fingers or toes (usually on both sides)
○ A nonspecific sign of pulmonary and cyanotic cardiovascular disorders

Assessment

History

○ Focus on cardiovascular and pulmonary history.
○ Ask about drug history.

Physical assessment

○ Perform a cardiopulmonary examination.
○ Evaluate the extent of clubbing in the fingers and toes. (See *Checking for clubbed fingers*.)

Assessment tip
Checking for clubbed fingers

To assess the patient for chronic tissue hypoxia, check his fingers for clubbing. Normally, the angle between the fingernail and the point where the nail enters the skin is about 160 degrees. Clubbing occurs when that angle increases to 180 degrees or more, as shown below.

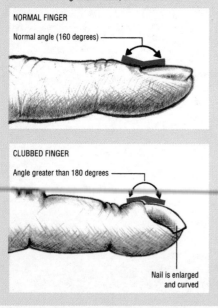

NORMAL FINGER

Normal angle (160 degrees)

CLUBBED FINGER

Angle greater than 180 degrees

Nail is enlarged and curved

Medical causes

Bronchiectasis

○ Clubbing occurs in the late stages.
○ A cough producing copious, foul-smelling, and mucopurulent sputum is a classic sign.
○ Hemoptysis and coarse crackles during inspiration are also characteristic.
○ Other signs and symptoms include weight loss, fatigue, weakness, exertional dyspnea, rhonchi, fever, malaise, and halitosis.

Bronchitis

○ Clubbing is a late sign.
○ Other findings include chronic productive cough, barrel chest, dyspnea, wheezing, use of accessory muscles, cyanosis, tachypnea, crackles, scattered rhonchi, and prolonged expiration.

Emphysema

○ Clubbing is a late sign.
○ Other signs and symptoms include anorexia, malaise, dyspnea, tachypnea, diminished breath sounds, accessory muscle use, barrel chest, a productive cough, peripheral cyanosis, and pursed-lip breathing.

Endocarditis

○ In subacute infective endocarditis, clubbing with fever, anorexia, pallor, weakness, night sweats, fatigue, tachycardia, and weight loss
○ Other findings: arthralgia, petechiae, murmurs, Osler's nodes, splinter hemorrhages, Janeway lesions, splenomegaly, and Roth's spots

Heart failure

○ Clubbing is a late sign with wheezing, dyspnea, and fatigue.
○ Other signs and symptoms include jugular vein distention, hepatomegaly, tachypnea, palpitations, dependent edema, weight gain, nausea, anorexia, chest tightness, slowed mental response, hypotension, diaphoresis, narrow pulse pressure, pallor, oliguria, a gallop rhythm, and crackles on inspiration.

Interstitial fibrosis

○ Clubbing occurs with advanced disease.
○ Intermittent chest pain, dyspnea, crackles, fatigue, weight loss, and cyanosis may also be present.

Lung abscess

○ Clubbing occurs initially but may reverse with resolution of the abscess.
○ Other findings include pleuritic chest pain; dyspnea; crackles; productive cough with a large amount of purulent, foul-smelling, often bloody sputum; and halitosis.

○ Weakness, fatigue, anorexia, headache, malaise, weight loss, and fever with chills may also be present.

Lung and pleural cancer
○ Clubbing is common.
○ Other signs and symptoms include hemoptysis, dyspnea, wheezing, chest pain, weight loss, anorexia, fatigue, and fever.

Nursing considerations

○ Don't mistake curved nails for clubbing.

Pediatric pointers
○ Clubbing usually occurs in children with cyanotic congenital heart disease or cystic fibrosis.
○ Surgical correction of heart defects may reverse clubbing.

Geriatric pointers
○ Arthritic deformities of the fingers or toes may disguise clubbing.

Patient teaching
○ Explain that clubbing may not disappear even if cause has been resolved.

Confusion

Overview

- Refers to the inability to think quickly and coherently
- May be temporary or irreversible
- Severe: Arises suddenly and is accompanied by hallucinations and psychomotor activity is classified as *delirium*
- Dementia: Long-term, progressive confusion with deterioration of all cognitive functions

Assessment

History

- Obtain a medical history, including head trauma or cardiopulmonary, metabolic, cerebrovascular, or neurologic disorders.
- Check with family members or friends about the onset and frequency of confusion.
- Ask what drugs the patient is taking and about alcohol use.
- Inquire about changes in his daily habits.

Physical assessment

- Assess for systemic disorders.
- Check vital signs, and assess for changes in blood pressure, temperature, and pulse.
- Perform a neurologic assessment to establish level of consciousness.

Medical causes

Alzheimer's disease

- Primary progressive dementia with insidious onset
- Initially characterized by loss of recent and remote memory and disorientation
- As disease progresses, impaired cognition, inability to concentrate, confusion, and severe deterioration in memory, language, and motor function

Brain tumor

- Is mild and difficult to detect in the early stages.
- Worsens as the tumor impinges on cerebral structures.
- Causes personality changes, bizarre behavior, sensory and motor deficits, visual field deficits, and aphasia.

Decreased cerebral perfusion

- Mild confusion is an early symptom; it may be insidious and fleeting or acute and permanent.
- Other findings include hypotension, tachycardia or bradycardia, irregular pulse, ventricular gallop, edema, and cyanosis.

Fluid and electrolyte imbalance

- The extent of imbalance determines the severity of confusion.
- Signs of dehydration may also be present.

Head trauma

- Confusion may occur at the time of injury, shortly afterward, or months or years afterward.
- Other signs and symptoms commonly include vomiting, severe headache, pupillary changes, and sensory and motor deficits.

Heatstroke

- Confusion gradually worsens as body temperature rises.
- Irritability and dizziness occur initially.
- Delirium, seizures, and loss of consciousness occur later.

Heavy metal poisoning

- Confusion, weakness, and drowsiness occur.
- Headache, vomiting, seizures, tremors, gait disturbances, and mental deterioration may also develop.

Hypothermia

- Confusion may be an early sign of hypothermia, and it progresses to stupor and coma as temperature drops.
- Other findings include slurred speech, cold and pale skin, hyperactive deep tendon reflexes, tachycardia, hypotension, and bradypnea.

Hypoxemia

- Confusion ranges from mild disorientation to delirium.
- In advanced stages of chronic pulmonary disorders, persistent confusion, severe dyspnea, disability, cor pulmonale, and severe respiratory failure occur.

Infection

- Severe generalized infection commonly produces delirium.
- Central nervous system (CNS) infections cause varying degrees of confusion, headache, and nuchal rigidity.

Metabolic encephalopathy

- Hyperglycemia and hypoglycemia can produce sudden confusion.
- Uremic and hepatic encephalopathies produce gradual confusion that may progress to seizures and coma.

Nutritional deficiencies

- Inadequate intake of thiamine, niacin, or vitamin B_{12} produces insidious, progressive confusion.
- Other CNS abnormalities may induce hallucinations and paranoia.

Seizure disorder

○ Mild to moderate confusion may immediately follow a seizure, disappearing within several hours.
○ The patient may have difficulty talking and may fall into a deep sleep after the seizures.

Thyroid hormone disorders

○ Hyperthyroidism produces mild to moderate confusion along with nervousness, inability to concentrate, weight loss, flushed skin, and tachycardia.
○ Hypothyroidism produces mild, insidious confusion and memory loss; weight gain; bradycardia; and fatigue.

Other causes

Alcohol

○ Intoxication causes confusion and stupor.
○ Alcohol withdrawal may cause delirium and seizures.

Drugs

○ Large doses of CNS depressants produce confusion.
○ Opioid and barbiturate withdrawal can cause confusion, possibly with delirium.
○ Other drugs that commonly cause confusion include lidocaine, digoxin, indomethacin, atropine, chloroquine, cimetidine, and cycloserine.

Nursing considerations

○ Keep the patient safe from injury, such as falls and getting lost.
○ Keep the patient calm and quiet.
○ Plan uninterrupted rest periods for the patient.
○ Correct the underlying cause of confusion.

Pediatric pointers

○ Confusion can't be determined in infants and very young children.
○ Older children with acute febrile illnesses commonly experience transient delirium or acute confusion.

Geriatric pointers

○ Elderly patients will typically become more confused and disoriented at the end of the day.

Patient teaching

○ Teach the patient how to orient himself.

Conjunctival injection

Overview

- Nonuniform redness of the conjunctiva
- May be diffuse, localized, or peripheral or may encircle a clear cornea
- A common ocular sign associated with inflammation

⭐ Emergency actions

To treat a chemical splash, first remove contact lenses. Then quickly irrigate the eye with normal saline solution. Evert the lids and wipe the fornices with a cotton-tipped applicator to remove foreign-body particles and as much of the chemical as possible.

Assessment

History

- Determine the onset, location, and duration of eye pain.
- Determine whether other signs or symptoms are present.
- Ask about a history of eye disease or trauma.

Physical assessment

- If the eyelids can be opened without applying pressure, test visual acuity and intraocular pressure (IOP).
- Determine location and severity of injection.
- Note any discharge, edema, ocular deviation, conjunctival follicles, ptosis, or exophthalmos.
- Test pupillary reaction to light.

Medical causes

Blepharitis

- Diffuse conjunctival injection occurs, and ulcerations that burn and itch appear on the eyelids.
- The patient may report a sensation of a foreign body in the eye.
- Rubbing of the eyes may lead to reddened rims or continuous blinking.

Chemical burns

- Diffuse conjunctival injection occurs, with severe pain being the most prominent symptom.
- Other findings include photophobia, blepharospasm, and decreased visual acuity in the affected eye; the cornea may appear gray; and differently sized pupils.

Conjunctival foreign bodies and abrasions

- Localized conjunctival injection occurs.
- Eye pain is sudden and severe.
- Increased tearing and photophobia may be present, but visual acuity usually isn't affected.

Conjunctivitis

- With allergic conjunctivitis, a milky, diffuse, peripheral conjunctival injection occurs.
- With bacterial conjunctivitis, diffuse peripheral conjunctival injection occurs along with a thick, purulent eye discharge that contains mucus threads.
- With fungal conjunctivitis, diffuse peripheral conjunctival injection occurs with photophobia and increased tearing, itching, and burning.
- With viral conjunctivitis, the conjunctival injection is brilliant red, diffuse, and peripheral.

Corneal abrasion

- Diffuse conjunctival injection is extremely painful, especially when the eyelids move over the abrasion.
- Other signs and symptoms include photophobia, excessive tearing, blurred vision, and a sensation of a foreign body in the eye.

Corneal erosion

- Diffuse conjunctival injection, severe, continuous pain, and photophobia develop.
- Reduced vision may occur.

Corneal ulcer

- Diffuse conjunctival injection increases around the cornea.
- Other signs and symptoms include severe photophobia, severe pain in and around the eye, markedly decreased visual acuity, and copious and purulent eye discharge and crusting.
- Corneal opacities and an abnormal pupillary response to light are associated with iritis.

Dacryoadenitis

- Diffuse conjunctival injection occurs with constant tearing.
- Pain over the temporal part of the eye; considerable lid swelling; and purulent eye discharge may be present.

Episcleritis

- Conjunctival injection is localized and raised and may be violet or purplish pink.
- Other signs and symptoms include deep pain, photophobia, increased tearing, and conjunctival edema.

Glaucoma

- Conjunctival injection is typically circumcorneal with acute angle-closure glaucoma.
- Accompanying signs and symptoms include severe eye pain, nausea, vomiting, severely elevated IOP,

blurred vision, and the perception of rainbow-colored halos around lights.
○ Corneas appear steamy because of corneal edema.
○ The pupil of the affected eye is moderately dilated and completely unresponsive to light.

Hyphema

○ Diffuse conjunctival injection occurs, possibly with lid and orbital edema.
○ Pain may be present in and around the eye.

Iritis

○ Marked conjunctival injection is found mainly around the cornea.
○ Other signs and symptoms include moderate to severe pain, photophobia, blurred vision, constricted pupils, and poor pupillary response to light.

Keratoconjunctivitis sicca

○ Severe diffuse conjunctival injection occurs.
○ Associated signs and symptoms include generalized eye pain along with burning, itching, a foreign-body sensation, excessive mucus secretion from the eye, absence of tears, and photophobia.

Lyme disease

○ Conjunctival injection occurs with diffuse urticaria, malaise, fatigue, headache, fever, chills, aches, and lymphadenopathy.
○ Other ocular signs and symptoms include pain, photophobia, conjunctivitis, and blurry or double vision.

Ocular lacerations and intraocular foreign bodies

○ Diffuse conjunctival injection may be increased in the area of injury.
○ Impaired visual acuity and moderate to severe pain vary with the type and extent of the injury.
○ Other findings include lid edema, photophobia, excessive tearing, and abnormal pupillary response.

Ocular tumors

○ If tumor is located in the orbit behind the globe, conjunctival injection may occur with exophthalmos.
○ Conjunctival edema, ocular deviation, and diplopia may occur with muscle involvement.

Uveitis

○ Diffuse conjunctival injection may be increased in the circumcorneal area.
○ Other findings include constricted, irregularly shaped pupils; blurred vision; tenderness; photophobia; and sudden, severe ocular pain.

Nursing considerations

○ Obtain cultures of any eye discharge; record its appearance, consistency, and amount.
○ If the patient has photophobia, darken his room.

Pediatric pointers

○ An infant can develop self-limited chemical conjunctivitis at birth from receiving silver nitrate eye drops.
○ An infant may develop bacterial conjunctivitis 2 to 5 days after birth caused by contamination from the birth canal.
○ An infant with congenital syphilis has prominent conjunctival injection and grayish pink corneas.

Patient teaching

○ Teach the patient techniques for reducing photophobia.
○ If visual acuity is impaired, help the patient to orient himself to his surroundings.
○ Instruct the patient in ways to avoid spreading infection.

Constipation

Overview

- Refers to small, infrequent, or difficult bowel movements
- Can lead to headache, anorexia, and abdominal discomfort
- Usually occurs when the urge to defecate is suppressed and the muscles associated with bowel movements remain contracted

Assessment

History

- Ask about frequency, size, and consistency of bowel movements.
- Determine the onset and location of associated pain.
- Find out about any changes in diet, eating habits, drug or alcohol use, or physical activity.
- Determine dietary fiber and fluid intake.
- Ask about recent emotional distress.
- Obtain a history of GI, rectoanal, neurologic, or metabolic disorders; abdominal surgery; or radiation therapy.
- Ask about the use of drugs, including over-the-counter preparations, such as laxatives, mineral oil, stool softeners, and enemas.

Physical assessment

- Inspect the abdomen for distention or scars from previous surgery.
- Auscultate for bowel sounds and characterize their motility.
- Percuss all four abdominal quadrants.
- Gently palpate for abdominal tenderness, a palpable mass, and hepatomegaly.
- Examine the rectum; inspect for inflammation, lesions, scars, fissures, and external hemorrhoids.
- Palpate the anal sphincter for laxity or stricture.
- Palpate for rectal masses and fecal impaction.
- Obtain a stool specimen and test it for occult blood.

Medical causes

Anal fissure

- Acute constipation usually develops from the fear of the severe tearing or burning pain associated with bowel movements.
- A few drops of blood may be reported on toilet tissue or underwear.

Anorectal abscess

- Constipation occurs with severe, throbbing, localized pain and tenderness at the abscess site.

- Localized inflammation, swelling, purulent drainage, fever, and malaise may also be present.

Diverticulitis

- Constipation or diarrhea occurs with left-lower-quadrant pain and tenderness.
- A tender, fixed, firm abdominal mass may be palpable.
- Mild nausea, flatulence, and a low-grade fever may develop.

Hemorrhoids

- Constipation occurs as the patient tries to avoid the severe pain of defecation.
- Bleeding may occur during defecation.

Hepatic porphyria

- Abdominal pain, which may be severe, colicky, localized, or generalized, precedes constipation.
- Other signs and symptoms include fever, sinus tachycardia, labile hypertension, excessive diaphoresis, severe vomiting, photophobia, urine retention, nervousness or restlessness, disorientation, absent or diminished deep tendon reflexes, and visual hallucinations.
- Areas exposed to light may develop skin lesions with itching, burning, erythema, altered pigmentation, and edema.
- If the disease is severe, delirium, coma, seizures, paraplegia, or complete flaccid paralysis may occur.

Hypercalcemia

- Usually occurs with anorexia, nausea, vomiting, polyuria, and polydipsia
- May occur with arrhythmias, bone pain, muscle weakness and atrophy, hypoactive deep tendon reflexes, and personality changes

Hypothyroidism

- Constipation occurs early and insidiously.
- Other signs and symptoms include fatigue, sensitivity to cold, anorexia with weight gain, menorrhagia, decreased memory, hearing impairment, muscle cramps, and paresthesia.

Intestinal obstruction

- With partial obstruction, constipation may alternate with leakage of liquid stools.
- With complete obstruction, obstipation may occur.
- Other signs and symptoms include episodes of colicky abdominal pain, abdominal distention, nausea, and vomiting.
- Hyperactive bowel sounds, visible peristaltic waves, a palpable abdominal mass, and abdominal tenderness may also develop.

Irritable bowel syndrome

- Chronic constipation occurs.

- Some patients report alternating constipation and diarrhea, an intense urge to defecate, and feelings of incomplete evacuation.
- Nausea and abdominal distention and tenderness may be triggered by stress; defecation usually produces relief.
- Stools are hard and dry and contain visible mucus.

Mesenteric artery ischemia
- Constipation is sudden.
- The patient can't expel stools or flatus.
- Initially, the abdomen is soft and nontender, but soon severe abdominal pain, tenderness, vomiting, and anorexia occur.
- Later, abdominal guarding, rigidity, and distention; tachycardia; syncope; fever; and signs of shock may be produced.
- A bruit may be heard.

Multiple sclerosis
- Constipation occurs with ocular disturbances, vertigo, and sensory disturbances.
- Other findings include motor weakness, seizures, paralysis, muscle spasticity, gait ataxia, intention tremor, hyperreflexia, dysarthria, and dysphagia.
- Urinary urgency, frequency, and incontinence as well as emotional instability may occur.

Spinal cord lesion
- Constipation may occur in addition to urine retention, sexual dysfunction, and pain.
- Motor weakness, paralysis, or sensory impairment below the level of the lesion may also occur.

Ulcerative colitis
- Constipation may occur in patients with chronic ulcerative colitis.
- Bloody diarrhea with pus, mucus, or both is the hallmark sign.
- Other signs and symptoms include hyperactive bowel sounds, cramping lower abdominal pain, tenesmus, anorexia, low-grade fever, nausea, and vomiting.
- Weight loss, weakness, and arthralgia are late findings.

Other causes

Diagnostic tests
- Retention of barium during certain GI studies can cause constipation.

Drugs
- Constipation may occur with the use of antacids containing aluminum or calcium, anticholinergics, drugs with anticholinergic effects, calcium channel blockers, opioid analgesics, and vinca alkaloids.
- Overusing laxatives or enemas can lead to constipation.

Surgery and radiation therapy
- Rectoanal surgery can traumatize nerves, resulting in constipation.
- Abdominal irradiation can cause intestinal stricture and constipation.

Nursing considerations
- If the patient has instructions for bed rest, reposition him frequently.
- Help the patient perform active or passive exercises.

Pediatric pointers
- In infants, causes include inadequate fluid intake, anal fissures, Hirschsprung's disease, and casein and calcium in cow's milk.
- In older children, causes include inadequate fiber intake, excessive intake of milk, bowel spasm, mechanical obstruction, hypothyroidism, reluctance to stop playing for bathroom breaks, and the lack of privacy in some school bathrooms.

Geriatric pointers
- Acute constipation is associated with structural abnormalities.
- Chronic constipation is chiefly caused by lifelong bowel and dietary habits and laxative use.

Patient teaching
- Encourage avoidance of straining, laxatives, and enemas.
- Explain the role of diet and fluid intake.
- Encourage the patient to exercise.
- Train him in relaxation techniques.
- Discuss and encourage abdominal toning exercises.

Costovertebral angle tenderness

Overview

- Indicates sudden distention of the renal capsule
- Accompanies unelicited, dull, constant flank pain in the costovertebral angle (CVA), just to the side of the spine and the 12th rib
- Elicited by percussing the CVA (see *Eliciting costovertebral angle tenderness*)
- Travels forward, below the ribs toward the umbilicus

Assessment

History

- Find out about other signs and symptoms of renal or urologic dysfunction.
- Ask about voiding habits and the onset and description of any recent changes.
- Obtain a personal or family history of urinary tract infections, congenital anomalies, calculi, other obstructive nephropathies or uropathies, or renovascular disorders.

Physical assessment

- Take vital signs.
- If the patient has hypertension and bradycardia, look for other autonomic effects of renal pain.
- Inspect, auscultate, and gently palpate the abdomen for clues to the underlying cause of CVA tenderness.
- Look for abdominal distention, hypoactive bowel sounds, and palpable masses.

Medical causes

Calculi

- CVA tenderness occurs with waves of waxing and waning flank pain that may radiate to the groin, testicles, suprapubic area, or labia.
- Nausea, vomiting, severe abdominal pain, abdominal distention, and decreased bowel sounds may also occur.

Perirenal abscess

- Exquisite CVA tenderness occurs.
- Severe flank pain, dysuria, persistent high fever, chills, erythema of the skin, and a palpable abdominal mass may be present.
- Flank pain may radiate to the groin or down the leg.

Pyelonephritis (acute)

- CVA tenderness occurs with persistent high fever, chills, flank pain, anorexia, nausea and vomiting, weakness, dysuria, hematuria, nocturia, urinary urgency and frequency, and tenesmus.

Renal artery occlusion

- The patient experiences flank pain and CVA tenderness.
- Other findings include severe, continuous upper abdominal pain; nausea; vomiting; hematuria; decreased bowel sounds; and high fever.

Nursing considerations

- Give drugs for pain.
- Monitor vital signs and fluid intake and urine output.
- Collect blood samples and urine specimens.

Assessment tip
Eliciting costovertebral angle tenderness

To elicit costovertebral angle (CVA) tenderness, have the patient sit upright facing away from you or have him lie in a prone position. Place the palm of your left hand over the left CVA, then strike the back of your left hand with the ulnar surface of your right fist (as shown below). Repeat this percussion technique over the right CVA. A patient with CVA tenderness will experience intense pain.

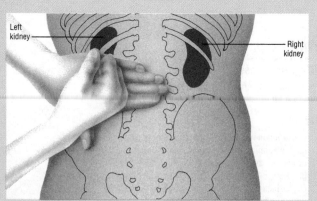

Left kidney

Right kidney

Pediatric pointers

○ An infant won't exhibit CVA tenderness; instead he'll display nonspecific signs and symptoms.

○ In older children, CVA tenderness has the same significance as in adults.

Geriatric pointers

○ Advanced age and cognitive impairment reduce an elderly patient's ability to perceive pain.

Patient teaching

○ Explain any dietary restrictions the patient needs.

○ Tell the patient to drink at least 2 qt (2 L) daily unless he's instructed otherwise.

○ Explain which signs and symptoms of kidney infection he should report.

○ Emphasize the importance of taking the full course of prescribed antibiotics.

Cough, barking

Overview

○ Resonant, brassy, and harsh cough
○ Part of a complex of signs and symptoms that characterize croup syndrome
○ Indicates edema of the larynx and surrounding tissue
○ Can lead to airway occlusion, a life-threatening emergency (see *Managing a barking cough*)

Assessment

History

○ Ask about the onset of cough and other associated signs and symptoms.
○ Find out about aggravating and alleviating factors.
○ Determine whether the child has a history of previous episodes of croup syndrome.

Physical assessment

○ Observe the child for signs of respiratory distress.
○ Note use of sternal or intercostal retractions or nasal flaring.
○ Observe skin for cyanosis and diaphoresis.
○ Take vital signs, noting respiratory rate and depth.
○ Auscultate the lungs.

Emergency actions
Managing a barking cough

If the child experiences edema, quickly evaluate his respiratory status. Then take his vital signs. Be particularly alert for tachycardia and signs of hypoxemia. Also, check for a decreased level of consciousness. Try to determine if the child has been playing with a small object that he may have aspirated.

Check for cyanosis in the lips and nail beds. Observe the patient for sternal or intercostal retractions or nasal flaring. Next, note the depth and rate of his respirations; they may become increasingly shallow as respiratory distress increases. Observe the child's body position. Is he sitting up, leaning forward, struggling to breathe? Observe his activity level and facial expression. As respiratory distress increases from airway edema, the child will become restless and have a frightened, wide-eyed expression. As air hunger continues, the child will become lethargic and difficult to arouse.

If the child shows signs of severe respiratory distress, try to calm him, maintain airway patency, and provide oxygen. Endotracheal intubation or a tracheotomy may be necessary.

Medical causes

Aspiration of foreign body

○ Sudden hoarseness occurs initially with partial obstruction of the upper airway, followed by barking cough and inspiratory stridor.
○ Other effects of this life-threatening condition include gagging, tachycardia, dyspnea, decreased breath sounds, wheezing, and cyanosis.

Epiglottiditis

○ A life-threatening childhood disorder — starts with a barking cough and a high fever at night.
○ The child is hoarse, dysphagic, dyspneic, and restless and appears extremely ill and panicky.
○ Cough may progress to severe respiratory distress with sternal and intercostal retractions, nasal flaring, cyanosis, and tachycardia.

Laryngotracheobronchitis (acute)

○ Fever, runny nose, poor appetite, and infrequent cough occur initially in infants ages 9 to 18 months.
○ When infection descends into the laryngotracheal area, barking cough, hoarseness, and inspiratory stridor occur.
○ As respiratory distress progresses, substernal and intercostal retractions, tachycardia, restlessness, cyanosis, irritability, paleness, and shallow, rapid respirations occur.

Spasmodic croup

○ Onset of a barking cough is abrupt and usually awakens a child from sleep.
○ The child may be hoarse, restless, and dyspneic, but without fever.
○ As the conditions worsens, the child may exhibit sternal and intercostal retractions, nasal flaring, tachycardia, cyanosis, and an anxious, frantic appearance.
○ Attacks subside with a few hours but tend to recur.

Nursing considerations

○ Don't inspect throat of a child with barking cough unless intubation equipment is available.
○ If the child isn't in severe respiratory distress, a neck X-ray may be needed to check for epiglottal edema.
○ A chest X-ray can rule out lower respiratory tract infection.
○ Depending on child's age and degree of respiratory distress, oxygen may be administered.
○ Rapid-acting epinephrine and a steroid may be needed.
○ Observe the child frequently, and if oxygen is used, monitor the level.

○ Maintain a calm, quiet environment and offer reassurance.
○ Encourage the parents to stay with the child.

Pediatric pointers

○ Because a child's airway is smaller in diameter than that of an adult, edema can rapidly lead to airway occlusion, a life-threatening emergency.

Patient teaching

○ Discuss with parents or caregiver methods of relieving subsequent attacks.

Cough, nonproductive

Overview

- The noisy, forceful expulsion of air from the lungs, but one that doesn't yield sputum
- Can cause airway collapse or rupture of alveoli or blebs
- May occur in paroxysms and can worsen by becoming more frequent
- May be acute (self-limiting) or chronic (see *Reviewing the cough mechanism*)

Assessment

History

- Ask about the onset, frequency, and description of cough.
- Ask about aggravating factors.
- Obtain smoking history.
- Find out the onset and location of associated pain.
- Obtain a history of surgery or trauma.
- Inquire about hypersensitivity to drugs, foods, pets, dust, or pollen.
- Find out which drugs the patient is taking.
- Ask about recent changes in appetite, weight, exercise tolerance, or energy level.
- Ask about recent exposure to irritating fumes, chemicals, or smoke.

Physical assessment

- Observe the patient, and note behavior, cyanosis, clubbed fingers, or edema.
- Observe for use of accessory muscles, and note retractions.
- Take the patient's vital signs, checking the depth and rhythm of respirations; note if wheezing occurs with breathing.
- Inspect the neck for distended veins and a deviated trachea.
- Check the skin, noting whether it's cool or warm, dry or clammy.
- Check the mouth and nose for congestion, inflammation, drainage, and signs of infection.
- Examine the chest, looking for abnormal chest wall configuration and motion.
- Auscultate for wheezing, crackles, rhonchi, pleural rubs, and decreased or absent breath sounds.
- Percuss for dullness, tympany, and flatness.

Medical causes

Airway occlusion

- Partial occlusion of the upper airway produces a sudden onset of dry, paroxysmal coughing.
- Other findings include gagging, wheezing, hoarseness, stridor, tachycardia, and decreased breath sounds.
- If choking on a foreign object, the patient may clutch his throat with thumb and fingers extended.

Anthrax (inhalation)

- Initial signs and symptoms include fever, chills, weakness, cough, and chest pain.
- Rapid deterioration marked by fever, dyspnea, stridor, and hypotension, generally leading to death within 24 hours, occurs in the second stage.

Aortic aneurysm (thoracic)

- A brassy cough occurs with dyspnea, hoarseness, wheezing, and a substernal ache in the shoulders, lower back, or abdomen.
- Other findings include facial or neck edema, neck vein distention, dysphagia, prominent veins over the chest, stridor, paresthesia, and neuralgia.

Asthma

- Attacks start with a nonproductive cough and mild wheezing.
- As the attack progresses, severe dyspnea, audible wheezing, chest tightness, and a cough that produces thick mucus develops.
- Other signs and symptoms include apprehension, rhonchi, prolonged expiration, intercostal and supraclavicular retractions on inspiration, accessory muscle use, flaring nostrils, tachypnea, tachycardia, diaphoresis, and flushing or cyanosis.

Atelectasis

- As lung tissue deflates, it stimulates cough receptors, causing a nonproductive cough.
- Other findings include pleuritic chest pain, anxiety, cyanosis, diaphoresis, dullness on percussion, inspiratory lag, substernal or intercostal retractions, decreased vocal fremitus, dyspnea, tachypnea, and tachycardia.
- Trachea may deviate toward the affected side.

Bronchitis (chronic)

- A nonproductive, hacking cough later becomes productive.
- Other findings include prolonged expiration, wheezing, dyspnea, accessory muscle use, barrel chest, cyanosis, tachypnea, crackles, and scattered rhonchi.
- Clubbing may occur in stages.

Bronchogenic carcinoma

○ Chronic, nonproductive cough, dyspnea, and vague chest pain are early indicators.
○ Wheezing, hemoptysis, and stridor may develop.

Common cold

○ Nonproductive, hacking cough progresses to a mix of sneezing, headache, malaise, fatigue, rhinorrhea, myalgia, arthralgia, nasal congestion, and sore throat.

Esophageal achalasia

○ Regurgitation and aspiration produce a dry cough.
○ Recurrent pulmonary infections and dysphagia may develop.
○ Weight loss, heartburn, and chest pain that increases after eating may be reported.

Esophageal diverticula

○ Nocturnal nonproductive cough, regurgitation and aspiration, dyspepsia, and dysphagia are characteristic.
○ Other findings include a swollen neck, a gurgling sound, halitosis, and weight loss.

Esophageal occlusion

○ Immediate nonproductive coughing and gagging accompanies a sensation of something stuck in the throat.
○ Other findings include neck or chest pain, dysphagia, and the inability to swallow.

Esophagitis with reflux

○ Regurgitation and aspiration produce a nonproductive night-time cough.
○ Other signs and symptoms include chest pain that mimics angina pectoris; heartburn that worsens if the patient lies down soon after eating; and increased salivation, dysphagia, hematemesis, and melena.

Hodgkin's disease

○ A crowing nonproductive cough may develop.
○ Painless swelling of cervical lymph nodes or, occasionally, the axillary, mediastinal, or inguinal nodes, is an early sign.
○ Pruritus is also an early sign.
○ Other findings include dyspnea, dysphagia, hepatosplenomegaly, edema, jaundice, nerve pain, and hyperpigmentation.

Hypersensitivity pneumonitis

○ Acute nonproductive cough, fever, dyspnea, and malaise occur 5 to 6 hours after exposure to an antigen.
○ Chest tightness and extreme fatigue may also occur.

Interstitial lung disease

○ Nonproductive cough and progressive dyspnea occur.

Reviewing the cough mechanism

Cough receptors are thought to be located in the nose, sinuses, auditory canals, nasopharynx, larynx, trachea, bronchi, pleurae, diaphragm, and possibly the pericardium and GI tract. When a cough receptor is stimulated, the vagus and glossopharyngeal nerves transmit the impulse to the "cough center" in the medulla. From there, the impulse is transmitted to the larynx and to the intercostal and abdominal muscles. Deep inspiration (1) is followed by closure of the glottis and the vocal cords (2), relaxation of the diaphragm, and contraction of the abdominal and intercostal muscles. The resulting increased pressure in the lungs opens the glottis to release the forceful, noisy expiration known as a cough (3).

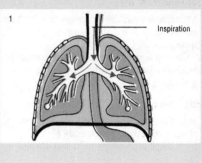

1
Inspiration

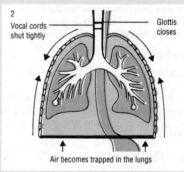

2
Vocal cords shut tightly
Glottis closes
Air becomes trapped in the lungs

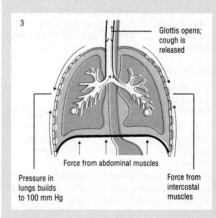

3
Glottis opens; cough is released
Force from abdominal muscles
Pressure in lungs builds to 100 mm Hg
Force from intercostal muscles

- Associated findings include cyanosis, clubbing, fine crackles, fatigue, chest pain, weight loss, and dyspnea on exertion.

Laryngeal tumor

- Mild, nonproductive cough; minor throat discomfort; and hoarseness are early signs.
- Dysphagia, dyspnea, cervical lymphadenopathy, stridor, and earache occur later.

Laryngitis

- In acute cases, a nonproductive cough occurs with localized pain, hoarseness, fever, and malaise.

Legionnaires' disease

- A nonproductive cough progresses to a cough that may produce mucoid, mucopurulent and bloody sputum.
- Prodromal signs and symptoms include malaise, headache, diarrhea, anorexia, diffuse myalgia, and generalized weakness.

Lung abscess

- Nonproductive coughing, weakness, dyspnea, and pleuritic chest pain occur initially.
- Later, cough produces purulent, foul-smelling sputum.
- Other signs and symptoms include diaphoresis, fever, headache, malaise, fatigue, crackles, decreased breath sounds, anorexia, and weight loss.

Mediastinal tumor

- Nonproductive cough, dyspnea, and retrosternal pain occur.
- Stertorous respirations with suprasternal retraction on inspiration, hoarseness, dysphagia, tracheal shift or tug, jugular vein distention, and facial or neck edema may develop.

Pleural effusion

- Nonproductive cough, dyspnea, pleuritic chest pain, and decreased chest motion are characteristic.
- Other findings include pleural rub, tachycardia, tachypnea, egophony, flatness on percussion, decreased or absent breath sounds, and decreased tactile fremitus.

Pneumonia

- Bacterial pneumonia causes nonproductive, hacking, painful cough that becomes productive.
- Other findings include shaking chills, headache, high fever, dyspnea, pleuritic chest pain, tachypnea, tachycardia, grunting respirations, nasal flaring, decreased breath sounds, fine crackles, rhonchi, and cyanosis.
- With mycoplasmal pneumonia, a nonproductive cough that may be paroxysmal arises 2 to 3 days after onset of malaise, headache, and sore throat.

- Viral pneumonia causes a nonproductive, hacking cough and gradual onset of malaise, headache, and low-grade fever.

Pneumothorax

- A life-threatening disorder — the patient exhibits dry cough and signs of respiratory distress.
- Other signs and symptoms include sudden, sharp chest pain that worsens with chest movement; subcutaneous crepitation; hyperresonance or tympany; decreased vocal fremitus; and decreased or absent breath sounds on the affected side.

Pulmonary edema

- Dry cough, exertional dyspnea, paroxysmal nocturnal dyspnea, orthopnea, tachycardia, tachypnea, dependent crackles, and ventricular gallop occur initially.
- Respirations become more rapid and labored, with diffuse crackles and coughing that produces frothy, bloody sputum as the condition worsens.

Pulmonary embolism

- A life-threatening disorder — dry cough, dyspnea, and pleuritic or anginal chest pain may occur suddenly.
- More commonly, the cough produces blood-tinged sputum.
- Tachycardia, low-grade fever, pleural rub, diffuse wheezing, dullness on percussion, and decreased breath sounds may also occur.

Sarcoidosis

- A nonproductive cough is accompanied by dyspnea, substernal pain, and malaise.
- Other signs and symptoms include fatigue, arthralgia, myalgia, weight loss, tachypnea, crackles, lymphadenopathy, hepatosplenomegaly, skin lesions, vision impairment, difficulty swallowing, and arrhythmias.

Severe acute respiratory syndrome

- A life-threatening disorder — severe acute respiratory syndrome begins with a fever; headache, malaise, dry nonproductive cough, and dyspnea also occur.

Sinusitis (chronic)

- Chronic nonproductive cough may develop from postnasal drip.
- Nasal mucosa may appear inflamed; nasal congestion with profuse drainage and a musty breath odor may occur.

Tracheobronchitis (acute)

- A secretions increase, a dry cough becomes productive.
- Chills, sore throat, slight fever, muscle and back pain, and substernal tightness generally precede the cough's onset.

Tularemia

○ Onset of fever, chills, headache, generalized myalgia, nonproductive cough, dyspnea, pleuritic chest pain, and empyema is abrupt.

Other causes

Diagnostic tests

○ Pulmonary function tests and bronchoscopy may stimulate cough receptors, triggering coughing.

Treatments

○ Suctioning or deep endotracheal or tracheal tube placement can trigger a paroxysmal or hacking cough.
○ Intermittent positive-pressure breathing or spirometry may cause a nonproductive cough.
○ Inhalants such as pentamidine may stimulate coughing.

Nursing considerations

○ A nonproductive, paroxysmal cough may induce life-threatening bronchospasm; the patient may need a bronchodilator.
○ Unless the patient has chronic obstructive pulmonary disease, give an antitussive and a sedative to suppress the cough.
○ Humidify the air in the patient's room.

Pediatric pointers

○ Sudden onset of paroxysmal nonproductive coughing may indicate aspiration of a foreign body.
○ Nonproductive coughing can result from asthma, bacterial pneumonia, acute bronchiolitis, acute otitis media, measles, cystic fibrosis, airway hyperactivity, or a foreign body in the external auditory canal; it may also be psychogenic.

Geriatric pointers

○ Nonproductive cough may indicate serious acute or chronic illness in elderly patients.

Patient teaching

○ Explain how to the use a respirator and humidifier.
○ Teach the patient to avoid respiratory irritants.
○ Explain how to treat productive and nonproductive coughs.
○ Explain the importance of adequate fluids and nutrition.
○ If the patient smokes, stress the importance of smoking cessation, and refer him to appropriate resources, support groups, and information to help him quit smoking.

Cough, productive

Overview

- A sudden, forceful, expulsion of air from the lungs with sputum, blood, or both
- An acute or chronic infection causes inflammation, edema, and increased mucus production
- Note sputum color, consistency, and odor

Emergency actions

If the patient has acute respiratory distress from thick or excessive secretions, bronchospasm, or fatigue, take vital signs and check the rate, depth, and rhythm of respirations. Keep the airway patent, and provide supplemental oxygen if he becomes restless or confused, or if his respirations become shallow, irregular, rapid, or slow. Look for stridor, wheezing, choking, gurgling, nasal flaring, and cyanosis.

Assessment

History

- Ask about the onset of coughing.
- Find out about the amount, color, odor, and consistency of the sputum.
- Note time of day and what aggravates and alleviates coughing and sputum production.
- Ask the patient to describe the sound of the cough.
- Note the location and severity of pain.
- Ask about weight and appetite changes, smoking and alcohol use, asthma, allergies, and respiratory problems.
- Obtain a drug history.
- Review his occupational history.

Physical assessment

- Examine the patient's mouth and nose for congestion, drainage, or inflammation.
- Note breath odor.
- Inspect the neck for distended veins, and palpate for tenderness and masses or enlarged lymph nodes.
- Observe the chest for accessory muscle use, retractions, and uneven chest expansion.
- Percuss the chest for dullness, tympany, or flatness.
- Auscultate for pleural rub and abnormal breath sounds.

Medical causes

Aspiration pneumonitis

- Pink, frothy, possibly purulent sputum
- Severe dyspnea, fever, tachypnea, fatigue, chest pain, halitosis, tachycardia, wheezing, and cyanosis

Asthma (acute)

- A life-threatening disorder — mucoid sputum and mucus plugs when dry cough becomes productive.
- As the attack progresses, severe dyspnea, audible wheezing, and chest tightness occur.
- Other signs and symptoms include apprehension, prolonged expirations, intercostal and supraclavicular retraction on inspiration, accessory muscle use, rhonchi, crackles, flaring nostrils, tachypnea, tachycardia, diaphoresis, and flushing or cyanosis.

Bronchiectasis

- Copious, mucopurulent, layered sputum (top: frothy; middle: clear; bottom: dense; purulent particles).
- Foul- or sickeningly sweet-smelling sputum
- Hemoptysis, persistent coarse crackles, wheezing, rhonchi, exertional dyspnea, weight loss, fatigue, malaise, weakness, fever, and late-stage clubbing.

Bronchitis (chronic)

- Cough is nonproductive initially.
- Mucoid sputum becomes purulent
- Coughing usually occurs when the patient is recumbent or rises from sleep.
- Other findings include prolonged expiration, use of accessory muscles, barrel chest, tachypnea, cyanosis, wheezing, exertional dyspnea, scattered rhonchi, coarse crackles, and late-stage clubbing.

Chemical pneumonitis

- Purulent sputum
- Dyspnea, wheezing, orthopnea, malaise, and crackles; mucus irritation of the conjunctivae, throat, and nose; laryngitis; and rhinitis

Common cold

- Mucoid or mucopurulent sputum
- Early: dry, hacking cough; sneezing; headache; malaise; fatigue; rhinorrhea; nasal congestion; sore throat; and myalgia

Legionnaires' disease

- Scant mucoid, nonpurulent, blood-streaked sputum
- Early: malaise, fatigue, weakness, anorexia, myalgia, and diarrhea
- Within 48 hours, turns to dry cough with a sudden high fever and chills
- Pleuritic pain, headache, tachypnea, tachycardia, nausea, vomiting, dyspnea, crackles, and confusion

Lung abscess (ruptured)

- Purulent, foul-smelling, blood-tinged sputum
- Diaphoresis, anorexia, clubbing, weight loss, weakness, fatigue, fever, chills, dyspnea, headache, malaise, pleuritic chest pain, and inspiratory crackles

Lung cancer

- Early: chronic cough that produces small amounts of purulent (or mucopurulent), blood-streaked sputum

- With bronchoalveolar cancer, large amounts of frothy sputum
- Dyspnea, anorexia, fatigue, weight loss, chest pain, fever, diaphoresis, wheezing, and clubbing

Plague

- Pulmonary signs and symptoms include productive cough, chest pain, tachypnea, dyspnea, hemoptysis, and increasing respiratory distress.
- Other findings include fever, chills, and swollen, inflamed, and tender lymph nodes.

Pneumonia

- Dry cough becomes productive.
- Other findings develop suddenly and include shaking chills, high fever, myalgia, pleuritic chest pain, tachycardia, tachypnea, dyspnea, cyanosis, diaphoresis, decreased breath sounds, crackles, and rhonchi.

Pulmonary edema

- A life-threatening disorder — early signs include exertional dyspnea; paroxysmal nocturnal dyspnea, followed by orthopnea; and nonproductive coughing that eventually produces frothy, bloody sputum.
- Other findings include fever, fatigue, tachycardia, tachypnea, crackles, and ventricular gallop.

Pulmonary embolism

- Cough may be nonproductive or may produce blood-tinged sputum.
- Usually, the first sign of this life-threatening disorder is severe dyspnea with angina or pleuritic chest pain.
- Severe anxiety, low-grade fever, tachycardia, tachypnea, and diaphoresis develop.
- Other findings include pleural rub, wheezing, crackles, chest dullness on percussion, decreased breath sounds, and signs of circulatory collapse.

Pulmonary emphysema

- Chronic cough produces scant, mucoid, translucent, grayish white sputum, which can become mucopurulent.
- Other findings include thin appearance, weight loss, accessory muscle use, tachypnea, grunting expirations through pursed lips, diminished breath sounds, exertional dyspnea, rhonchi, barrel chest, anorexia, and late clubbing.

Pulmonary tuberculosis

- Mild to severe productive cough with scant and mucoid or copious and purulent sputum
- Hemoptysis, malaise, dyspnea, pleuritic chest pain, night sweats, fatigue, and weight loss

Silicosis

- A productive cough with mucopurulent sputum is the earliest sign.
- Exertional dyspnea, tachypnea, weight loss, fatigue, weakness, recurrent respiratory infections, and end-inspiratory crackles develop.

Tracheobronchitis

- After the onset of chills, sore throat, fever, muscle and back pain, and substernal tightness, cough becomes productive.
- Sputum is mucoid, mucopurulent, or purulent.
- Other findings include rhonchi, wheezes, crackles, fever, and bronchospasm.

Other causes

Diagnostic tests

- Bronchoscopy and pulmonary function tests

Drugs

- Expectorants increase productive coughing.

Respiratory therapy

- Incentive spirometry, intermittent positive-pressure breathing, and nebulizer therapy

Nursing considerations

- Give a mucolytic and an expectorant to increase productive coughing.
- Increase the patient's fluid intake to thin secretions.
- Give a bronchodilator to relieve bronchospasm and open airways.
- If an infection is present, give antibiotics.
- Humidify the air to relieve mucous membrane irritation and loosen secretions.
- Provide pulmonary physiotherapy to loosen secretions.
- Provide rest periods.
- Collect sputum specimens for culture and sensitivity testing.

Pediatric pointers

- A child with a productive cough can quickly develop airway occlusion and respiratory distress.
- Causes of a productive cough in children include asthma, bronchiectasis, bronchitis, acute bronchiolitis, cystic fibrosis, and pertussis.
- High humidity can induce bronchospasm in a hyperactive child or overhydration in an infant.

Geriatric pointers

- May mean serious acute or chronic illness

Patient teaching

- Refer patient to resources to quit smoking.
- Teach him coughing and deep-breathing techniques.
- Teach the patient and caregiver to use chest percussion to loosen secretions.
- Explain infection control techniques.
- Explain how he can avoid respiratory irritants.

Crackles

Overview

- Also known as *rales* or *crepitations*
- The nonmusical clicking or rattling noises heard during auscultation of breath sounds
- Can be on one or both sides, moist- or dry-sounding.
- Usually occur during inspiration and recur constantly from one respiratory cycle to the next
- Indicate abnormal movement of air through fluid-filled airways

Emergency actions

Take vital signs, and examine the patient for signs of respiratory distress or airway obstruction. Check the depth and rhythm of respirations. Check for increased accessory muscle use and chest-wall motion, retractions, stridor, or nasal flaring. Provide supplemental oxygen. An endotracheal intubation may be necessary.

Assessment

History

- Ask about the onset, duration, and description of cough and pain.
- Note the sputum's consistency, amount, odor, and color.
- Obtain a medical history, including cancer, respiratory or cardiovascular problems, surgery, or trauma.
- Find out about smoking and alcohol use.
- Obtain a drug and occupational history.
- Inquire about recent weight loss, anorexia, nausea, vomiting, fatigue, weakness, vertigo, hoarseness, difficulty swallowing, and syncope.
- Determine exposure to respiratory irritants.

Physical assessment

- Examine the nose and mouth for signs of infection.
- Note breath odor.
- Check the neck for masses, tenderness, lymphadenopathy, swelling, or venous distention.
- Inspect the chest for abnormal configuration or uneven expansion.
- Percuss the chest for dullness, tympany, or flatness.
- Auscultate the lungs for other abnormal, diminished, or absent breath sounds.
- Listen for abnormal heart sounds.
- Check the hands and feet for edema or clubbing.

Medical causes

Acute respiratory distress syndrome

- A life-threatening disorder — diffuse, fine to coarse crackles are usually heard in the dependent portions of the lungs.
- Other findings include cyanosis, nasal flaring, tachypnea, tachycardia, grunting respirations, rhonchi, dyspnea, anxiety, and decreased level of consciousness.

Asthma (acute)

- Dry, whistling crackles occur.
- Dry cough and mild wheezing progress to severe dyspnea, audible wheezing, chest tightness, and productive cough.
- Other findings include apprehension, prolonged expirations, rhonchi, intercostal and supraclavicular retractions, accessory muscle use, flaring nostrils, tachypnea, tachycardia, diaphoresis, and flushing or cyanosis.

Bronchiectasis

- Persistent, coarse crackles are heard over the affected area of the lung.
- Chronic cough that produces copious amounts of mucopurulent sputum accompanies crackles.
- Other characteristics include halitosis, wheezing, exertional dyspnea, rhonchi, weight loss, fatigue, malaise, weakness, recurrent fever, and late clubbing.

Bronchitis (chronic)

- Coarse crackles are usually heard at the lung base.
- Prolonged expirations, wheezing, rhonchi, exertional dyspnea, tachypnea, cyanosis, clubbing, and persistent, productive cough also occur.

Chemical pneumonitis

- Diffuse, fine to coarse, moist crackles can be heard.
- Other findings include a productive cough with purulent sputum, dyspnea, wheezing, orthopnea, fever, malaise, and mucous membrane irritation.

Interstitial fibrosis of the lungs

- Cellophane-like crackles can be heard over all lobes.
- Nonproductive cough, dyspnea, fatigue, weight loss, cyanosis, pleuritic chest pain, nasal flaring, and cyanosis occur as the disease progresses.

Legionnaires' disease

- Diffuse moist crackles can be heard.
- Cough produces scant mucoid, nonpurulent, possibly blood-streaked sputum.
- Early signs and symptoms include malaise, fatigue, weakness, anorexia, myalgia, and diarrhea.
- Dry cough and sudden high fever with chills develop within 24 hours of onset.

○ Other signs and symptoms include pleuritic chest pain, headache, tachypnea, tachycardia, nausea, vomiting, dyspnea, confusion, flushing, diaphoresis, and prostration.

Lung abscess

○ Fine to medium and moist inspiratory crackles occur.
○ Other findings include sweats, anorexia, weight loss, fever, fatigue, weakness, dyspnea, clubbing, pleuritic chest pain, pleural rub, and a cough that produces large amounts of foul-smelling, purulent, bloody sputum.

Pneumonia

○ Bacterial pneumonia produces diffuse fine crackles.
○ Other findings include sudden onset of shaking chills, high fever, tachypnea, pleuritic chest pain, cyanosis, grunting respirations, nasal flaring, decreased breath sounds, myalgia, headache, tachycardia, dyspnea, diaphoresis, rhonchi, and a dry cough that becomes productive.
○ Mycoplasmal pneumonia produces medium to fine crackles.
○ Viral pneumonia causes gradually developing, diffuse crackles.

Pulmonary edema

○ A life-threatening disorder—moist, bubbling crackles on inspiration are one of the first signs.
○ Other findings include exertional dyspnea; paroxysmal nocturnal dyspnea, then orthopnea; tachycardia; tachypnea; ventricular gallop; and coughing that's initially nonproductive but later produces frothy, bloody sputum.

Pulmonary embolism

○ Fine to coarse crackles occur in this life-threatening disorder.
○ Severe dyspnea is usually the first sign and may be accompanied by angina or pleuritic chest pain.
○ Cough may be nonproductive or produce blood-tinged sputum.
○ Acute anxiety, low-grade fever, tachycardia, tachypnea, and diaphoresis develop.
○ Other findings include pleural rub, wheezing, chest dullness on percussion, decreased breath sounds, and signs of circulatory collapse.

Pulmonary tuberculosis

○ Fine crackles occur after coughing.
○ Sputum may be scant and mucoid or copious and purulent.
○ Other signs and symptoms include hemoptysis, malaise, dyspnea, pleuritic chest pain, fatigue, night sweats, weakness, weight loss, and amphoric breath sounds.

Sarcoidosis

○ The patient has fine, basilar, end-inspiratory crackles.

○ Other signs and symptoms include malaise, fatigue, weakness, weight loss, cough, dyspnea, and tachypnea.

Silicosis

○ End-inspiratory, fine crackles are heard at the lung bases.
○ Productive cough with mucopurulent sputum is the earliest sign.
○ Other signs and symptoms include exertional dyspnea, tachypnea, weight loss, fatigue, weakness, and recurrent respiratory infections.

Tracheobronchitis

○ Moist or coarse crackles occur.
○ Other signs and symptoms include productive cough, chills, sore throat, slight fever, muscle and back pain, substernal tightness, rhonchi, and wheezes.
○ With severe disease, moderate fever and bronchospasm occur.

Nursing considerations

○ Elevate the head of the bed to ease the patient's breathing.
○ Administer fluids and humidified air to liquefy secretions and relieve mucous membrane inflammation
○ Administer oxygen.
○ If crackles result from cardiogenic pulmonary edema, give a diuretic.
○ Turn the patient every 1 to 2 hours, and encourage deep breathing.
○ Plan daily rest periods for him.

Pediatric pointers

○ Pneumonias produce diffuse, sudden crackles.
○ Esophageal atresia and tracheoesophageal fistula can cause bubbling, moist crackles.
○ Pulmonary edema causes fine crackles.
○ Bronchiectasis produces moist crackles.
○ Cystic fibrosis produces widespread, fine to coarse inspiratory crackles in infants.
○ Sickle cell anemia may produce crackles with pulmonary infection or infarction.

Geriatric pointers

○ Crackles that clear after deep breathing may indicate mild basilar atelectasis.
○ Auscultate lung bases before and after auscultating apices.

Patient teaching

○ Teach the patient effective coughing techniques.
○ Teach him to avoiding respiratory irritants.
○ Stress the importance of quitting smoking, and refer him to appropriate resources to help him quit smoking.

Crepitation, subcutaneous

Overview

○ Results from trapping of air or gas bubbles in the subcutaneous tissue
○ A crackling sound on palpation
○ Bubbles that feel like small, unstable nodules
○ Edema in affected area
○ If edema affects the neck or upper chest, life-threatening airway occlusion

⚡ Emergency actions

For signs of respiratory distress, quickly test for Hamman's sign. (See Testing for Hamman's sign.*) Endotracheal intubation, an emergency tracheotomy, or chest tube insertion will be needed. Provide supplemental oxygen, and start an I.V. line to administer fluids and medications. Connect the patient to a cardiac monitor.*

Assessment

History

○ Ask if the patient is having difficulty breathing.

Assessment tip
Testing for Hamman's sign

To test for Hamman's sign, help the patient assume a left-lateral recumbent position. Then place your stethoscope over the precordium. If you hear a loud crunching sound that synchronizes with his heartbeat, the patient has a positive Hamman's sign.

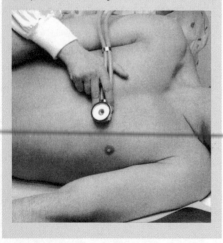

○ Ask about the onset, location, and severity of any associated pain.
○ Obtain a medical and surgical history, including recent thoracic surgery, diagnostic tests, and respiratory therapy as well as trauma or chronic pulmonary disease.

Physical assessment

○ Palpate the affected skin to evaluate the location and text of crepitus.
○ Palpate frequently to determine if the subcutaneous crepitation is increasing.
○ Perform abbreviated cardiac, pulmonary, and GI assessments as the patient's condition allows.
○ When the patient is stabilized, perform a complete physical examination.

Medical causes

Orbital fracture

○ Subcutaneous crepitation of the eyelid and orbit develops.
○ Periorbital ecchymosis is the most common sign.
○ Other findings include facial and eyelid edema, diplopia, a hyphema, impaired extraocular movements, and a dilated or unreactive pupil on the affected side.

Pneumothorax

○ Subcutaneous crepitation occurs in the upper chest and neck in severe cases.
○ One-sided chest pain increases on inspiration.
○ Other findings include dyspnea, anxiety, restlessness, tachypnea, cyanosis, tachycardia, accessory muscle use, asymmetrical chest expansion, decreased or absent breath sounds on the affected side, and a nonproductive cough.

Rupture of the esophagus

○ Subcutaneous crepitation may be palpable in the neck, chest wall, or supraclavicular fossa, but it doesn't always occur.
○ With cervical esophagus rupture, findings include excruciating pain in the neck or supraclavicular area, resistance to passive neck movement, local tenderness, soft-tissue swelling, dysphagia, odynophagia, and orthostatic vertigo.
○ With life-threatening rupture of the intrathoracic esophagus, findings include a positive Hamman's sign; severe retrosternal, epigastric, neck, or scapular pain; edema of the chest wall and neck; dyspnea; tachypnea; asymmetrical chest movement; nasal flaring; cyanosis; diaphoresis; tachycardia; hypotension; dysphagia; and fever.

Rupture of trachea or major bronchus

○ A life-threatening disorder — abrupt subcutaneous crepitation of the neck and anterior chest wall occurs.
○ Other findings include severe dyspnea with nasal flaring, tachycardia, accessory muscle use, hypotension, cyanosis, extreme anxiety, hemoptysis, and mediastinal emphysema with a positive Hamman's sign.

Other causes

Diagnostic tests

○ Endoscopic tests can rupture or perforate respiratory or GI organs, producing subcutaneous crepitation.

Respiratory treatments

○ Intermittent positive-pressure breathing and mechanical ventilation can rupture alveoli, producing subcutaneous crepitation.

Thoracic surgery

○ If air escapes into the tissue in the area of the incision, subcutaneous crepitation can occur.

Nursing considerations

○ Monitor vital signs frequently, especially respirations.
○ Look for signs of respiratory distress and airway obstruction.
○ Tell the patient that the affected tissues will eventually absorb the air or gas bubbles, decreasing subcutaneous crepitation.
○ Provide reassurance to reduce anxiety.

Pediatric pointers

○ Children may develop subcutaneous crepitation in the neck from ingestion of corrosive substances that perforate the esophagus.

Patient teaching

○ Explain diagnostic tests and procedures the patient needs.
○ Explain the signs and symptoms of subcutaneous crepitation to report

Cyanosis

Overview

O Refers to a bluish or bluish black discoloration of the skin and mucous membranes.
O Results from excessive concentration of unoxygenated hemoglobin in the blood.
O Classified as central (inadequate oxygenation of systemic arterial blood) or peripheral (sluggish peripheral circulation).
O Isn't always an accurate gauge of oxygenation.

⚡ Emergency actions

If sudden, localized cyanosis occurs with other signs of arterial occlusion, protect the affected limb from injury, but don't massage it. If central cyanosis stems from a pulmonary disorder or shock, perform a rapid evaluation. Take immediate steps to maintain an airway, assist breathing, and monitor circulation.

Assessment

History

O Obtain a medical history, including cardiac, pulmonary, and hematologic disorders, and previous surgery.
O Evaluate the patient's mental status while obtaining his history.
O Ask about the onset, aggravating and alleviating factors, and characteristics of the cyanosis.
O Ask about other signs and symptoms.

Physical assessment

O Take vital signs, measure oxygen saturation, and evaluate respiratory rate and rhythm.
O Check for nasal flaring and accessory muscle use.
O Inspect the skin, lips, and nail bed color and mucous membranes.
O Inspect for asymmetrical chest expansion or barrel chest.
O Inspect the abdomen for ascites.
O Palpate peripheral pulses, test capillary refill, and note edema.
O Percuss and palpate for liver enlargement and tenderness.
O Percuss the lungs for dullness or hyperresonance.
O Auscultate for decreased or adventitious breath sounds.
O Auscultate heart rate and rhythm.
O Auscultate abdominal aorta and femoral arteries for bruits.

Medical causes

Arteriosclerotic occlusive disease (chronic)

O Peripheral cyanosis occurs in the legs whenever they're in a dependent position.
O Other signs and symptoms include intermittent claudication and burning pain at rest, paresthesia, pallor, muscle atrophy, weak leg pulses, and impotence.
O Leg ulcers and gangrene are late signs.

Bronchiectasis

O Chronic central cyanosis develops.
O The classic sign is chronic productive cough with copious, foul-smelling, mucopurulent sputum, or hemoptysis.
O Other findings include dyspnea, recurrent fever and chills, weight loss, malaise, clubbing, and signs of anemia.

Buerger's disease

O Exposure to cold initially causes the feet to become cold, cyanotic, and numb; later, they redden, become hot, and tingle.
O Intermittent claudication of the instep is characteristic.
O Other findings include weak peripheral pulses and, in later stages, ulceration, muscle atrophy, and gangrene.

Chronic obstructive pulmonary disease

O Chronic central cyanosis occurs in advanced stages.
O Exertion aggravates cyanosis.
O Other findings include exertional dyspnea, productive cough with thick sputum, anorexia, weight loss, pursed-lip breathing, tachypnea, accessory muscle use, and wheezing.
O Barrel chest and clubbing are late signs.

Heart failure

O Acute or chronic cyanosis may occur (late sign).
O With left-sided heart failure, central cyanosis occurs with tachycardia, fatigue, dyspnea, cold intolerance, orthopnea, cough, ventricular or atrial gallop, and crackles.
O With right-sided heart failure, peripheral cyanosis occurs with fatigue, peripheral edema, ascites, jugular vein distention, and hepatomegaly.

Peripheral arterial occlusion (acute)

O Acute cyanosis of arm or leg occurs.
O Cyanosis is accompanied by sharp or aching pain that worsens with movement.
O Paresthesia, weakness, decreased or absent pulse, and pale, cool skin occur in the affected extremity.

Pneumonia

○ Acute central cyanosis is usually preceded by fever, shaking chills, cough with purulent sputum, crackles, rhonchi, and pleuritic chest pain that's exacerbated by deep inspiration.

○ Other signs and symptoms include tachycardia, dyspnea, tachypnea, diminished breath sounds, diaphoresis, myalgia, fatigue, headache, and anorexia.

Pneumothorax

○ Acute central cyanosis is a cardinal sign.

○ Other signs and symptoms include sharp chest pain that's exacerbated by movement, deep breathing, and coughing; asymmetrical chest movement; and shortness of breath.

○ Rapid, shallow respirations; weak, rapid pulse; pallor; jugular vein distention; anxiety; and absence of breath sounds over the affected lobe may also occur.

Polycythemia vera

○ Ruddy complexion that can appear cyanotic is characteristic.

○ Other signs and symptoms include hepatosplenomegaly, headache, dizziness, fatigue, blurred vision, chest pain, intermittent claudication, and coagulation defects.

Pulmonary edema

○ Acute central cyanosis occurs.

○ Other signs and symptoms include dyspnea; orthopnea; frothy, blood-tinged sputum; tachycardia; tachypnea; crackles; ventricular gallop; cold, clammy skin; hypotension; weak, thready pulse; and confusion.

Pulmonary embolism

○ Acute central cyanosis occurs when a large embolus obstructs pulmonary circulation.

○ Other signs and symptoms include syncope, jugular vein distention, dyspnea, chest pain, tachycardia, paradoxical pulse, dry cough or productive cough with blood-tinged sputum, fever, restlessness, and diaphoresis.

Raynaud's disease

○ Exposure to cold or stress causes the fingers or hands to blanch, turn cold, then become cyanotic, and finally to redden with return of normal temperature.

○ Numbness and tingling may also develop.

Shock

○ Acute peripheral cyanosis develops in the hands and feet.

○ Feet may be cold, clammy, and pale.

○ Other characteristic signs and symptoms include lethargy, confusion, increased capillary refill, tachypnea, hyperpnea, hypotension, and a rapid, weak pulse.

Nursing considerations

○ Provide supplemental oxygen to improve oxygenation.

○ Deliver small doses of oxygen of 2 L/minute to patients with chronic obstructive pulmonary disease (COPD); use a low-flow oxygen rate for mild COPD exacerbations.

○ For acute situations, a high-flow oxygen rate may be needed initially; in working with a patient who has COPD, remember to be attentive to his respiratory drive and adjust the amount of oxygen accordingly.

○ Position the patient comfortably to ease breathing.

○ Give a diuretic, bronchodilator, antibiotic, or cardiac drug, as needed.

○ Provide rest periods to prevent dyspnea.

Pediatric pointers

○ Central cyanosis may result from cystic fibrosis, asthma, airway obstruction, acute laryngotracheobronchitis, epiglottiditis, or congenital heart defects.

○ Cyanosis around the mouth may precede generalized cyanosis.

○ Acrocyanosis may occur in infants because of excessive crying or exposure to cold.

Geriatric pointers

○ Because of reduced tissue perfusion in elderly people, peripheral cyanosis can occur even with a slight decrease in cardiac output or systemic blood pressure.

Patient teaching

○ Instruct the patient to seek medical attention if cyanosis occurs.

○ Discuss the safe use of oxygen in the home.

Decerebrate posture

Overview

- Also known as *decerebrate rigidity* or *abnormal extensor reflex*
- Characterized by internally rotated and extended arms, pronated wrists, flexed fingers, stiffly extended legs, and forced plantar flexion of the feet
- Indicates upper brain stem damage
- May occur spontaneously or be elicited by noxious stimuli

⭐ Emergency actions

Check if the patient's airway is patent. Insert an artificial airway if needed and prevent aspiration. (If you suspect spinal cord injury, don't disrupt spinal alignment.) Suction as needed. Give supplemental oxygen. Intubation and mechanical ventilation may be required. Keep emergency resuscitation equipment handy.

Assessment

History

- Determine when the patient's level of consciousness (LOC) began to deteriorate.
- Ask if onset was abrupt or gradual and occurred with other signs or symptoms.
- Obtain a medical history, asking about diabetes, liver disease, cancer, blood clots, and aneurysm.
- Ask about recent trauma or accident.

Physical assessment

- Take vital signs.
- Determine LOC using the Glasgow Coma Scale.
- Evaluate pupils for size, equality, and response to light.
- Test deep tendon reflexes and cranial nerve reflexes.
- Check for doll's eye reflex.

Medical causes

Brain stem infarction

- Coma may occur with decerebrate posture.
- Other findings vary with the severity of infarct and may include cranial nerve palsies, cerebellar ataxia, and sensory loss.
- Absence of doll's eye sign, a positive Babinski's reflex, and flaccidity occur with deep coma.

Brain stem tumor

- Decerebrate posture is a late sign that occurs with coma.

- Earlier findings include hemiparesis or quadriparesis, cranial nerve palsies, vertigo, dizziness, ataxia, and vomiting.

Cerebral lesion

- Increased intracranial pressure (ICP) may produce decerebrate posture, a late sign.
- Related findings include coma, abnormal pupil size and response to light, and the classic triad of increased ICP: bradycardia, increasing systolic blood pressure, and widening pulse pressure.

Hepatic encephalopathy

- A late sign in this disorder, decerebrate posture occurs with coma resulting from increased ICP and ammonia toxicity.
- Related findings include fetor hepaticus, a positive Babinski's reflex and hyperactive deep tendon reflexes.

Hypoglycemic encephalopathy

- Decerebrate posture and coma may occur.
- Low glucose levels are characteristic.
- Other findings include dilated pupils, slow respirations, and bradycardia.
- Muscle spasms, twitching, and seizures progress to flaccidity.

Hypoxic encephalopathy

- Decerebrate posturing occurs.
- Related findings include coma, positive Babinski's reflex, absence of doll's eye sign, hypoactive deep tendon reflexes, fixed pupils, and respiratory arrest.

Pontine hemorrhage

- Decerebrate posture occurs rapidly along with coma in this life-threatening disorder.
- Other findings include paralysis, absence of doll's eye sign, a positive Babinski's reflex, and small, reactive pupils.

Posterior fossa hemorrhage

- Decerebrate posturing occurs with vomiting, headache, vertigo, ataxia, stiff neck, drowsiness, papilledema, and cranial nerve palsies.
- Eventually, coma and respiratory arrest may occur.

Other causes

Diagnostic tests

- Removing spinal fluid during a lumbar puncture may cause the brain stem to compress, causing decerebrate posture and coma.

Nursing considerations

- Monitor neurologic status and vital signs.

○ Look for symptoms of increased ICP and neurologic deterioration.

Pediatric pointers
○ Children younger than age 2 may not display decerebrate posture because of nervous system immaturity.
○ In children, the most common cause of decerebrate posture is head injury.

Patient teaching
○ Explain that decerebrate posture is a reflex response.
○ Provide emotional support to the patient and his family.

Decorticate posture

Overview

- Decorticate posture signals corticospinal damage, usually from stroke or head injury.
- It's characterized by adducted arms, flexion of the elbows, flexed wrists and fingers on the chest, and extended and internally rotated legs with plantar flexion of the feet.
- It may occur spontaneously or be elicited by noxious stimuli.
- The intensity of the stimulus, the duration of the posture, and the frequency of spontaneous episodes depend on the severity and location of cerebral injury.
- Decorticate posture carries a more favorable prognosis than decerebrate posture. (See *Differentiating decerebrate from decorticate postures.*)

 Emergency actions

Obtain vital signs and evaluate level of consciousness (LOC). Maintain a patent airway and prevent aspiration (If you suspect spinal cord injury, don't disrupt spinal alignment.) Intubation and mechanical ventilation may be required.

Assessment

History

- Check for symptoms, such as headache, dizziness, nausea, changes in vision, and numbness or tingling, and ask when they began.
- Obtain a medical history, asking about cerebrovascular disease, cancer, meningitis, encephalitis, upper respiratory tract infection, bleeding or clotting disorders, or recent trauma.

Physical assessment

- Test motor and sensory functions.
- Evaluate pupil size, equality, and response to light.
- Test cranial nerve function and deep tendon reflexes.
- Do a complete neurologic examination.

Medical causes

Brain abscess

- Decorticate posture may occur along with aphasia, behavioral changes, altered vital signs, decreased LOC, hemiparesis, headache, dizziness, seizures, nausea, and vomiting.

Brain tumor

- Decorticate posture results from increased intracranial pressure (ICP).

Assessment tip
Differentiating decerebrate from decorticate postures

Decerebrate posture results from damage to the upper brain stem. In this posture, the arms are adducted and extended, with the wrists pronated and the fingers flexed. The legs are stiffly extended, with plantar flexion of the feet.

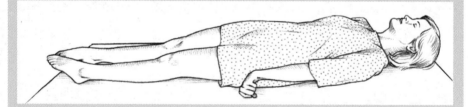

Decorticate posture results from damage to one or both corticospinal tracts. In this posture, the arms are adducted and flexed, with the wrists and fingers flexed on the chest. The legs are stiffly extended and internally rotated, with plantar flexion of the feet.

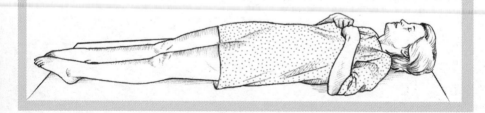

○ Related findings include headache, behavioral changes, memory loss, diplopia, blurred vision or vision loss, seizures, ataxia, apraxia, aphasia, sensory loss, paresthesia, vomiting, papilledema, and signs of hormonal imbalance.

Head injury

○ Decorticate posture may result, depending on the injury.
○ Related findings include headache, nausea, vomiting, dizziness, irritability, decreased LOC, aphasia, hemiparesis, seizures, and pupillary dilation.

Stroke

○ A stroke involving the cerebral cortex produces decorticate posture on one side of the body.
○ Other findings include hemiplegia, dysarthria, dysphagia, sensory loss, apraxia, agnosia, aphasia, memory loss, decreased LOC, homonymous hemianopia, and blurred vision.

Nursing considerations

○ Monitor neurologic status and vital signs frequently to detect signs of deterioration.
○ Look for other signs of increased ICP.

Pediatric pointers

○ Decorticate posture is an unreliable sign before age 2 because of nervous system immaturity.
○ In children, decorticate posture usually results from head injury.

Patient teaching

○ Explain the signs and symptoms of decreased LOC and seizures.
○ Discuss the patient's or caregiver's quality-of-life concerns.
○ Provide needed referrals.
○ Explain to the caregiver how to keep the patient safe, especially during seizure.

Deep tendon reflexes, hyperactive

Overview

- Sharply tapping the muscle's tendon of insertion induces abnormally brisk muscle contractions in response to sudden stretch.
- Deep tendon reflexes (DTRs) are graded as brisk or pathologically hyperactive.

Assessment

History

- Obtain a medical history, including spinal cord injury, other trauma, or prolonged exposure to cold, wind, or water.
- Ask a women if she's pregnant.
- Determine the onset and progression of other signs and symptoms, including paresthesia, vomiting, and altered bladder habits.

Physical assessment

- Evaluate level of consciousness (LOC).
- Test motor and sensory function in the limbs.
- Check for ataxia or tremors and for speech and visual deficits.
- Test for Chvostek's sign, Trousseau's sign and carpopedal spasm.
- Take vital signs.

Medical causes

Amyotrophic lateral sclerosis

- Generalized hyperactive DTRs accompany weakness of the hands and forearms and spasticity of the legs.
- Atrophy of the neck and tongue muscles, fasciculations, weakness of the legs, and bulbar signs eventually develop.

Brain tumor

- Hyperactive DTRs occur on the side opposite the lesion.
- Related findings include one-sided paresis or paralysis, visual field deficits, spasticity, and a positive Babinski's reflex

Hepatic encephalopathy

- Generalized hyperactive DTRs occur late in comatose stage.
- Other findings include a positive Babinski's reflex, fetor hepaticus, and coma.

Hypocalcemia

- Onset of generalized hyperactive DTRs may be gradual or sudden.
- Related findings include paresthesia, muscle twitching and cramping, positive Chvostek's and Trousseau's signs, carpopedal spasm, tetany, abdominal cramps, muscle cramps, arrhythmias, and diarrhea.

Hypomagnesemia

- Onset of generalized hyperactive DTRs is gradual.
- Other findings include muscle cramps, hypotension, tachycardia, paresthesia, ataxia, tetany, seizures, positive Chvostek's sign, confusion, and arrhythmias.

Hypothermia

- Mild hypothermia produces generalized hyperactive DTRs.
- Other findings include shivering, fatigue, weakness, lethargy, slurred speech, ataxia, muscle stiffness, arrhythmias, diuresis, hypotension, and cold, pale skin.

Multiple sclerosis

- Hyperactive DTRs are preceded by weakness and paresthesia in arms and legs.
- Other findings include clonus and a positive Babinski's reflex.
- Ataxia, diplopia, vertigo, vomiting, and urine retention or incontinence occur later.

Preeclampsia

- Onset of generalized hyperactive DTRs is gradual.
- Other findings include increased blood pressure; abnormal weight gain; edema of the face, fingers, and abdomen; albuminuria; oliguria; severe headache; blurred or double vision; epigastric pain; nausea and vomiting; irritability; cyanosis; shortness of breath; and crackles.
- If the condition progresses to eclampsia, seizures may occur.

Spinal cord lesion

- Incomplete lesions cause hyperactive DTRs below the lesion.
- In a traumatic lesion, hyperactive DTRs follow resolution of spinal shock.
- In a neoplastic lesion, hyperactive DTRs gradually replace normal DTRs.
- Other findings include paralysis and sensory loss below the level of the lesion, urine retention and overflow incontinence, and alternating constipation and diarrhea.
- A lesion at or above T6 may produce autonomic hyperreflexia with diaphoresis and flushing above the lesion, headache, nasal congestion, nausea, hypertension, and bradycardia.

Stroke

○ If the origin of the corticospinal tracts is affected, hyperactive DTRs on the side opposite the lesion suddenly occur.
○ Other findings include anesthesia, visual field deficits, spasticity, a positive Babinski's reflex, and one-sided paresis or paralysis.

Tetanus

○ Sudden onset of generalized hyperactive DTRs
○ Tachycardia, diaphoresis, low-grade fever, painful and involuntary muscle contractions, trismus (lockjaw), and *risus sardonicus* (a masklike grin)

Nursing considerations

○ If motor weakness is present, perform range-of-motion exercises.
○ Reposition the patient frequently, provide a special mattress, massage his back, and ensure adequate nutrition.
○ Give a muscle relaxant and a sedative to relieve severe muscle contractions.
○ Keep emergency resuscitation equipment on hand.
○ Provide a quiet, calm atmosphere to reduce neuromuscular excitability.
○ Assist with activities of daily living.

Pediatric pointers

○ Cerebral palsy typically causes hyperactive DTRs in children.
○ Reye's syndrome in stage II causes generalized hyperactive DTRs; in stage V, DTRs are absent.
○ Hyperreflexia may be normal in neonates.

Patient teaching

○ Explain to the caregiver the procedures and treatments that the patient may need.
○ Discuss safety measures that need to be taken.
○ Provide emotional support.

Deep tendon reflexes, hypoactive

Overview

○ Abnormally diminished muscle contractions in response to sudden stretch after sharply tapping the muscle's tendon of insertion
○ Result from damage to the reflex arc involving the specific muscle, the peripheral nerve, the nerve roots, or the spinal cord
○ An important sign of many disorders, especially when they appear with other neurologic signs

Assessment

History

○ Obtain a medical history.
○ Ask about other signs and symptoms.
○ Take a family and drug history.

Documenting deep tendon reflexes

To record the patient's deep tendon reflex scores, draw a stick figure and enter the rating on the drawing for each reflex. The figure shown here indicates hypoactive deep tendon reflexes in the legs; the other reflexes are normal.

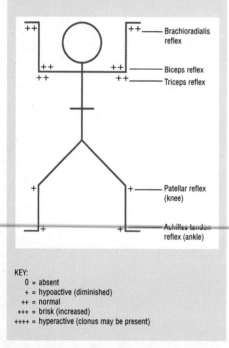

KEY:
    0 = absent
    + = hypoactive (diminished)
    ++ = normal
    +++ = brisk (increased)
    ++++ = hyperactive (clonus may be present)

Physical assessment

○ Assess level of consciousness and speech.
○ Test motor function in the limbs.
○ Palpate for muscle atrophy or increased mass.
○ Test sensory function, assessing for paresthesia.
○ Observe gait and coordination.
○ Check for Romberg's sign.
○ Check for signs of vision and hearing loss.
○ Take vital signs.
○ Monitor for increased heart rate and blood pressure.
○ Inspect the skin for pallor, dryness, flushing, and diaphoresis.
○ Auscultate for hypoactive bowel sounds.
○ Palpate for bladder distention.
○ Document the muscles in which deep tendon reflexes (DTRs) are lessened. (See *Documenting deep tendon reflexes*.)

Medical causes

Botulism

○ Generalized hypoactive DTRs accompany progressive descending muscle weakness.
○ Early findings include blurred vision, double vision, anorexia, nausea, vomiting, vertigo, hearing loss, dysarthria, and dysphagia.
○ Respiratory distress and severe constipation may develop.

Cerebellar dysfunction

○ Hypoactive DTRs occur with other findings depending on the cause and location of the dysfunction.

Guillain-Barré syndrome

○ Hypoactive DTRs progress rapidly from hypotonia to areflexia.
○ Muscle weakness begins in the legs and then extends to the arms and, possibly, to the trunk and neck, peaking in 10 to 14 days and then resolving.
○ Weakness may progress to total paralysis.
○ Other findings include cranial nerve palsies, pain, paresthesia, and signs of autonomic dysfunction.

Peripheral neuropathy

○ Progressive hypoactive DTRs.
○ Motor weakness, sensory loss, paresthesia, tremors, and possible autonomic dysfunction.

Polymyositis

○ Hypoactive DTRs with muscle weakness, pain, stiffness, spasms and, possibly, increased size or atrophy

Spinal cord lesions

○ Transient hypoactive DTRs or areflexia below the lesion.
○ Quadriplegia or paraplegia, flaccidity, loss of sensation, and pale, dry skin below the level of the lesion.

○ Other characteristic findings include urine retention with overflow incontinence, hypoactive bowel sounds, constipation, and genital reflex loss.

Other causes

Drugs

○ Barbiturates and paralyzing drugs, such as pancuronium and curare, may cause hypoactive DTRs.

Nursing considerations

○ If the patient has sensory deficits, protect him from heat, cold, and pressure.
○ Keep the skin clean and dry.
○ Reposition the patient frequently.
○ Encourage range-of-joint-motion exercises.
○ Provide a balanced diet with increased protein and fluids.

Pediatric pointers

○ Hypoactive DTRs commonly occur in children with muscular dystrophy, Friedreich's ataxia, syringomyelia, and spinal cord injury.
○ Hypoactive DTRs accompany progressive muscular atrophy, which affects preschoolers and adolescents.

Geriatric pointers

○ Reduced DTRs occur because of a decrease in the number of nerve axons and demyelination of axons in elderly patients.

Patient teaching

○ Teach skills that can help with independence in daily life.
○ Discuss safety measures, including walking with assistance.

Diaphoresis

Overview

- Refers to profuse sweating
- Can produce more than 1 L of sweat per hour
- Represents an autonomic nervous system response to physical or psychogenic stress or to fever or high environmental temperature

Assessment

History

- Ask the patient to describe his chief complaint.
- Note when diaphoresis occurs (day or night).
- Investigate other signs and symptoms.
- Find out about recent travel or exposure to high environmental temperatures or to pesticides.
- Ask about recent insect bites.
- Obtain a medical history, asking about partial gastrectomy or drug or alcohol abuse.
- Take a drug history.

Physical assessment

- Inspect the trunk, extremities, palms, soles, and forehead to determine the extent of diaphoresis.
- Observe for flushing, abnormal skin texture or lesions, and an increased amount of coarse body hair.
- Note poor skin turgor and dry mucous membranes.
- Look for splinter hemorrhages and Plummer's nails.
- Evaluate mental status.
- Take vital signs.
- Observe for fasciculations and flaccid paralysis.
- Assess for seizures.
- Note the patient's facial expression and examine the eyes.
- Auscultate breath sounds.
- Palpate for lymphadenopathy and hepatosplenomegaly.

Medical causes

Acquired immunodeficiency syndrome

- Night sweats may occur early as a manifestation of the disease or from an opportunistic infection.
- Other findings include fever, fatigue, lymphadenopathy, anorexia, weight loss, diarrhea, and a persistent cough.

Acromegaly

- Diaphoresis measures disease activity.
- Other findings include a hulking appearance; an enlarged supraorbital ridge and thickened ears and nose; warm, oily skin; enlarged hands, feet, and jaw; joint pain; weight gain; hoarseness; increased coarse body hair; elevated blood pressure; and visual field deficits or blindness.

Anxiety disorders

- Diaphoresis occurs on the palms, soles, and forehead
- Palpitations, tachycardia, tachypnea, tremors, and GI distress
- Fear, difficulty concentrating, and behavior changes

Autonomic hyperreflexia

- Profuse diaphoresis above the injury, pounding headache, blurred vision, and dramatically elevated blood pressure occur after spinal shock in spinal cord injury above T6.
- Other findings include flushing, restlessness, nausea, nasal congestion, and bradycardia.

Heart failure

- In left-sided heart failure, diaphoresis follows fatigue, dyspnea, orthopnea, and tachycardia.
- In patients with right-sided heart failure, diaphoresis follows jugular vein distention and dry cough.
- Other findings include tachypnea, cyanosis, edema, crackles, ventricular gallop, and anxiety.

Heat exhaustion

- Profuse diaphoresis, fatigue, weakness, and anxiety may occur initially, progressing to circulatory collapse and shock.
- Other findings include ashen gray appearance, dilated pupils, and normal or subnormal temperature.

Hodgkin's disease

- Early findings may include night sweats, fever, fatigue, pruritus, and weight loss.
- Initial sign is usually painless swelling of a cervical lymph node.

Hypoglycemia

- Rapidly induced hypoglycemia may cause diaphoresis, irritability, tremors, hypotension, blurred vision, tachycardia, hunger, and loss of consciousness.
- Confusion, motor weakness, hemiplegia, seizures, or coma may also occur.

Infective endocarditis (subacute)

- Generalized night sweats occur early.
- A sudden change in a murmur or a new murmur is a classic sign.
- Other findings include intermittent low-grade fever, weakness, fatigue, petechiae, splinter hemorrhages, weight loss, anorexia, and arthralgia.

Liver abscess

- Common diaphoresis, right-upper-quadrant pain, weight loss, fever, chills, nausea, vomiting, and anemia
- Possible jaundice, chalk-colored stools, and dark urine

Lung abscess

- Commonly, drenching night sweats
- Characteristically, a cough producing copious purulent, foul-smelling, bloody sputum
- Fever with chills, pleuritic chest pain, dyspnea, weakness, anorexia, weight loss, headache, malaise, clubbing, tubular or amorphic breath sounds, and dullness on percussion

Malaria

- Profuse diaphoresis marks the third stage of paroxysmal malaria, after chills (first stage) and high fever (second stage).
- Headache, arthralgia, and hepatosplenomegaly may occur.
- Severe malaria may progress to delirium, seizures, and coma.

Myocardial infarction

- Diaphoresis with acute, substernal, radiating chest pain in this life-threatening condition
- Anxiety, dyspnea, nausea, vomiting, tachycardia, blood pressure change, crackles, pallor, and clammy skin

Opioid and alcohol withdrawal syndromes

- Generalized diaphoresis occurs with dilated pupils, tachycardia, tremors, and altered mental status.
- Other findings include severe muscle cramps, paresthesia, tachypnea, altered blood pressure, nausea, vomiting, and seizures.

Pheochromocytoma

- Common diaphoresis
- Chiefly, persistent or paroxysmal hypertension
- Headache, palpitations, tachycardia, anxiety, tremors, paresthesia, abdominal pain, tachypnea, nausea, vomiting, and orthostatic hypotension

Pneumonia

- Intermittent, generalized diaphoresis accompanies fever and chills.
- Other findings include pleuritic pain, tachypnea, dyspnea, productive cough, headache, fatigue, myalgia, abdominal pain, anorexia, and cyanosis.

Relapsing fever

- Profuse diaphoresis marks resolution of the crisis stage of relapsing fever, which produces attacks of high fever, myalgia, headache, arthralgia, diarrhea, vomiting, coughing, and eye or chest pain.
- Febrile attack abruptly terminates in chills with tachycardia and tachypnea.
- Diaphoresis, flushing, and hypotension may then lead to circulatory collapse and death.

Tetanus

- Profuse sweating is accompanied by low-grade fever, tachycardia, and hyperactive deep tendon reflexes.

- Early restlessness, pain, and stiffness in the jaw, abdomen, and back progresses to spasms from lockjaw, risus sardonicus, dysphagia, and opisthotonos.

Thyrotoxicosis

- Diaphoresis with heat intolerance, weight loss despite increased appetite, tachycardia, palpitations, an enlarged thyroid gland, dyspnea, nervousness, diarrhea, tremors, Plummer's nails and, exophthalmos

Other causes

Drugs

- Aspirin or acetaminophen poisoning cause diaphoresis.
- Sympathomimetics, antipyretics, thyroid hormones, corticosteroids, and certain antipsychotics may cause diaphoresis.

Pesticide poisoning

- Toxic effects of pesticide poisoning are diaphoresis, nausea, vomiting, diarrhea, blurred vision, miosis, and excessive lacrimation and salivation.

Nursing considerations

- Sponge the face and body.
- Change wet clothes and sheets.
- To prevent skin irritation, dust skin folds in the groin and axillae and under pendulous breasts with cornstarch.
- Replace fluids and electrolytes.
- Monitor urine output.
- Encourage oral fluids high in electrolytes.
- Keep the room temperature moderate.

Pediatric pointers

- Diaphoresis in children commonly results from environmental heat, overdressing, drug withdrawal from the mother's addiction, heart failure, thyrotoxicosis, and the effects of such drugs as antihistamines, ephedrine, haloperidol, and thyroid hormone.
- Sweat glands function immaturely in infants.

Geriatric pointers

- In tuberculosis, fever and night sweats may not occur in elderly patients, who instead may exhibit a change in activity or weight.
- Elderly patients may not exhibit diaphoresis because of a decreased sweating mechanism, increasing the risk for developing heatstroke.

Patient teaching

- Explain proper skin care.
- Explain the disease process.
- Discuss the importance of fluid replacement and how to make sure fluid intake is adequate.

Diarrhea

Overview

- Increase in the volume of stools
- May be acute or chronic
- Can cause life-threatening fluid and electrolyte imbalances

Emergency actions

If diarrhea is profuse, check for signs of shock. If they occur, place the patient in the supine position and elevate his legs 20 degrees. Insert an I.V. line for fluid replacement and monitor for electrolyte imbalances. Keep emergency resuscitation equipment handy.

Assessment

History

- Check for other signs and symptoms (pain, cramps, difficulty breathing, weakness, fatigue).
- Find out about his drug history.
- Ask about recent GI surgery or radiation therapy.
- Review his diet and ask about food allergies.
- Ask about possible stress factors.

Physical assessment

- Check skin turgor and mucous membranes.
- Take blood pressure with the patient lying, sitting, and standing.
- Inspect the abdomen for distention, and palpate for tenderness.
- Percuss the abdomen for tympany.
- Auscultate bowel sounds.
- Take the patient's temperature and note any chills.
- Look for a rash.

Medical causes

Anthrax, GI

- Later signs and symptoms are severe bloody diarrhea, abdominal pain, and hematemesis.
- Decreased appetite, nausea, vomiting, and fever occur initially.

Clostridium difficile infection

- The patient may have soft, unformed stools or watery diarrhea that may be foul-smelling or bloody.
- Other features include abdominal pain, cramping, and tenderness; fever; and a white blood cell count as high as 20,000/µl.
- Toxic megacolon, colonic perforation, or peritonitis may develop in severe cases.

Crohn's disease

- Diarrhea is accompanied by abdominal pain, with guarding and tenderness and nausea.
- Fever, chills, anorexia, weakness, and weight loss may also develop.

Escherichia coli 0157:H7

- Watery or bloody diarrhea, nausea, vomiting, fever, and abdominal cramps occur.

Infections

- Acute viral, bacterial, and protozoan infections cause the sudden onset of watery diarrhea with abdominal pain, cramps, nausea, vomiting, and fever.
- Chronic tuberculosis and fungal and parasitic infections produce a less severe but more persistent diarrhea, along with epigastric distress, vomiting, weight loss, and passage of blood and mucus.

Intestinal obstruction

- Diarrhea occurs along with abdominal pain with tenderness and guarding, nausea and, possibly, distention.
- Other findings include borborygmi and rushes on auscultation and vomiting of fecal material.

Irritable bowel syndrome

- Diarrhea alternates with constipation or normal bowel function.
- Related findings include abdominal pain, tenderness, and distention; dyspepsia; passage of mucus and pasty pencil-like stools; and nausea.

Ischemic bowel disease

- A life-threatening disorder — bloody diarrhea occurs with abdominal pain.
- Other findings include abdominal distention, nausea, vomiting and, if severe, shock.

Lactose intolerance

- Diarrhea occurs within hours of ingesting milk or milk products.
- Other findings include cramps, abdominal pain, borborygmi, bloating, nausea, and flatus.

Large-bowel cancer

- Bloody diarrhea is seen with a partial obstruction.
- Other findings include abdominal pain, anorexia, weight loss, weakness, fatigue, and exertional dyspnea.

Lead poisoning

- Diarrhea alternates with constipation.
- Other effects include abdominal pain, anorexia, nausea, vomiting, a metallic taste, headache, dizziness, and a bluish gingival lead line.

Listeriosis

- Diarrhea occurs along with fever, myalgias, abdominal pain, nausea and vomiting.

○ Fever, headache, nuchal rigidity and altered level of consciousness may occur if infection spreads to the nervous system and causes meningitis.

Malabsorption syndrome

○ Diarrhea occurs after meals along with steatorrhea, abdominal distention, and muscle cramps.
○ Other findings include anorexia, weight loss, bone pain, anemia, weakness, fatigue, bruising, and night blindness.

Pseudomembranous enterocolitis

○ A life-threatening disorder — copious watery, green, foul-smelling, bloody diarrhea rapidly precipitates signs of shock.
○ Other findings include colicky abdominal pain, distention, fever, and dehydration.

Q Fever

○ Diarrhea occurs along with fever, chills, severe headache, malaise, chest pain, and vomiting.
○ Hepatitis and pneumonia may occur in severe cases.
○ Prolonged fever, night sweats, chills, fatigue, and dyspnea may occur in chronic Q fever.

Rotavirus gastroenteritis

○ Fever, nausea, and vomiting are followed by diarrhea.

Thyrotoxicosis

○ Diarrhea accompanies diaphoresis, dyspnea, tachycardia, nervousness, tremors, palpitations, heat intolerance, weight loss despite increased appetite, and, possibly, exophthalmos.

Ulcerative colitis

○ Recurrent bloody diarrhea with pus or mucus is a characteristic sign.
○ Other features include tenesmus, hyperactive bowel sounds, cramping, lower abdominal pain, low-grade fever, anorexia, nausea, and vomiting.
○ Weight loss, anemia, and weakness are late findings.

Other causes

Drugs

○ Many antibiotics, herbal remedies, and laxative abuse cause diarrhea.
○ Other drugs that may cause diarrhea include antacids containing magnesium, colchicine, guanethidine, lactulose, dantrolene, ethacrynic acid, mefenamic acid, methotrexate, metyrosine and, in high doses, cardiac glycosides and quinidine.

Treatments

○ Gastrectomy, gastroenterostomy, or pyloroplasty may produce diarrhea.
○ High-dose radiation therapy may produce enteritis, leading to diarrhea.

Nursing considerations

○ Administer an analgesic and an opiate to decrease intestinal motility, unless the patient has a possible or confirmed stool infection.
○ Clean the perineum thoroughly to prevent skin breakdown.
○ Quantify the amount of liquid stools and monitor intake and output.
○ Monitor electrolyte levels and hematocrit.
○ Administer I.V. fluid replacements.

Pediatric pointers

○ Diarrhea in children commonly results from infection.
○ Chronic diarrhea may result from malabsorption syndrome, an anatomic defect, or allergies.
○ Diarrhea can quickly cause life-threatening dehydration in children.

Geriatric pointers

○ In an elderly patient with new-onset segmental colitis, consider ischemia before assuming Crohn's disease.

Patient teaching

○ Emphasize the importance of maintaining adequate hydration.
○ Explain any foods or liquids the patient should avoid.
○ Discuss stress-reduction techniques.
○ Refer for counseling as needed.
○ Discuss the importance of medical follow-up with inflammatory bowel disease.

Diplopia

Overview

- Refers to double vision or seeing one object as two
- Results when extraocular muscles fail to work together, causing images to fall on the wrong parts of the retinas
- Can occur in one eye or in both eyes

Assessment

History

- Ask about other symptoms, including severe headache, neurologic symptoms, and eye pain.
- Ask about the onset and ask for a description of the diplopia.
- Obtain a medical history, asking about hypertension; diabetes mellitus; allergies; thyroid, neurologic, or muscular disorders; extraocular muscle disorders; trauma; or eye surgery.

Physical assessment

- Perform a neurologic examination.
- Evaluate level of consciousness (LOC); pupil size, equality, and response to light; and motor and sensory function.
- Take vital signs.
- Observe the patient for ocular deviation, ptosis, proptosis, lid edema, and conjunctival injection.
- Distinguish monocular from binocular diplopia.
- Test visual acuity and extraocular muscles (See *Testing extraocular muscles.*)

Medical causes

Brain tumor

- Diplopia may be an early symptom.
- Other signs and symptoms vary with tumor size and location but may include eye deviation, emotional lability, decreased LOC, headache, vomiting, seizures, hearing loss, visual field defects, abnormal pupillary responses, nystagmus, motor weakness, and paralysis.

Diabetes mellitus

- Sudden diplopia with intense periorbital pain or head pain may be a long-term effect.

Encephalitis

- A brief episode of diplopia and eye deviation may occur initially.
- Sudden onset of high fever, severe headache, and vomiting are early findings.
- As inflammation progresses, decreased LOC, seizures, ataxia, and paralysis indicate meningeal irritation.

Head injury

- Diplopia may occur in potentially life-threatening head injuries depending on the site and extent of injury.
- Other findings include eye deviation, pupillary changes, headache, decreased LOC, altered vital signs, nausea, vomiting, and motor weakness or paralysis.

Intracranial aneurysm

- A life-threatening condition — diplopia and eye deviation occur initially, possibly with ptosis and a dilated pupil on the affected side.
- A recurrent, severe, one-sided, frontal headache develops.
- Other findings include neck and spinal pain and rigidity, decreased LOC, tinnitus, dizziness, nausea, vomiting, and muscle weakness or paralysis on one side.

Multiple sclerosis

- Diplopia, a common early symptom, is usually accompanied by blurred vision and paresthesia.
- As the disease progresses, findings include nystagmus, constipation, muscle weakness, paralysis, spasticity, hyperreflexia, intention tremor, gait ataxia, dysphagia, dysarthria, impotence, emotional lability, and urinary frequency, urgency, and incontinence.

Myasthenia gravis

- Diplopia and ptosis occur initially and may worsen throughout the day.
- As the disorder progresses, other muscles are involved, resulting in blank facial expression; nasal voice; difficulty making fine hand movements, chewing, and swallowing; and possibly life-threatening respiratory muscle weakness.

Ophthalmologic migraine

- Diplopia occurs and persists for days after the headache.
- Other findings include severe, one-sided pain; ptosis; irritability; depression; slight confusion; and extraocular muscle palsies.

Orbital blowout fracture

- Monocular diplopia affecting the upward gaze usually occurs.
- With marked periorbital edema, diplopia may affect other directions of gaze.
- Periorbital ecchymoses occurs, but visual acuity is unaffected.
- Other findings include eyelid edema, subcutaneous crepitation of the eyelid and orbit, dilated and unreactive pupil, and hyphema.

The coordinated action of six muscles controls eyeball movements. To test the function of each muscle and the cranial nerve (CN) that innervates it, ask the patient to look in the direction you indicate (each of which you select as shown below). The six directions you can test make up the cardinal positions of gaze. The patient's inability to turn the eye in the designated direction indicates muscle weakness or paralysis.

SR — superior rectus (CN III)
IR — inferior rectus (CN III)
MR — medial rectus (CN III)
LR — lateral rectus (CN VI)
IO — inferior oblique (CN III)
SO — superior oblique (CN IV)

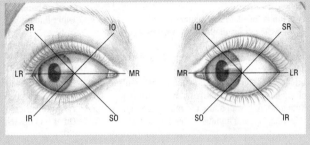

Orbital cellulitis

○ Diplopia develops suddenly.
○ Other findings are eye deviation and pain, purulent drainage, lid edema, chemosis and redness, proptosis, nausea, and fever.

Orbital tumors

○ Diplopia can occur, possibly with proptosis and blurred vision.
○ One or both eyes may appear prominent and the patient may report pain, redness, and swelling of the affected eye.

Stroke

○ If stroke affects the vertebrobasilar artery, diplopia occurs.
○ Other features include one-sided motor weakness or paralysis, ataxia, decreased LOC, dizziness, aphasia, visual field deficits, slurred speech, and dysphagia.

Thyrotoxicosis

○ Diplopia beginning in the upper field of gaze accompanies exophthalmos.
○ Other findings include impaired eye movement, excessive tearing, lid edema, and inability to close the lids.
○ Other characteristic findings include tachycardia, palpitations, weight loss, diarrhea, tremors, an enlarged thyroid gland, dyspnea, nervousness, diaphoresis, and heat intolerance.

Transient ischemic attack

○ Diplopia, dizziness, tinnitus, hearing loss, and numbness may occur.

Nursing considerations

○ Monitor vital signs and neurologic status.
○ Provide a safe environment.
○ Institute seizure precautions, if needed.

Pediatric pointers

○ School-age children who complain of double vision require a careful examination to rule out serious disorders such as a brain tumor.

Patient teaching

○ Explain the safety measures that are needed.
○ Teach the patient skills of ambulation with assistance.
○ Provide an orientation to room and meal tray.

Dizziness

Overview

- Sensation of imbalance or faintness
- May be associated with giddiness, weakness, confusion, and blurred or double vision
- Commonly from inadequate blood flow and oxygen supply to the cerebrum and spinal cord
- Commonly confused with vertigo, a sensation of revolving in space — or of surroundings revolving about oneself — with nausea, vomiting, nystagmus, staggering gait, and tinnitus or hearing loss

✦ Emergency actions

Ensure the patient's safety and prevent falls. Determine the severity and onset of the dizziness and ask if he has a headache or blurred vision. Take his blood pressure and check for orthostatic hypotension. Determine if he's at risk for hypoglycemia. Have him lie down, and recheck vital signs every 15 minutes. Start an I.V. line; give drugs as needed.

Assessment

History

- Obtain a medical history, noting diabetes mellitus, head injury, anxiety disorders, and cardiovascular, pulmonary, and kidney disease.
- Take a drug history and determine whether the patient is taking antihypertensives.
- Determine the onset and characteristics of dizziness.
- Ask about emotional stress.
- Ask about other signs and symptoms, such as palpitations, chest pain, diaphoresis, shortness of breath, and chronic cough.

Physical assessment

- Check neurologic vital signs, including level of consciousness (LOC), motor and sensory functions, and reflexes.
- Inspect for poor skin turgor and dry mucous membranes.
- Auscultate heart rate and rhythm.
- Inspect for barrel chest, clubbing, cyanosis, and accessory muscle use.
- Auscultate breath and heart sounds.
- Check for orthostatic hypotension.
- Palpate for edema and capillary refill time.

Medical causes

Anemia

- Dizziness is aggravated by postural changes or exertion.

- Other findings include pallor, dyspnea, fatigue, tachycardia, and bounding pulse.

Cardiac arrhythmias

- Dizziness lasts for several seconds or longer and may precede fainting.
- Other findings include palpitations; irregular, rapid, or thready pulse; hypotension; weakness; blurred vision; paresthesia, and confusion.

Carotid sinus hypersensitivity

- Brief episodes of dizziness usually result in fainting.
- Episode is preceded by stimulation of one or both carotid arteries.
- Other findings include sweating, nausea, and pallor.

Generalized anxiety disorder

- Continuous dizziness may intensify as the disorder worsens.
- Other findings include persistent anxiety, insomnia, difficulty concentrating, fidgeting, cold and clammy hands, dry mouth, frequent urination, tachycardia, tachypnea, diaphoresis, palpitations, and irritability.

Hypertension

- Dizziness may precede fainting or may be relieved by rest.
- Other signs and symptoms include headache, blurred vision, and retinal changes.

Hyperventilation syndrome

- Dizziness lasting a few minutes
- With frequent hyperventilation, dizziness between episodes
- Apprehension, diaphoresis, pallor, dyspnea, chest tightness, palpitations, trembling, fatigue, and peripheral and circumoral paresthesia

Hypoglycemia

- Dizziness, headache, clouding of vision, restlessness, and mental status changes can result from fasting hypoglycemia.
- Other findings include irritability, trembling, hunger, cold sweats, and tachycardia.

Hypovolemia

- Dizziness is caused by a lack of circulating volume.
- Other findings include orthostatic hypotension, thirst, poor skin turgor, and flattened neck veins.

Orthostatic hypotension

- Dizziness may terminate in fainting or disappear with rest.
- Related findings include dim vision, spots before the eyes, pallor, diaphoresis, hypotension, tachycardia, and signs of dehydration.

Panic disorder

- Dizziness may accompany acute attacks of panic.

○ Other findings include anxiety, dyspnea, palpitations, chest pain, a choking or smothering sensation, vertigo, paresthesia, hot and cold flashes, diaphoresis, and trembling or shaking.

Postconcussion syndrome

○ Dizziness, headache, emotional lability, alcohol intolerance, fatigue, anxiety and, possibly, vertigo occur 1 to 3 weeks after a head injury.

Rift Valley fever

○ Typical signs and symptoms include dizziness, fever, myalgia, weakness, and back pain.

Transient ischemic attack

○ Dizziness of varying severity, diplopia, blindness or visual field deficits, ptosis, tinnitus, hearing loss, paresis, and numbness occur.

Other causes

Drugs

○ Antihistamines, antihypertensives, anxiolytics, central nervous system depressants, decongestants, opioids, and vasodilators commonly cause dizziness.
○ Herbal remedies such as St. John's wort can produce dizziness.

Nursing considerations

○ If the patient is dizzy, provide for his safety.

Pediatric pointers

○ If you suspect dizziness, assess for vertigo, a more common symptom in children.

Patient teaching

○ Teach the patient how to control dizziness.

Doll's eye reflex, absent (Negative oculocephalic reflex)

Overview

- Doll's eye reflex is tested by rapid, gentle turning of the patient's head from side to side, noting the position of the eyes with each head turn.
- In a normal reflex, the patient's eyes will deviate in the direction opposite the head turn, and then return to the middle gaze.
- In a negative reflex, the eyes remain fixed in the center. (See *Testing for doll's eye sign.*)
- Absent doll's eye reflex is an indicator of injury to the midbrain or pons, involving cranial nerves III and VI.
- Absent doll's eye reflex is necessary for diagnosis of brain death.

Assessment

History

- Obtain a medical history from the patient's family.
- Ask about a drug history.

Physical assessment

- Evaluate level of consciousness (LOC) using the Glasgow Coma Scale.
- Note decerebrate or decorticate posture.
- Examine the pupils for size, equality, and response to light.

- Check for signs of increased intracranial pressure (ICP).

Medical causes

Brain stem infarction

- Absent doll's eye sign occurs with coma.
- Other findings include limb paralysis, cranial nerve palsies, cerebellar ataxia, variable sensory loss, a positive Babinski's reflex, decerebrate posture, and muscle flaccidity.

Brain stem tumors

- Absent doll's eye sign accompanies coma.
- Sign may be preceded by hemiparesis, nystagmus, extraocular nerve palsies, facial pain or sensory loss, facial paralysis, diminished corneal reflex, tinnitus, hearing loss, dysphagia, drooling, vertigo, ataxia, and vomiting.

Central midbrain infarction

- Coma, Weber's syndrome (oculomotor palsy with contralateral hemiplegia), contralateral ataxic tremor, nystagmus, and pupillary abnormalities may accompany absent doll's eye sign.

Cerebellar lesion

- If the lesion progresses to coma, absent doll's eye sign occur.
- Coma may be preceded by headache, nystagmus, ocular deviation to the side of the lesion, unequal pupils, dysarthria, dysphagia, ipsilateral facial paresis, cerebellar ataxia, and signs of increasing ICP.

Assessment tip
Testing for doll's eye sign

To evaluate the patient's oculocephalic reflex, hold the upper eyelids open and quickly (but gently) turn the head from side to side, noting eye movements with each head turn.

With absent doll's eye sign, the eyes remain fixed in midposition.

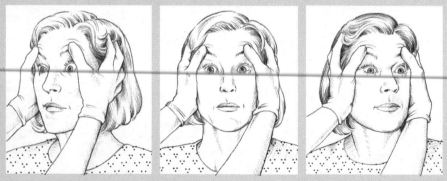

Pontine hemorrhage

○ A life-threatening disorder — absent doll's eye sign and coma develop within minutes.
○ Other ominous signs, such as complete paralysis, decerebrate posture, a positive Babinski's reflex, and small, reactive pupils, may then accompany a rapid progression to death.

Posterior fossa hematoma

○ Absent doll's eye sign and coma occur, preceded by headache, vomiting, drowsiness, confusion, unequal pupils, dysphagia, cranial nerve palsies, stiff neck, and cerebellar ataxia.

Other causes

Drugs

○ Barbiturates may produce severe central nervous depression, resulting in coma and absent doll's eye sign.

Nursing considerations

○ To reduce the risk of spinal cord damage, don't attempt to elicit doll's eye sign in a comatose patient with suspected cervical spine injury.
○ If you suspect cervical spine injury, don't turn the patient's head to elicit the sign. Instead, use the cold caloric test by injecting cold water into the ear.
○ Monitor vital signs and neurologic status.
○ Provide emotional support to the family.

Pediatric pointers

○ Doll's eye sign isn't present for the first 10 days after birth and may be irregular until age 2.
○ Absent doll's eye sign in children may accompany coma from head injury, near-drowning or suffocation, or brain stem astrocytoma.

Dysarthria

Overview

- Poorly articulated speech
- Speech characterized by slurring and labored, irregular rhythm
- Results from damage to brain stem that affects cranial nerves IX, X, or XII

⭐ Emergency actions

Assess the patient for difficulty swallowing. Withhold food and fluids. Determine respiratory rate and depth and measure vital capacity. Assess blood pressure and heart rate. Ensure a patent airway and place the patient in Fowler's position. Suction his mouth and oropharynx, and administer oxygen as necessary. Keep emergency resuscitation equipment nearby. If progressive respiratory muscle weakness occurs, intubate and start mechanical ventilation.

Assessment

History

- Ask about the onset and characteristics of dysarthria.
- Obtain a drug and alcohol history.
- Obtain a medical history, including seizures.

Physical assessment

- Check the patient's dentures for proper fit.
- Have the patient produce a few simple sounds and words.
- Compare muscle strength and tone in the limbs on one side of the body with the other.
- Assess the patient's tactile sense.
- Test deep tendon reflexes, and note gait ataxia.
- Assess cerebellar function.
- Test visual fields and ask about double vision.
- Check for signs of facial weakness.
- Determine level of consciousness (LOC) and mental status.

Medical causes

Alcoholic cerebellar degeneration

- Chronic, progressive dysarthria occurs.
- Other findings include ataxia, diplopia, ophthalmoplegia, hypotension, and altered mental status.

Amyotrophic lateral sclerosis

- Dysarthria occurs and worsens as the disease progresses.
- Other findings include dysphagia; difficulty breathing; muscle atrophy and weakness, especially in the hands and feet; fasciculations; spasticity; hyperactive deep tendon reflexes in the legs; and excessive drooling.

Basilar artery insufficiency

- Dysarthria is with diplopia, vertigo, facial numbness, ataxia, paresis, and visual field loss, lasting from minutes to hours.

Botulism

- Dysarthria, dysphagia, diplopia, and ptosis are characteristic signs.
- Early findings include dry mouth, sore throat, weakness, vomiting, and diarrhea.
- Later, descending weakness or paralysis of muscles in the extremities and trunk causes hyporeflexia and dyspnea.

Manganese poisoning

- Progressive dysarthria is accompanied by weakness, fatigue, confusion, hallucinations, drooling, hand tremors, limb stiffness, spasticity, gross rhythmic movements of the trunk and head, and propulsive gait.

Mercury poisoning

- Progressive dysarthria is accompanied by fatigue, depression, lethargy, irritability, confusion, ataxia, tremors, and changes in vision, hearing, and memory.

Multiple sclerosis

- Dysarthria may occur with nystagmus, blurred or double vision, dysphagia, ataxia, and intention tremor.
- Other findings include paresthesia, spasticity, hyperreflexia, muscle weakness or paralysis, constipation, emotional lability, and urinary frequency, urgency, and incontinence.

Myasthenia gravis

- Dysarthria, associated with a nasal voice, worsens during the day and may temporarily improve with short rest periods.
- Other findings include dysphagia, drooling, facial weakness, diplopia, ptosis, dyspnea, and muscle weakness.

Olivopontocerebellar degeneration

- Dysarthria, a major sign of this disorder, accompanies cerebellar ataxia and spasticity.
- Other findings include abnormal eye movement, sexual dysfunction, bowel and bladder problems, and difficulty swallowing.

Parkinson's disease

- Dysarthria and a monotone voice occur.
- Other findings include muscle rigidity, bradykinesia, involuntary tremor usually beginning in the fingers, difficulty walking, muscle weakness, stooped posture, masklike facies, dysphagia, and drooling.

Stroke (brain stem)

○ Dysarthria that's most severe at onset of the stroke occurs with dysphonia and dysphagia.
○ Other findings include facial weakness, diplopia, hemiparesis, spasticity, drooling, dyspnea, and decreased LOC.

Stroke (cerebral)

○ Weakness produces dysarthria that's most severe at onset of the stroke.
○ Other findings include dysphagia, drooling, dysphonia, hemianopsia, aphasia, spasticity, and hyperreflexia.

Other causes

Drugs

○ Large doses of anticonvulsants and barbiturates can cause dysarthria.

Nursing considerations

○ Consult with a speech pathologist as needed.
○ Give drugs and treatments as needed.
○ Assess swallow and gag reflexes before feeding the patient.
○ Give the patient time to express himself and encourage the use of gestures.

Pediatric pointers

○ Dysarthria usually results from brain stem glioma; it may also result from cerebral palsy.
○ Because dysarthria is difficult to detect in infants and young children, look for other neurologic deficits.

Patient teaching

○ Explain different ways in which the patient can communicate.
○ Encourage the patient to express his feelings.

Dyspepsia

Overview

- A feeling of uncomfortable fullness after meals
- Other findings: belching, heartburn and, possibly, cramping and abdominal distention
- Altered gastric secretions leading to excess stomach acidity

Assessment

History

- Ask about the onset, duration, and description of dyspepsia.
- Ask about alleviating and aggravating factors.
- Ask the patient about nausea, vomiting, melena, hematemesis, cough, chest pain, or urine changes.
- Obtain a drug and surgical history.
- Obtain a medical history, including renal, cardiovascular, or pulmonary disease.
- Ask about an unusual or overwhelming amount of emotional stress.

Physical assessment

- Inspect the abdomen for distention, ascites, scars, obvious hernias, jaundice, uremic frost, and bruising.
- Auscultate for bowel sounds and characterize their motility.
- Percuss then palpate the abdomen, noting any tenderness, pain, organ enlargement, or tympany.
- Auscultate for gallops and crackles.
- Percuss the lungs to detect consolidation.
- Note peripheral edema and swelling of lymph nodes.

Medical causes

Cholelithiasis

- Dyspepsia may occur, typically after intake of fatty foods.
- Other findings include diaphoresis, tachycardia, chills, low-grade fever, petechiae, bleeding tendencies, jaundice with pruritus, dark urine, clay-colored stools, and biliary colic.

Cirrhosis

- Dyspepsia is relieved by ingestion of an antacid.
- Other GI effects include anorexia, nausea, vomiting, flatulence, weight loss, jaundice, hepatomegaly, ascites, diarrhea, constipation, abdominal distention, and epigastric or right-upper-quadrant pain

Duodenal ulcer

- Dyspepsia ranges from a vague fullness or pressure to a boring or aching sensation.

- Symptom occurs 1½ to 3 hours after eating and is relieved by ingestion of food or antacids.
- Pain may awaken the patient at night with heartburn and fluid regurgitation.

Gastric dilation (acute)

- A life-threatening disorder — epigastric fullness is an early symptom.
- Dyspepsia, nausea, vomiting, upper abdominal distention, succussion splash, and apathy occur.
- Dehydration and gastric bleeding may also occur.

Gastric ulcer

- Dyspepsia and heartburn occur after eating.
- Epigastric pain is a characteristic symptom that may occur with vomiting, fullness, weight loss, GI bleeding, and abdominal distention and may not be relieved by food.

Gastritis (chronic)

- Dyspepsia is relieved by antacids; lessened by smaller, more frequent meals; and aggravated by spicy foods or excessive caffeine.
- Other findings include anorexia, a feeling of fullness, vague epigastric pain, belching, nausea, and vomiting.

GI cancer

- Chronic dyspepsia occurs along with anorexia, fatigue, jaundice, melena, hematemesis, constipation, weight loss, weakness, syncope, and abdominal pain.

Heart failure

- In right-sided heart failure, transient dyspepsia may occur with chest tightness and pain or ache in the right upper quadrant.
- Other findings include hepatomegaly, anorexia, nausea, vomiting, bloating, ascites, tachycardia, jugular vein distention, tachypnea, dyspnea, orthopnea, edema, and fatigue.

Hepatitis

- Before an attack, moderate to severe dyspepsia along with fever, malaise, arthralgia, coryza, myalgia, nausea, vomiting, an altered sense of taste or smell, and hepatomegaly occur.
- Jaundice marks the onset of an attack with continuing dyspepsia, anorexia, irritability, and severe pruritus.
- As jaundice clears, dyspepsia and other GI effects also diminish.

Hiatal hernia

- Dyspepsia occurs with heartburn and retrosternal or substernal chest pain.

Pancreatitis (chronic)

- A feeling of fullness or dyspepsia may occur with epigastric pain that radiates to the back or through the abdomen.

○ Other findings include anorexia, nausea, vomiting, jaundice, dramatic weight loss, Turner's or Cullen's sign, hyperglycemia, and steatorrhea.

Uremia

○ Dyspepsia may be the earliest and most important GI complaint.
○ Other GI findings include anorexia, nausea, vomiting, bloating, diarrhea, abdominal cramps, epigastric pain, and weight gain.
○ As the disease progresses, the patient may experience edema, pruritus, pallor, hyperpigmentation, uremic frost, ecchymoses, irritability, drowsiness, muscle twitching, seizures, and oliguria.

Other causes

Drugs

○ Antibiotics, antihypertensives, corticosteroid, diuretics, nonsteroidal anti-inflammatory drugs, and many other drugs may cause dyspepsia.

Surgery

○ After GI surgery, postoperative gastritis can cause dyspepsia.

Nursing considerations

○ Give an antacid 30 minutes before or 1 hour after a meal.
○ Provide food to relieve dyspepsia.
○ If drugs cause dyspepsia, give them after meals.

Pediatric pointers

○ Dyspepsia may occur in adolescents with peptic ulcer disease, but isn't relieved by food.
○ Dyspepsia may occur with congenital pyloric stenosis, but projectile vomiting after meals is more common.
○ Lactose intolerance may also cause dyspepsia.

Geriatric pointers

○ Most elderly patients with chronic pancreatitis have less severe pain than younger adults; some have no pain at all.

Patient teaching

○ Discuss the importance of small, frequent meals.
○ Describe foods or liquids the patient should avoid.
○ Discuss stress reduction techniques the patient can use.

Dysphagia

Overview

- Refers to difficulty swallowing, the most common symptom of esophageal disorders
- Classified by three phases: transfer (phase 1), transport (phase 2), or entrance (phase 3)
- Increases the risk of choking and aspiration and may lead to malnutrition and dehydration

⚡ Emergency actions

If the patient has signs of respiratory distress, such as dyspnea and stridor, suspect an airway obstruction and quickly perform abdominal thrusts. Administer oxygen and insert an endotracheal tube.

Assessment

History

- Ask about the onset and description of pain.
- Determine aggravating and alleviating factors.
- Ask about recent vomiting, regurgitation, weight loss, anorexia, hoarseness, dyspnea, or cough.

Physical assessment

- Evaluate swallowing and cough reflexes.
- If a good swallow or cough reflex is present, check the gag reflex.
- Listen to the patient's speech for signs of muscle weakness.
- Check the mouth for dry mucous membranes and thick, sticky secretions.
- Observe for tongue and facial weakness and obstructions.
- Assess for disorientation.

Medical causes

Achalasia

- Gradually developing Phase 3 dysphagia, precipitated or exacerbated by stress
- Dysphagia preceded by esophageal colic
- Regurgitation of undigested food, especially at night, causing wheezing, coughing, choking, and halitosis
- Later, weight loss, cachexia, hematemesis, and heartburn

Airway obstruction

- Phase 2 dysphagia with gagging and dysphonia
- When hemorrhage obstructs the trachea, painless rapid-onset dysphagia
- When inflammation causes the obstruction, painful slow-onset dysphagia
- Signs of respiratory distress with life-threatening upper airway obstruction

Amyotrophic lateral sclerosis

- Dysphagia, muscle weakness and atrophy, fasciculations, dysarthria, dyspnea, shallow respirations, tachypnea, slurred speech, hyperactive deep tendon reflexes, and emotional lability

Botulism

- Dysphagia (phase 1) and dysuria usually within 36 hours of toxin ingestion
- Blurred or double vision, dry mouth, sore throat, nausea, vomiting, and diarrhea
- Gradual symmetrical descending weakness or paralysis

Bulbar paralysis

- Painful and progressive phase 1 dysphagia with drooling, difficulty chewing, dysarthria, and nasal regurgitation
- Arm and leg spasticity, hyperreflexia, and emotional lability

Esophageal cancer

- Painless dysphagia (phases 2 and 3) with weight loss are the earliest and most common findings.
- As the cancer advances, dysphagia becomes painful and is accompanied by steady chest pain, cough with hemoptysis, hoarseness, and sore throat.
- Other findings include nausea, vomiting, fever, hiccups, hematemesis, melena, and halitosis.

Esophageal diverticulum

- Phase 3 dysphagia when the enlarged diverticulum obstructs the esophagus
- Regurgitation, chronic cough, hoarseness, chest pain, and halitosis

Esophageal obstruction by foreign body

- Sudden onset of phase 2 or 3 dysphagia with gagging, coughing, and esophageal pain
- If the obstruction compresses the trachea, dyspnea

Esophageal spasm

- Phase 2 dysphagia for solids and liquids occurs along with substernal chest pain.
- Pain may radiate and be relieved by drinking water.
- Bradycardia may occur.

Esophageal stricture

- Phase 3 dysphagia occurs, possibly with drooling, tachypnea, and gagging.
- With chemical ingestion, burns, ulcers, or erythema of the lips and mouth may develop.

Esophagitis

- Corrosive esophagitis, resulting from ingestion of alkalis or acids, causes severe phase 3 dysphagia with marked salivation, hematemesis, tachypnea, fever, and intense pain in the mouth and chest that's aggravated by swallowing.

- Candidal esophagitis causes phase 2 dysphagia, sore throat and, possibly, retrosternal pain on swallowing.
- With reflux esophagitis, phase 3 dysphagia is a late symptom with heartburn; regurgitation; vomiting; a dry, nocturnal cough; and substernal chest pain.

Hypocalcemia

- Phase 1 dysphagia with numbness and tingling in the nose, ears, fingertips, and toes, and around the mouth
- Tetany with carpopedal spasms, muscle twitching, and laryngeal spasms

Laryngeal cancer (extrinsic)

- Phase 2 dysphagia and dyspnea develop late.
- Other findings include muffled voice, stridor, pain, halitosis, weight loss, ipsilateral otalgia, chronic cough, and cachexia.

Lead poisoning

- Painless, progressive dysphagia
- A lead line on the gums, metallic taste, papilledema, ocular palsy, footdrop or wristdrop, mental impairment, seizures, and signs of hemolytic anemia

Lower esophageal ring

- Phase 3 dysphagia occurs with feeling of a foreign body in the lower esophagus that may be relieved by drinking water or vomiting.

Myasthenia gravis

- Painless phase 1 dysphagia after ptosis and diplopia
- Masklike facies, nasal voice, nasal regurgitation, shallow respirations, dyspnea, and head bobbing

Oral cavity tumor

- Painful phase 1 dysphagia with hoarseness and ulcerating lesions
- Abnormal taste or bleeding in the mouth or dentures that no longer fit

Parkinson's disease

- Late, painless progressive phase 1 dysphagia, causing choking
- Bradykinesia, tremors, muscle rigidity, dysarthria, masklike facies, muffled voice, increased salivation and lacrimation, constipation, stooped posture, propulsive gait, and incontinence

Pharyngitis (chronic)

- Painful phase 2 dysphagia with a dry, sore throat; cough; and thick mucus and sensation of fullness in the throat

Progressive systemic sclerosis

- Preceded by Raynaud's phenomenon, mild dysphagia worsening until only liquids can be swallowed
- Heartburn, weight loss, abdominal distention, diarrhea, and malodorous, floating stools

- Joint pain and stiffness, masklike facies, thickening of the skin that progresses to taut, shiny skin

Rabies

- A life-threatening disorder — phase 2 dysphagia of liquids
- Signs of dehydration, drooling, hydrophobia, and progressive flaccid paralysis that leads to vascular collapse, coma, and death

Tetanus

- Phase 1 dysphagia about a week after the unimmunized patient receives a puncture wound
- Marked muscle hypotonicity, hyperactive deep tendon reflexes, tachycardia, diaphoresis, drooling, trismus (lockjaw), risus sardonicus, opisthotonos, boardlike abdominal rigidity, seizures, and low-grade fever

Other causes

Procedures

- Recent tracheostomy, or repeated or prolonged intubation may cause temporary dysphagia.

Radiation therapy

- Radiation therapy for oral cancer may cause scant salivation and temporary dysphagia.

Nursing considerations

- Stimulate salivation by talking about food, adding a lemon slice or dill pickle to food tray, and providing mouth care.
- With decreased salivation, moisten food with liquid.
- Give an anticholinergic or antiemetic to control excess salivation.
- Consult with the dietitian to select foods with distinct temperatures and textures.
- Consult a therapist to assess the patient's aspiration risk and to begin exercises to aid swallowing.

Pediatric pointers

- Coughing, choking, or regurgitation during feeding suggests dysphagia.
- Dysphagia in children may result from corrosive esophagitis, esophageal obstruction by a foreign body (most common), and congenital anomalies.

Geriatric pointers

- In patients older than age 50, dysphagia is typically the first complaint in cases of head or neck cancer.

Patient teaching

- Discuss easy-to-swallow foods.
- Explain measures the patient can take to reduce the risk of choking and aspiration.

Dyspnea

Overview

- Shortness of breath
- Indicates cardiopulmonary dysfunction
- Arises suddenly or slowly and subsides rapidly or persists for years

Emergency actions

Look for signs of respiratory distress. Give oxygen if needed. Ensure patent I.V. access and begin cardiac and oxygen saturation monitoring. Insert a chest tube for severe pneumothorax and for continuous positive airway pressure. Intubation and mechanical ventilation may be needed.

Assessment

History

- Ask about the onset and progression.
- Determine aggravating and alleviating factors.
- Ask the patient if he has a cough.
- Obtain a history, including trauma, upper respiratory tract infection, deep vein phlebitis, orthopnea, paroxysmal nocturnal dyspnea, fatigue, smoking, or exposure to occupational hazards.
- Ask about current orthopnea, paroxysmal nocturnal dyspnea, or progressive fatigue.

Physical assessment

- Look for pursed-lip exhalation, clubbing, peripheral edema, barrel chest, diaphoresis, jugular vein distention, and edema.
- Take vital signs.
- Auscultate for crackles, egophony, bronchophony, abnormal heart sounds or rhythms, and whispered pectoriloquy.
- Palpate the abdomen for hepatomegaly.

Medical causes

Acute respiratory distress syndrome

- A life-threatening condition — acute dyspnea usually first complaint
- Progressive respiratory distress with restlessness, anxiety, decreased mental acuity, tachycardia, and crackles and rhonchi
- Cyanosis, tachypnea, motor dysfunction, intercostal and suprasternal retractions, and shock

Amyotrophic lateral sclerosis

- Slow-onset dyspnea worsening with time
- Dysphagia, dysarthria, muscle weakness and atrophy, fasciculations, shallow respirations, tachypnea, and emotional lability

Anemia

- Gradual dyspnea
- Fatigue, weakness, syncope, tachycardia, tachypnea, restlessness, and anxiety
- Pallor, inability to concentrate, irritability, dysphagia, smooth tongue, and spoon-shaped and brittle nails

Anthrax (inhalation)

- A life-threatening disorder — dyspnea occurs in the second stage, with fever, stridor and hypotension
- Fever, chills, weakness, cough, and chest pain

Asthma

- Dyspneic attacks with audible wheezing, dry cough, accessory muscle use, nasal flaring, intercostal and supraclavicular retractions, tachypnea, tachycardia, diaphoresis, prolonged expiration, flush or cyanosis, and apprehension

Cor pulmonale

- Chronic dyspnea begins gradually with exertion and progressively worsens until it occurs at rest.
- Other findings include chronic productive cough, wheezing, tachypnea, jugular vein distention, edema, fatigue, weakness, and hepatomegaly.

Emphysema

- Progressive exertional dyspnea occurs.
- Other findings include barrel chest, accessory muscle use, diminished breath sounds, anorexia, weight loss, malaise, peripheral cyanosis, tachypnea, pursed-lip breathing, prolonged expiration, a chronic and productive cough, and late clubbing.

Flail chest

- Sudden dyspnea is accompanied by paradoxical chest movement, severe chest pain, hypotension, tachypnea, tachycardia, and cyanosis.
- Bruising and decreased or absent breath sounds occur over the affected side.

Guillain-Barré syndrome

- Slowly worsening dyspnea with fatigue, ascending muscle weakness and paralysis following a fever and upper respiratory tract infection
- Facial diplegia, dysphagia or dysarthria and, less commonly, weakness of the muscles supplied by cranial nerve XI

Heart failure

- Gradual dyspnea with orthopnea, tachypnea, tachycardia, palpitations, ventricular gallop, fatigue, dependent edema, jugular vein distention, paroxysmal nocturnal dyspnea, hepatosplenomegaly, cough, and weight gain

Inhalation injury

- Sudden dyspnea or over several hours with sooty or bloody sputum, persistent cough, and oropharyngeal edema

○ Orofacial burns, singed nasal hairs, crackles, rhonchi, wheezing, and signs of respiratory distress

Lung cancer

○ Slow-developing and progressively worsening dyspnea
○ Fever, hemoptysis, productive cough, wheezing, clubbing, pain, weight loss, anorexia, and pleural rub

Myasthenia gravis

○ Bouts of dyspnea with difficulty chewing and swallowing
○ With myasthenic crisis, acute respiratory distress with shallow respirations and tachypnea

Myocardial infarction

○ Sudden dyspnea with crushing substernal chest pain that may radiate to the back, neck, jaw, and arms
○ Nausea, vomiting, diaphoresis, vertigo, tachycardia, anxiety, and pale, cool, clammy skin

Plague

○ A life-threatening disorder—dyspnea, a productive cough, chest pain, tachypnea, hemoptysis, increasing respiratory distress, and cardiopulmonary insufficiency
○ Chills, fever, headache, and myalgia at the onset

Pleural effusion

○ Dyspnea develops slowly and progressively worsens.
○ Initial findings include pleural friction rub and pleuritic pain, worsening cough, and deep breathing.
○ Other findings include dry cough, dullness on percussion, tachycardia, tachypnea, weight loss, fever, and decreased breath sounds.

Pneumonia

○ Sudden dyspnea with fever, shaking chills, pleuritic chest pain, and a productive cough
○ Fatigue, headache, myalgia, anorexia, abdominal pain, crackles, rhonchi, tachycardia, tachypnea, cyanosis, decreased breath sounds, and diaphoresis

Pneumothorax

○ Acute dyspnea that's unrelated to the severity of pain
○ Sudden, stabbing chest pain radiating to the arms, face, back, or abdomen
○ Anxiety, restlessness, dry cough, cyanosis, tachypnea, decreased or absent breath sounds on the affected side, splinting, and accessory muscle use

Pulmonary edema

○ Acute dyspnea preceded by signs of heart failure
○ Tachycardia, tachypnea, crackles, ventricular gallop, thready pulse, hypotension, diaphoresis, cyanosis, marked anxiety, and a cough that's dry or productive of copious amounts of pink, frothy sputum

Pulmonary embolism

○ A life-threatening disorder—acute dyspnea usually with sudden pleuritic chest pain

○ Tachycardia, low-grade fever, tachypnea, pleural rub, crackles, diffuse wheezing, dullness on percussion, nonproductive cough or productive cough with blood-tinged sputum, decreased breath sounds, diaphoresis, anxiety and, with a massive embolism, signs of shock

Severe acute respiratory syndrome

○ A life-threatening disorder—fever with headache; malaise; a dry, nonproductive cough; and dyspnea

Shock

○ A life-threatening disorder— sudden dyspnea that worsens progressively
○ Severe hypotension, tachypnea, tachycardia, decreased peripheral pulses, decreased mental acuity, restlessness, anxiety, and cool, clammy skin

Tuberculosis

○ Dyspnea with chest pain, crackles, and productive cough
○ Night sweats, fever, anorexia, weight loss, palpitations on mild exertion, and dullness on percussion

Tularemia

○ Dyspnea with fever, chills, headache, generalized myalgia, pleuritic chest pain, empyema, and a nonproductive cough
○ Diaphoresis, weight loss, and a red spot on the skin that becomes an ulcer

Nursing considerations

○ Monitor the patient closely.
○ Position the patient comfortably, usually in high Fowler's or forward-leaning position.
○ Administer oxygen if needed.
○ Give a bronchodilator, an antiarrhythmic, a diuretic, and an analgesic as needed.

Pediatric pointers

○ Suspect dyspnea in an infant who breathes costally, an older child who breathes abdominally, or any child who uses his neck or shoulder muscles to help him breathe.
○ Acute epiglottiditis and laryngotracheobronchitis can cause severe dyspnea in a child.

Geriatric pointers

○ An older patient with dyspnea from chronic illness may not be aware of a significant change in his breathing pattern.

Patient teaching

○ Teach the patient about pursed-lip, diaphragmatic breathing, and chest splinting.
○ Instruct the patient to avoid chemical irritants, pollutants, and people with respiratory infections.

Dysuria

Overview

- Painful or difficult urination
- Commonly accompanied by urinary frequency, urgency, or hesitancy
- Important clue about cause: when and how the pain began

Assessment

History

- Ask about the onset, severity, and location of dysuria.
- Find out about aggravating and alleviating factors.
- Obtain a medical history, including urinary or genital tract infections, invasive procedures, intestinal disease, and menstrual disorders and vaginal discharge.
- Note the use of products that irritate the urinary tract.

Physical assessment

- Ask the patient to void before beginning your examination.
- Inspect the urethral meatus for discharge, irritation, and other abnormalities.
- Percuss over the kidneys and costovertebral angle.
- Percuss the bladder.
- Palpate the kidneys and bladder. (See *Palpating the kidneys.*)
- Perform a pelvic or rectal examination, if needed.

Medical causes

Appendicitis

- Occasionally, dysuria persists throughout voiding and is accompanied by bladder tenderness.
- Characteristic findings include periumbilical abdominal pain that shifts to McBurney's point, anorexia, nausea, vomiting, constipation, slight fever, abdominal rigidity and rebound tenderness, and tachycardia.

Bladder cancer

- Dysuria throughout voiding is a late symptom.
- Other findings include urinary frequency and urgency, nocturia, hematuria, and perineal, back, or flank pain.

Cystitis

- Dysuria throughout voiding, urinary frequency, nocturia, straining to void, and hematuria are common.
- Bacterial cystitis may produce urinary urgency, perineal and lower back pain, suprapubic discomfort, fatigue, and low-grade fever.

- Chronic interstitial cystitis produces cystitis at the end of voiding.
- Viral cystitis causes severe dysuria with gross hematuria, urinary urgency, and fever.
- In tubercular cystitis, findings also include urinary urgency, flank pain, fatigue, and anorexia.

Diverticulitis

- Inflammation near the bladder may cause dysuria throughout voiding.
- Other effects include urinary frequency and urgency, nocturia, hematuria, fever, abdominal pain and tenderness, perineal pain, constipation or diarrhea and, possibly, an abdominal mass.

Paraurethral gland inflammation

- Dysuria throughout voiding occurs with urinary frequency and urgency, diminished urine stream, mild perineal pain and, occasionally, hematuria.

Prostatitis

- Acute prostatitis causes dysuria throughout or toward the end of voiding.
- Other findings include a diminished urine stream, urinary frequency and urgency, hematuria, suprapubic fullness, fever, chills, fatigue, myalgia, nausea, vomiting, and constipation.
- With chronic prostatitis, urethral narrowing causes dysuria throughout voiding; urinary frequency and urgency; diminished urine stream; perineal, back, and buttocks pain; urethral discharge; nocturia; and, at times, hematospermia and ejaculatory pain.

Pyelonephritis (acute)

- Dysuria occurs throughout voiding.
- Other symptoms include high fever, costovertebral angle tenderness, flank pain, urinary urgency and frequency, nausea, vomiting, anorexia, and hematuria.

Reiter's syndrome

- Dysuria occurs 1 to 2 weeks after sexual contact with infected person.
- A mucopurulent discharge, urinary urgency and frequency, meatal swelling and redness, suprapubic pain, anorexia, weight loss, and low-grade fever occur initially.
- Hematuria, conjunctivitis, arthritic symptoms, a papular rash, and oral and penile lesions may follow.

Urethral syndrome

- In sexually active women, dysuria throughout voiding may occur with urinary frequency, diminished urine stream, suprapubic aching and cramping, tenesmus, and lower back and flank pain.

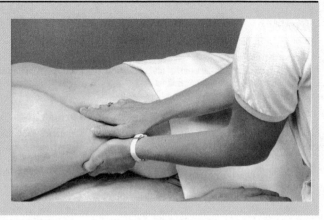

To palpate the kidneys, first have the patient lie in a supine position. To palpate the right kidney, stand on his right side. Place your left hand under his back and your right hand on his abdomen.

Instruct him to inhale deeply, so his kidney moves downward. As he inhales, press up with your left hand and down with your right, as shown.

Urethritis

○ In sexually active men, dysuria occurs throughout voiding and is accompanied by a reddened meatus and copious, yellow, purulent discharge (gonorrheal infection) or white or clear mucoid discharge (non-gonorrheal infection).

Urinary obstruction

○ Dysuria occurs throughout voiding, with diminished urine stream, urinary frequency and urgency, and a sensation of fullness or bloating in the lower abdomen or groin.
○ With complete obstruction, bladder distention develops and dysuria precedes voiding.

Vaginitis

○ Dysuria occurs throughout voiding along with urinary frequency and urgency, nocturia, hematuria, perineal pain, and vaginal discharge and odor.

Other causes

Chemical irritants

○ Bubble bath, bath salts, feminine deodorants, and spermicides can cause dysuria.

Drugs

○ Monoamine oxidase inhibitors and metyrosine can cause dysuria.

Nursing considerations

○ Monitor vital signs and intake and output.
○ Give drugs as needed.

Geriatric pointers

○ Elderly patients may underreport urinary-related symptoms.
○ Older men have an increased incidence of nonsexual urinary tract infections.
○ Postmenopausal women have an increased incidence of noninfectious dysuria.

Patient teaching

○ Explain the importance of increased fluid intake.
○ Emphasize the importance of frequent urination.
○ Teach the patient to perform proper perineal care.
○ Discourage the use of bubble baths and vaginal deodorants.
○ Discuss the importance of taking prescribed drugs as instructed.

Earache

Overview

- Known as *otalgia*
- Caused by disorders of the external and middle ear from infection, obstruction, or trauma
- Ranges from a feeling of fullness or blockage to deep, boring pain

Assessment

History

- Ask about the onset and description of the pain.
- Inquire about recent head cold or problems with mouth, sinuses, or throat.
- Find out about aggravating and alleviating factors.
- Ask about itching, drainage, ringing noises, dizziness, vertigo, and pain when mouth opens.
- Ask about recent airplane travel, travel to high altitudes, or scuba diving.
- Obtain a medical history, including head colds or problems with the eyes, mouth, teeth, jaw, sinuses, and throat.

Physical assessment

- Inspect external ear for redness, drainage, swelling, or deformity.
- Apply pressure to mastoid process and tragus to check for tenderness.
- Using an otoscope, examine external auditory canal for lesions, bleeding or other discharge, impacted cerumen, foreign bodies, tenderness, or swelling. (See *Using an otoscope*.)
- Examine the tympanic membrane.
- Perform tests for hearing loss.

Medical causes

Abscess (extradural)

- Severe earache is accompanied by persistent ipsilateral headache, malaise, hearing loss, and recurrent mild fever.

Barotrauma (acute)

- Earache ranges from mild pressure to severe pain.
- Tympanic membrane ecchymoses or bleeding into the tympanic cavity may occur.

Cerumen impaction

- Produces blockage or fullness in the ear accompanied by partial hearing loss, itching, dizziness, and ringing in the ear.

Chondrodermatitis nodularis chronica

- Small, painful, indurated areas develop along the upper rim of the auricle.
- Lesion may have a central core with scaly discharge.

Frostbite

- Burning or tingling pain may occur in the ear, followed by numbness.
- Ear appears mottled and gray or white and turns purplish as it warms.

Furunculosis

- Infected hair follicles in the outer ear canal may produce severe, localized ear pain from a pus-filled furuncle.
- Pain is aggravated by jaw movement and relived by rupture or incision of the furuncle.
- Other findings include pinna tenderness, swelling of the auditory meatus, partial hearing loss, and a feeling of fullness in the ear canal.

Herpes zoster oticus

- Burning or stabbing pain typically in the ear vesicles.
- Other findings include hearing loss; vertigo; transitory, ipsilateral, facial paralysis; partial loss of taste; tongue vesicles; and nausea and vomiting.

Mastoiditis (acute)

- Dull ache behind the ear is accompanied by low-grade fever and purulent discharge.
- Eardrum appears dull and edematous and may perforate, and soft tissue near the eardrum may sag.

Ménière's disease

- A sensation of fullness may occur in the affected ear with severe vertigo, tinnitus, and sensorineural hearing loss.
- Other findings include nausea, vomiting, diaphoresis, and nystagmus.

Middle ear tumor

- Deep, boring ear pain and facial paralysis are late signs.
- Hearing loss and facial nerve dysfunction may develop.

Otitis externa (acute)

- Initially, pain is mild to moderate and occurs with tragus manipulation.
- Later, ear pain intensifies, causing the side of the head to ache.
- Other findings include fever; sticky yellow or purulent discharge; partial hearing loss; a feeling of blockage; swelling of the tragus, external meatus, and external ear canal; reddened eardrum; lymphadenopathy; dizziness; and malaise.

When the patient reports an earache, use an otoscope to inspect the ear structures closely. Follow these techniques to obtain the best view and ensure the patient's safety.

Child younger than age 3
To inspect a young child's ear, grasp the lower part of the auricle and pull it down and back to straighten the upward S curve of the external canal. Then gently insert the speculum into the canal no more than ½″ (1.3 cm).

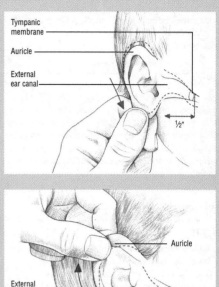

Adult
To inspect an adult's ear, grasp the upper part of the auricle and pull it up and back to straighten the external canal. Then insert the speculum about 1″ (2.5 cm). Also use this technique for children age 3 and older.

Otitis media (acute)

○ Acute serous otitis media may cause a feeling of fullness in the ear, hearing loss, and a vague sensation of top-heaviness.
○ Acute suppurative otitis media involves severe, deep, throbbing ear pain, hearing loss, and fever.

Petrositis

○ Infection produces deep ear pain with headache and pain behind the eye.
○ Other findings include diplopia, loss of lateral gaze, vomiting, sensorineural hearing loss, vertigo, and, possibly, nuchal rigidity.

Temporomandibular joint infection

○ Ear pain is referred from the jaw joint.
○ Pain is aggravated by pressure on the joint with jaw movement and may radiate to the temporal area or entire side of the head.

Nursing considerations

○ Give an analgesic.
○ Apply heat to relieve discomfort.
○ Instill eardrops.

Pediatric pointers

○ Common causes of earache in children are acute otitis media and insertion of foreign bodies that become lodged or cause infection.
○ In a child not old enough to speak, ear tugging and crying may indicate an earache.

Patient teaching

○ Teach the patient or caregiver to instill eardrops correctly.
○ Explain the importance of taking prescribed antibiotics correctly.
○ Explain ways to avoid vertigo.
○ Instruct the patient or caregiver about ways to avoid ear trauma.

Edema, generalized

Overview

- Excessive accumulation of interstitial fluid throughout the body
- Chronic and progressive

✦ Emergency actions

If the patient has severe edema, take his vital signs and determine the degree of pitting. Check for jugular vein distention and cyanotic lips. Auscultate the lungs and heart. Look for signs of heart failure or pulmonary congestion. Place the patient in Fowler's position and prepare to administer oxygen and an I.V. diuretic. Have emergency resuscitation equipment nearby.

Assessment

History

- Note the onset, location, and description of edema.
- Ask about shortness of breath or pain.
- Obtain a medical history, including previous burns and cardiac, renal, hepatic, endocrine, and GI disorders.
- Find out about recent weight gain and urine output changes.
- Ask the patient to describe his diet.
- Obtain a drug history.

Physical assessment

- Compare the patient's arms and legs for symmetrical edema.
- Note ecchymoses and cyanosis.
- Assess the back, sacrum, and hips of a bedridden patient for dependent edema.
- Palpate peripheral pulses, noting any coolness in hands and feet.
- Perform complete cardiac and respiratory assessments.

Medical causes

Angioneurotic edema or angioedema

- Recurrent attacks of acute, painless, nonpitting edema involve the skin and mucous membranes.
- Abdominal pain, nausea, vomiting, and diarrhea accompany visceral edema.
- Dyspnea and stridor accompany life-threatening laryngeal edema.

Burns

- Severe generalized edema may occur within 2 days of a major burn.

- Depending on the degree of edema, signs and symptoms of reduced or absent circulation and airway obstruction may occur.

Cirrhosis

- Edema is a late sign.
- Other findings include abdominal pain, anorexia, nausea, vomiting, hepatomegaly, ascites, jaundice, pruritus, bleeding tendencies, musty breath, lethargy, mental changes, and asterixis.

Heart failure

- Severe, generalized pitting edema may follow leg edema.
- Edema may improve with exercise or elevation of limbs and is worst at the end of day.
- Other classic late findings include hemoptysis, cyanosis, clubbing, crackles marked hepatosplenomegaly, and a ventricular gallop.

Myxedema

- Generalized nonpitting edema is accompanied by dry, flaky, inelastic, waxy, pale skin; puffy face; and upper eyelid droop.
- Other findings include masklike facies, hair loss or coarsening, hoarseness, weight gain, fatigue, cold intolerance, bradycardia, constipation, abdominal distention, menorrhagia, impotence, and infertility.

Nephrotic syndrome

- Edema is initially localized around the eyes, and then becomes generalized and pitting.
- Anasarca develops in severe cases.
- Other common findings include ascites, anorexia, fatigue, malaise, depression, and pallor.

Pericardial effusion

- Generalized pitting edema may be most prominent in arms and legs.
- Other findings include chest pain, dyspnea, orthopnea, nonproductive cough, pericardial friction rub, jugular vein distention, dysphagia, and fever.

Renal failure

- Generalized pitting edema occurs as a late sign.
- With chronic renal failure, edema is less likely to become generalized; its severity depends on the degree of fluid overload.
- Other findings include oliguria, anorexia, nausea, vomiting, drowsiness, confusion, hypertension, dyspnea, crackles, dizziness, and pallor.

Septic shock

- A life-threatening disorder — a late sign, generalized edema typically develops rapidly.
- Edema is pitting, moderately severe and other findings include cool skin, hypotension, oliguria, anxiety, and signs of respiratory failure.

Other causes

Drugs

○ Drugs that cause sodium retention — such as anti-hypertensives, corticosteroids, androgenic and ana-bolic steroids, estrogens, and nonsteroidal anti-inflammatory drugs — may aggravate or cause generalized edema.
○ In patients with cardiac or renal disease, I.V. saline solution infusions and enteral feedings may cause sodium and fluid overload, resulting in generalized edema.

Treatments

○ Enteral feedings and I.V. saline solution infusions may cause sodium and fluid overload.

Nursing considerations

○ Position the patient with his limbs above heart level to promote drainage.
○ Periodically reposition the patient.
○ If the patient develops dyspnea, lower the limbs, elevate the head of the bed, and administer oxygen.
○ Prevent skin breakdown by placing a pressure mattress on the patient's bed.
○ Restrict fluids and sodium, and administer a diuretic or I.V. albumin.
○ Monitor intake and output and daily weight.
○ Monitor electrolyte levels.

Pediatric pointers

○ Renal failure typically causes generalized edema; kwashiorkor causes massive generalized edema.

Geriatric pointers

○ Use caution when giving I.V. fluids or drugs that can raise sodium levels.

Patient teaching

○ Explain signs and symptoms of edema that the patient should report.
○ Discuss foods and fluids the patient should avoid.

Edema of the arm

Overview

○ Results from excess interstitial fluid in the arm
○ Signals localized fluid imbalance between the vascular and interstitial spaces

 Emergency actions

Remove rings, bracelets, and watches from the affected arm. With neuromuscular compromise, elevate the arm.

Assessment

History

○ Ask when the edema began.
○ Find out about arm pain, numbness, or tingling.
○ Find out what alleviates and aggravates the edema.
○ Take a medical history, noting recent injury, I.V. therapy, surgery, or radiation therapy.

Physical assessment

○ Compare the size and symmetry of arms and test for pitting. (See *Differentiating between pitting and nonpitting edema.*)
○ Examine and compare the color and temperature of both arms.
○ Look for erythema, ecchymoses, and wounds.
○ Palpate both arms and compare their pulses.
○ Look for arm tenderness and decreased sensation or mobility.

Medical causes

Angioneurotic edema

○ Sudden, painless, nonpruritic edema affects hands, feet, eyelids, lips, face, neck, or viscera.

Arm trauma

○ Severe edema in the entire arm
○ Ecchymoses or superficial bleeding, pain or numbness, deformity if the arm is fractured, and possibly, paralysis

Burns

○ Within two days of injury, mild to severe edema, pain, and tissue damage may develop.

> **Assessment tip**
> ### Differentiating between pitting and nonpitting edema
>
> To distinguish pitting from nonpitting edema, press your finger against a swollen area for 5 seconds, then quickly remove it.
>
> With **pitting edema,** pressure forces fluid into the underlying tissues, causing an indentation that slowly fills. To determine the severity of pitting edema, estimate the indentation's depth in centimeters: 1+ (1 cm), 2+ (2 cm), 3+ (3 cm), or 4+ (4 cm).
>
> With **nonpitting edema,** pressure leaves no indentation because fluid has coagulated in the tissues. Typically, the skin feels unusually tight and firm.

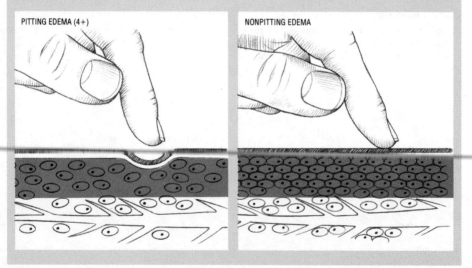

PITTING EDEMA (4+)   NONPITTING EDEMA

○ Depending on the burn degree, the arm may have erythema; blisters; white, brown, or leathery tissue; or charring.

Envenomation

○ Initially, edema may develop around the bite or sting and quickly spread to the entire arm.
○ Pain, erythema, pruritus, and paresthesia may occur.
○ Later, nausea, vomiting, weakness, muscle cramps, fever, chills, hypotension, headache develop.
○ In severe cases, dyspnea, seizures, and paralysis occur.

Superior vena cava syndrome

○ Edema in both arms usually progresses slowly and is accompanied by edema in the face and neck.
○ Other findings include dilated veins over edematous area, headache, vertigo, and vision disturbances.

Thrombophlebitis

○ Arm edema, pain, and warmth may occur.
○ Cyanosis, fever, chills, and malaise also occur with deep vein thrombosis.
○ Redness, tenderness, and induration along the vein occur with superficial vein thrombosis.

Other causes

Treatments

○ Infiltration of I.V. fluid into the interstitial tissue may cause localized arm edema.
○ Axillary node dissection and mastectomy that disrupts lymphatic drainage may cause edema of the entire arm.
○ Radiation therapy for breast cancer may cause arm edema.

Nursing considerations

○ Elevate the arm and frequently reposition the patient.
○ Use bandages and dressings as needed to promote drainage.
○ Care for the patient's skin to prevent breakdown of skin and formation of pressure ulcers.
○ Give an analgesic and anticoagulant as needed.

Pediatric pointers

○ Arm edema rarely occurs in children, but it may result from burns or crush injuries.

Patient teaching

○ Instruct the patient in postoperative arm care.
○ Teach the patient arm exercises that will help to prevent lymphedema.

Edema of the face

Overview

○ Involves localized or generalized facial swelling
○ May extend to neck and upper arms

⚡ Emergency actions

If a patient has facial edema from burns or recent exposure to an allergen, quickly assess his respiratory system. If you detect respiratory distress, give epinephrine. For patients with absent breath sounds and cyanosis, tracheal intubation, cricothyroidotomy, or tracheotomy may be needed. Always administer oxygen.

Assessment

History

○ Ask about the onset (sudden or gradual) and description of facial edema.
○ Ask about changes in urine color or output.
○ Note changes in appetite.
○ Take a drug history.
○ Ask about recent facial trauma.

Physical assessment

○ Describe severity, pitting, and location of edema. (See *Recognizing angioneurotic edema.*)
○ Take vital signs.
○ Assess neurologic condition.
○ Examine the oral cavity.
○ Visualize the oropharynx and look for soft-tissue swelling.

Medical causes

Abscess (periodontal)

○ Edema of the side of the face, pain, warmth, erythema, and purulent discharge around the affected tooth occur.
○ Gums may be bright red and inflamed.

Abscess (peritonsillar)

○ Facial edema with severe throat pain, neck swelling, drooling, cervical adenopathy, fever, chills, and malaise

Allergic reaction

○ Facial edema may develop.
○ With life-threatening anaphylaxis, angioneurotic facial edema may occur with urticaria and flushing.
○ Airway edema causes hoarseness, stridor, bronchospasm, dyspnea, tachypnea and, possibly, signs of shock.

Chalazion

○ Localized swelling and tenderness of the affected eyelid with a small red lump on the conjunctiva
○ Tearing and photophobia

Conjunctivitis

○ Eyelid edema, excessive tearing, and itchy, burning eyes
○ Thick purulent discharge, crusty eyelids, conjunctival injection and, with corneal involvement, photophobia and pain

Corneal ulcers (fungal)

○ Red, edematous eyelids with conjunctival injection, intense pain, photophobia, severely impaired visual acuity, and copious, purulent eye discharge
○ A dense, central ulcer grows slowly, is whitish gray, and is surrounded by progressively clearer rings

Dacryocystitis

○ Prominent eyelid edema with constant tearing, pain, tenderness, and purulent discharge

Facial burns

○ Extensive edema may develop, impairing respiration.
○ Additional findings include singed nasal hairs and eyebrows, red mucosa, sooty sputum, and signs of respiratory distress.

Facial trauma

○ Extent of edema and other findings vary with the type of injury.
○ Contusion may cause localized edema; nasal or maxillary fractures cause more generalized edema.

Herpes zoster ophthalmicus

○ Edematous and red eyelids with excessive tearing and a serous discharge
○ Severe facial pain occurring several days before vesicles erupt, fever, and malaise

Hordeolum

○ Localized eyelid edema, erythema, photophobia, foreign-body sensation, and pain

Malnutrition

○ Facial edema followed by swelling of the feet and legs
○ Muscle atrophy and weakness; anorexia; diarrhea; lethargy; dry, wrinkled skin; sparse, brittle hair; and slowed pulse and respiratory rates.

Myxedema

○ Generalized facial edema with waxy, dry skin; hair loss or coarsening; upper eyelid drooping, and other signs of hypothyroidism

Nephrotic syndrome

○ Periorbital edema is typically the first sign and precedes dependent and abdominal edema.

○ Other findings include weight gain, nausea, anorexia, lethargy, fatigue, and pallor.

Orbital cellulitis

○ Sudden onset of periorbital edema
○ Purulent discharge, hyperemia, exophthalmos, conjunctival injection, impaired extraocular movements, fever, and extreme orbital pain

Preeclampsia

○ Edema of the face, hands, and ankles is an early sign.
○ Other characteristics include excessive weight gain, severe headache, blurred vision, hypertension, and midepigastric pain.

Rhinitis (allergic)

○ Red, edematous eyelids are accompanied by paroxysmal sneezing, itchy nose and eyes, and profuse, watery rhinorrhea.
○ Other findings include nasal congestion, excessive tearing, headache, sinus pain, malaise, and fever.

Sinusitis

○ Frontal sinusitis causes edema of the forehead and eyelids.
○ Maxillary sinusitis produces edema in the maxillary area as well as malaise, gingival swelling, and trismus.
○ Findings common to both include facial pain, fever, nasal congestion, purulent nasal discharge, and red, swollen nasal mucosa.

Superior vena cava syndrome

○ Gradually developing facial and neck edema with thoracic vein or jugular vein distention
○ Headache, vision disturbances, and vertigo

Other causes

Diagnostic tests

○ Allergic reaction to contrast media may produce facial edema.

Drugs

○ Long-term use of glucocorticoids and allergic reactions to drugs (such as aspirin, antipyretics, penicillin, and sulfa preparations) may produce facial edema.
○ Ingestion of the fruit pulp of ginkgo biloba can cause severe erythema and edema and the rapid formation of vesicles.

Surgery and transfusion

○ Cranial, nasal, or jaw surgery may cause facial edema.
○ A blood transfusion that causes an allergic reaction may cause facial edema.

Most dramatic in the lips, eyelids, and tongue, angioneurotic edema typically results from an allergic reaction. It's characterized by rapid onset of painless, nonpitting, subcutaneous swelling that usually resolves in 1 to 2 days. This type of edema may also involve the hands, feet, genitalia, and viscera; laryngeal edema may cause life-threatening airway obstruction.

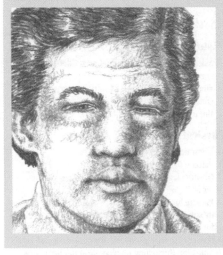

Nursing considerations

○ Administer an analgesic for pain.
○ Apply a topical drug to reduce itching.
○ Apply cold compresses to the eyes.
○ Elevate the head of the bed to help drain the accumulated fluid.

Pediatric pointers

○ Children are more likely to develop periorbital edema because of lower periorbital tissue pressure.

Patient teaching

○ Explain the risks of delayed allergy symptoms.
○ Explain which signs and symptoms the patient or caregiver should report.
○ Discuss ways to avoid allergens and insect bites or stings.
○ Emphasize the importance of having an anaphylaxis kit and medical identification bracelet.

Edema of the leg

Overview

- Results when excess interstitial fluid accumulates in one or both legs
- May be slight or dramatic, pitting or nonpitting, and affect just the foot or extend to the thigh

Assessment

History

- Ask about the onset (gradual or sudden) and description of edema.
- Find out about recent leg injury, surgery, or illness.
- Obtain a drug history.
- Inquire about a history of cardiovascular disease.

Physical assessment

- Examine legs for pitting edema.
- Palpate or auscultate peripheral pulses.
- Observe leg color and look for unusual vein patterns.
- Palpate for warmth, tenderness, and cords, and gently squeeze the calf muscle against the tibia to check for deep pain.
- If edema is only in one leg, look for Homans' sign.
- Note skin thickening or ulceration in edematous areas.

Medical causes

Burns

- Two days or less after injury, mild to severe edema, pain, and tissue damage may occur.
- Depending on the degree of the burn, the leg may have erythema; blisters; white, brown, or leathery tissue; or charring.

Cellulitis

- Pitting edema and orange peel skin with erythema, warmth, and tenderness in the infected area

Envenomation

- Mild to severe localized edema may develop suddenly at the site of bite or sting.
- Other findings include erythema, pain, urticaria, pruritus, and a burning sensation.
- Late signs include nausea, vomiting, weakness, muscle cramps, fever, chills, hypotension, headache and, in severe cases, dyspnea, seizures, and paralysis.

Heart failure

- Edema in both legs is an early sign of right-sided heart failure.
- Pitting ankle edema signals more advanced heart failure.
- Other findings include weight gain, anorexia, nausea, chest tightness, hypotension, pallor, tachypnea, exertional dyspnea, orthopnea, paroxysmal nocturnal dyspnea, palpitations, ventricular gallop, and crackles.

Hypoproteinemia

- Edema in both legs occurs with muscle weakness; lethargy; anorexia; diarrhea; apathy; dry, wrinkled skin; and signs of anemia.

Leg trauma

- Mild to severe localized edema may form at the site of the trauma.
- Ecchymoses or bleeding pain or numbness, and paralysis may occur.
- Deformity may be present if a fracture has occurred.

Nephrotic syndrome

- Edema in both legs occurs with polyuria and eyelid edema.
- Generalized pitting edema may occur as well as ascites, fatigue, malaise, depression, and pallor.

Osteomyelitis

- If the lower leg is affected, localized, mild to moderate edema develops and may spread to the adjacent joint.
- Edema follows fever, localized tenderness, and pain that increases with leg movement.

Rupture of popliteal cyst

- Onset of calf pain and edema is sudden, usually occurring after walking or exercising.

Thrombophlebitis

- Mild to moderate edema occurs.
- Severe pain, warmth, and cyanosis in the affected leg as well as fever, chills, and malaise occur with deep vein thrombosis.
- Pain, warmth, redness, tenderness, and induration along the affected vein occur with superficial thrombophlebitis.

Venous insufficiency (chronic)

- Moderate to severe edema in one or both legs occurs; initially, edema is soft and pitting; later, it's hard.
- Other signs include darkened skin and painless stasis ulcers around the ankles.

Other causes

Coronary artery bypass surgery

- Venous insufficiency in one leg may follow saphenous vein retrieval.

Drugs

○ Hormonal contraceptives, lithium, nonsteroidal anti-inflammatory drugs, vasodilators, and drugs that cause sodium retention can cause leg edema.

Nursing considerations

○ Have the patient avoid prolonged sitting or standing.
○ Elevate his legs as needed.
○ Give an analgesic and antibiotic as needed.
○ Monitor intake and output, and check weight and leg circumference daily to detect changes.
○ Monitor for skin breakdown.

Pediatric pointers

○ Leg edema is uncommon but may result from osteomyelitis, leg trauma, or heart failure.

Patient teaching

○ Teach the proper application of antiembolism stockings or bandages.
○ Instruct the patient in appropriate leg exercises.
○ Explain the foods or fluids the patient should avoid.

Epistaxis

Overview

- Also called *nosebleed* and occurs in the anterior-inferior nasal septum (most commonly) or at the point where the inferior turbinates meet the nasopharynx
- Usually from only one nostril, bleeding may be mild to severe, even life-threatening

✦ Emergency actions

If the patient has severe epistaxis, quickly take vital signs and look for signs of hypovolemic shock. Insert a large-gauge I.V. line for fluid and blood replacement. Unless you suspect a nasal fracture, control bleeding by pinching the nares closed, then place gauze under the nose.

- Have a hypovolemic patient lie down and turn his head to the side to prevent aspiration. If the patient isn't hypovolemic, have him sit upright and tilt his head forward. Check airway patency. If the patient is unstable, begin cardiac monitoring and give oxygen.

Assessment

History

- Ask about recent trauma or surgery.
- Obtain a description of past nosebleeds.
- Take a medical history, including hypertension, bleeding or liver disorders, and other recent illnesses.
- Find out what drugs the patient is taking, especially anti-inflammatory drugs and anticoagulants.

Physical assessment

- Inspect for other signs of bleeding.
- Look for trauma injuries.

Medical causes

Aplastic anemia

- Nosebleeds are accompanied by ecchymoses, retinal hemorrhages, menorrhagia, petechiae, and signs of GI bleeding.
- Fatigue, dyspnea, headache, tachycardia, and pallor may also occur.

Biliary obstruction

- Bleeding tendencies, including epistaxis
- Colicky right-upper-quadrant pain after eating fatty food, nausea, vomiting, fever, flatulence, and jaundice

Cirrhosis

- Epistaxis and other bleeding tendencies are late signs.
- Other late findings include ascites, abdominal pain, shallow respirations, hepatomegaly or splenomegaly, and fever.
- The patient may also exhibit muscle atrophy, pruritus, extremely dry skin, abnormal pigmentation, spider angiomas, jaundice, and central nervous system disturbances.

Coagulation disorders

- Epistaxis, ecchymoses, petechiae, menorrhagia, GI bleeding, and bleeding from the gums, mouth, and I.V. puncture sites may occur.

Glomerulonephritis (chronic)

- Nosebleeds, hypertension, proteinuria, hematuria, headache, edema, oliguria, hemoptysis, nausea, vomiting, pruritus, dyspnea, malaise, and fatigue

Hepatitis

- Epistaxis occurs along with jaundice, clay-colored stools, pruritus, hepatomegaly, abdominal pain, fever, fatigue, weakness, dark amber urine, anorexia, nausea, and vomiting.

Hypertension

- Severe hypertension can produce extreme epistaxis with dizziness, a throbbing headache, anxiety, peripheral edema, nocturia, nausea, vomiting, drowsiness, and mental impairment.

Infectious mononucleosis

- Blood may ooze from the nose.
- Characteristic findings include sore throat, cervical lymphadenopathy, and a fluctuating fever that peaks in the evening.

Influenza

- A slow, oozing nosebleed may occur with dry cough, chills, fever, malaise, myalgia, sore throat, hoarseness or loss of voice, conjunctivitis, facial flushing, headache, rhinitis, and rhinorrhea.

Leukemia

- With acute leukemia, sudden epistaxis is accompanied by high fever and other types of abnormal bleeding.
- Other findings include weakness, pallor, chills, recurrent infections, low-grade fever, dyspnea, fatigue, malaise, tachycardia, palpitations, a systolic ejection murmur, and abdominal or bone pain.
- With chronic leukemia, epistaxis is a late sign that may be accompanied by other bleeding, extreme fatigue, weight loss, hepatosplenomegaly, bone tenderness, macular or nodular skin lesions, pallor, weakness, dyspnea, tachycardia, palpitations, and headache.

Maxillofacial injury

○ Severe epistaxis may occur with facial pain, swelling, open-bite malocclusion or inability to open the mouth, diplopia, conjunctival hemorrhage, lip edema, and buccal, mucosal, and soft palatal ecchymoses.

Nasal fracture

○ One or both nostrils may bleed.
○ Nasal swelling, periorbital ecchymoses and edema, pain, nasal deformity, and crepitation of the nasal bones may also occur.

Polycythemia vera

○ Spontaneous epistaxis is a common sign.
○ Other findings include bleeding gums; ecchymoses; ruddy cyanosis of the face, nose, ears, and lips; headache; dizziness; vision disturbances; hypertension; chest pain; splenomegaly; epigastric pain; pruritus; dyspnea; and congestion of the conjunctiva, retina, and oral mucous membranes.

Renal failure

○ Epistaxis can occur as well as oliguria or anuria, weight loss, anorexia, abdominal pain, diarrhea, nausea, vomiting, tissue wasting, dry mucous membranes, uremic breath, Kussmaul's respirations, deteriorating mental condition, and tachycardia.

Sarcoidosis

○ Oozing epistaxis may occur along with a nonproductive cough, substernal pain, malaise, and weight loss.
○ Other findings include tachycardia, arrhythmias, parotid enlargement, cervical lymphadenopathy, skin lesions, hepatosplenomegaly, and arthritis in the ankles, knees, and wrists.

Sinusitis (acute)

○ Bloody or blood-tinged nasal discharge may become purulent and copious 48 hours of onset.
○ Other findings include nasal congestion, pain, tenderness, malaise, headache, low-grade fever, and red, edematous nasal mucosa.

Skull fracture

○ Epistaxis is direct or indirect, depending on the type of fracture.
○ With severe skull fracture, findings include severe headache, decreased level of consciousness, hemiparesis, dizziness, seizures, projectile vomiting, and decreased pulse and respirations.
○ With a basilar fracture, findings include raccoon eyes; Battle's sign; bleeding from the pharynx, ears, and conjunctiva; and leakage of cerebrospinal fluid or brain tissue from the nose or ears.
○ With a sphenoid fracture blindness may also occur.
○ With a temporal fracture, deafness in one ear or facial paralysis may also occur.

Systemic lupus erythematosus

○ Oozing epistaxis occurs.
○ Characteristic findings include butterfly rash, lymphadenopathy, joint pain and stiffness, anorexia, nausea, vomiting, myalgia, and weight loss.

Other causes

Chemical irritants

○ Some chemicals, such as phosphorus, sulfuric acid, ammonia, printer's ink, and chromates, irritate the nasal mucosa, producing epistaxis.

Drugs

○ Anticoagulants or anti-inflammatory drugs can cause epistaxis.
○ Frequent cocaine use may also cause epistaxis.

Vigorous nose blowing

○ Vigorous nose blowing may rupture superficial blood vessels and cause epistaxis.

Nursing considerations

○ Monitor for signs of hypovolemic shock.
○ If external pressure doesn't control the bleeding, insert cotton saturated with a vasoconstrictor and local anesthetic into the nose.
○ If bleeding persists, insert anterior or posterior nasal packing.
○ Administer humidified oxygen by face mask to a patient with posterior packing.

Pediatric pointers

○ Children are more likely to experience anterior nosebleeds.
○ Causes of epistaxis include nose picking, allergic rhinitis, biliary atresia, cystic fibrosis, hereditary afibrinogenemia, nasal trauma from foreign body, and rubeola.

Geriatric pointers

○ Elderly patients are more likely to have posterior nosebleeds.

Patient teaching

○ Teach the patient or caregiver pinching pressure techniques.
○ Discuss ways to prevent nosebleeds.

Erectile dysfunction

Overview

- Inability to achieve and maintain penile erection sufficient to complete satisfactory sexual intercourse
- May be primary or secondary
- Occurs when psychological, vascular, neurologic, or hormonal dysfunction occurs

Assessment

History

- Obtain a psychosocial history.
- Review the patient's medical history, noting diabetes mellitus, hypertension, heart disease, urologic disease, and neurologic disease.
- Ask about the patient's surgical history, including neurologic, hormonal, vascular, and urologic surgery.
- Find out about recent trauma and its severity, other findings, and treatment.
- Ask about alcohol and drug use or abuse.
- Ask about diet, smoking, and exercise.
- Find out about onset, quality, aggravating and alleviating factors, and progression of impotence.
- Inspect and palpate the genitalia and prostate for structural abnormalities.
- Assess sensory function in the perineum.
- Test motor strength and deep tendon reflexes.
- Note neurologic deficits.
- Take vital signs.
- Palpate pulses for quality.
- Note cyanosis and cool extremities.
- Auscultate for abdominal, aortic, femoral, carotid, or iliac bruits.
- Palpate for thyroid gland enlargement.

Medical causes

Central nervous system disorders

- Spinal cord lesions from trauma produce sudden impotence.
- Complete lesion above S2 causes loss of voluntary erectile control but not reflex erection and reflex ejaculation.
- Complete lesion in the lumbosacral spinal cord causes loss of reflex ejaculation and reflex erection.
- Degenerative disease of the brain and spinal cord cause progressive impotence.

Endocrine disorders

- Testicular or pituitary dysfunction may cause impotence from deficient androgens.

- Adrenocortical and thyroid disease and chronic hepatitis may cause impotence by affecting hormone regulation.

Penile disorders

- In Peyronie's disease a bent penis makes erection painful and penetration difficult.
- Phimosis prevents erection until circumcision releases constricted foreskin.
- Other inflammatory, infectious, or destructive diseases of the penis may cause impotence.

Peripheral neuropathy

- Progressive impotence occurs.
- Other findings include bladder distention with overflow incontinence, orthostatic hypotension, syncope, paresthesia and other sensory disturbances, muscle weakness, and leg atrophy.

Psychological distress

- Diverse psychological causes can result in impotence.

Trauma

- Traumatic injury involving the penis, urethra, prostate, perineum, or pelvis can cause sudden impotence.

Vascular disorders

- Advanced atherosclerosis, Leriche's syndrome, and arteriosclerosis, thrombosis, or embolization of smaller vessels supplying the penis can result in impotence.

Other causes

Alcohol and drugs

- Alcoholism and drug abuse are linked to erectile dysfunction, as are many prescription drugs, especially antihypertensives.

Surgery

- Surgical injury to the penis, bladder neck, urinary sphincter, rectum, or perineum can cause impotence, as can injury to local nerves or blood vessels.

Nursing considerations

- Help the patient feel comfortable about discussing his sexuality.
- Discuss counseling for the patient and his partner.
- Provide care for treatments, such as surgical revascularization, drug-induced erection, surgical repairs, and penile prosthesis.
- Provide emotional support and encourage the patient to talk about his feelings.

Geriatric pointers

○ Keep in mind that sexual performance doesn't normally decline with aging and that elderly patients can be capable of and interested in sexual activity.

Patient teaching

○ Explain which treatment options are available to the patient.
○ Explain the importance of routine follow-up for treatment of medical conditions.
○ Discuss with the patient the importance of communicating with his sexual partner.

Erythema

Overview

- Refers to red skin caused by dilated or congested blood vessels
- A common sign of skin inflammation or irritation
- Color ranges from bright red in acute conditions to pale violet or brown in chronic conditions
- Blanches momentarily when pressure is applied, distinguishing it from purpura (redness from bleeding into the skin), which doesn't blanch with pressure

⭐ Emergency actions

If the patient has sudden erythema with rapid pulse, dyspnea, hoarseness, and agitation, quickly take his vital signs and treat him for anaphylactic shock. Provide respiratory support and give epinephrine.

Assessment

History

- Ask about the onset and duration of erythema.
- Obtain a medical history, including recent fever, upper respiratory tract infection, skin disease, allergies, or asthma.
- Ask about pain or itching.
- Note recent fall or injury.
- Ask about exposure to anyone with a rash.
- Take a drug history, including recent immunizations.
- Review food intake and exposure to chemicals.

Physical assessment

- Assess the extent, distribution, and intensity of erythema.
- Look for edema and other skin lesions.
- Examine the affected area for warmth.
- Gently palpate the affected area to check for tenderness or crepitus.

Medical causes

Allergic reactions

- Localized reaction produces erythema, hivelike eruptions, and edema.
- With life-threatening anaphylaxis, erythema is sudden and accompanied by flushing; facial edema; diaphoresis; weakness; bronchospasm with tachypnea and dyspnea; shock; and airway edema with hoarseness and stridor.

Burns

- With thermal burns, erythema and swelling appear first, possibly followed by blisters.

- Burns from ultraviolet rays cause delayed erythema and tenderness.

Candidiasis

- If the skin is affected, erythema and a scaly, papular rash under breasts or at axillae, neck, umbilicus, or groin develop.
- Small pustules occur at the periphery of the rash.

Cellulitis

- Erythema, tenderness, and edema occur.
- Pain and warmth develop at the site of the infection.

Dermatitis

- With atopic dermatitis, erythema and intense pruritus precede the development of small papules that may redden, weep, scale, and lichenify.
- Contact dermatitis produces erythema and vesicles, blisters, or ulcerations.
- With seborrheic dermatitis, erythema appears with dull-red or yellow lesions that are sharply marginated and may be ring-shaped and covered with greasy scales.

Erysipelas

- Reddish, well-demarcated, tender, warm areas occur most commonly on the face and neck.
- Other findings include fever, chills, local adenopathy, malaise, headache, and sore throat.

Erythema annulare centrifugum

- Small, pink infiltrated papules appear on the trunk, buttocks, and inner thighs, slowing spreading at the margins and clearing in the center.
- Other findings include itching, scaling, and tissue hardening.

Erythema marginatum rheumaticum

- Erythematous lesions are superficial, flat, and slightly hardened.
- Lesions shift, spread rapidly, and may last for hours or days.

Erythema multiforme

- In minor form, urticarial red-pink, iris-shaped, localized lesions that burn or itch typically occur on flexor surfaces of extremities.
- Early findings include mild fever, cough, and sore throat.
- In major form, blisters on the lips, tongue, and buccal mucosa and sore throat precede development of widespread erythematous, symmetrical, bullous lesions.
- Early findings include cough, vomiting, diarrhea, coryza, and epistaxis.
- Late findings include fever, prostration, conjunctivitis, vulvitis, balanitis, and difficulty with oral intake because of oral lesions.

Erythema nodosum

○ Tender erythematous nodules develop suddenly in crops on the shins, knees, and ankles.
○ Other findings include mild fever, chills, malaise, muscle and joint pain, and swollen feet and ankles.

Gout

○ Tight, erythematous skin is seen over inflamed, edematous joint.
○ The metatarsophalangeal joint of the great toe usually becomes inflamed first, followed by the instep, ankle, heel, knee, or wrist joint.

Liver disease (chronic)

○ Local vasodilation and palmar erythema occur along with jaundice, pruritus, spider angiomas, xanthomas, and characteristic systemic signs.

Lupus erythematosus

○ Characteristic erythematous butterfly rash develops.
○ Rash may range from a blush with swelling to a scaly, sharply demarcated, macular rash with plaques that may spread to the forehead, chin, ears, chest, and other sun-exposed body parts.
○ Acute onset of erythema may accompany photosensitivity and mucous membrane ulcers in systemic lupus erythematosus.

Psoriasis

○ Silvery white scales with a thickened erythematous base affect the elbows, knees, chest, scalp, and intergluteal folds.
○ Fingernails become thick and pitted.

Rheumatoid arthritis

○ During flare-ups, erythema, heat, swelling, pain, and stiffness occur at affected joints.
○ Early findings include malaise, fatigue, myalgia, and morning stiffness.
○ Muscle atrophy, palmar erythema, edema, mottled skin, and structural deformities occur as the disease progresses.

Rosacea

○ Scattered erythema develops across the center of the face.
○ Superficial telangiectases, papules, pustules, and nodules follow.

Rubella

○ Flat solitary lesions form a blotchy pink erythematous rash that spreads rapidly to the trunk and extremities and clears in 4 to 5 days.
○ Small red lesions may appear on the soft palate.
○ Other findings include fever, headache, malaise, sore throat, a gritty eye sensation, lymphadenopathy, joint pain, and coryza.

Staphylococcal scalded skin syndrome

○ Occurring mainly in infants and small children, erythema and widespread exfoliation of superficial epidermal layers occur.
○ Other findings include low-grade fever and irritability.

Thrombophlebitis

○ Erythema may develop over the inflamed vein.
○ Fever, chills, and malaise may accompany severe, localized pain, warmth, and induration; distal edema; and a positive Homans' sign.

Other causes

Drugs

○ Many drugs commonly cause erythema.

Radiation therapy

○ Radiation therapy may produce dull erythema and edema within 24 hours.

Nursing considerations

○ Monitor and replace fluids and electrolytes.
○ Withhold drugs until the cause of erythema is identified.
○ Give an antibiotic and topical or systemic corticosteroid.
○ To relieve itching skin, give soothing baths or apply open wet dressings containing starch, bran, or sodium bicarbonate.
○ Give an antihistamine and an analgesic as needed.
○ Keep erythematous legs elevated above heart level.
○ For a burn patient with erythema, immerse the affected area in cold water, or apply a sheet soaked in cold water.

Pediatric pointers

○ Neonates may develop a pink papular rash during the first 4 days after birth, which spontaneously disappears.
○ Infections and other disorders can cause erythema in neonates and infants.
○ Roseola, rubeola, scarlet fever, granuloma annulare, and cutis marmorata cause erythema in children.

Geriatric pointers

○ Well-defined purple macules or patches, usually on the back of the hands and on the forearms, may result from blood leaking through fragile capillaries.

Patient teaching

○ Teach the patient to recognize the signs and symptoms of flare-ups of disease.
○ Stress the avoidance of sun exposure and use of sunblock.
○ Teach the patient methods to relieve itching.

Exophthalmos

Overview

- Also known as *proptosis*
- Abnormal protrusion of one or both eyeballs
- May be sudden or gradual, mild or dramatic

Assessment

History

- Ask about the onset of exophthalmos.
- Find out if the patient has pain and its quality, quantity, and duration.
- Inquire about recent sinus infection or vision problems.
- Obtain a medical history, including thyroid disease.
- Ask about recent injury or trauma.

Physical assessment

- Take vital signs, noting fever.
- Evaluate severity of exophthalmos with exophthalmometer and assess for unilateral exophthalmos. (See *Detecting unilateral exophthalmus*.)
- If eyes bulge severely, look for cloudiness on the cornea, which may indicate ulcer formation.
- Describe any eye discharge and observe for ptosis.

Assessment tip

Detecting unilateral exophthalmos

If one of the patient's eyes seems more prominent than the other, examine both eyes from above the patient's head. Look down across his face, gently draw his lids up, and compare the relationship of the corneas to the lower lids. Abnormal protrusion of one eye suggests unilateral exophthalmos.

Don't perform this test if you suspect eye trauma.

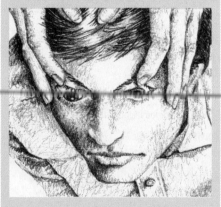

- Check visual acuity, with and without correction.
- Palpate the thyroid for enlargement or goiter.

Medical causes

Foreign body in eye

- Exophthalmos may accompany eye pain, redness, and tearing.
- Loss of vision or blurred vision occurs in the affected eye.

Hemangioma

- Exophthalmos is progressive and may be mild or severe.
- Other findings include ptosis, limited extraocular movements, and blurred vision.

Lacrimal gland tumor

- Exophthalmos usually develops slowly in one eye, displacing it downward toward the nose.
- Ptosis, eye deviation, and pain may develop.

Optic nerve meningioma

- Exophthalmos in one eye and a swollen temple are common.
- Impaired visual acuity, visual field deficits, and headache may occur.

Orbital cellulitis

- An ocular emergency — onset of exophthalmos in one eye, which may be mild or severe, is sudden.
- Other findings include fever, eye pain, headache, malaise, conjunctival injection, tearing, eyelid edema and erythema, purulent discharge, and impaired extraocular movements.

Orbital choristoma

- Progressive exophthalmos may occur with diplopia and blurred vision.
- A mass may be visible in the orbital area.

Orbital emphysema

- Exophthalmos in one eye, crepitation on palpation of the globe, and orbital pressure occur.

Parasite infestation

- Painless, progressive exophthalmos develops in one eye and may spread to the other eye.
- Other findings include limited extraocular movement, diplopia, eye pain, and impaired visual acuity.

Scleritis (posterior)

- Onset of mild to severe exophthalmos in one eye is gradual.
- Other findings include severe eye pain, diplopia, papilledema, limited extraocular movement, and impaired visual acuity.

Thyrotoxicosis

○ Exophthalmos (a classic sign) usually in both eyes, progressive, and severe.
○ Ptosis, increased tearing, lid lag and edema, photophobia, conjunctival injection, diplopia, and decreased visual acuity
○ Enlarged thyroid gland, nervousness, heat intolerance, weight loss despite increased appetite, sweating, diarrhea, tremors, palpitations, and tachycardia

Nursing considerations

○ Provide privacy and emotional support.
○ Protect the eye from trauma.
○ Don't place a gauze eye pad or other objects over the affected eye.
○ If a slit-lamp examination is needed, explain the procedure to the patient.
○ If needed, refer the patient to ophthalmologist for a complete examination.

Pediatric pointers

○ Rhabdomyosarcoma produces rapid onset of exophthalmos.
○ In Hand-Schüller-Christian syndrome, exophthalmos typically accompanies signs of diabetes insipidus and bone destruction.

Patient teaching

○ Explain ways to protect the eye from trauma, wind, and dust.
○ Explain the proper application of lubricants to the eye.

Eye discharge

Overview

- Excretion of any substance other than tears
- Usually occurs with conjunctivitis

Assessment

History

- Determine the onset and description of eye drainage.
- Assess the location and description of pain, if needed.
- Inquire about additional signs and symptoms, including burning, tearing, sensitivity to light, and the sensation of something foreign in the eye.

Physical assessment

- Take vital signs.
- Inspect the eye discharge, noting the amount, color, consistency, and source. (See *Assessing the source of eye discharge*.)
- Test visual acuity, with and without correction.
- Examine external eye structures, beginning with the unaffected eye, to prevent cross-contamination.
- Observe for eyelid edema, entropion, crusts, lesions, and trichiasis.
- Ask the patient to blink; watch for impaired lid movement.
- If eyes seem to bulge, measure them with an exophthalmometer.
- Test the six fields of gaze.
- Examine for conjunctival injection and follicles and for corneal cloudiness or white lesions.

Medical causes

Conjunctivitis

- *Allergic:* With itching and tearing, both eyes excrete a ropy discharge.
- *Bacterial:* Moderate, greenish white purulent or mucopurulent discharge may form sticky crusts on the eyelids during sleep.
- *Viral:* A serous, clear discharge and preauricular adenopathy are usually present.
- *Fungal:* Copious, thick, purulent discharge makes the eyelids crusty and sticky.
- *Inclusion:* Scant mucoid discharge in both eyes is accompanied by pseudoptosis and conjunctival follicles.

Corneal ulcers

- Copious, purulent eye discharge from one eye occurs along with crusty, sticky eyelid.
- Severe pain, photophobia, conjunctival injection, and impaired visual acuity may occur.
- A bacterial corneal ulcer may cause an irregular gray-white area on the cornea, blurred vision, and pupil constriction.
- Fungal corneal ulcers also result in eyelid edema and erythema; and a painless, dense, whitish gray central ulcer that develops slowly and may be surrounded by progressively clearer rings.

Dacryocystitis

- Scant but continuous purulent discharge is produced that's easily expressed from the tear sac.
- Additional findings include excessive eye tearing, and pain, tenderness, and erythema near the tear sac.

Herpes zoster ophthalmicus

- Moderate to copious serous eye discharge accompanies excessive tearing.

Assessment tip
Assessing the source of eye discharge

Eye discharge can come from the tear sac, punctum, meibomian glands, or canaliculi. If the patient reports a discharge that isn't immediately apparent, you can express a sample by pressing your fingertip lightly over these structures. Then characterize the discharge, and note its source.

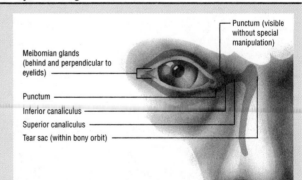

Meibomian glands (behind and perpendicular to eyelids)

Punctum

Inferior canaliculus

Superior canaliculus

Tear sac (within bony orbit)

Punctum (visible without special manipulation)

○ Other findings include eyelid edema and erythema; conjunctival injection, eye pain, and severe facial pain that occurs several days before vesicles erupt; and a white, cloudy cornea.

Keratoconjunctivitis sicca

○ Excessive, continuous mucoid discharge and insufficient tearing occur.
○ Other findings include eye pain, itching, burning, a foreign-body sensation, dramatic conjunctival injection, and difficulty closing the eye.

Meibomianitis

○ A continuous frothy, foul-smelling, cheesy yellow eye discharge may be produced.
○ The eye appears chronically red, with inflamed lid margins.

Orbital cellulitis

○ A purulent eye discharge may be present, but exophthalmos is the obvious sign.
○ Other findings include eyelid edema, conjunctival injection, headache, orbital pain, impaired visual acuity, limited extraocular movement, and fever.

Psoriasis vulgaris

○ Substantial mucous discharge and redness occur in both eyes.
○ Lesions occur on the eyelids but may extend to the conjunctiva, causing irritation, excessive tearing, and a foreign-body sensation.

Nursing considerations

○ Apply warm soaks to soften crusts on the eyelids and lashes.
○ Gently wipe the eyes with a soft gauze pad.
○ Carefully dispose of used dressings, tissues, and cotton swabs.
○ Sterilize ophthalmic equipment after use.

Pediatric pointers

○ In children, eye discharge usually results from eye trauma, eye infection, or upper respiratory tract infection.
○ In infants, prophylactic eye drops (silver nitrate) commonly cause eye irritation and discharge.

Patient teaching

○ Instruct the patient or caregiver about measures to prevent the spread of infection.

Eye pain

Overview

○ Burning, throbbing, aching, stabbing, or foreign-body sensation in eye

✦ Emergency actions

If the patient has eye pain caused by a chemical burn, remove contact lenses and irrigate the eye with at least 1 L of normal saline solution. Evert lids and wipe fornices. If the patient has eye pain from acute angle-closure glaucoma, intervene to decrease intraocular pressure (IOP). If drug treatment doesn't reduce IOP, the patient needs laser iridotomy or surgical peripheral iridectomy to save vision.

Assessment

History

○ Ask about the onset, description, and duration of pain.
○ Find out about other symptoms, such as burning, itching, or discharge.
○ Ask about recent trauma, surgery, or headaches.

Physical assessment

○ If you suspect trauma, don't manipulate the eye.
○ Carefully assess the lids and conjunctivae for redness, inflammation, and swelling.
○ Examine the eyes for ptosis and exophthalmos.
○ Test visual acuity, with and without correction
○ Assess extraocular movements.
○ Characterize any discharge.

Medical causes

Blepharitis

○ Burning pain in both eyelids, itching, sticky discharge, and conjunctival injection occur.
○ Other findings include foreign-body sensation, lid ulcerations, and loss of eyelashes.

Burns

○ With chemical burns, sudden and severe eye pain may occur with erythema and blistering of the face and lids, photophobia, miosis, conjunctival injection, and blurred vision.
○ With ultraviolet radiation burns, moderate to severe pain occurs about 12 hours after exposure along with photophobia and vision changes.

Chalazion

○ Localized pain, tenderness, redness, conjunctival injection, swelling, and a small red lump develop on the eyelid.

Conjunctivitis

○ *Allergic:* causes mild, burning, pain in both eyes with itching, conjunctival injection, and a ropy discharge.
○ *Bacterial:* causes pain when it affects the cornea and may produce burning, a foreign-body sensation, conjunctival injection, and a purulent discharge.
○ *Fungal:* if the cornea is affected, may cause pain with itching, burning, conjunctival injection, photophobia, and a thick, purulent discharge.
○ *Viral:* produces itching, red eyes, foreign-body sensation, visible conjunctival follicles, and eyelid edema.

Corneal abrasions

○ Eye pain is characterized by a foreign-body sensation.
○ Other findings include excessive tearing, photophobia, and conjunctival injection.

Corneal erosion (recurrent)

○ Severe pain occurs on waking and continues during the day along with conjunctival injection and photophobia.

Corneal ulcers

○ Severe eye pain may occur with purulent eye discharge, sticky eyelids, photophobia, conjunctival injection, and impaired visual acuity.
○ Bacterial corneal ulcers also produce a grayish white, irregularly shaped ulcer on the cornea, and pupil constriction.
○ Fungal corneal ulcers produce eyelid edema and erythema, and a dense, cloudy, central ulcer surrounded by progressively clearer rings.

Dacryocystitis

○ Pain and tenderness occur near the tear sac.
○ Other findings include excessive tearing, a purulent discharge, eyelid edema, and swelling of the lacrimal punctum area.

Foreign body in cornea or conjunctiva

○ Sudden severe pain is common, but vision usually remains intact.
○ Other findings include excessive tearing, photophobia, miosis, a foreign-body sensation, a dark speck on the cornea, and dramatic conjunctival injection.

Glaucoma

○ *Open-angle glaucoma* may cause mild aching in the eyes as well as halo vision, loss of peripheral vision, and reduced visual acuity that's uncorrected with glasses.
○ *Angle-closure glaucoma* is characterized by blurred vision and sudden, excruciating pain in and around the eye that may be accompanied by nausea, vomiting, halo vision, rapidly decreasing visual acuity, and a fixed, nonreactive pupil.

Herpes zoster ophthalmicus

○ Ocular and facial pain occur days before vesicles erupt.
○ Other findings include red, swollen eyelids; excessive tearing; a serous eye discharge; conjunctival injection; and a white, cloudy cornea.

Hordeolum

○ Localized eye pain, burning, and discomfort increases as the stye grows.
○ Eyelid erythema and edema are also common.

Hyphema

○ Sudden pain in and around the eye occurs after eye injury or surgery.
○ Orbital and lid edema, conjunctival injection, nausea, and visual impairment may develop.

Keratoconjunctivitis sicca

○ Chronic burning pain occurs in both eyes.
○ Other findings include itching, a foreign-body sensation, photophobia, dramatic conjunctival injection, difficulty moving the eyelids, excessive mucoid discharge, and inadequate tearing.

Lacrimal gland tumor

○ Tumor produces eye pain, impaired visual acuity, and some degree of exophthalmos.
○ Ptosis and eye deviation may also occur.

Ocular laceration and intraocular foreign bodies

○ Penetrating eye injuries usually cause mild to severe eye pain and impaired visual acuity.
○ Eyelid edema, conjunctival injection, and an abnormal pupillary response may also occur.

Optic cellulitis

○ Dull, aching pain occurs in the affected eye.
○ Other findings include exophthalmos, eyelid edema and erythema, purulent discharge, impaired extraocular movement and, possibly, decreased visual acuity and fever.

Optic neuritis

○ Pain in and around the eye occurs with eye movement.
○ Severe vision loss, tunnel vision, and sluggish pupillary response may develop.

Orbital floor fracture

○ Eye pain and dramatic eyelid edema occur, possibly with exophthalmos and diplopia.
○ Other findings include reduced vision, ecchymoses, and ptosis.

Orbital pseudotumor

○ Deep, boring eye pain and diplopia may occur.
○ Prominent exophthalmos and lateral ocular deviation are more characteristic.

Uveitis

○ With anterior uveitis, onset of severe pain is sudden with dramatic conjunctival injection, photophobia, and a small, nonreactive pupil.
○ With posterior uveitis, onset of pain is insidious, with gradual blurring of vision and distorted pupil shape.
○ With lens-induced uveitis, moderate eye pain occurs with conjunctival injection, pupil constriction, and impaired visual acuity.

Other causes

Treatments

○ Contact lenses may cause eye pain and a foreign-body sensation.
○ Ocular surgery may produce eye pain, ranging from a mild ache to a severe pounding or stabbing sensation.

Nursing considerations

○ To reduce eye pain, provide a darkened, quiet environment and have the patient close his eyes.

Pediatric pointers

○ Trauma and infection are the most common causes of eye pain in children.
○ Tightly shutting or frequently rubbing the eyes may be nonverbal clues to eye pain.

Geriatric pointers

○ Glaucoma, which can cause eye pain, is a disease most commonly found in older patients.

Patient teaching

○ Stress the importance of following instructions for drug therapy.
○ Give the patient careful instructions about eye protection.
○ Explain that the patient should seek medical attention for eye pain.

Facial pain

Overview

- May result from various neurologic, vascular, or infectious disorders
- May be referred from the ears, nose, paranasal sinuses, teeth, neck, and jaw
- Is typically paroxysmal and intense

Assessment

History

- Ask about onset, description, location, and duration.
- Determine what alleviates or aggravates the pain.
- Obtain a medical and dental history, noting previous head trauma, dental disease, and infection.

Physical assessment

- Inspect the ear for vesicles and changes in the tympanic membrane.
- Inspect the nose for deformity or asymmetry and characterize any secretions.
- Palpate the sinuses for tenderness and swelling.
- Evaluate oral hygiene.
- Ask about sensitivity to hot, cold, or sweet liquids or foods.
- Have the patient open and close his mouth as you palpate the temporomandibular joint.
- Assess cranial nerves V and VII. (See *Major nerve pathways of the face.*)

Medical causes

Angina pectoris

- Jaw pain may be described as burning, squeezing, or tightness.
- Pain may radiate to the left arm, neck, and shoulder blade.

Dental caries

- Caries in the mandibular molars can produce ear, preauricular, and temporal pain.
- Caries in the maxillary teeth can produce maxillary, orbital, retro-orbital and parietal pain.

Herpes zoster oticus

- Severe pain localizes around the ear, followed by the appearance of vesicles in the ear.
- Eye pain may occur with corneal and scleral damage and impaired vision.

Multiple sclerosis

- Facial pain may resemble that of trigeminal neuralgia.
- Pain is accompanied by jaw and facial weakness.
- Other findings include visual blurring, diplopia, and nystagmus; sensory impairment; generalized muscle weakness and gait abnormalities; urinary disturbances; and emotional lability.

Ocular glaucoma

- Periorbital pain appears late.
- Other findings include loss of peripheral vision, reduced visual acuity (especially at night), and seeing halos around lights.

Postherpetic neuralgia

- Burning, itching, prickly pain that worsens with contact or movement and persists along any of the three trigeminal nerve divisions.
- Mild hypoesthesia or paresthesia and vesicles affect the area before the onset of pain.

Sinusitis (acute)

- Acute maxillary sinusitis produces pressure, fullness, or burning pain over cheekbone and upper teeth and around eyes that worsens with bending over.
- Acute frontal sinusitis produces severe pain above or around the eyes that worsens when the patient is in a supine position.
- Acute ethmoid sinusitis produces pain at or around the inner corner of the eye.
- Acute sphenoid sinusitis produces a persistent, deep-seated pain behind the eyes or nose or on the top of the head that increases with bending forward.

Sinusitis (chronic)

- Chronic maxillary sinusitis produces a chronic toothache or a feeling of pressure below the eyes.
- Chronic ethmoid sinusitis is characterized by nasal congestion and discharge and discomfort at medial corners of eyes.
- Chronic frontal sinusitis produces a persistent low-grade pain above the eyes.
- Chronic sphenoid sinusitis produces a persistent low-grade, diffuse headache or retro-orbital discomfort.

Sphenopalatine neuralgia

- Deep, boring pain occurs below the ear and may radiate to the eye, ear, cheek, nose, palate, maxillary teeth, temple, neck, shoulder, or back of head.
- Attacks bring increased tearing and salivation, rhinorrhea, a sensation of fullness in the ear, tinnitus, vertigo, taste disturbance, pruritus, and shoulder stiffness or weakness.

Temporal arteritis

- Pain occurs behind one eye or in scalp, jaw, tongue, or neck.
- A typical episode consists of a severe throbbing or boring temporal headache with redness, swelling, and nodulation of the temporal artery.

Cranial nerve V has three branches. The *ophthalmic branch* supplies sensation to the anterior scalp, forehead, upper nose, and cornea. The *maxillary branch* supplies sensation to the midportion of the face, lower nose, upper lip, and mucous membrane of the anterior palate. The *mandibular branch* supplies sensation to the lower face, lower jaw, mucous membrane of the cheek, and base of the tongue.

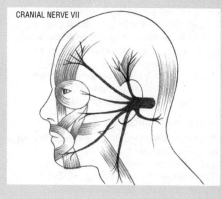

CRANIAL NERVE V

Cranial nerve VII innervates the facial muscles. Its motor branch controls the muscles of the forehead, eye orbit, and mouth.

CRANIAL NERVE VII

Temporomandibular joint syndrome

- An intermittent severe, dull ache or intense spasm, usually on one side, radiates to the cheek, temple, lower jaw, or ear.
- Other findings include trismus, malocclusion, and clicking, crepitus, and tenderness of the joint.

Trigeminal neuralgia

- Paroxysms of intense pain shoot along the three branches of the trigeminal nerve.
- May be triggered by touching the nose, cheek, or mouth; exposure to hot or cold; consuming hot or cold foods or beverages; or even smiling and talking.

Patient teaching

- Teach the patient about triggers to avoid.
- Explain which signs and symptoms to report.

Nursing considerations

- Give drugs for pain.
- Apply direct heat or give a muscle relaxant.
- Provide a humidifier, vaporizer, or decongestant to relieve nasal or sinus congestion.

Pediatric pointers

- Look for subtle signs of pain, such as facial rubbing, irritability, or poor eating habits.

Fatigue

Overview

- A feeling of excessive tiredness, lack of energy, or exhaustion, with a strong desire to rest or sleep
- Reflects hypermetabolic and hypometabolic states in which nutrients needed for cellular energy and growth are lacking

Assessment

History

- Review the pattern, onset, and duration of fatigue.
- Ask if the patient has other symptoms.
- Inquire about viral or bacterial illness or stress.
- Ask about nutrition and appetite or weight changes.
- Review the medical and psychiatric history for disorders that produce fatigue.
- Ask about a family history of chronic disorders.
- Obtain a drug and alcohol history.
- Ask about carbon monoxide exposure.

Physical assessment

- Observe the patient's general appearance for overt signs of depression or organic illness.
- Evaluate mental status.
- Take vital signs.
- Perform a complete physical examination.

Medical causes

Acquired immunodeficiency syndrome

- Fatigue, fever, night sweats, weight loss, diarrhea, and a cough may develop.
- Signs of opportunistic infection and malnutrition may be apparent.

Adrenocortical insufficiency

- Mild fatigue initially appears after exertion and stress; later it becomes more severe and persistent.
- Other findings include weakness, weight loss, nausea, vomiting, anorexia, abdominal pain, chronic diarrhea, hyperpigmentation, orthostatic hypotension, and a weak, irregular pulse.

Anemia

- Fatigue after mild activity (common first symptom)
- Listlessness, irritability, inability to concentrate, pallor, tachycardia, and dyspnea

Anxiety

- Chronic anxiety invariably produces fatigue characterized as nervous exhaustion.

- Other findings include apprehension, indecisiveness, restlessness, insomnia, trembling, and increased muscle tension.

Cancer

- Unexplained fatigue is typically the earliest sign.
- Other findings vary with the type of cancer and may include pain, nausea, vomiting, anorexia, weight loss, abnormal bleeding, and a palpable mass.

Chronic fatigue syndrome

- Incapacitating fatigue
- Sore throat, myalgia, low-grade fever, painful lymph nodes, sleep disturbances, and cognitive dysfunction

Chronic obstructive pulmonary disease

- Progressive fatigue and dyspnea are the earliest symptoms.
- Other findings include a chronic and productive cough, weight loss, barrel chest, cyanosis, slight dependent edema, and poor exercise tolerance.

Depression

- Persistent fatigue unrelated to exertion accompanies chronic depression.
- Other somatic complaints include headache, anorexia, constipation, and sexual dysfunction.
- Other findings include insomnia, slowed speech, agitation or bradykinesia, irritability, loss of concentration, feelings of worthlessness, and persistent thoughts of death.

Diabetes mellitus

- Insidious or abrupt fatigue
- Weight loss, blurred vision, polyuria, polydipsia, and polyphagia

Heart failure

- Persistent fatigue and lethargy are characteristic.
- Left-sided heart failure produces exertional and paroxysmal nocturnal dyspnea, orthopnea, and tachycardia.
- Right-sided heart failure produces jugular vein distention and possibly a slight but persistent nonproductive cough.

Hypercortisolism

- Fatigue from sleep disturbances
- Characteristic signs: truncal obesity with slender extremities, buffalo hump, moon face, purple striae, acne, hirsutism, increased blood pressure, and muscle weakness.

Hypopituitarism

- Slowly developing fatigue, lethargy, and weakness
- Irritability, anorexia, amenorrhea or impotence, decreased libido, hypotension, dizziness, headache, vision disturbances, and cold intolerance

Hypothyroidism

○ Fatigue occurs early with forgetfulness, cold intolerance, weight gain, metrorrhagia, and constipation.
○ Other findings include coarse hair and alopecia; anorexia; edema; dry, flaky skin; and thinning nails.

Infection

○ With chronic infection, fatigue is typically the most prominent symptom.
○ With acute infection, brief fatigue typically accompanies headache, anorexia, arthralgia, chills, and fever.

Lyme disease

○ Fatigue, malaise, headache, fever, chills, expanding red rash, and muscle and joint aches occur.
○ In later stages, arthritis, fluctuating meningoencephalitis, and cardiac abnormalities may occur.

Malnutrition

○ Easy fatigability, lethargy, and apathy
○ Weight loss, muscle wasting, pallor, edema, cold sensation, and dry, flaky skin

Myasthenia gravis

○ Easy fatigability and muscle weakness, which worsen as the day progresses, are classic symptoms.
○ Symptoms worsen with exertion and subside with rest.

Myocardial infarction

○ Fatigue can be severe but is typically overshadowed by chest pain.
○ Other findings include dyspnea, anxiety, pallor, cold sweat, increased or decreased blood pressure, and abnormal heart sounds.

Narcolepsy

○ Hypersomnia, hypnagogic hallucinations, cataplexy, sleep paralysis, insomnia, and fatigue are common.

Renal failure

○ Sudden fatigue occurs with drowsiness and lethargy.
○ Other findings include oliguria, ammonia breath odor, nausea, vomiting, diarrhea or constipation, dry skin and mucous membranes, muscle twitching, changes in personality and LOC, seizures, and coma.
○ Chronic renal failure causes insidious fatigue and lethargy with marked changes in all body systems.

Restrictive lung disease

○ Chronic fatigue may accompany dyspnea, cough, cyanosis, and rapid, shallow respirations.

Rheumatoid arthritis

○ Fatigue, weakness, and anorexia precede joint pain, tenderness, warmth, swelling, and morning stiffness.
○ Other findings include enlarged lymph nodes, fever, leukopenia, subcutaneous nodules, pericarditis, and Raynaud's phenomenon.

Systemic lupus erythematosus

○ Fatigue occurs with generalized aching, malaise, low-grade fever, headache, and irritability.
○ Other findings include joint pain and stiffness, butterfly rash, photosensitivity, Raynaud's phenomenon, patchy alopecia, and mucous membrane ulcers.

Thyrotoxicosis

○ Fatigue may occur with enlarged thyroid gland, tachycardia, palpitations, tremors, weight loss despite increased appetite, diarrhea, dyspnea, nervousness, diaphoresis, heat intolerance, amenorrhea, and exophthalmos.

Valvular heart disease

○ Progressive fatigue and a cardiac murmur are common and accompanied by exertional dyspnea, cough, and hemoptysis.

Other causes

Carbon monoxide poisoning

○ Fatigue occurs with headache, dyspnea, and confusion and can progress to unconsciousness and apnea.

Drugs

○ Antihypertensives and sedatives may cause fatigue.
○ In the patient taking digoxin, fatigue may signal toxicity.

Nursing considerations

○ Help the patient determine and pace activities.
○ Encourage rest periods.
○ Take measures to reduce pain and nausea.
○ If fatigue results from a psychogenic cause, refer the patient for psychological counseling.

Pediatric pointers

○ Fatigue occurs normally during accelerated growth phases.
○ Consider depression as a cause.
○ In a pubescent child, consider drug abuse.

Geriatric pointers

○ Fatigue may be insidious and mask more serious underlying conditions in this age-group.

Patient teaching

○ Educate the patient about lifestyle modifications, including diet and exercise.
○ Stress the importance of pacing his activities and planning rest periods.
○ Discuss stress management techniques.

Fecal incontinence

Overview

○ Refers to the involuntary passage of feces
○ Follows any loss or impairment of external anal sphincter control
○ May be temporary or permanent, with sudden or gradual onset

Assessment

History

○ Ask about the onset, duration, and severity of fecal incontinence.
○ Note a discernible pattern.
○ Note the frequency, consistency, and volume of stools.
○ Obtain a medical history, focusing on GI, neurological, and psychological disorders.

Physical assessment

○ If a brain or spinal cord lesion is the suspected cause, perform a neurologic examination. (See *How the nervous system controls defecation.*)
○ If a GI disturbance seems likely, inspect, auscultate, percuss, and palpate the abdomen.
○ Inspect the anal area for excoriation or infection.
○ Check for fecal impaction.

Medical causes

Dementia

○ Fecal as well as urinary incontinence may occur.
○ Other findings include impaired judgment and abstract thinking, amnesia, emotional lability, hyperactive deep tendon reflexes (DTRs), aphasia or dysarthria, and diffuse choreoathetoid movements.

Gastroenteritis

○ Temporary fecal incontinence may occur with explosive diarrhea.
○ Other findings include nausea, vomiting, headache, myalgia, hyperactive bowel sounds, and colicky, peristaltic abdominal pain.

Head trauma

○ Fecal incontinence can occur.
○ Other findings depend on the location and severity of the injury and may include decreased level of consciousness, seizures, vomiting, and motor and sensory impairments.

Inflammatory bowel disease

○ Nocturnal fecal incontinence may occur with diarrhea.

○ Other findings include abdominal pain, anorexia, weight loss, blood in stool, and hyperactive bowel sounds.

Multiple sclerosis

○ Fecal incontinence is a variable sign.
○ Other findings include muscle weakness, ataxia, and paralysis; gait disturbances; sensory impairment; blurred vision, diplopia, or nystagmus; urinary disturbances; and emotional lability.

Rectovaginal fistula

○ Fecal incontinence occurs with uninhibited passage of flatus.

Spinal cord lesions

○ Fecal incontinence occurs that may be permanent, depending on the severity of the lesion.
○ Other findings include motor and sensory disturbances below the level of the lesion.

Stroke

○ Temporary fecal incontinence occurs that resolves when muscle tone and DTRs are restored.
○ Persistent fecal incontinence reflects extensive neurologic damage.
○ Other findings include urinary incontinence, hemiplegia, dysarthria, aphasia, sensory losses, reflex changes, and visual field deficits.

Tabes dorsalis

○ This late sign of syphilis may result in fecal incontinence.
○ Other findings include urinary incontinence, ataxic gait, paresthesia, loss of DTRs and temperature sensation, severe flashing pain, Charcot's joints, Argyll Robertson pupils, and impotence.

Other causes

Drugs

○ Chronic laxative abuse may cause insensitivity to a fecal mass or loss of the colonic defecation reflex.

Surgery

○ Pelvic, prostate, or rectal surgery occasionally produces temporary fecal incontinence.

Nursing considerations

○ Maintain proper hygiene, including control of odors.
○ Take measures to allay the patient's embarrassment.
○ Encourage Kegel exercises to strengthen abdominal and perirectal muscles for the patient with intermittent or temporary incontinence.
○ Provide bowel retraining for the neurologically capable patient.

Three neurologic mechanisms normally control defecation: the intrinsic defecation reflex in the colon, the parasympathetic defecation reflex involving sacral segments of the spinal cord, and voluntary control. Here's how they interact. When the rectum is distended by feces, this activates the relatively weak intrinsic reflex, causing afferent impulses to spread through the myenteric plexus, starting peristalsis in the descending and sigmoid colon and in the rectum. The feces move toward the anus, causing receptive relaxation of the internal anal sphincter.

To complete defecation, the parasympathetic reflex magnifies the intrinsic reflex. Stimulation of afferent nerves in the rectal wall sends impulses through the spinal cord and back to the descending and sigmoid colon, rectum, and anus to intensify peristalsis. (See illustration.)

However, when the feces move and the sphincter relaxes, this may cause the external anal sphincter to immediately contract and the feces to be temporarily retained. At this point, conscious control of the external sphincter either prevents or permits defecation. Except in infants or neurologically impaired patients, this voluntary mechanism further contracts the sphincter to prevent defecation at inappropriate times, or relaxes it and allows defecation to occur.

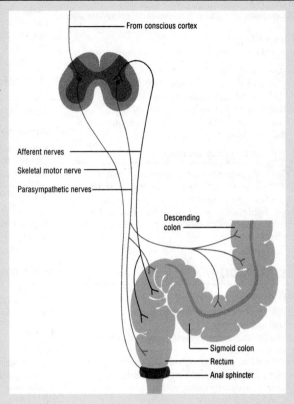

Pediatric pointers

○ Fecal incontinence is normal in infants and may occur temporarily in young children who experience psychological regression from stress or a physical illness with diarrhea.
○ Fecal incontinence may also result from myelomeningocele.

Geriatric pointers

○ Age-related changes affecting smooth muscle cells of the colon may change GI motility and lead to fecal incontinence, but disease must still be ruled out.

Patient teaching

○ Instruct the patient in the essential techniques of bowel retraining.
○ Explain how to do Kegel exercises.
○ Teach the patient how to maintain proper hygiene.

Fever

Overview

- Also called *pyrexia*
- Classified as low (oral reading of 99° to 100.4° F [37.2° to 38° C]), moderate (100.5° to 104° F [38.1° to 40° C]), or high (above 104° F)
- May also be classified as remittent, intermittent, sustained, relapsing, or undulant

Emergency actions

If a patient's fever is higher than 106° F (41.1° C), take the other vital signs and determine level of consciousness (LOC). Give an antipyretic and begin rapid cooling measures. To prevent a cooling response, constantly monitor the patient's rectal temperature.

Assessment

History

- Ask about the onset of fever, temperature pattern, and highest reading.
- Inquire about other symptoms, such as chills, fatigue, or pain.
- Obtain a medical history, including immunosuppressive treatments or disorders, infection, trauma, surgery, diagnostic testing, and use of anesthesia or other drugs.
- Ask about recent travel.

Physical assessment

- Take vital signs.
- Let the history findings direct your physical examination (may range from brief evaluation of one body system to comprehensive review of all systems).

Medical causes

Anthrax, cutaneous

- Fever may occur with lymphadenopathy, malaise, and headache.
- A small, painless or pruritic, macular or papular lesion develops, changing to a vesicle in 1 to 2 days, and then into a painless ulcer with a characteristic black, necrotic center.

Anthrax, GI

- Fever, loss of appetite, nausea, and vomiting occur after eating contaminated food.
- Abdominal pain, severe bloody diarrhea, and hematemesis may also develop.

Anthrax, inhalation

- Initially, fever, chills, weakness, cough, and chest pain occur.
- Abrupt deterioration—marked by fever, dyspnea, stridor, and hypotension—occurs in the second stage, generally leading to death within 24 hours.

Escherichia coli 0157:H7

- Fever, bloody diarrhea, nausea, vomiting, and abdominal cramps occur.

Immune complex dysfunction

- Fever usually remains low and may be remittent, intermittent, or sustained.
- Other findings depend on the specific disease.

Infectious and inflammatory disorders

- Fever varies depending on the disorder and may be remittent, intermittent, sustained, or relapsing.
- Fever may occur abruptly or insidiously.
- Other findings involve every body system.

Neoplasms

- Prolonged fever of varying elevations occurs.
- Other findings include nocturnal diaphoresis, anorexia, fatigue, malaise, and weight loss.

Plague

- Bubonic form causes fever, chills, and swollen, inflamed, and tender lymph nodes near the bite.
- Pneumonic form manifests as a sudden onset of chills, fever, headache, and myalgia.
- Other findings of pneumonic form include productive cough, chest pain, tachypnea, dyspnea, hemoptysis, increasing respiratory distress, and cardiopulmonary insufficiency.

Rhabdomyolysis

- Fever, muscle weakness or pain, nausea, vomiting, malaise, or dark reddish brown urine result.

Severe acute respiratory syndrome

- Disease generally begins with fever greater than 100.4° F (38° C).
- Other symptoms include headache, malaise, a dry nonproductive cough, and dyspnea.

Smallpox

- Initial findings include high fever, malaise, prostration, severe headache, backache, and abdominal pain.
- A maculopapular rash develops on the mucosa of the mouth, pharynx, face, and forearms and then spreads to the trunk and legs.
- Within 2 days, the rash becomes vesicular and later pustular; by day 8 or 9 crusts form that later separate, leaving a scar.

Thermoregulatory dysfunction

○ Sudden onset of fever that rises rapidly and remains as high as 107° F (41.7° C) occurs in life-threatening disorders.
○ Low or moderate fever appears in dehydrated patients.
○ Prolonged high fever produces vomiting, anhidrosis, decreased LOC, and hot, flushed skin.

Tularemia

○ Onset of fever, chills, headache, generalized myalgia, nonproductive cough, dyspnea, pleuritic chest pain, and empyema is abrupt.

West Nile encephalitis

○ Fever, headache, body aches, skin rash, and swollen lymph nodes occur.
○ Severe infection is marked by high fever, headache, neck stiffness, stupor, disorientation, coma, tremors, seizures, and paralysis.

Other causes

Drugs

○ Fever can accompany chemotherapy.
○ Drugs that impair sweating, such as anticholinergics, phenothiazines, and monoamine oxidase inhibitors, can result in fever.
○ Hypersensitivity to antifungals, sulfonamides, penicillins, cephalosporins, tetracyclines, barbiturates, phenytoin, quinidine, iodides, phenolphthalein, methyldopa, procainamide, and some antitoxins can cause fever and rash.
○ Muscle relaxants and inhaled anesthetics and muscle relaxants can trigger malignant hyperthermia.
○ Toxic doses of salicylates, amphetamines, and tricyclic antidepressants can cause fever.

Nursing considerations

○ Regularly monitor and record temperature.
○ Increase fluid and nutritional intake.
○ Maintain stable room temperature.
○ Provide frequent bedding and clothing changes.
○ Give antipyretics according to a regular dosage schedule to minimize chills and diaphoresis.

Pediatric pointers

○ Infants and young children experience higher and more prolonged fevers, more rapid temperature increases, and greater temperature fluctuations.
○ Common pediatric causes of fever include varicella, croup syndrome, dehydration, meningitis, mumps, otitis media, pertussis, roseola infantum, rubella, rubeola, tonsillitis, and adverse reactions to immunizations and antibiotics.
○ Be aware that seizures commonly accompany extremely high fever in children.

Geriatric pointers

○ Elderly patients may have impaired thermoregulatory mechanisms, making temperature change a much less reliable measure of disease severity than other measures.

Patient teaching

○ Instruct the patient about the proper way to take oral temperature measurement at home.
○ Emphasize the importance of increased fluid intake (unless contraindicated).
○ Discuss the use of antipyretics.

Flank pain

Overview

○ Indicates renal and upper urinary tract disease or trauma
○ May range from a dull ache to a severe stabbing or throbbing pain
○ May be in one or both flanks, constant or intermittent

Emergency actions

If the patient has suffered trauma, quickly look for a visible or palpable flank mass, other injuries, costovertebral angle (CVA) tenderness, hematuria, Turner's sign, and signs of shock. If one or more signs of shock are present, insert an I.V. line to allow fluid or drug infusion. Insert an indwelling urinary catheter to monitor urine output and evaluate hematuria.

Assessment

History

○ Ask about the onset, location, intensity, pattern, and duration of pain.
○ Ask what alleviates or aggravates the pain.
○ Explore precipitating events to pain.
○ Ask about the patient's normal fluid intake and urine output and recent changes.
○ Obtain a medical history, including urinary tract infection (UTI), obstruction, renal disease, or recent streptococcal infection.

Physical assessment

○ Palpate the flank area and percuss the CVA.

Medical causes

Bladder cancer

○ Dull, constant flank pain radiating to the legs, back, and perineum
○ The first signs: gross, painless, intermittent hematuria, usually with clots
○ Urinary frequency and urgency, nocturia, dysuria, or pyuria; bladder distention; pain in the bladder, rectum, pelvis, back, or legs, diarrhea, vomiting, and sleep disturbances

Calculi

○ Intense colicky pain in one flank radiates from the CVA.
○ Other findings include nausea, vomiting, CVA tenderness, hematuria, hypoactive bowel sounds, and signs and symptoms of UTI.

Cystitis (bacterial)

○ Flank pain as well as perineal, lower back, and suprapubic pain
○ Dysuria, nocturia, hematuria, urinary frequency and urgency, tenesmus, fatigue, and low-grade fever

Glomerulonephritis (acute)

○ Constant and moderately intense flank pain
○ Most commonly, moderate facial and generalized edema, hematuria, oliguria or anuria, and fatigue
○ Low-grade fever, malaise, nausea, vomiting, dyspnea, tachypnea, and crackles

Obstructive uropathy

○ With acute obstruction, flank pain may be excruciating.
○ With gradual obstruction, pain is typically a dull ache.
○ Other findings include nausea, vomiting, abdominal distention, anuria alternating with periods of oliguria and polyuria, and hypoactive bowel sounds.
○ A palpable abdominal mass, CVA tenderness, and bladder distention vary with the site and cause of the obstruction.

Pancreatitis (acute)

○ Flank pain may develop as severe epigastric or left-upper-quadrant pain that radiates to the back.
○ A severe attack causes extreme pain, nausea, persistent vomiting, abdominal tenderness and rigidity, hypoactive bowel sounds, restlessness, low-grade fever, tachycardia, hypotension, and positive Turner's and Cullen's signs.

Papillary necrosis (acute)

○ Intense flank pain with renal colic, CVA tenderness, and abdominal pain and rigidity
○ Oliguria or anuria, hematuria, and pyuria, with fever, chills, vomiting, and hypoactive bowel sounds

Perirenal abscess

○ Intense pain in one flank and CVA tenderness accompany dysuria, persistent high fever, and chills.

Polycystic kidney disease

○ Dull, aching, pain in both flanks is an early symptom.
○ Pain may become severe and colicky if cysts rupture and clots migrate or cause obstruction.
○ Early findings include polyuria, increased blood pressure, and signs of UTI.
○ Late findings include hematuria, and perineal, lower back, and suprapubic pain.

Pyelonephritis (acute)

○ Intense, constant flank pain develops.
○ Typical urinary features include dysuria, nocturia, hematuria, urgency, frequency, and tenesmus.

○ Other common findings include persistent high fever, chills, anorexia, weakness, fatigue, myalgia, abdominal pain, and CVA tenderness.

Renal cancer

○ The classic triad: pain in one flank that's dull and vague, gross hematuria, and a palpable flank mass
○ Signs of advanced disease: weight loss, leg edema, nausea, and vomiting
○ Fever, increased blood pressure, and urine retention

Renal infarction

○ Constant, severe pain in one flank and tenderness typically accompany persistent, severe upper abdominal pain.
○ Other findings include CVA tenderness, anorexia, nausea, vomiting, fever, hypoactive bowel sounds, hematuria, and oliguria or anuria.

Renal trauma

○ Variable flank pain is common.
○ A visible or palpable flank mass and CVA or abdominal pain, which may be severe and radiate to the groin, may also develop.
○ Other findings include hematuria, oliguria, abdominal distention, Turner's sign, hypoactive bowel sounds, nausea, vomiting and, with severe injury, signs of shock.

Renal vein thrombosis

○ Severe pain in one flank and lower back pain with CVA and epigastric tenderness are typical.
○ Other findings include fever, hematuria, and leg edema.

Nursing considerations

○ Give drugs for pain.
○ Continue to monitor vital signs.
○ Maintain a precise record of intake and output.

Pediatric pointers

○ Transillumination of the abdomen and flanks may help in assessment of bladder distention and identification of masses in children.
○ Common causes of flank pain in children include obstructive uropathy, acute poststreptococcal glomerulonephritis, infantile polycystic kidney disease, and nephroblastoma.

Patient teaching

○ Explain the importance of increased fluid intake (unless contraindicated).
○ Explain the signs and symptoms to report.
○ Emphasize the importance of taking drugs as prescribed.
○ Stress the importance of keeping follow-up appointments.

Flatulence

Overview

- Sensation of gaseous abdominal fullness
- Reflects slowed intestinal motility, excessive swallowing of air, or increased intraluminal gas production

Assessment

History
- Determine the duration and amount of flatulence.
- Ask about other signs, including belching, snoring, and overly rapid speech.
- Inquire about unusual emotional stress.
- Obtain a medical history, including GI disorders and systemic illnesses.

Physical assessment
- Inspect the abdomen for distention.
- Auscultate for abnormal bowel sounds.
- Percuss for increased tympany from gas accumulation.
- Palpate for tenderness and masses.

Medical causes

Cirrhosis
- Early and insidious flatulence
- Anorexia, dyspepsia, nausea, vomiting, diarrhea or constipation, dull right-upper-quadrant pain, hepatomegaly, splenomegaly, fatigue, and malaise.

Teaching a patient to follow an antiflatulence diet

To help the patient reduce gas, tell him to follow these dietary suggestions:
- Avoid these vegetables and fruits: broccoli, brussels sprouts, cabbage, cauliflower, cucumbers, dried beans, green peppers, kohlrabi, lettuce, lima beans, melons, onions, peas, prunes, radishes, and raw apples.
- Avoid all fatty foods, such as red meats, fried foods, and pastries.
- Avoid foods and beverages that contain excess air, including souffles, carbonated drinks, and milk shakes.
- If you have lactose intolerance, avoid milk, cheese, ice cream, and all other dairy products.
- Don't overeat, eat too rapidly, or eat while under emotional stress.
- Don't drink large amounts of liquids with meals.
- Don't take laxatives.

Colon cancer
- Flatulence may be accompanied by abdominal distention and tympany on percussion.
- Other findings include abdominal pain, anorexia, weight loss, malaise, and altered bowel habits.

Crohn's disease
- Flatulence accompanies abdominal pain, cramps, and tenderness; diarrhea; low-grade fever; nausea; and melena.

Irritable bowel syndrome
- Chronic flatulence, belching, and excessive flatus
- Chronic constipation, but diurnal diarrhea may occur, and intermittent lower abdominal pain that abates with defecation of passage of flatus

Lactose intolerance
- Flatulence develops within several hours after the ingestion of dairy products.
- Other findings include cramping, abdominal pain, and diarrhea.

Malabsorption syndromes
- Flatulence may occur.
- Other findings include abdominal pain, anorexia, weight loss, and passage of bulky, oily, malodorous, or watery stools.
- With severe malabsorption, muscle wasting and weakness, skeletal pain, edema, ecchymoses, and ulceration of the tongue may occur.

Other causes

Abdominal surgery
- When peristalsis resumes, gas accumulation produces flatulence.

Herbal products
- Some herbal products such as garlic can cause flatulence.

Nursing considerations

- Encourage frequent repositioning, ambulation, and normal fluid intake, as permitted, to prevent gas buildup.
- Position the patient on his left side to aid expulsion of gas.
- Insert rectal tube if needed.
- Give an enema, suppository, antiflatulent, or anticholinergic.
- Provide a diet that excludes gaseous foods. (See *Teaching a patient to follow an antiflatulence diet.*)

Pediatric pointers

○ Stomachache commonly results from flatulence.
○ Children may be more sensitive to flatus-producing foods and aerophagia.

Geriatric pointers

○ Increased flatulence may result from poor dentition, leading to poor mastication of food, poor dietary intake, and decreased GI motility.

Patient teaching

○ Explain ways to reduce flatulence.
○ If the patient is lactose intolerant, explain which foods he should avoid.

Footdrop

Overview

- Plantar flexion of foot with the toes bent toward the instep
- Results from weakness or paralysis of dorsiflexor muscles of foot and ankle
- A characteristic sign of certain peripheral nerve or motor neuron disorders; may also result from prolonged immobility when inadequate support, improper positioning, or infrequent passive exercise produces shortening of the Achilles tendon

Assessment

History

- Ask about the onset, duration, and character of footdrop.
- Determine what alleviates or aggravates footdrop.
- Ask about weakness or tiredness.

Physical assessment

- Assess muscle tone and strength in feet and legs; compare findings on both sides.
- Assess deep tendon reflexes (DTRs) in both legs.
- Assess the patient's gait.

Medical causes

Guillain-Barré syndrome

- Footdrop and steppage gait result from profound muscle weakness.
- Weakness begins in the legs and extends to the arms and face within 72 hours, possibly progressing to total motor paralysis and respiratory failure.
- Other findings include transient paresthesia, hypoactive DTRs, hypernasality, dysphagia, diaphoresis, tachycardia, orthostatic hypotension, and incontinence.

Herniated lumbar disk

- Footdrop and steppage gait may result from leg muscle weakness and atrophy.
- The most pronounced finding is lower back pain that may radiate to the buttocks, legs, and feet.
- Other findings include sciatic pain, muscle spasms, sensorimotor loss, paresthesia, hypoactive DTRs, and fasciculations.

Multiple sclerosis

- Footdrop may develop suddenly or slowly, producing steppage gait.
- Muscle weakness ranges from minor fatigability to paraparesis with urinary urgency and constipation.

- Other findings include facial pain, vision disturbances, paresthesia, lack of coordination, and loss of vibration and position sensation in the ankles and toes.

Myasthenia gravis

- Footdrop and limb weakness are common.
- Typically, muscle function worsens throughout the day and with exercise and improves with rest; condition may progress to skeletal and respiratory muscle paralysis.
- Weak eye closure, ptosis, and diplopia may develop.

Peroneal muscle atrophy

- Footdrop, ankle instability, and steppage gait occur.
- Foot, peroneal, and ankle dorsiflexor muscles are affected first.
- Other early findings include paresthesia, aching, and cramping in the feet and legs, with coldness, swelling, and cyanosis.
- As the disease progresses, leg muscles become weak with hypoactive or absent DTRs.
- Later, atrophy and sensory loss spread to the arms.

Peroneal nerve trauma

- Sudden footdrop resolving with the release of peroneal nerve compression
- Ipsilateral steppage gait, muscle weakness, and sensory loss over the lateral surface of the calf and foot

Poliomyelitis

- Footdrop, producing a steppage gait
- Fever, asymmetrical muscle weakness, paresthesia, hypoactive or absent DTRs, and permanent muscle paralysis and atrophy

Polyneuropathy

- Footdrop and steppage gait with muscle weakness, that progresses to flaccid paralysis
- Muscle atrophy; hypoactive or absent DTRs; paresthesia, hyperesthesia, or anesthesia and loss of vibration sensation in the hands and feet; glossy skin; and anhidrosis

Spinal cord trauma

- Sudden and possibly permanent footdrop
- ONeck and back pain; paresthesia, sensory loss, and muscle weakness, atrophy, or paralysis distal to the injury; asymmetrical or absent DTRs; and fecal and urinary incontinence

Stroke

- Footdrop with arm and leg weakness or paralysis
- Paresthesia, dysphagia, visual field defects, diplopia, bowel and bladder changes, personality changes, amnesia, aphasia, dysarthria, and decreased level of consciousness

Nursing considerations

○ Anticipate physical therapy, in-shoe splints, or leg braces.
○ Perform range-of-motion exercises and use positioning aids to help prevent footdrop in the immobilized patient.

Pediatric pointers

○ Common causes of footdrop in children include spinal birth defects and degenerative disorders.

Patient teaching

○ Explain the use of assistive devices.
○ Emphasize the safety measures the patient should take — such as asking for assistance with activities.

Gallop, atrial (S₄)

Overview

- Also known as *presystolic gallop*
- Refers to a fourth (S₄) heart sound heard or palpated before the S₁
- Originates from left atrial contraction
- A low-pitched sound best heard with the bell of the stethoscope pressed lightly against the cardiac apex (see *Locating heart sounds*)

Emergency actions

If the patient has chest pain, suspect myocardial ischemia. Take vital signs and assess for signs of heart failure. Connect the patient to the cardiac monitor, obtain an electrocardiogram, and administer oxygen and an antianginal. If the patient has dyspnea, elevate the head of the bed. If you detect coarse crackles, give oxygen and diuretics. If the patient has bradycardia, give atropine and tell the patient he may need a pacemaker.

Assessment

History

- Obtain a medical history, including hypertension, angina, cardiomyopathy, or valvular stenosis.
- Ask about the frequency and severity of anginal attacks.

Physical assessment

- Take vital signs.
- Perform a complete cardiopulmonary examination.

Medical causes

Anemia

- An atrial gallop may accompany increased cardiac output.
- Other findings may include fatigue, pallor, dyspnea, tachycardia, a bounding pulse, crackles, and a systolic bruit over the carotid arteries.

Angina

- An intermittent atrial gallop typically occurs during an attack.
- The gallop may be accompanied by paradoxical S₂ or a new murmur.
- Other findings include chest tightness, pressure, aching, or burning that radiates to the neck, jaw, left shoulder, and arm; dyspnea; tachycardia; increased blood pressure; diaphoresis; dizziness; nausea; and vomiting.

Aortic insufficiency (acute)

- Atrial gallop is accompanied by a soft, short diastolic murmur along the left sternal border.
- S₂ may be soft or absent and a soft, short midsystolic murmur may be heard over the second right intercostal space.
- Other findings include tachycardia, dyspnea, jugular vein distention, crackles, cool extremities, and angina.

Aortic stenosis

- Atrial gallop occurs with severe valvular obstruction.
- Auscultation reveals a harsh, crescendo-decrescendo (louder-then-softer), systolic-ejection murmur.
- Angina and syncope are principal findings.
- Other findings include crackles, palpitations, fatigue, and diminished carotid pulses.

Assessment tip
Locating heart sounds

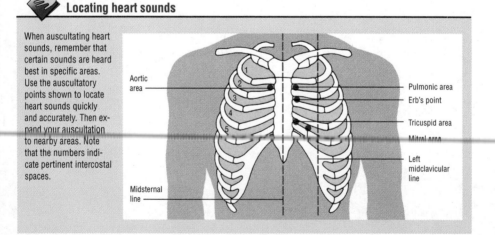

When auscultating heart sounds, remember that certain sounds are heard best in specific areas. Use the auscultatory points shown to locate heart sounds quickly and accurately. Then expand your auscultation to nearby areas. Note that the numbers indicate pertinent intercostal spaces.

Aortic area

Midsternal line

Pulmonic area
Erb's point
Tricuspid area
Mitral area

Left midclavicular line

Atrioventricular block

○ First-degree atrioventricular (AV) block may cause an atrial gallop accompanied by a faint S_1, but the patient remains asymptomatic.
○ Second-degree AV block produces an atrial gallop.
○ Third-degree AV block produces an atrial gallop that varies in intensity with S_1.
○ Other findings include hypotension, light-headedness, dizziness, angina, and syncope.

Cardiomyopathy

○ Atrial gallop, dyspnea, orthopnea, crackles, fatigue, syncope, chest pain, palpitations, edema, jugular vein distention, S_3, and transient or sustained bradycardia, usually associated with tachycardia

Hypertension

○ Atrial gallop is an early sign.
○ The patient may be asymptomatic or may experience headache, weakness, epistaxis, tinnitus, dizziness, and fatigue.

Mitral insufficiency

○ Atrial gallop with an S_3
○ A harsh holosystolic murmur, fatigue, dyspnea, tachypnea, orthopnea, tachycardia, crackles, and jugular vein distention.

Myocardial infarction

○ Atrial gallop signifies a life-threatening myocardial infarction (MI) and may persist after the infarction heals.
○ Crushing substernal chest pain may radiate to the back, neck, jaw, shoulder, and left arm.
○ Other findings include dyspnea, restlessness, anxiety, a feeling of impending doom, diaphoresis, pallor, clammy skin, nausea, vomiting, and increased or decreased blood pressure.

Pulmonary embolism

○ A life-threatening disorder; right-sided atrial gallop heard along the lower left sternal border with a loud pulmonic closure sound
○ Tachycardia, tachypnea, fever, chest pain, diaphoresis, syncope, cyanosis, and a nonproductive or productive cough with blood-tinged sputum

Thyrotoxicosis

○ Atrial gallop and S_3
○ Tachycardia, bounding pulse, wide pulse pressure, palpitations, weight loss despite increased appetite, diarrhea, tremors, an enlarged thyroid gland, dyspnea, nervousness, difficulty concentrating, heat intolerance, exophthalmos, weakness, fatigue, and muscle atrophy

Nursing considerations

○ Monitor for signs and symptoms of heart failure.
○ Give drugs and oxygen.

Pediatric pointers

○ May occur normally, especially after exercise or may result from congenital heart disease

Geriatric pointers

○ May occur normally in elderly patients

Patient teaching

○ Discuss with the patient ways to reduce his cardiac risk.
○ Teach the patient the correct way to measure his pulse rate.
○ Emphasize conditions that require medical attention.
○ Stress the importance of follow-up appointments.

Gallop, ventricular (S₃)

Overview

○ Refers to a third heart sound (S_3) after the S_2
○ May be physiologic or pathologic
○ Associated with rapid ventricular filling in early diastole
○ Best heard along the lower left sternal border or over the xiphoid region on inspiration (right-sided) or at the apex on expiration (left-sided)

Assessment

History

○ Ask about location, frequency, and duration of chest pain and what aggravates and alleviates it.
○ Ask about palpitations, dizziness, syncope, difficulty breathing, or cough.
○ Obtain a medical history, including cardiac disorders.
○ Obtain a drug history.

Physical assessment

○ Auscultate for murmurs or abnormalities in S_1 and S_2. (See *Auscultating the heart.*)
○ Listen for pulmonary crackles.
○ Assess peripheral pulses.
○ Palpate the liver.
○ Assess for jugular vein distention and peripheral edema.

Medical causes

Aortic insufficiency

○ In acute cases, ventricular and atrial gallops may occur with a soft, short diastolic murmur.

Assessment tip
Auscultating the heart

Follow these tips when you auscultate a patient's heart:
● Concentrate as you listen for each sound.
● Avoid auscultating through clothing or wound dressings because they can block sound.
● Avoid picking up extraneous sounds by keeping the stethoscope tubing off the patient's body and other surfaces.
● Until you become proficient at auscultation and can examine a patient quickly, explain to him that even though you may listen to his chest for a long period, it doesn't mean that anything is wrong.
● Ask the patient to breathe normally and to hold his breath periodically to enhance sounds that may be difficult to hear.

○ Other findings in acute disease include tachycardia, dyspnea, jugular vein distention, and crackles.
○ In chronic cases, a ventricular gallop and a high-pitched, blowing, decrescendo diastolic murmur occur.
○ Other findings of chronic disease include tachycardia, palpitations, angina, fatigue, dyspnea, orthopnea, and crackles.

Cardiomyopathy

○ Ventricular gallop is common.
○ Other alternating pulse and altered S_1 and S_2 signal advanced heart disease.
○ Other findings include fatigue, dyspnea, orthopnea, chest pain, palpitations, syncope, crackles, peripheral edema, jugular vein distention, and an atrial gallop.

Heart failure

○ Ventricular gallop is a classic sign.
○ Other sinus tachycardia indicates severe heart failure.
○ Other findings of left-sided heart failure include fatigue, exertional dyspnea, paroxysmal nocturnal dyspnea, orthopnea, and a dry cough.
○ Jugular vein distention occurs with right-sided heart failure.
○ Other late findings include tachypnea, chest tightness, palpitations, anorexia, nausea, dependent edema, weight gain, slowed mental response, hepatomegaly, and pallor.

Mitral insufficiency

○ In acute cases, ventricular gallop may be accompanied by an early or holosystolic decrescendo murmur at the apex, an atrial gallop, and a widely split second heart sound.
○ Other findings of acute disease include tachycardia, tachypnea, orthopnea, dyspnea, crackles, jugular vein distention, and fatigue.
○ In chronic cases, ventricular gallop is progressively severe and accompanied by fatigue, exertional dyspnea, and palpitations.

Thyrotoxicosis

○ Ventricular and atrial gallops may occur.
○ Important findings include an enlarged thyroid gland, weight loss despite increased appetite, heat intolerance, diaphoresis, nervousness, tremors, tachycardia, palpitations, diarrhea, and dyspnea.

Nursing considerations

○ Assess for tachycardia, dyspnea, crackles, and jugular vein distention.
○ To prevent pulmonary edema, give oxygen, diuretics, and other drugs, such as digoxin and angiotensin-converting enzyme inhibitors.

Pediatric pointers

○ Ventricular gallop is normally heard in children but may accompany congenital abnormalities associated with heart failure or result from sickle cell anemia.

Patient teaching

○ Explain dietary and fluid restrictions the patient needs.
○ Stress the importance of scheduled rest periods.
○ Explain signs and symptoms of fluid overload that the patient should report.
○ Teach the patient how to measure and monitor his daily weight.

Genital lesions, male

Overview

- Include warts, papules, ulcers, scales, and pustules
- May be painful or painless, singular or multiple
- May result from infection, neoplasms, parasites, allergy, or drugs

Assessment

History

- Ask about the onset and description of lesions.
- Obtain a description of drainage, itching, or pain.
- Take a sexual history, including frequency of relations, number of sexual partners, and pattern of condom use.

Physical assessment

- Observe the patient for tight clothing.
- Examine the skin, noting location, size, color, and pattern of lesions. (See *Recognizing common genital lesions in men and boys.*)
- Palpate for nodules, masses, and tenderness.
- Look for bleeding, edema, or signs of infection.
- Take vital signs.

Medical causes

Balanitis and balanoposthitis

- Painful ulceration on the glans, foreskin, or penile shaft occurs.
- Prepuce irritation and soreness, followed by a foul discharge and edema, precede ulceration by 2 to 3 days.
- Other findings include fever with chills, malaise, and dysuria.

Bowen's disease

- Painless, premalignant lesion that appears as a brownish red, raised, scaly, indurated plaque with well-defined borders occurs, usually on the penis or scrotum.

Candidiasis

- Erythematous, weepy, circumscribed lesions usually appear under the prepuce.
- Vesicles and pustules may also develop.

Chancroid

- One or more lesions erupt on the groin, inner thigh, or penis.
- Lesions progress from a reddened area to a small papule, then to a pustule that ulcerates.
- Ulcer is painful, deep, bleeds easily, and has a purulent gray or yellow exudate.

- Inguinal lymph nodes enlarge, become tender, and may drain pus.

Folliculitis and furunculosis

- Folliculitis may cause red, pointed lesions that are tender and swollen with central pustules.
- If folliculitis progresses to furunculosis, lesions become hard, painful nodules that may enlarge and rupture.

Genital herpes

- Fluid-filled vesicles develop on the glans penis, foreskin, or shaft.
- Vesicles are painless at first but may rupture into shallow, painful ulcers with redness, edema, and dysuria.

Genital warts

- Tiny red or pink painless swellings develop on the subpreputial sac or urethral meatus and spread to the perineum and perianal area.
- Warts may grow, become pedunculated, cauliflower-like, and malodorous.

Lichen planus

- Small, shiny, polygonal, violet papules with white, lacy, milky striations develop on the glans penis.
- Papules may be linear or coalesce into plaques.
- Other findings include pruritus, distorted nails, and alopecia.

Pediculosis pubis

- Erythematous, itching papules develop in the pubic area and around anus, abdomen, and thigh.
- Other features include grayish white specks (lice eggs) attached to hair shafts, and skin irritation.

Psoriasis

- Red, raised, scaly plaques may develop on the penis.
- Other features include itching, pain from dry, cracked, encrusted lesions; nail pitting; and joint stiffness.

Scabies

- Crusted lesions or large papules appear on the glans and shaft of the penis and on the scrotum.
- Nocturnal itching is typical, causing excoriation.

Seborrheic dermatitis

- Erythematous, dry or moist greasy scaling papules and yellow crusts that form annular plaques develop on the shaft of the penis, scrotum, groin, scalp, chest, eyebrows, back, axillae, and umbilicus.

Syphilis

- Small, red, fluid-filled chancres may erupt on the genitalia 2 to 4 weeks after exposure.
- Chancres erode to form painless, firm, indurated, shallow ulcers with clear bases and scant, yellow serous discharge.

Tinea cruris

○ Sharply defined, slightly raised, scaling patches typically develop on the inner thigh or groin.
○ Pruritus may be severe.

Urticaria

○ Pruritic hives may appear on the genitalia, especially on foreskin or shaft of penis.

Other causes

Drugs

○ Phenolphthalein, barbiturates, and certain broad-spectrum antibiotics may cause a fixed drug eruption and a genital lesion.

Nursing considerations

○ Screen every patient with penile lesions for sexually transmitted diseases (STDs).
○ Provide emotional support, especially if cancer is suspected.

Pediatric pointers

○ In infants, contact dermatitis may cause red, weepy, excoriated lesions.
○ The spirochete that causes syphilis can pass through the placenta, producing congenital syphilis.
○ In children, impetigo may cause pustules with thick, yellow, weepy crusts.
○ Children with STDs must be evaluated for sexual abuse.
○ Adolescents ages 15 to 19 have a high incidence of STDs.

Geriatric pointers

○ Older patients may have different symptoms of STDs from younger patients because of other disease, decreased immunity, poor hygiene, and poor symptom reporting

Patient teaching

○ Explain the use of ointments and creams.
○ Explain methods to relieve crusting and itching.
○ Emphasize the lesion changes the patient should report.
○ Discuss and teach the proper use of condoms.

Recognizing common genital lesions in men and boys

Various lesions may affect male genitalia. Some of the more common lesions and their causes appear below.

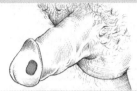

A *fixed drug eruption* causes a bright red to purplish lesion on the glans penis.

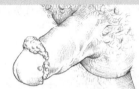

Genital warts are marked by clusters of flesh-colored papillary growths that may be barely visible or several inches in diameter.

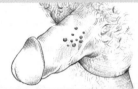

Genital herpes begins as a swollen, slightly pruritic wheal and later becomes a group of small vesicles or blisters on the foreskin, glans, or penile shaft.

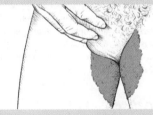

Tinea cruris (commonly known as "jock itch") produces itchy patches of well-defined, slightly raised, scaly lesions that usually affect the inner thighs and groin.

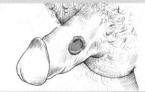

A *chancroid* causes a painful ulcer that's usually less than ¾" (2 cm) in diameter and bleeds easily. The lesion may be deep and covered by a gray or yellow exudate at its base.

Gum bleeding

Overview

- Results from dental disorders
- Ranges from slight oozing to life-threatening hemorrhage

![star] **Emergency actions**

If the patient has profuse bleeding in his mouth, check for airway patency and look for signs of cardiovascular collapse. Apply suction to remove pooled blood. Apply direct pressure to the bleeding site. Insert an airway, administer I.V. fluids, and collect serum samples.

Assessment

History

- Ask about the onset and description of the bleeding.
- Obtain a personal or family history of bleeding tendencies.
- Obtain a dental history and assess oral hygienic practices.
- Obtain a medical history, including liver or spleen disease.
- Review diet and alcohol use.
- Obtain a drug history.

Physical assessment

- Have the patient remove his dentures.
- Examine the gums.
- Check for inflammation, pockets around teeth, swelling, retraction, hypertrophy, discoloration, and gum hyperplasia.
- Note obvious decay, discoloration, foreign material, and absence of teeth.

Medical causes

Agranulocytosis

- Spontaneous gum bleeding and other systemic hemorrhages may occur.
- Signs of infection, such as fever and chills, may develop.
- Oral and perianal lesions are rough-edged with a gray or black membrane.

Aplastic anemia

- Profuse or scant gum bleeding may follow trauma.
- Other findings include other signs of bleeding, weakness, fatigue, shortness of breath, headache, pallor, and fever.
- Eventually, tachycardia and signs of heart failure develop.

Cirrhosis

- Gum bleeding, epistaxis, and other bleeding tendencies
- Ascites, hepatomegaly, pruritus, and jaundice
- Abdominal pain, anorexia, fatigue, nausea, vomiting, and weakness

Gingivitis

- Gums become bulbous, reddened, and edematous and bleed easily with slight trauma.
- With acute necrotizing ulcerative gingivitis, bleeding is spontaneous and gums are painful.
- A characteristic grayish yellow pseudomembrane develops over punched-out gum erosions.
- Other findings include halitosis, headache, malaise, fever, and cervical adenopathy.

Hemophilia

- Mild hemophilia causes easy bruising, hematomas, epistaxis, bleeding gums, and prolonged bleeding during and after surgery.
- Moderate disease produces more frequent episodes of abnormal bleeding.
- Severe disease causes spontaneous or severe bleeding after minor trauma, resulting in painful joints, peripheral neuropathies, anemia, shock, and even death.

Leukemia

- Early: easy gum bleeding with gum swelling, necrosis, and petechiae
- Acute leukemia: severe prostration marked by high fever, bleeding tendencies, dyspnea, tachycardia, palpitations, and abdominal or bone pain.
- Chronic leukemia: insidious development produces less-severe bleeding tendencies.
- Late: confusion, headaches, vomiting, seizures, papilledema, and nuchal rigidity

Periodontal disease

- Gum bleeding typically occurs after chewing, toothbrushing, or gum probing but may also occur spontaneously.
- Other findings include unpleasant taste with halitosis, facial pain, loose teeth, pus-filled pockets around the teeth, and dental calculi and plaque.

Pernicious anemia

- Gum bleeding and a sore tongue make eating painful.
- Other findings include weakness, paresthesia, altered bowel and bladder habits, personality changes, ataxia, tinnitus, dyspnea, and tachycardia.

Polycythemia vera

- Engorged gums ooze blood after even slight trauma.
- The gums and tongue are a deep red-violet.
- Other findings include headache, dyspnea, dizziness, fatigue, paresthesia, tinnitus, double or blurred vi-

sion, aquagenic pruritus, epigastric distress, weight loss, ruddy cyanosis, ecchymoses, and hepatosplenomegaly.

Thrombocytopenia

○ Blood oozes between the teeth and gums.
○ Severe bleeding may follow minor trauma.
○ Other findings include large blood-filled bullae in the mouth, petechiae, ecchymoses, epistaxis, hematuria, malaise, fatigue, weakness, and lethargy.

Thrombocytopenic purpura (idiopathic)

○ Profuse gum bleeding occurs.
○ Spontaneous hemorrhagic skin lesions range from pinpoint petechiae to massive hemorrhages.
○ Other findings include the tendency to bruise easily, petechiae on the oral mucosa, melena, epistaxis, and hematuria.

Vitamin K deficiency

○ Gums bleed when the teeth are brushed.
○ Other signs include ecchymoses, epistaxis, hematuria, hematemesis, melena, and focal neurologic deficits.

Other causes

Chemical irritants

○ Occupational exposure to benzene may irritate the gums, resulting in bleeding.

Drugs

○ Warfarin and heparin interfere with blood clotting and may cause gum bleeding.
○ Abuse of aspirin and nonsteroidal anti-inflammatory drugs may alter platelets, causing bleeding gums.

Nursing considerations

○ Anticipate a blood or blood-product transfusion.
○ When providing mouth care, avoid using lemon-glycerin swabs, which may burn or dry the gums.

Pediatric pointers

○ In neonates, bleeding gums may result from vitamin K deficiency.
○ In infants who primarily drink cow's milk and don't receive vitamin supplements, bleeding gums can result from vitamin C deficiency.

Geriatric pointers

○ In patients who have no teeth, constant gum trauma and bleeding may result from using a dental prosthesis.

Patient teaching

○ Instruct the patient in proper mouth and gum care.

○ Discuss situations that require medical attention.
○ Emphasize the importance of seeking regular dental care.

Gynecomastia

Overview

- Increased breast size in men from excessive mammary gland development
- Usually in both breasts and may be associated with breast tenderness and milk secretion

Assessment

History

- Ask about the onset of breast enlargement.
- Inquire about tenderness, discharge, testicular mass or pain, loss of libido, decreased potency, and loss of chest, axillary, or facial hair.
- Ask about recent nipple piercing.
- Obtain a drug history.

Physical assessment

- Examine the breasts for asymmetry, dimpling, abnormal pigmentation, or ulceration.
- Observe the testicles for size and symmetry; palpate to detect nodules, tenderness, or unusual consistency.
- Look for normal penile development after puberty, and note hypospadias.

Medical causes

Adrenal carcinoma

- Estrogen production by an adrenal tumor may produce a feminizing syndrome in men characterized by gynecomastia, loss of libido, impotence, testicular atrophy, and reduced facial hair growth.

Breast cancer

- Painful gynecomastia develops rapidly in the affected breast.
- Hard, stony breast lump may be palpated.
- Other findings include changes in breast symmetry, skin thickening, peau d'orange, nipple changes, and a watery, bloody, or purulent discharge.

Cirrhosis

- Gynecomastia, a late sign, is accompanied by testicular atrophy, decreased libido, and loss of facial, chest, and axillary hair.
- Other late findings include mental changes, bleeding tendencies, spider angiomas, palmar erythema, severe pruritus, dry skin, fetor hepaticus, enlarged superficial abdominal veins, jaundice, and hepatomegaly.

Hypothyroidism

- Gynecomastia with bradycardia, cold intolerance, weight gain despite anorexia, and mental dullness
- Periorbital edema; puffy face, hands, and feet; brittle, sparse hair; and dry, pale, cool, doughy skin.

Klinefelter's syndrome

- Painless gynecomastia first appears during adolescence.
- Before puberty, abnormally small testicles and slight mental deficiency appear.
- After puberty, sparse facial hair, a small penis, decreased libido, and impotence occur.

Malnutrition

- Painful gynecomastia in one breast when the malnourished patient begins to take nourishment again
- Apathy; muscle wasting; weakness; limb paresthesia; anorexia; nausea; vomiting; diarrhea; dull, sparse, dry hair; brittle nails; dark, swollen cheeks and lips; dry, flaky skin; edema; and hepatomegaly.

Pituitary tumor

- Gynecomastia with galactorrhea, impotence, and decreased libido
- Enlarged hands and feet, coarse facial features with prognathism, voice deepening, weight gain, increased blood pressure, diaphoresis, heat intolerance, hyperpigmentation, thick and oily skin, and paresthesia or sensory loss and muscle weakness in the limbs

Renal failure (chronic)

- Gynecomastia with decreased libido and impotence
- Ammonia breath odor, oliguria, fatigue, decreased mental acuity, seizures, muscle cramps, peripheral neuropathy, anorexia, nausea, vomiting, constipation or diarrhea, bleeding tendencies, yellow-brown or bronze skin, high blood pressure, and uremic frost

Testicular failure (secondary)

- Gynecomastia appears after normal puberty.
- Other signs and symptoms include sparse facial hair, decreased libido, impotence, and testicular atrophy.

Testicular tumor

- Gynecomastia, nipple tenderness, and decreased libido
- A firm mass and a heavy sensation in the scrotum

Thyrotoxicosis

- Gynecomastia may occur with loss of libido and impotence.
- Important findings include tachycardia, palpitations, weight loss despite increased appetite, diarrhea, tremors, an enlarged thyroid gland, dyspnea, nervousness, diaphoresis, heat intolerance, and exophthalmos.

Other causes

Drugs

○ Antihypertensives, cyproterone, cimetidine, estrogens and drugs with estrogen-like effects, flutamide, ketoconazole, spironolactone, phenothiazines, and tricyclic antidepressants may cause gynecomastia.
○ Regular use of alcohol, marijuana, or heroin reduces plasma testosterone levels, resulting in gynecomastia.

Treatments

○ Gynecomastia may follow major surgery, testicular irradiation, or starting hemodialysis for chronic renal failure.

Nursing considerations

○ Apply cold compresses to the breasts.
○ Give analgesics.
○ Tamoxifen, an antiestrogen, or testolactone may be helpful.
○ If drug treatment fails, surgical removal of breast tissue may be needed.
○ Provide emotional support.

Pediatric pointers

○ In neonates, gynecomastia may be associated with galactorrhea, disappearing within a few weeks of birth.
○ Most boys have physiologic gynecomastia at some time during adolescence, usually around age 14.

Patient teaching

○ Explain treatments and procedures the patient needs.

Halitosis

Overview

○ Unpleasant, disagreeable, or offensive breath odor

Assessment

History

○ Ask about the onset and characteristics of halitosis.
○ Find out about associated bad taste, difficulty swallowing or chewing, reflux, regurgitation, pain, tenderness, flatus, or cough.
○ Determine the pattern and characteristics of bowel movements.
○ Inquire about smoking or tobacco habits.
○ Obtain a description of diet and daily oral hygiene.
○ Obtain a medical history, including chronic disorders and respiratory tract infection.

Physical assessment

○ Examine the mouth, throat, and nose for lesions, bleeding, drainage, obstruction, and signs of infection.
○ Percuss and palpate over the sinuses for tenderness.
○ Auscultate the lungs for abnormal breath sounds.
○ Auscultate the abdomen for bowel sounds; percuss, noting any tympany.
○ Take vital signs.

Medical causes

Bowel obstruction

○ Fecal halitosis is a late sign.
○ Other findings of a small-bowel obstruction include vomiting, constipation, abdominal distention, and intermittent periumbilical cramping pain.
○ Constant lower abdominal pain may occur with large-bowel obstruction.

Bronchiectasis

○ Foul or putrid halitosis is typical.
○ Some patients may have a sickeningly sweet breath odor.
○ Other findings include exertional dyspnea, fatigue, malaise, weakness, weight loss, crackles, late clubbing, and a chronic productive cough with copious, foul-smelling, mucopurulent sputum.

Common cold

○ A musty breath odor may be present.
○ Other findings include a dry, hacking cough with sore throat, sneezing, nasal congestion with rhinorrhea, headache, malaise, fatigue, and aching joints and muscles.

Esophageal cancer

○ Halitosis may accompany dysphagia, hoarseness, chest pain, and weight loss.
○ Nocturnal regurgitation and cachexia are late signs.

Gastric cancer

○ Late halitosis.
○ Chronic dyspepsia unrelieved by antacids, a vague feeling of fullness, nausea, anorexia, fatigue, pallor, weakness, altered bowel habits, weight loss, muscle wasting, and, if bleeding occurs, hematemesis and melena.

Gastrocolic fistula

○ A fecal breath odor is preceded by intermittent diarrhea.

Gingivitis

○ Halitosis may occur along with red, edematous, bleeding gums.
○ Acute necrotizing ulcerative gingivitis causes fetid breath.
○ Other findings of acute necrotizing ulcerative gingivitis include ulcers that may become covered with gray exudate, fever, cervical adenopathy, headache, and malaise.

Hepatic encephalopathy

○ Late fetor hepaticus (a musty, sweet, or mousy [new-mown hay] breath odor).
○ Coma, asterixis, and hyperactive deep tendon reflexes.

Lung abscess

○ Putrid halitosis develops along with a productive cough with copious, purulent, often bloody sputum.
○ Other findings include fever with chills, dyspnea, headache, anorexia, malaise, pleuritic chest pain, asymmetrical chest movement, weight loss, and temporary clubbing.

Ozena

○ Musty or fetid breath odor occurs along with thick, green mucus and progressive anosmia.

Periodontal disease

○ Halitosis occurs with a bad taste in the mouth, bleeding gums, and pus-filled pockets around the teeth.
○ Related findings include facial pain, headache, and loose teeth covered by calculi and plaque.

Pharyngitis (gangrenous)

○ Halitosis occurs with an extremely sore throat.
○ Other findings include a foul taste in the mouth, choking sensation, fever, cervical lymphadenopathy, and a swollen, red, ulcerated pharynx.

Renal failure (chronic)

○ A urinous or ammonia breath odor is produced.

○ Related findings include signs of anemia, emotional lability, lethargy, irritability, decreased mental acuity, coarse muscular twitching, peripheral neuropathies, muscle wasting, anorexia, signs of GI bleeding, ecchymoses, yellow-brown or bronze skin, pruritus, anuria, and increased blood pressure.

Sinusitis

○ Acute sinusitis causes purulent nasal discharge that leads to halitosis.
○ Related findings of acute sinusitis include a characteristic postnasal drip, nasal congestion, sore throat, cough, malaise, headache, facial pain and tenderness, and fever.
○ Chronic sinusitis causes continuous mucopurulent discharge and musty breath odor.
○ Related findings of the chronic condition include postnasal drip, nasal congestion, and a chronic, nonproductive cough.

Other causes

Drugs

○ Drugs that may cause halitosis include triamterene, inhaled anesthetics, paraldehyde, and any drugs known to cause metabolic acidosis such as nitroprusside.

Nursing considerations

○ To enhance appetite, provide oral hygiene before meals.

Pediatric pointers

○ In children, halitosis commonly results from physiologic causes, such as continual mouth breathing and thumb or blanket sucking.
○ Phenylketonuria may produce a musty or mousy odor.

Geriatric pointers

○ Dental caries, dry mouth, and poor oral hygiene can cause halitosis in elderly patients.

Patient teaching

○ Teach the patient about proper oral hygiene.

Headache

Overview

- The most common neurologic symptom
- May be localized or generalized, producing mild to severe pain
- May be described as vascular, muscle-contraction, or a combination of both
- About 90% are benign

Assessment

History

- Ask about the characteristics and location of the headache.
- Find out about precipitating or alleviating factors.
- Obtain a drug and alcohol history.
- Find out about recent head trauma, nausea, vomiting, photophobia, or vision changes.
- Ask about associated drowsiness, confusion, dizziness, or seizures.

Physical assessment

- Evaluate level of consciousness (LOC).
- Check vital signs.
- Be alert for signs of increased intracranial pressure (ICP).
- Check pupil size and response to light.
- Note any neck stiffness.

Medical causes

Brain abscess

- Headache is localized to the abscess site and intensifies over a few days.
- Straining aggravates headache.
- Accompanying findings include nausea, vomiting, focal or generalized seizures, changes in LOC and, depending on the location of the abscess, aphasia, impaired visual acuity, hemiparesis, ataxia, tremors, and personality changes.

Brain tumor

- Headache is localized near the tumor site but becomes generalized as the tumor grows.
- Pain is usually intermittent, deep-seated, dull, and most intense in the morning; aggravating factors include coughing, stooping, Valsalva's maneuver, and changes in head position; and alleviating factors include sitting and rest.
- Other findings include personality changes, altered LOC, motor and sensory dysfunction, and signs of increased ICP.

Cerebral aneurysm (ruptured)

- A life-threatening condition — headache is sudden and excruciating and usually peaks within minutes of the rupture.
- The patient may lose consciousness immediately or display a variably altered LOC.
- Depending on the location and severity of the bleeding, other findings may include nausea, vomiting, nuchal rigidity, blurred vision, and hemiparesis.

Encephalitis

- A severe, generalized headache is characteristic.
- Within 48 hours, the patient's LOC typically deteriorates.
- Other findings include fever, nuchal rigidity, irritability, seizures, nausea, vomiting, photophobia, cranial nerve palsies, and focal neurologic deficits.

Epidural hemorrhage (acute)

- A progressively severe headache with nausea, vomiting, bladder distention, confusion, and rapid decrease in LOC
- Unilateral seizures, hemiparesis, hemiplegia, high fever, decreased pulse rate and bounding pulse, widened pulse pressure, increased blood pressure, a positive Babinski's reflex, and decerebrate posture

Glaucoma (acute angleclosure)

- Excruciating headache as well as acute eye pain, blurred vision, halo vision, nausea, and vomiting may occur in this ophthalmic emergency.
- Other findings include conjunctival injection, a cloudy cornea, and a moderately dilated, fixed pupil.

Hypertension

- A slightly throbbing occipital headache on awakening may occur; severity decreases during the day (if diastolic pressure remains greater than 120 mm Hg, the headache is constant).
- Other findings include atrial gallop, restlessness, confusion, nausea, vomiting, blurred vision, seizures, and altered LOC.

Influenza

- A severe generalized or frontal headache usually begins suddenly.
- Accompanying findings include stabbing retro-orbital pain, weakness, myalgia, fever, chills, coughing, rhinorrhea, and hoarseness.

Intracerebral hemorrhage

- A severe generalized headache may develop.
- Signs and symptoms vary with the size and location of the hemorrhage and may include altered LOC, hemiplegia, hemiparesis, abnormal pupil size and response, aphasia, dizziness, nausea, vomiting, seizures, decreased sensation, irregular respirations, positive Babinski's reflex, decorticate or decerebrate posture, and increased blood pressure.

Meningitis

○ Onset of a severe, constant, generalized headache is sudden.
○ Headache worsens with movement.
○ Other findings include altered LOC, seizures, fever, chills, nuchal rigidity, ocular palsies, facial weakness, hearing loss, positive Kernig's sign and Brudzinski's sign, hyperreflexia, opisthotonos, and signs of increased ICP.

Plague

○ Pneumonic form results in sudden onset of headache, chills, fever, myalgia, productive cough, chest pain, tachypnea, dyspnea, hemoptysis, respiratory distress, and cardiopulmonary insufficiency.

Postconcussional syndrome

○ A generalized or localized headache may develop 1 to 30 days after head trauma and last for 2 to 3 weeks.
○ Pain may be aching, pounding, pressing, stabbing, or throbbing.
○ Other findings include giddiness or dizziness, blurred vision, fatigue, insomnia, inability to concentrate, noise and alcohol intolerance, fever, chills, malaise, chest pain, nausea, vomiting, and diarrhea.

Severe acute respiratory syndrome

○ A potentially life-threatening illness — symptoms include fever, headache, malaise, a dry nonproductive cough, and dyspnea.

Sinusitis (acute)

○ A dull periorbital headache is usually aggravated by bending over or touching the face and is relieved by sinus drainage.
○ Fever, sinus tenderness, nasal turbinate edema, sore throat, malaise, cough, and nasal discharge may develop.

Smallpox

○ Initial signs and symptoms include severe headache, backache, abdominal pain, high fever, malaise, prostration, and a maculopapular rash on the mucosa of the mouth, pharynx, face, and forearms, and then the trunk and legs.
○ Rash becomes vesicular, then pustular, and finally forms a crust and scab, leaving a pitted scar.

Subarachnoid hemorrhage

○ A sudden, violent headache occurs along with nuchal rigidity, nausea and vomiting, seizures, dizziness, ipsilateral pupil dilation, and altered LOC that may progress to coma.
○ Other findings include positive Kernig's sign and Brudzinski's sign, photophobia, blurred vision, fever, hemiparesis, hemiplegia, sensory disturbances, aphasia, and signs of increased ICP.

Subdural hematoma

○ Headache develops and LOC decreases.
○ In acute cases, findings include drowsiness, confusion, and agitation that may progress to coma, and later signs of increased ICP and focal neurologic deficits.
○ In chronic cases, pounding headache fluctuates in severity and is located over the hematoma.
○ Giddiness, personality changes, confusion, seizures, and progressively worsening LOC may develop weeks or months after the trauma.

Temporal arteritis

○ A throbbing unilateral headache in the temporal or frontotemporal region may be accompanied by vision loss, hearing loss, confusion, and fever.
○ The temporal arteries are tender, swollen, nodular and, possibly, erythematous.

Tularemia

○ Onset of headache is abrupt.
○ Other findings include fever, chills, myalgia, nonproductive cough, dyspnea, pleuritic chest pain, and empyema.

Other causes

Diagnostic tests

○ Lumbar puncture or myelogram may produce a throbbing frontal headache that worsens on standing.

Drugs

○ Indomethacin, vasodilators, and drugs with a vasodilating effect may produce headaches.
○ Withdrawal from vasopressors may also result in headaches.

Nursing considerations

○ Monitor vital signs and LOC.
○ Watch for change in the headache's severity or location.
○ Administer an analgesic, darken the room, and minimize stimuli to ease the headache.

Pediatric pointers

○ In children older than age 3, headache is the most common symptom of a brain tumor.
○ Suspect a headache if a young child is banging or holding his head.

Patient teaching

○ Explain the signs of reduced LOC and seizures that the patient or his caregivers should report.
○ Explain ways to maintain a safe, quiet environment and reduce environmental stress.
○ Discuss the use of analgesics.

Hearing loss

Overview

- May be temporary, permanent and partial, or complete
- Classified as conductive (resulting from external or middle ear disorders), sensorineural (resulting from disorders of the inner ear or of the eighth cranial nerve), mixed (resulting from a combination of conductive and sensorineural factors), or functional (resulting from psychological factors)

Assessment

History

- Ask for a description of the hearing loss.
- Obtain a medical history, including chronic ear infections, ear surgery, ear or head trauma, and recent upper respiratory tract infection.
- Obtain a drug history.
- Ask for a description of the occupational environment.
- Ask about other signs and symptoms, such as pain; discharge; ringing, buzzing, hissing, or other noises; and dizziness.

Physical assessment

- Inspect the external ear for inflammation, boils, foreign bodies, and discharge.

Assessment tip
Using an otoscope

Inserting the speculum
Before inserting the speculum into the patient's ear, straighten the ear canal by grasping the auricle and pulling it up and back, as shown below.

Positioning the scope
To examine the ear's external canal, hold the otoscope with the handle parallel to the patient's head, as shown below. Bracing your hand firmly against the patient's head keeps you from hitting the canal with the speculum.

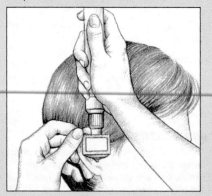

Viewing the structures
When the otoscope is positioned properly, you should see the tympanic membrane structures shown here.

- Pars flaccida
- Short process of malleus
- Handle of malleus
- Umbo
- Annulus
- Light reflex
- Pars tensa

Weber's test and the Rinne test can help determine whether the patient's hearing loss is conductive or sensorineural. Weber's test evaluates bone conduction of sound; the Rinne test, bone and air conduction. Using a 512-Hz tuning fork, perform these preliminary tests as described below.

Weber's test

Place the base of a vibrating tuning fork firmly against the midline of the patient's skull at the forehead. Ask if the tone is heard equally well in both ears. If so, the test is graded midline—a normal finding. In an abnormal Weber's test (graded right or left), the sound is louder in the impaired ear, suggesting a conductive hearing loss in that ear or the sound is louder in the normal ear, suggesting sensorineural loss in the other ear.

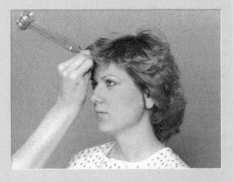

Rinne test

Hold the base of a vibrating tuning fork against the patient's mastoid process to test bone conduction (BC) of the sound. Then quickly move the vibrating fork to a position in front of the ear canal to test air conduction (AC) of the sound. Ask the patient to tell you which location has the louder or longer sound. Repeat the procedure for the other ear. Normally, AC sound lasts longer than BC sound (a positive Rinne test). Also, AC sound is normally louder than BC sound. In conductive hearing loss, BC sound is as long as or longer than AC sound, a negative Rinne test. In sensorineural loss, AC sound is longer than BC sound, but BC sound is louder.

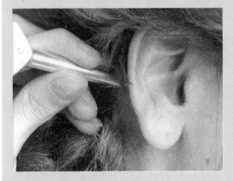
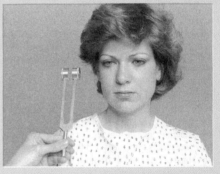

Conductive hearing loss causes:
- abnormal Weber's test result
- negative Rinne test result (BC sounds longer than AC)
- normal ability to discriminate sounds with decreased ability to detect low tones
- the patient to speak in a quiet voice.

Sensorineural hearing loss causes:
- positive Rinne test (AC sounds longer than BC)
- poor hearing in noisy areas
- difficulty hearing high-frequency sounds
- the patient to complain that others mumble or shout
- tinnitus
- the patient to speak in a loud voice.

○ Apply pressure to the tragus and mastoid to elicit tenderness.

○ During otoscopic examination, note color change, perforation, bulging, or retraction of tympanic membrane. (See *Using an otoscope.*)

○ Evaluate hearing acuity.

○ Perform the Weber's test and Rinne test. (See *Differentiating conductive from sensorineural hearing loss.*)

Medical causes

Acoustic neuroma

- Unilateral, progressive, sensorineural hearing loss occurs.
- Tinnitus, vertigo, and facial paralysis may develop.

Adenoid hypertrophy

- Gradual conductive hearing loss
- Ear discharge, mouth breathing, and a sensation of ear fullness

Allergies

- Conductive hearing loss may result.
- Other findings include ear pain or a feeling of fullness, nasal congestion, and conjunctivitis.

Cholesteatoma

- Gradual hearing loss may be accompanied by vertigo and facial paralysis.
- Examination reveals eardrum perforation, pearly white balls in the ear canal, and discharge.

External ear canal tumor (malignant)

- Progressive conductive hearing loss occurs with deep, boring ear pain; purulent discharge; and facial paralysis.

Furuncle

- Reversible conductive hearing loss may occur.
- Other findings include a sense of fullness in the ear, pain on palpation of the tragus or auricle and, with boil rupture, pain relief and a purulent, necrotic discharge.

Glomus jugulare tumor

- Mild, unilateral conductive hearing loss becomes progressively more severe.
- Other findings include tinnitus that sounds like a heartbeat, gradual congestion in the affected ear, throbbing or pulsating discomfort, bloody otorrhea, facial nerve paralysis, and vertigo.

Head trauma

- Sudden conductive or sensorineural hearing loss
- Headache and bleeding from the ear
- Neurologic findings dependent on the type of trauma

Hypothyroidism

- Reversible sensorineural hearing loss may occur.
- Other findings include bradycardia, weight gain despite anorexia, mental dullness, cold intolerance, facial edema, brittle hair, and dry, pale, cool and doughy skin.

Ménière's disease

- Intermittent, unilateral sensorineural hearing loss that involves only low tones progresses to constant hearing loss that involves other tones.

- Other findings include intermittent severe vertigo, nausea, vomiting, a sensation of fullness in the ear, a roaring or hollow-seashell tinnitus, diaphoresis, and nystagmus.

Osteoma

- Sudden or intermittent conductive hearing loss occurs.

Otitis externa

- Conductive hearing loss is characteristic.
- Acute form produces pain, headache on the affected side, low-grade fever, lymphadenopathy, itching, and a foul-smelling sticky yellow discharge.
- Malignant form involves visible debris in the ear canal, pruritus, tinnitus, and severe ear pain.

Otitis media

- In acute and chronic forms, hearing loss develops gradually.
- Other findings of the acute form include upper respiratory tract infection with sore throat, cough, nasal discharge, headache, dizziness, a sensation of fullness in the ear, intermittent or constant ear pain, fever, nausea, and vomiting.
- Other findings of the chronic form include a perforated tympanic membrane, purulent ear drainage, earache, nausea, and vertigo.
- Serous form produces a stuffy feeling in the ear and pain that worsens at night.

Otosclerosis

- Unilateral conductive hearing loss usually begins in early 20s and may gradually progress to bilateral mixed loss.
- Tinnitus and the ability to hear better in a noisy environment may occur.

Skull fracture

- Sudden unilateral sensorineural hearing loss may occur if the auditory nerve is damaged.
- Accompanying findings include ringing tinnitus, blood behind the tympanic membrane, and scalp wounds.

Temporal arteritis

- Unilateral sensorineural hearing loss may occur along with throbbing unilateral facial pain, pain behind the eye, temporal or frontotemporal headache and, occasionally, vision loss.
- Other findings include malaise, anorexia, weight loss, weakness, low-grade fever, and myalgia.
- Examination may reveal a nodular, swollen artery.

Temporal bone fracture

- Sudden unilateral sensorineural hearing loss is accompanied by hissing tinnitus.
- Other findings may include a perforated tympanic membrane, loss of consciousness, Battle's sign, and facial paralysis.

Tuberculosis

○ Eardrum perforation, mild conductive hearing loss, and cervical lymphadenopathy may occur if infection spreads to the ear.
○ Other findings include chest pain, crackles, dyspnea, fever, and tachypnea.

Tympanic membrane perforation

○ Abrupt hearing loss occurs with ear pain, tinnitus, vertigo, and a sensation of fullness in the ear.

Other causes

Drugs

○ Chloroquine, cisplatin, vancomycin, and aminoglycosides may cause irreversible hearing loss.
○ Loop diuretics, quinine, quinidine, and high doses of erythromycin or salicylates may cause reversible hearing loss.

Radiation therapy

○ Radiation of the middle ear, thyroid, face, skull, or nasopharynx may cause eustachian tube dysfunction, resulting in hearing loss.

Surgery

○ Myringotomy, myringoplasty, simple or radical mastoidectomy, or fenestrations may cause scarring that result in hearing loss.

Nursing considerations

○ When talking, face the patient and speak slowly.
○ Don't shout, smoke, eat, or chew gum when talking.

Pediatric pointers

○ Hereditary disorders cause hearing loss in half of deaf infants.
○ Congenital sensorineural hearing loss may be caused by nonhereditary disorders, maternal use of ototoxic drugs, birth trauma, and anoxia.
○ Causes of unilateral sensorineural hearing loss include mumps, meningitis, measles, influenza, and acute febrile illness.
○ Disorders that can produce congenital conductive hearing loss include atresia and ossicle malformation.
○ Serous otitis media commonly causes bilateral conductive hearing loss in children.
○ Conductive hearing loss may occur in children who put foreign objects in their ears.

Geriatric pointers

○ In older patients, presbycusis may be aggravated by exposure to noise as well as other factors.

Patient teaching

○ Explain the importance of ear protection and avoidance of loud noise.
○ Stress the importance of following instructions for taking prescribed antibiotics.

Hematemesis

Overview

- Usually indicates GI bleeding above the ligament of Treitz
- May be life-threatening if massive (500 to 1,000 ml of blood)
- Bright red or blood-streaked vomitus: fresh or recent bleeding
- Dark red, brown, or black vomitus: blood retained in the stomach or partially digested

⭐ Emergency actions

If the patient has massive hematemesis, check vital signs. If you detect signs of shock, place the patient in a supine position and elevate his feet. Start a large-bore I.V. line for emergency fluid replacement. Send a blood sample for typing and cross-matching, hemoglobin level, and hematocrit; administer oxygen. Emergency endoscopy may be necessary to locate the source of bleeding. Prepare to insert a nasogastric (NG) tube for suction or iced lavage.

Assessment

History

- Ask about the onset, amount, color, and consistency of vomitus.
- Ask for a description of stools.
- Inquire about associated nausea, flatulence, diarrhea, or weakness.
- Obtain a medical history, including ulcers or liver or coagulation disorders.
- Find out about alcohol use.
- Obtain a drug history, including aspirin and other nonsteroidal anti-inflammatory drugs (NSAIDs).

Physical assessment

- Check for orthostatic hypotension.
- Obtain other vital signs.
- Inspect the mucous membranes, nasopharynx, and skin for signs of bleeding.
- Palpate the abdomen for tenderness, pain, or masses.
- Note lymphadenopathy.

Medical causes

Anthrax (GI)

- Signs and symptoms may progress to hematemesis, abdominal pain, and severe bloody diarrhea.
- Initial findings include loss of appetite, nausea, vomiting, and fever.

Coagulation disorders

- GI bleeding and moderate to severe hematemesis may occur.
- Other findings vary with the specific coagulation disorder and may include epistaxis and ecchymoses.

Esophageal cancer

- Hematemesis, a late sign, with steady chest pain that radiates to the back
- Substernal fullness, severe dysphagia, nausea, vomiting with nocturnal regurgitation and aspiration, hemoptysis, fever, hiccups, sore throat, melena, and halitosis

Esophageal injury by caustic substances

- Hematemesis occurs with epigastric and anterior or retrosternal chest pain that's intensified by swallowing.

Esophageal rupture

- Severity of hematemesis depends on the cause of the rupture.
- Severe retrosternal, epigastric, neck, or scapular pain accompanied by chest and neck edema may occur.
- Other findings include subcutaneous crepitation in the chest wall, supraclavicular fossa, and neck; and signs of respiratory distress.

Esophageal varices (ruptured)

- A life-threatening condition — coffee-ground or massive, bright red vomitus may occur.
- Other findings include signs of shock, abdominal distention, and melena or painless hematochezia, ranging from slight oozing to massive rectal hemorrhage.

Gastric cancer

- Painless bright red or dark brown vomitus is a late sign.
- Related findings include upper-abdominal discomfort, anorexia, mild nausea, and chronic dyspepsia unrelieved by antacids and exacerbated by food.
- Late findings include fatigue, weakness, weight loss, feelings of fullness, melena, altered bowel habits, and signs of malnutrition.

Gastritis (acute)

- Hematemesis and melena are the most common signs.
- Other features include mild epigastric discomfort, nausea, fever, malaise, and, with massive blood loss, signs of shock.

GI leiomyoma

- Hematemesis occurs, possibly with dysphagia and weight loss.

Mallory-Weiss syndrome

- Hematemesis and melena may occur.

○ Signs of shock may accompany severe bleeding.

Peptic ulcer

○ Hematemesis, possibly life-threatening, may occur.
○ Other features include melena or hematochezia, chills, fever, and signs of shock.

Other causes

Treatments

○ Nose or throat surgery, and traumatic nasogastric or endotracheal intubation may cause hematemesis.

Nursing considerations

○ Monitor vital signs; watch for signs of shock.
○ Check stools for occult blood.
○ Keep accurate intake and output records.
○ Place the patient on bed rest in a low or semi-Fowler's position.
○ Keep suctioning equipment nearby; use as needed.
○ Provide frequent oral hygiene.
○ Give a histamine-2 blocker I.V.; vasopressin may be required for variceal hemorrhage.

Pediatric pointers

○ Hematemesis may be related to foreign-body ingestion.
○ Hemorrhagic disease and esophageal erosion may cause hematemesis in infants.

Geriatric pointers

○ Hematemesis may be caused by a vascular anomaly, an aortoenteric fistula, or upper GI cancer.
○ Chronic obstructive pulmonary disease, chronic liver or renal failure, and chronic NSAID use predispose elderly people to hemorrhage caused by coexisting ulcerative disorders.

Patient teaching

○ Explain foods or fluids the patient should avoid.
○ Stress the importance of avoiding the use of alcohol.

Hematochezia

Overview

- Passage of bloody stools
- Usually develops abruptly and indicates bleeding below the ligament of Treitz
- May precipitate life-threatening hypovolemia

⭐ Emergency actions

If the patient has severe hematochezia, check vital signs for signs of shock. Place the patient in a supine position and elevate his feet. Prepare to administer oxygen, and start a large-bore I.V. line for emergency fluid replacement. Obtain a blood sample for typing and crossmatching, hemoglobin level, and hematocrit. Insert a nasogastric tube. Iced lavage may be indicated to control bleeding. Endoscopy may be necessary to detect the source of the bleeding.

Assessment

History

- Ask about the onset, amount, color, and consistency of stools.
- Find out about associated signs and symptoms.
- Obtain a medical history, including GI and coagulation disorders.
- Determine the use of GI irritants, such as alcohol, aspirin, and other NSAIDs.

Physical assessment

- Check for orthostatic hypotension.
- Examine the skin for petechiae or spider angiomas.
- Palpate the abdomen for tenderness, pain, or masses.
- Note lymphadenopathy.
- Perform a digital rectal examination to detect rectal masses or hemorrhoids.

Medical causes

Anal fissure

- Slight hematochezia occurs; blood may streak the stools or appear on toilet tissue.
- Severe rectal pain occurs, leading to reluctance to defecate and thus to constipation.

Anorectal fistula

- Blood, pus, mucus, and occasionally stools may drain from an anorectal fistula.
- Other findings include rectal pain and pruritus.

Coagulation disorders

- GI bleeding marked by moderate to severe hematochezia may occur.

- Other findings vary with the specific coagulation disorder but may include epistaxis and purpura.

Colitis

- Ischemic colitis commonly causes slight or massive hematochezia; severe, cramping lower abdominal pain; abdominal distention and tenderness; absent bowel sounds; and hypotension.
- Ulcerative colitis typically causes hematochezia that may also contain mucus.
- Other findings of ulcerative colitis include abdominal cramps, fever, tenesmus, anorexia, nausea, vomiting, hyperactive bowel sounds, tachycardia and, later, weight loss and weakness.

Colon cancer

- Bright red rectal bleeding with or without pain occurs.
- With a left colon tumor, early signs of obstruction occur; later, obstipation, diarrhea or ribbon-shaped stools, and pain relieved by passage of stools or flatus occurs.
- With a right colon tumor, melena, abdominal aching, pressure, and dull cramps occur; later, weakness, fatigue, diarrhea, anorexia, weight loss, anemia, vomiting, abdominal mass, and signs of obstruction develop.

Colorectal polyps

- Intermittent hematochezia occurs.

Crohn's disease

- Hematochezia isn't common unless the perineum is involved.
- If rectal bleeding occurs, it's likely to be massive.
- Chief clinical features include fever, abdominal distention and pain with guarding, diarrhea, hyperactive bowel sounds, anorexia, nausea, and fatigue.

Diverticulitis

- Mild to moderate rectal bleeding occurs after the patient feels the urge to defecate.
- Other findings include left-lower-quadrant pain that's relieved by defecation, alternating episodes of constipation and diarrhea, anorexia, nausea, vomiting, rebound tenderness, and a distended, tympanic abdomen.

Dysentery

- Bloody diarrhea is common.
- Abdominal pain or cramps, tenesmus, fever, nausea, and signs of dehydration may occur.

Esophageal varices (ruptured)

- A life-threatening condition — hematochezia ranges from slight rectal oozing to grossly bloody stools.
- Other findings include hematemesis, melena, and signs of shock.

Food poisoning (staphylococcal)

○ Bloody diarrhea may occur 1 to 6 hours after ingesting food toxins.
○ Accompanying findings include nausea, vomiting, prostration, and severe, cramping abdominal pain.

Hemorrhoids

○ Hematochezia may accompany external hemorrhoids, causing painful defecation, possibly leading to constipation.
○ Internal hemorrhoids usually produce chronic bleeding with bowel movements, leading to signs of anemia.

Peptic ulcer

○ Hematochezia, hematemesis, or melena may occur.
○ Other findings include pain relieved by food or antacids, chills, fever, nausea, vomiting, and signs of dehydration and shock.

Small-intestine cancer

○ Slight hematochezia or blood-streaked stools
○ Colicky pan, postprandial vomiting, weight loss, anorexia, and fever

Ulcerative proctitis

○ The patient has an intense urge to defecate, but passes only bright red blood, pus, or mucus.
○ Constipation and tenesmus may develop.

Other causes

Diagnostic tests

○ Certain procedures, especially colonoscopy, polypectomy, and proctosigmoidoscopy may cause rectal bleeding.

Heavy metal poisoning

○ Heavy metal poisoning may cause bloody diarrhea accompanied by cramping abdominal pain, nausea, vomiting, tachycardia, hypotension, seizures, paresthesia, depressed or absent deep tendon reflexes, and an altered level of consciousness.

Nursing considerations

○ Place the patient on bed rest.
○ Check vital signs frequently, watching for signs of shock.
○ Monitor intake and output hourly.
○ Visually examine stools and test them for occult blood.
○ If necessary, send a stool sample to the laboratory to check for parasites.

Pediatric pointers

○ Hematochezia may result from structural and inflammatory disorders.

○ In children, ulcerative colitis typically produces chronic signs and symptoms.
○ Suspect sexual abuse in all cases of rectal bleeding in children.

Geriatric pointers

○ Hematochezia should be evaluated using colonoscopy after ruling out perirectal lesions as the cause of bleeding.

Patient teaching

○ Explain the signs and symptoms the patient should report.
○ Teach the patient about ostomy self-care.
○ Discuss proper bowel elimination habits.
○ Explain dietary recommendations and restrictions.

Hematuria

Overview

- Abnormal presence of blood in urine
- A cardinal sign of renal and urinary tract disorders
- May be microscopic or macroscopic
- Classified as initial (occurring at the start of urination), terminal (occurring at the end of urination), or total (occurring throughout urination)

Assessment

History

- Ask about the onset, description, and severity.
- Find out about associated pain or burning.
- Obtain a medical history, including renal, urinary, prostatic, or coagulation disorders, and recent abdominal or flank trauma.
- Find out about recent strenuous exercise.
- Take a drug history, noting anticoagulants or aspirin.

Physical assessment

- Percuss the palpate the abdomen and flanks.
- Percuss the costovertebral angle (CVA) to elicit tenderness.
- Check the urinary meatus for bleeding or other abnormalities.
- Using a chemical reagent strip, test a urine specimen for protein.
- Perform a vaginal or digital rectal examination.

Medical causes

Bladder cancer

- Gross hematuria with pain in bladder, rectum, pelvis, flank, back, or leg
- Nocturia, dysuria, urinary frequency and urgency, vomiting, diarrhea, and insomnia

Bladder trauma

- Hematuria with lower abdominal pain
- Anuria despite a strong urge to void; swelling of the scrotum, buttocks, or perineum; and signs of shock

Calculi

- Bladder calculi: gross hematuria, pain that's referred to the lower back or penile or vulvar area, and bladder distention
- Renal calculi: microscopic or gross hematuria, but the cardinal sign is colicky pain that travels from the CVA to the flank, suprapubic region, and external genitalia when a calculus is passed; nausea; vomiting; restlessness; fever; chills; and abdominal distention

Coagulation disorders

- Macroscopic hematuria (first sign of hemorrhage)
- Epistaxis, purpura, and signs of GI bleeding

Cystitis

- Bacterial cystitis usually produces macroscopic hematuria with urinary urgency and frequency, dysuria, perineal and lumbar pain, suprapubic discomfort, and nocturia.
- Chronic interstitial cystitis occasionally causes grossly bloody hematuria with urinary frequency, dysuria, nocturia, and tenesmus.
- Viral cystitis usually produces hematuria, urinary urgency and frequency, dysuria, nocturia, tenesmus, and fever.

Glomerulonephritis

- With acute form, gross hematuria tapers off to microscopic hematuria and red cell casts.
- Other acute findings include oliguria or anuria, proteinuria, mild fever, fatigue, flank and abdominal pain, edema, increased blood pressure, nausea, vomiting, and crackles.
- Chronic form causes hematuria accompanied by proteinuria, generalized edema, and increased blood pressure.

Nephritis (interstitial)

- Microscopic hematuria is typical, but some patients may develop gross hematuria.
- Other findings include fever, maculopapular rash, and oliguria or anuria.

Nephropathy (obstructive)

- Microscopic or macroscopic hematuria with colicky flank and abdominal pain, CVA tenderness, and anuria or oliguria that alternates with polyuria

Polycystic kidney disease

- Microscopic or gross hematuria
- Increased blood pressure, polyuria, dull flank pain, and signs of urinary tract infection
- Later, a swollen, tender abdomen and lumbar pain that's aggravated by exertion and relieved by lying down

Prostatic hyperplasia (benign)

- Macroscopic hematuria with significant obstruction
- Early: diminished urinary stream, tenesmus, and a feeling of incomplete voiding
- Urinary hesitancy, frequency, and incontinence; nocturia; perineal pain; an enlarged prostate on rectal palpation; and constipation.

Prostatitis

- Macroscopic hematuria at the end of urination
- Urinary frequency and urgency and dysuria followed by visible bladder distention
- Acute form: fatigue, malaise, myalgia, arthralgia, fever, chills, nausea, vomiting, perineal and lower

back pain, decreased libido, and a tender, swollen, firm prostate on palpation
○ Chronic form: persistent urethral discharge, dull perineal pain, ejaculatory pain, and decreased libido

Pyelonephritis (acute)

○ Microscopic or macroscopic hematuria progresses to grossly bloody hematuria.
○ After the infection resolves, microscopic hematuria may persist for a few months.
○ Related findings include persistent high fever, flank pain, CVA tenderness, shaking chills, weakness, nausea, vomiting, anorexia, fatigue, dysuria, urinary frequency and urgency, nocturia, and tenesmus.

Renal cancer

○ Classic triad: grossly bloody hematuria; dull, aching flank pain; and a smooth, firm, palpable flank mass
○ Colicky pain accompanying the passage of clots, CVA tenderness, fever, and increased blood pressure
○ In advanced disease, weight loss, nausea, vomiting, and leg edema with varicoceles

Renal infarction

○ Gross hematuria
○ Constant, severe flank and upper abdominal pain with CVA tenderness, anorexia, nausea, and vomiting
○ Oliguria or anuria, proteinuria, hypoactive bowel sounds, fever, and increased blood pressure

Renal papillary necrosis (acute)

○ Grossly bloody hematuria
○ Intense flank pain, CVA tenderness, abdominal rigidity and colicky pain, oliguria or anuria, pyuria, fever, chills, hypertension, arthralgia, vomiting, and hypoactive bowel sounds

Renal trauma

○ Microscopic or gross hematuria
○ Flank pain, a palpable flank mass, oliguria, hematoma or ecchymoses over the upper abdomen or flank, nausea, vomiting, hypoactive bowel sounds and, in severe trauma, signs of shock

Renal tuberculosis

○ Gross hematuria is commonly the first sign.
○ Accompanying findings include urinary frequency, dysuria, pyuria, tenesmus, colicky abdominal pain, lumbar pain, and proteinuria.

Renal vein thrombosis

○ Grossly bloody hematuria
○ With abrupt venous obstruction, severe flank and lumbar pain and epigastric and CVA tenderness
○ Fever, pallor, proteinuria, peripheral edema, and oliguria or anuria if obstruction is bilateral

Sickle cell anemia

○ Gross hematuria

○ Pallor, dehydration, chronic fatigue, tachycardia, heart murmurs, polyarthralgia, leg ulcers, dyspnea, chest pain, impaired growth and development, hepatomegaly, and jaundice

Systemic lupus erythematosus

○ Gross hematuria and proteinuria if the kidneys are involved.
○ Joint pain and stiffness, butterfly rash, photosensitivity, Raynaud's phenomenon, seizures, psychoses, recurrent fever, lymphadenopathy, oral or nasopharyngeal ulcers, anorexia, and weight loss.

Urethral trauma

○ Initial hematuria with blood at the urinary meatus, local pain, and penile or vulvar ecchymoses

Other causes

Diagnostic tests and treatments

○ Renal biopsy and biopsy or manipulative instrumentation of the urinary tract may result in hematuria.
○ Kidney transplant may cause hematuria.

Drugs

○ Anticoagulants, aspirin toxicity, analgesics, cyclophosphamide, metyrosine, phenylbutazone, penicillin, rifampin, and thiabendazole

Nursing considerations

○ Check vital signs frequently.
○ Monitor intake and output, including the amount and pattern of hematuria.
○ If the patient has an indwelling urinary catheter in place, ensure its patency; irrigate if necessary.
○ Administer analgesics as indicated.

Pediatric pointers

○ Common causes of hematuria in children include congenital anomalies, birth trauma, hematologic disorders, certain neoplasms, allergies, and foreign bodies in the urinary tract.

Geriatric pointers

○ Evaluation of hematuria should include a urine culture, excretory urography or sonography, and consultation with a urologist.

Patient teaching

○ Instruct the patient in three-glass technique for collecting serial urine specimens.
○ Emphasize increasing fluid intake.

Hemianopsia

Overview

○ Vision loss in one-half the visual field of one or both eyes (see *Recognizing visual field defects*)
○ Caused by a lesion affecting the optic chiasm, tract, or radiation

Assessment

History

○ Ask about associated headache, dysarthria, seizures, hallucinations, or loss of color vision.
○ Determine the onset of neurologic symptoms.
○ Obtain a medical history, noting eye disorders, hypertension, diabetes mellitus, and recent head trauma.

Physical assessment

○ Take vital signs.
○ Evaluate level of consciousness (LOC).
○ Check pupillary reaction.
○ Evaluate for ptosis or facial or extremity weakness.
○ Assess visual fields and plot areas of vision loss.

Medical causes

Carotid artery aneurysm

○ Contralateral or bilateral defects in visual fields may occur with hemiplegia, decreased LOC, headache, aphasia, behavior disturbances, and unilateral hypoesthesia.

Occipital lobe lesion

○ Incomplete homonymous hemianopsia, scotomas, and impaired color vision are the most common symptoms.
○ Visual hallucinations that appear in the defective field or move toward it from the intact field may occur.

Parietal lobe lesion

○ Homonymous hemianopsia and sensory deficits occur.
○ Apraxia and visual or tactile agnosia may also develop.

Pituitary tumor

○ Complete or partial bitemporal hemianopsia first occurs in the upper visual fields but later can progress to blindness.
○ Related findings include blurred vision, diplopia, and headache.

Stroke

○ Hemianopsia can result when stroke affects any part of the optic pathway.
○ Other findings vary with the location and size of the stroke and may include decreased LOC, intellectual deficits, personality changes, emotional lability, hemiplegia, dysarthria, dysphagia, ataxia, sensory loss, apraxia, aphasia, blurred vision, urine retention or incontinence, headache, and seizures.

Nursing considerations

○ To avoid startling the patient, approach him from the unaffected side.
○ Position the bed so that the patient's unaffected side faces the door.
○ Remove objects that could cause falls, and alert the patient to other possible hazards.
○ Place personal objects within field of vision; avoid putting dangerous objects where the patient can't see them.

Pediatric pointers

○ The most common cause of hemianopsia in children is brain tumors.

Patient teaching

○ Discuss compensation techniques.
○ Stress safety measures.

Lesions of the optic pathways cause visual field defects. The lesion's site determines the type of defect. For example, a lesion of the optic chiasm involving only those fibers that cross over to the opposite side causes bitemporal hemianopsia—visual loss in the temporal half of each field. However, a lesion of the optic tract or a complete lesion of the optic radiation produces visual loss in the same half of each field—either left or right homonymous hemianopsia.

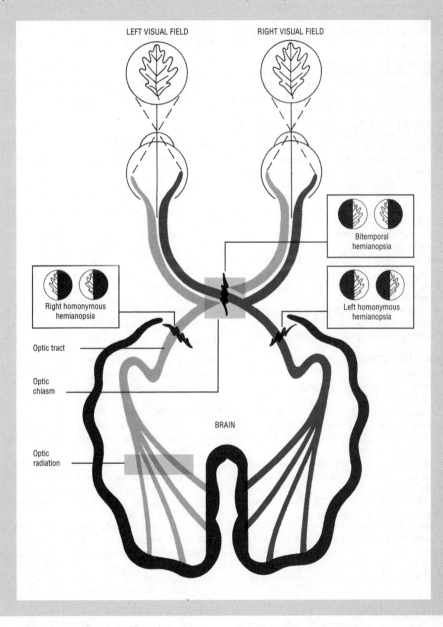

Hemoptysis

Overview

- Expectoration of blood or bloody sputum from the lungs or tracheobronchial tree (see *Identifying hemoptysis*)
- Usually results from chronic bronchitis, lung cancer, or bronchiectasis

⭐ Emergency actions

If the patient coughs up a copious amount of blood, endotracheal intubation may be required. Suction frequently to remove blood. Lavage may be necessary to loosen tenacious secretions or clots. Massive hemoptysis can cause airway obstruction and asphyxiation. Insert an I.V. line for fluid replacement, drug administration, and blood transfusion if needed. Bronchoscopy should be performed to identify the bleeding site. Monitor vital signs to detect shock.

Assessment

History

- Ask about the onset and extent of hemoptysis.
- Obtain a medical history of cardiac, pulmonary, bleeding disorders, recent infection, and exposure to tuberculosis.
- Obtain a drug history, including anticoagulants.
- Obtain a smoking history.
- Ask about the date and results of the last tine test.

Physical assessment

- Take vital signs.
- Examine the nose, mouth, and pharynx for sources of bleeding.
- Inspect the chest; look for abnormal movement during breathing and use of accessory muscles.
- Observe respiratory rate, depth, and rhythm.
- Examine skin for lesions.
- Palpate the chest for diaphragm level and for tenderness, respiratory excursion, fremitus, and abnormal pulsations.
- Percuss the chest for flatness, dullness, resonance, hyperresonance, and tympany.
- Auscultate for breath sounds.
- Auscultate for heart murmurs, bruits, and pleural rubs.
- Obtain sputum sample, examine it for quantity, amount of blood, and color, odor, and consistency.

Medical causes

Bronchial adenoma

- Recurring hemoptysis occurs along with a chronic cough and local wheezing.

- Recurrent infection, dyspnea, and wheezing may also occur.

Bronchiectasis

- Hemoptysis from blood-tinged sputum to blood
- Chronic cough, coarse crackles, late clubbing, fever, weight loss, fatigue, weakness, malaise, dyspnea on exertion, and copious, foul-smelling, and purulent sputum

Bronchitis (chronic)

- A productive cough leads to production of blood-streaked sputum.
- Accompanying findings include dyspnea, prolonged expirations, wheezing, scattered rhonchi, accessory muscle use, barrel chest, tachypnea, and late clubbing.

Coagulation disorders

- Hemoptysis with multisystem hemorrhaging and purpuric lesions

Laryngeal cancer

- Hemoptysis occurs, but hoarseness is the usual early sign.
- Other findings include dysphagia, dyspnea, stridor, cervical lymphadenopathy, and neck pain.

Lung abscess

- Blood-streaked sputum
- Fever, chills, diaphoresis, anorexia, dyspnea, pleuritic or dull chest pain, clubbing, and a cough with purulent, foul-smelling sputum

Lung cancer

- Recurring hemoptysis (an early sign)
- A productive cough, dyspnea, fever, anorexia, weight loss, wheezing, and chest pain (a late sign)

Pneumonia

- *Klebsiella* pneumonia produces dark brown or red tenacious sputum that the patient has difficulty expelling from his mouth.
- Abrupt onset with chills, fever, dyspnea, productive cough, severe pleuritic chest pain, cyanosis, tachycardia, decreased breath sounds, and crackles
- Pneumococcal pneumonia causes pinkish or rust-colored mucoid sputum.
- Onset is marked by sudden shaking chills, a rapidly rising temperature, tachycardia, and tachypnea.
- Severe, stabbing, pleuritic chest pain; rapid, shallow, grunting respirations with splinting; dyspnea; accessory muscle use; crackles; malaise; weakness; myalgia; prostration; and a productive cough

Pulmonary contusion

- Cough and hemoptysis after blunt chest trauma
- Dyspnea, tachypnea, chest pain, tachycardia, hypotension, crackles, decreased or absent breath

sounds over the affected area and, possibly, severe respiratory distress

Pulmonary edema

○ A life-threatening condition — frothy, blood-tinged pink sputum accompanies severe dyspnea, orthopnea, gasping, anxiety, cyanosis, diffuse crackles, a ventricular gallop, and cold, clammy skin.
○ Other findings include tachycardia, lethargy, arrhythmias, tachypnea, hypotension, and a thready pulse.

Pulmonary embolism with infarction

○ A life-threatening disorder — hemoptysis is common.
○ Typically initial symptoms include dyspnea and anginal or pleuritic chest pain.

Pulmonary hypertension (primary)

○ Hemoptysis, exertional dyspnea, and fatigue are common, but generally develop late.
○ Other findings include arrhythmias, syncope, cough, hoarseness, and angina-like pain that occurs with exertion and may radiate to the neck.

Pulmonary tuberculosis

○ Blood-streaked or blood-tinged sputum commonly occurs in pulmonary tuberculosis.
○ Accompanying findings include chronic productive cough, fine crackles after coughing, dyspnea, dullness to percussion, increased tactile fremitus, amphoric breath sounds, night sweats, malaise, fatigue, fever, anorexia, weight loss, and pleuritic chest pain.

Silicosis

○ A productive cough with mucopurulent sputum becomes blood-streaked, and, occasionally, massive hemoptysis may occur.
○ Other findings include exertional dyspnea, tachypnea, weight loss, fatigue, weakness, and fine, end-inspiratory crackles.

Systemic lupus erythematosus

○ Pleuritis and pneumonitis may cause hemoptysis.
○ Related findings include a butterfly rash, nondeforming joint pain and stiffness, photosensitivity, Raynaud's phenomenon, convulsions or psychoses, anorexia with weight loss, and lymphadenopathy.

Other causes

Diagnostic tests

○ Lung or airway injury from bronchoscopy, laryngoscopy, mediastinoscopy, or lung biopsy may cause bleeding and hemoptysis.

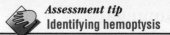

Assessment tip
Identifying hemoptysis

These guidelines will help you distinguish hemoptysis from epistaxis, hematemesis, and brown, red, or pink sputum.

Hemoptysis
Usually frothy because it's mixed with air, blood is typically bright red with an alkaline pH (tested with nitrazine paper). Hemoptysis is strongly suggested by the presence of respiratory signs and symptoms, including a cough, a tickling sensation in the throat, and blood produced from repeated coughing episodes. (You can rule out epistaxis because the patient's nasal passages and posterior pharynx are usually clear.)

Hematemesis
The usual site of hematemesis is the GI tract; the patient vomits or regurgitates coffee-ground-like material that contains food particles, tests positive for occult blood, and has an acid pH. However, he may vomit bright red blood or swallowed blood from the oral cavity and nasopharynx. After an episode of hematemesis, the patient may have stools with traces of blood. Many patients with hematemesis also complain of dyspepsia.

Brown, red, or pink sputum
Brown, red, or pink sputum can result from oxidation of inhaled bronchodilators. Sputum that looks like old blood may result from rupture of an amebic abscess into the bronchus. Red or brown sputum may occur in a patient with pneumonia caused by the enterobacterium *Serratia marcescens*. Currant-jelly–like sputum occurs with *Klebsiella* infections.

Nursing considerations

○ If necessary to protect the nonbleeding lung, place the patient in the lateral decubitus position, with the suspected bleeding lung facing down.
○ Monitor the patient's respiratory status closely.

Pediatric pointers

○ Hemoptysis in children may stem from Goodpasture's syndrome or cystic fibrosis.

Geriatric pointers

○ If the patient is receiving anticoagulants, determine any changes that need to be made in diet or medications because these factors may affect clotting.

Patient teaching

○ Explain the importance of reporting recurrent episodes.
○ Give the patient instructions for providing sputum samples.

Hepatomegaly

Overview

- Refers to enlargement of the liver
- Indicates potentially reversible primary or secondary liver disease
- May be confirmed by palpation, percussion, or radiologic tests

Assessment

History

- Ask about alcohol use.
- Determine exposure to hepatitis.
- Obtain a drug history.
- Ask about the location and description of any associated abdominal pain.

Physical assessment

- Inspect the skin and sclerae for jaundice, dilated veins, scars from previous surgery, and spider angiomas.
- Inspect the contour of the abdomen and measure abdominal girth.
- Percuss the liver. (See *Percussing the liver for size and position.*)
- During deep inspiration, palpate the liver's edge.
- Take vital signs.
- Assess nutritional status.
- Evaluate level of consciousness (LOC).
- Watch for personality changes, irritability, agitation, memory loss, inability to concentrate, poor mentation, and — in a severely ill patient — coma.

Medical causes

Cirrhosis

- In late cirrhosis, liver becomes enlarged, nodular, and hard.
- Other late findings affect all body system and include jaundice and abdominal distention.

Diabetes mellitus

- Hepatomegaly, and right-upper-quadrant tenderness along with polydipsia, polyphagia, and polyuria may occur in overweight patients with poorly controlled diabetes.

Heart failure

- Hepatomegaly occurs along with jugular vein distention, cyanosis, nocturia, dependent edema of the legs and sacrum, steady weight gain, confusion and, possibly, nausea, vomiting, abdominal discomfort, and anorexia.
- Massive right-sided failure may cause anasarca, oliguria, severe weakness, and anxiety.
- If left-sided failure precedes right-sided failure, findings include dyspnea, orthopnea, paroxysmal nocturnal dyspnea, tachypnea, arrhythmias, tachycardia, and fatigue.

Hepatitis

- Hepatomegaly occurs in the icteric phase and continues during the recovery phase.
- Early findings include nausea, vomiting, fatigue, malaise, photophobia, sore throat, cough, and headache.
- Other findings of the icteric phase include liver tenderness, slight weight loss, dark urine, clay-colored stools, jaundice, pruritus, right-upper-quadrant pain, and splenomegaly.

Assessment tip
Percussing the liver for size and position

With your patient in a supine position, begin at the right iliac crest to percuss up the right midclavicular line (MCL), as shown here. The percussion note becomes dull when you reach the liver's inferior border — usually at the costal margin but sometimes at a lower point in a patient with liver disease. Mark this point and then percuss down from the right clavicle, again along the right MCL. The liver's superior border usually lies between the fifth and seventh intercostal spaces. Mark the superior border.

The distance between the two marked points represents the approximate span of the liver's right lobe, which normally ranges from 2¼″ to 4¾″ (5.5 to 12 cm).

Next, assess the liver's left lobe similarly, percussing along the sternal midline. Again, mark the points where you hear dull percussion notes. Also, measure the span of the left lobe, which normally ranges from 1½″ to 3⅛″ (4 to 8 cm). Record your findings for use as a baseline.

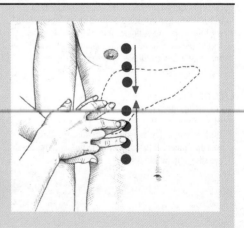

Leukemia and lymphomas

○ Moderate to massive hepatomegaly, splenomegaly, and abdominal discomfort are common.
○ General findings include malaise, low-grade fever, fatigue, weakness, tachycardia, weight loss, bleeding disorders, and anorexia.

Liver cancer

○ Primary tumors cause irregular, nodular, firm hepatomegaly, with pain or tenderness in the right upper quadrant and a friction rub or bruit over the liver.
○ Other findings include weight loss, anorexia, cachexia, nausea, vomiting, peripheral edema, ascites, jaundice, and a palpable right-upper-quadrant mass.
○ Metastatic liver tumors cause hepatomegaly, but accompanying signs and symptoms reflect the primary cancer.

Mononucleosis (infectious)

○ Hepatomegaly may occur.
○ Prodromal symptoms include headache, malaise, and fatigue.
○ After 3 to 5 days, findings include sore throat, cervical lymphadenopathy, temperature fluctuations, stomatitis, palatal petechiae, periorbital edema, splenomegaly, exudative tonsillitis, pharyngitis, and a maculopapular rash.

Obesity

○ Hepatomegaly may occur along with respiratory difficulties, cardiovascular disease, diabetes, renal disease, gallbladder disease, and psychological difficulties.

Pancreatic cancer

○ Hepatomegaly accompanies anorexia, weight loss, abdominal or back pain, and jaundice.
○ Other findings include nausea, vomiting, fever, fatigue, weakness, pruritus, and skin lesions.

Patient teaching

○ Explain the treatment plan for underlying disorder.
○ Stress the avoidance of alcohol and people with infections.
○ Emphasize personal hygiene.
○ Discuss the importance of pacing activities and rest periods.

Nursing considerations

○ Provide bed rest, relief from stress, and adequate nutrition.
○ Monitor and restrict dietary protein as needed.
○ Give hepatotoxic drugs or drugs metabolized by the liver in very small doses, if at all.

Pediatric pointers

○ Childhood hepatomegaly may stem from Reye's syndrome, biliary atresia, rare disorders, or poorly controlled type 1 diabetes mellitus.

Hirsutism

Overview

- Refers to excessive growth of coarse body hair in females
- Involves excessive androgen production or an increased sensitivity of the skin to androgens
- May be mild, moderate, or severe
- Virilization caused by extremely high androgen levels (see *Recognizing signs of virilization*)

Assessment

History
- Ask about the onset of hirsutism.
- Inquire about the use of hair removal techniques.
- Obtain a menstrual history.
- Obtain a drug history, including drugs containing an androgen or progestin compound.

Physical assessment
- Examine the hirsute areas.

Assessment tip
Recognizing signs of virilization

Excessive androgen levels produce severe hirsutism and other marked signs of virilization. As you examine your patient, look for the signs of virilization shown in the figure below.

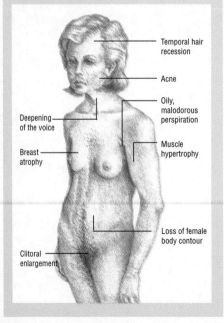

- Temporal hair recession
- Acne
- Oily, malodorous perspiration
- Muscle hypertrophy
- Deepening of the voice
- Breast atrophy
- Loss of female body contour
- Clitoral enlargement

- Observe the patient for obesity.
- Observe for signs of virilization.
- Examine the distribution pattern of hair.

Medical causes

Acromegaly
- Hirsutism may be accompanied by enlarged hands and feet, coarsened facial features, prognathism, increased diaphoresis, oily skin, fatigue, weight gain, heat intolerance, and lethargy.

Adrenocortical carcinoma
- Hirsutism progresses rapidly.
- Truncal obesity, buffalo hump, moon face, oligomenorrhea, amenorrhea, muscle wasting, and thin skin with purple striae develop.
- Other findings include muscle weakness, excessive diaphoresis, poor wound healing, weakness, fatigue, hypertension, hyperpigmentation, and personality changes.

Androgen overproduction by ovaries
- Hirsutism and anovulation occur with other signs of virilization.

Cushing's syndrome
- Hair growth increases on the face, abdomen, breasts, chest, or upper thighs.
- Other findings include truncal obesity, buffalo hump, moon face, thin skin, purple striae, ecchymoses, petechiae, muscle wasting and weakness, poor wound healing, hypertension, weakness, fatigue, excessive diaphoresis, hyperpigmentation, menstrual irregularities, and personality changes.

Hyperprolactinemia
- Hirsutism, hypogonadism, galactorrhea, amenorrhea, and acne develop.
- Infertility may be present.
- Visual field defects may occur if a pituitary tumor is the cause.

Idiopathic hirsutism
- Excess hair at puberty, increasing in early adulthood
- Acne, obesity, infrequent menses or anovulation, and thick, oily skin

Ovarian tumor
- If tumor produces androgens, rapidly progressing hirsutism may occur with amenorrhea and rapidly developing virilization.

Polycystic ovary disease
- Hirsutism after onset of menstrual irregularities.
- Obesity, amenorrhea, oligomenorrhea, menometrorrhagia, infertility, and acne.

Other causes

Drugs

○ Aminoglutethimide, cyclosporine, drugs containing androgens or progestins, glucocorticoids, metoclopramide, and minoxidil can result in hirsutism.

Nursing considerations

○ Prepare the patient for tests to determine blood levels of luteinizing hormone, follicle-stimulating hormone, prolactin, and other hormones.
○ Encourage verbalization of concerns about self-image.

Pediatric pointers

○ Hirsutism can stem from congenital adrenal hyperplasia.
○ Hirsutism that occurs at or after puberty commonly results from polycystic ovary disease.

Geriatric pointers

○ Hirsutism can occur after menopause if peripheral conversion of estrogen is poor.

Patient teaching

○ Explain the cause of the patient's hirsutism.
○ Explain the treatment.
○ Discuss hair removal techniques.

Hoarseness

Overview

○ Characterized as a rough or harsh sound to the voice
○ May be acute or chronic

Assessment

History

○ Ask about the onset of hoarseness.
○ Inquire about associated shortness of breath, sore throat, dry mouth, cough, or difficulty swallowing dry food.
○ Find out about exposure to fire within the past 48 hours or overuse of voice.
○ Obtain a medical history, including cancer, rheumatoid arthritis, or aortic aneurysm.
○ Find out about alcohol and smoking habits.

Physical assessment

○ Inspect the oral cavity and pharynx for redness or exudate.
○ Palpate the neck for masses and the cervical lymph nodes and the thyroid gland for enlargement.
○ Palpate the trachea.
○ Ask the patient to stick out his tongue; if he can't, he may have paralysis from cranial nerve involvement.
○ Examine the eyes for corneal ulcers and enlarged lacrimal ducts.
○ Examine for dilated jugular and chest veins.
○ Take vital signs.
○ Inspect for asymmetrical chest expansion or signs of respiratory distress.
○ Auscultate for crackles, rhonchi, wheezing, and tubular sounds.
○ Percuss the chest for dullness.

Medical causes

Gastroesophageal reflux

○ Hoarseness, sore throat, cough, throat clearing, and feeling of a lump in the throat may occur.
○ The arytenoid tissue and vocal cords may appear red and swollen.

Hypothyroidism

○ Hoarseness may occur early.
○ Other findings include fatigue, cold intolerance, coarse hair, alopecia, weight gain despite anorexia, menorrhagia, thinning nails, and dry, flaky skin.

Laryngeal cancer

○ Hoarseness is an early sign but may not occur until later in cancer of other laryngeal areas.

○ Other features include a long history of smoking, minor throat discomfort, otalgia, hemoptysis, and a mild, dry cough.

Laryngeal leukoplakia

○ Hoarseness is common, especially in smokers.
○ Mild, moderate, or severe dysphagia may also occur.

Laryngitis

○ Persistent hoarseness may be the only sign of chronic form.
○ With acute laryngitis, hoarseness or complete loss of voice develops suddenly.
○ Related findings include pain (especially during swallowing or speaking), cough, fever, profuse diaphoresis, sore throat, and rhinorrhea.

Thoracic aortic aneurysm

○ Hoarseness may occur with thoracic aortic aneurysm.
○ The most common symptom is penetrating pain that's especially severe when the patient is supine.
○ Related findings include brassy cough, dyspnea, and a substernal aching in the shoulders, lower back or abdomen.

Tracheal trauma

○ Hoarseness occurs with hemoptysis, dysphagia, neck pain, airway occlusion, and respiratory distress.
○ Cervical spine injuries may also be present.

Vocal cord paralysis

○ Hoarseness and vocal weakness with vocal cord paralysis
○ Signs of head or neck trauma and dysphagia

Vocal cord polyps or nodules

○ Raspy hoarseness accompanies chronic cough and crackling voice.

Other causes

Inhalation injury

○ Inhalation injury from a fire or explosion produces hoarseness, coughing, singed nasal hairs, orofacial burns, soot-stained sputum and, possibly, respiratory distress.

Treatments

○ Prolonged intubation may cause temporary hoarseness.
○ Surgical trauma to the laryngeal nerve may cause temporary or permanent vocal cord paralysis.

Nursing considerations

○ Observe the patient for stridor.
○ When hoarseness lasts for longer than 2 weeks, indirect or fiber-optic laryngoscopy is indicated.

Pediatric pointers

○ In children, hoarseness may result from congenital anomalies.
○ In prepubescent boys, hoarseness can stem from juvenile papillomatosis of the upper respiratory tract.
○ In infants and young children, hoarseness commonly stems from croup.

Patient teaching

○ Explain the importance of resting the voice.
○ Teach the patient alternative ways to communicate.
○ Stress the avoidance of alcohol, smoking, and second-hand smoke.

Homans' sign

Overview

○ Positive Homans' sign reflects deep calf pain that results from strong and abrupt dorsiflexion of ankle. (See *Eliciting Homans' sign.*)
○ Positive Homans' sign results from venous thrombosis or inflammation of calf muscles.
○ Positive sign is an unreliable indicator of venous disorders.
○ If deep vein thrombosis is suspected, sign should be elicited very carefully to avoid dislodging a clot and possibly causing pulmonary embolism.

Assessment

History

○ Ask about signs and symptoms of deep vein thrombosis or thrombophlebitis.
○ Ask about associated shortness of breath or chest pain.
○ Inquire about predisposing events, such as leg injury, recent surgery, childbirth, use of hormonal contraceptives, associated diseases, and prolonged inactivity.

Physical assessment

○ Inspect and palpate the calf for warmth, tenderness, redness, swelling, and a palpable vein.
○ Measure circumferences of both calves.

Medical causes

Deep vein thrombophlebitis

○ Positive Homans' sign and calf tenderness may be the only signs.
○ Other findings include severe pain, heaviness, warmth, and swelling of the affected leg; visible, engorged superficial veins or palpable, cordlike veins; and fever, chills, and malaise.

Deep vein thrombosis

○ Positive Homans' sign occurs with tenderness over the deep calf veins, slight edema of the calves and thighs, a low-grade fever, and tachycardia.

Assessment tip
Eliciting Homans' sign

To elicit Homans' sign, first support the patient's thigh with one hand and his foot with the other. Bend his leg slightly at the knee; then firmly and abruptly dorsiflex the ankle. Resulting deep calf pain indicates a positive Homans' sign. (The patient may also resist ankle dorsiflexion or flex the knee involuntarily if Homans' sign is positive.)

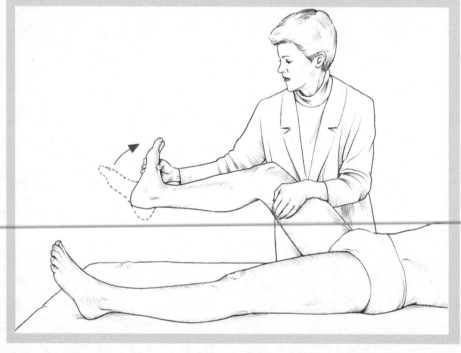

○ Cyanosis and cool skin in the affected leg may occur with venous obstruction.

Popliteal cyst (ruptured)

○ Positive Homans' sign and sudden onset of calf tenderness, swelling, and redness are produced.
○ Bruising may be observed on the popliteal space and calf.

Nursing considerations

○ Place the patient on bed rest with the affected leg elevated above heart level.
○ Apply warm, moist compresses to the affected area.
○ Administer analgesics as needed.
○ Have the patient keep the affected leg elevated while sitting and avoid crossing his legs at the knees.
○ Administer anticoagulants and thrombolytic therapy, as ordered, for thrombophlebitis.

Pediatric pointers

○ Homans' sign is seldom assessed in children.

Patient teaching

○ Explain the signs of prolonged clotting time the patient should report, if anticoagulant is ordered.
○ Stress the importance of follow-up appointments.
○ Emphasize the avoidance of alcohol.
○ Explain necessary dietary restrictions (green leafy vegetables).
○ Explain drugs the patient will need.
○ Explain the use of elastic support stockings.
○ Discuss the importance of checking with the physician before taking any new drugs.

Hyperpnea

Overview

- Refers to breathing at normal or increased rate with marked chest expansion during inhalation
- May result in hyperventilation
- May be a sign of a life-threatening condition (see *Managing hyperpnea*)
- Known as *Kussmaul's respirations* when it's a compensatory mechanism in metabolic acidosis

Assessment

History

- Ask about recent illnesses or infections.
- Find out about the ingestion of aspirin or other drugs or inhalation of drugs or chemicals.
- Obtain a medical history, including diabetes mellitus, renal disease, or pulmonary conditions.
- Ask about associated signs and symptoms, such as thirst, hunger, nausea, vomiting, severe diarrhea, or upper respiratory tract infection.

Physical assessment

- Assess level of consciousness (LOC).
- Observe for clues to abnormal breathing pattern.
- Examine for cyanosis, restlessness, and anxiety.
- Observe for intercostal and abdominal retractions, accessory muscle use, and diaphoresis.
- Inspect for draining wounds or signs of infection.
- Take vital signs, including oxygen saturation.
- Auscultate the heart and lungs.
- Assess for dehydration.

Medical causes

Head injury

- Hyperpnea
- Signs of increased intracranial pressure; loss of consciousness; soft-tissue injury or bony deformity of the face, head, or neck; facial edema; cloudy or bloody drainage from the mouth, nose, or ears; raccoon eyes; Battle's sign; an absent doll's eye sign; and motor and sensory disturbances

Hyperventilation syndrome

- Acute anxiety triggers episodic hyperpnea.
- Other findings include agitation, vertigo, syncope, pallor, circumoral and peripheral cyanosis, muscle twitching, carpopedal spasm, weakness, and arrhythmias.

Hypoxemia

- Many pulmonary disorders that cause hypoxemia may cause hyperpnea and episodes of hyperventilation with chest pain, dizziness, and paresthesia.
- Other findings include dyspnea, cough, crackles, rhonchi, wheezing, and decreased breath sounds.

Ketoacidosis

- In alcoholic ketoacidosis, Kussmaul's respirations begin abruptly and are accompanied by vomiting for several days, fruity breath odor, dehydration, abdominal pain and distention, and absent bowel sounds.
- In diabetic ketoacidosis, a potentially life-threatening disorder, Kussmaul's respirations occur with polydipsia, polyphagia, and polyuria.
- Other findings of diabetic ketoacidosis include fruity breath odor, orthostatic hypotension, weakness, decreased LOC, nausea, vomiting, anorexia, abdominal pain, and a rapid, thready pulse.
- In starvation ketoacidosis, a life-threatening disorder, Kussmaul's respirations occur gradually and may be accompanied by cachexia, dehydration, decreased LOC, bradycardia, and a history of severely limited food intake.

Renal failure

- Life-threatening acidosis and Kussmaul's respirations can occur.
- Other findings include oliguria or anuria, uremic fetor, severe pruritus, uremic frost, purpura, ecchymoses, nausea, vomiting, weakness, burning in the legs and feet, diarrhea or constipation, altered LOC, seizures, and yellow, dry, scaly skin.

Sepsis

- Severe infection may cause acidosis, resulting in Kussmaul's respirations.
- Other findings include tachycardia, fever or a low temperature, chills, headache, lethargy, profuse diaphoresis, anorexia, cough, change in mental status, and signs of infection.

Shock

- A life-threatening condition — Kussmaul's respirations, hypotension, tachycardia, narrowed pulse pressure, weak pulse, dyspnea, oliguria, anxiety, restlessness, stupor that can progress to coma, and cool, clammy skin
- External or internal bleeding (in hypovolemic shock), chest pain, arrhythmias, and signs of heart failure (in cardiogenic shock); high fever and chills (in septic shock); or stridor (in anaphylactic shock)

Carefully examine the patient with hyperpnea for related signs of life-threatening conditions, such as increased intracranial pressure (ICP), metabolic acidosis, diabetic ketoacidosis, and uremia. Be prepared for rapid interventions.

Increased ICP

If you observe hyperpnea in a patient who has signs of head trauma (soft-tissue injury, edema, or ecchymoses on the face or head) from a recent accident and has lost consciousness, act quickly to prevent further brain stem injury and irreversible deterioration. Take the patient's vital signs, noting bradycardia, increased systolic blood pressure, and widening pulse pressure—signs of increased ICP.

Examine his pupillary reaction. Elevate the head of the bed 30 degrees (unless you suspect spinal cord injury), insert an artificial airway, and administer oxygen. Connect the patient to a cardiac monitor and continuously observe his respiratory pattern. (Irregular respirations signal deterioration.) Start an I.V. line at a slow infusion rate and prepare to administer an osmotic diuretic, such as mannitol, to decrease cerebral edema. Obtain a blood sample for arterial blood gas analysis to help guide treatments.

Metabolic acidosis

If the patient with hyperpnea doesn't have a head injury, his increased respiratory rate probably indicates metabolic acidosis. Suspect shock if the patient has cold, clammy skin. Palpate for a rapid, thready pulse and take his blood pressure, noting hypotension. Elevate the patient's legs 30 degrees, apply pressure dressings to any obvious hemorrhage, start several large-bore I.V. lines, and prepare to administer fluids, vasopressors, and blood transfusions.

A patient with hyperpnea who has a history of alcohol abuse, is vomiting profusely, has diarrhea or profuse abdominal drainage, has ingested an overdose of aspirin, or is cachectic and has a history of starvation may also have metabolic acidosis. Inspect his skin for dryness and poor turgor, indicating dehydration. Take his vital signs, looking for low-grade fever and hypotension. Start an I.V. line for fluid replacement. Draw blood for electrolyte studies, and prepare to administer sodium bicarbonate.

Diabetic ketoacidosis

If the patient has a history of diabetes mellitus, is vomiting, and has a fruity breath odor (acetone breath), suspect diabetic ketoacidosis. Catheterize him to monitor increased urine output, and infuse normal saline solution. Perform a fingerstick to estimate blood glucose levels with a reagent strip. Obtain a urine specimen to test for glucose and acetone, and draw blood for glucose and ketone tests. Also, administer fluids, insulin, potassium, and sodium bicarbonate I.V.

Uremia

If the patient has a history of renal disease, an ammonia breath odor (uremic fetor), and a fine, white powder on his skin (uremic frost), suspect uremia. Start an I.V. line at a slow rate, and prepare to administer sodium bicarbonate. Monitor his electrocardiogram for arrhythmias due to hyperkalemia. Monitor his serum electrolyte, blood urea nitrogen, and creatinine levels as well until hemodialysis or peritoneal dialysis begins.

Other causes

Drugs

○ Toxic levels of salicylates, ammonium chloride, acetazolamide, and other carbonic anhydrase inhibitors can cause Kussmaul's respirations.
○ Ingestion of methanol and ethylene glycol can also cause Kussmaul's respirations.

Nursing considerations

○ Monitor vital signs, including oxygen saturation.
○ Observe for increasing respiratory distress or an irregular respiratory pattern.
○ Start an I.V. line for administration of fluids, blood transfusions, and vasopressor drugs, as ordered.
○ Prepare to give ventilatory support.

Pediatric pointers

○ Hyperpnea in a child indicates the same metabolic or neurologic causes as in an adult.
○ The most common cause of metabolic acidosis in a child is diarrhea.

Patient teaching

○ Teach the patient how to monitor his blood glucose level.
○ Stress the importance of compliance with diabetes therapy, if applicable.
○ Explain fluids and foods the patient should avoid.
○ Discuss pulmonary hygiene.
○ Teach the patient ways to avoid respiratory infections.
○ Emphasize the importance of alcohol use cessation and provide information about groups or other resources that can help.

Insomnia

Overview

- Inability to fall asleep, remain asleep, or feel refreshed by sleep
- May have a physiologic or pathophysiologic cause

Assessment

History

- Obtain a sleep history.
- Determine when the onset of insomnia occurred.
- Obtain a drug history, noting the use of central nervous system stimulants.
- Ask about the use of caffeine and caffeinated beverages.
- Obtain a medical history of chronic or acute conditions, including painful or pruritic conditions.
- Ask about alcohol use.
- Determine emotional status and stress factors.
- Obtain a psychosocial history, noting factors such as frequent travel, exercise, and personal or job-related problems.

Physical assessment

- Perform a complete physical assessment.
- Pay close attention to findings that suggest a neurologic, cardiac, respiratory, or endocrine disorder.

Medical causes

Alcohol withdrawal syndrome

- Insomnia may persist for up to 2 years.
- Other early effects include excessive diaphoresis, tachycardia, hypertension, tremors, restlessness, irritability, headache, nausea, flushing, and nightmares.
- Progression to alcohol withdrawal delirium produces confusion, disorientation, paranoia, delusions, hallucinations, and seizures.

Depression

- Chronic insomnia occurs with difficulty falling asleep, waking and being unable to fall back to sleep, or waking early in the morning.
- Related findings include dysphoria, decreased appetite with weight loss or increased appetite with weight gain, and psychomotor agitation or retardation.
- The patient also experiences loss of interest in usual activities, feelings of worthlessness and guilt, fatigue, difficulty concentrating, indecisiveness, and recurrent thoughts of death.

Generalized anxiety disorder

- Chronic insomnia occurs with fatigue, restlessness, diaphoresis, dyspepsia, high resting pulse and respiratory rates, and signs of apprehension.

Nocturnal myoclonus

- Involuntary and fleeting muscle jerks of the legs occur every 20 to 40 seconds, disturbing sleep.
- The patient reports poor sleep and daytime somnolence.

Pain

- Conditions that cause pain can also cause insomnia.
- Behavioral responses include altered body position, moaning, grimacing, withdrawal, crying, restlessness, muscle twitching, and immobility.
- With mild or moderate pain, findings include pallor, elevated blood pressure, dilated pupils, skeletal muscle tension, dyspnea, tachycardia, and diaphoresis.
- With severe and deep pain, findings include pallor, decreased blood pressure, bradycardia, nausea, vomiting, weakness, dizziness, and loss of consciousness.

Pruritus

- Insomnia results because of scratching.

Sleep apnea syndrome

- Sleep is disturbed by apneic periods that end with a series of gasps and arousal.
- With central sleep apnea, respiratory movement ceases for the apneic period.
- With obstructive sleep apnea, upper airway obstruction blocks incoming air, but breathing movements continue.
- Other findings include morning headache, daytime fatigue, hypertension, ankle edema, and personality changes.

Thyrotoxicosis

- Difficulty falling asleep and then sleeping for only a brief period is a characteristic symptom.
- Other findings include dyspnea, tachycardia, palpitations, atrial or ventricular gallop, weight loss despite increased appetite, diarrhea, tremors, nervousness, diaphoresis, hypersensitivity to heat, an enlarged thyroid gland, and exophthalmos.

Other causes

Drugs

- Use of, abuse of, or withdrawal from sedatives or hypnotics may produce insomnia.
- Central nervous system stimulants may also produce insomnia.

Tips for relieving insomnia

Common problems	Causes	Interventions
Acroparesthesia	Improper positioning may compress superficial (ulnar, radial, and peroneal) nerves, disrupting circulation to the compressed nerve. This causes numbness, tingling, and stiffness in an arm or leg.	Teach the patient to assume a comfortable position in bed with his limbs unrestricted. If he tends to awaken with a numb arm or leg, tell him to massage and move it until sensation returns completely and then to assume an unrestricted position.
Anxiety	Physical and emotional stress produces anxiety, which causes autonomic stimulation.	Encourage the patient to discuss his fears and concerns and teach him relaxation techniques, such as guided imagery and deep breathing. Give a mild sedative, such as temazepam or another sedative hypnotic, before bedtime. Emphasize that these drugs are to be used for the short-term only.
Dyspnea	With many cardiac and pulmonary disorders, a recumbent position and inactivity cause restricted chest expansion, secretion pooling, and pulmonary vascular congestion, leading to coughing and shortness of breath.	Elevate the head of the bed or provide at least two pillows or a reclining chair to help the patient sleep. Suction him when he awakens and encourage deep breathing and incentive spirometry every 2 to 4 hours. Also, provide supplementary oxygen by nasal cannula. If the patient is pregnant, encourage her to sleep on her left side at a comfortable elevation.
Pain	Chronic or acute pain can prevent or disrupt sleep.	Give drugs for pain 20 minutes before bedtime, and teach deep, even, slow breathing to promote relaxation. If the patient has back pain, help him lie on his side with his legs flexed. If he has epigastric pain, encourage him to take an antacid before bedtime and to sleep with the head of the bed elevated. If he has incisions, instruct him to splint during coughing or movement.
Pruritus	A localized skin infection or a systemic disorder, such as liver failure, may produce intensely annoying itching, even during the night.	Wash the patient's skin with a mild soap and water and dry the skin thoroughly. Apply moisturizing lotion on dry, unbroken skin and an antipruritic such as calamine lotion on pruritic areas. Administer diphenhydramine or hydroxyzine, as ordered, to help minimize itching.
Restless leg	Excessive exercise during the day may cause tired, aching legs at night, requiring movement for relief.	Help the patient exercise his legs gently by slowly walking with him around the room and down the hall. If ordered, administer a muscle relaxant such as diazepam.

Nursing considerations

○ Prepare the patient for tests to evaluate his insomnia.
○ Institute measures to help relieve insomnia. (See *Tips for relieving insomnia*.)

Pediatric pointers

○ Insomnia in early childhood may develop along with separation anxiety (ages 2 to 3), after a stressful or tiring day, or during illness or teething.
○ In children ages 6 to 11, insomnia usually reflects residual excitement from the day's activities.

Geriatric pointers

○ Sleep patterns of older people are marked by frequent awakenings, diminished stage III and stage IV non-rapid eye movement time, increased time spent awake at night, and more frequent daytime naps.

Patient teaching

○ Teach the patient techniques to increase comfort and relaxation.
○ Discuss the appropriate use of tranquilizers or sedatives.
○ Refer the patient to counseling or sleep disorder clinic as needed.

Intermittent claudication

Overview

○ Cramping limb pain
○ Brought on by exercise; relieved by 1 to 2 minutes of rest
○ May be acute or chronic

Emergency actions

If the patient has sudden intermittent claudication with severe or aching leg pain at rest, check the temperature and color of his leg and palpate femoral, popliteal, posterior tibial, and dorsalis pedis pulses. Suspect acute arterial occlusion if pulses are absent; if the leg feels cold and looks pale, cyanotic, or mottled; and if paresthesia and pain are present.

Mark areas of pallor, cyanosis, or mottling, and reassess frequently. Don't elevate the leg. Protect it, allowing nothing to press on it. Start an I.V. line, and administer an anticoagulant and analgesics. Anticipate diagnostic tests and, possibly, surgery.

Assessment

History

○ Ask the patient how far he can walk before pain occurs, how long it takes for pain to subside, and recent changes in pain pattern and characteristics.
○ Explore risk factors, such as smoking, diabetes, hypertension, and hyperlipidemia.
○ Ask about associated signs and symptoms, such as paresthesia in the affected limb and visible changes in the color of the fingers.

Physical assessment

○ Palpate lower extremity pulses.
○ Note color and temperature differences between the legs and compared with the arms.
○ Auscultate for bruits over major arteries.
○ Elevate the affected leg for 2 minutes and assess color changes, note how long it takes for color to return when legs are dependent.
○ Examine the feet, toes, and fingers for ulceration.
○ Inspect the hands and lower legs for small, tender nodules and erythema along blood vessels.
○ If the patient has arm pain, inspect the arms for a change in color (to white) on elevation.
○ Palpate and compare upper extremity pulses.

Medical causes

Aortic arteriosclerotic occlusive disease

○ Intermittent claudication occurs in the buttock, hip, thigh, and calf, along with absent or diminished femoral pulses.
○ Other findings include bruits over the femoral and iliac arteries, pallor and coolness of the affected limb on elevation, and profound limb weakness.

Arterial occlusion (acute)

○ Intense intermittent claudication occurs.
○ The limb is cool, pale, and cyanotic with absent pulses below the occlusion.
○ Other findings include paresthesia, paresis, increased capillary refill time, and a sensation of cold in the affected limb.

Arteriosclerosis obliterans

○ Intermittent claudication appears in the calf.
○ Related findings include diminished or absent popliteal and pedal pulses, coolness in the affected limb, pallor on elevation, and profound limb weakness with continuing exercise.
○ Other findings include numbness, paresthesia and, in more severe disease, pain in the toes or foot while at rest, ulceration, and gangrene.

Buerger's disease

○ Intermittent claudication of the instep is typical.
○ Early signs include migratory superficial nodules and erythema along extremity blood vessels and migratory venous phlebitis.
○ With exposure to cold, feet initially become cold, cyanotic, and numb; later, they redden, become hot, and tingle.
○ Other findings include impaired peripheral pulses, paresthesia of the hands and feet, and migratory superficial thrombophlebitis.

Leriche's syndrome

○ Arterial occlusion causes intermittent claudication of the hip, thigh, buttocks, and calf and impotence in men.
○ Other findings include bruits, global atrophy, absent or diminished pulses, gangrene of the toes, and legs that become cool and pale with elevation.

Neurogenic claudication

○ Pain from intermittent claudication requires a longer rest time than pain from vascular claudication.
○ Other findings include paresthesia, weakness and clumsiness when walking, and hypoactive deep tendon reflexes after walking.

Nursing considerations

○ Encourage the patient to exercise.

○ Advise the patient to avoid prolonged sitting or standing as well as crossing his legs at the knees.

Pediatric pointers

○ Intermittent claudication rarely occurs in children.
○ Intermittent claudication may develop in children with coarctation of the aorta; however, extensive compensatory collateral circulation typically prevents manifestation of this sign.

Patient teaching

○ Discuss the risk factors for intermittent claudication.
○ Stress the importance of inspecting his legs and feet for ulcers.
○ Explain ways the patient can protect his extremities from injury and elements.
○ Teach the patient the signs and symptoms he should report.

Jaundice

Overview

- Yellow discoloration of skin, mucous membranes, or sclerae of the eyes
- Indicates excessive levels of bilirubin in the blood
- Also known as *icterus*
- Easier to detect in natural light

Assessment

History

- Ask about the onset of jaundice.
- Inquire about associated pruritus, clay-colored stools, dark urine, fatigue, fever, chills, GI signs or symptoms, and cardiopulmonary symptoms.
- Obtain a medical history, including cancer; liver, pancreatic or gallbladder disease; hepatitis; or gallstones.
- Ask about drug and alcohol use.
- Find out about recent weight loss.

Physical assessment

- Perform the physical examination in a room with natural light.
- Rule out hypercarotenemia.
- Inspect the skin for texture, dryness, hyperpigmentation, spider angiomas, petechiae, and xanthomas.
- Note clubbed fingers and gynecomastia.
- Palpate the abdomen for tenderness, pain, and swelling.
- Palpate and percuss the liver and spleen for enlargement.
- Test for ascites.
- Auscultate for arrhythmias, murmurs, or gallops.
- Palpate lymph nodes for swelling.
- Obtain baseline data on mental status.

Medical causes

Carcinoma

- Cancer of the hepatopancreatic ampulla produces fluctuating jaundice, occult bleeding, mild abdominal pain, recurrent fever, weight loss, pruritus, back pain, and chills.
- Hepatic cancer produces jaundice, right-upper-quadrant discomfort and tenderness, nausea, weight loss, slight fever, ascites, edema, and an irregular, nodular, firm, enlarged liver.
- With pancreatic cancer, progressive jaundice may be the only sign; other findings include weight loss, back or abdominal pain, anorexia, nausea, vomiting, fever, steatorrhea, fatigue, weakness, diarrhea, pruritus, and skin lesions.

Cholangitis

- Jaundice along with right-upper-quadrant pain and high fever with chills make up Charcot's triad.
- Other findings include pruritus and acholic or hypocholic stools.

Cholecystitis

- Nonobstructive jaundice occurs.
- Biliary colic typically peaks abruptly, persisting for 2 to 4 hours, then localizes to the right upper quadrant and becomes constant.
- Other findings include nausea, vomiting, fever, profuse diaphoresis, chills, tenderness on palpation, a positive Murphy's sign, and abdominal distention and rigidity.

Cholelithiasis

- Jaundice and biliary colic are common.
- Pain is severe and steady in the right upper quadrant or epigastrium, radiates to the right scapula or shoulder, and intensifies over several hours.
- Accompanying findings include nausea, vomiting, tachycardia, restlessness and, if the common bile duct is occluded, fever, chills, jaundice, clay-colored stools, and abdominal tenderness.

Cholestasis

- Prolonged attacks of jaundice (sometimes spaced several years apart) are accompanied by pruritus.
- Other findings include fatigue, nausea, weight loss, anorexia, pale stools, and right-upper-quadrant pain.

Cirrhosis

- With Laënnec's cirrhosis, mild to moderate jaundice occurs with pruritus; common early findings include ascites, weakness, leg edema, nausea, vomiting, diarrhea or constipation, anorexia, massive hematemesis, weight loss, and right-upper-quadrant pain.
- With primary biliary cirrhosis, fluctuating jaundice may appear years after the onset of other findings, such as pruritus that worsens at bedtime (commonly the first sign), weakness, fatigue, weight loss, and vague abdominal pain.

Glucose-6-phosphate dehydrogenase deficiency

- Jaundice occurs along with pallor, dyspnea, tachycardia, malaise, and hepatosplenomegaly.

Heart failure

- Jaundice occurs with severe right-sided heart failure.
- Other findings of right-sided failure include jugular vein distention, cyanosis, dependent edema, weight gain, weakness, confusion, hepatomegaly, nausea, vomiting, abdominal discomfort, anorexia, and ascites (a late sign).

Hemolytic anemia (acquired)

- Prominent jaundice appears with dyspnea, fatigue, pallor, tachycardia, and palpitations.

O With rapid hemolysis, chills, fever, irritability, headache, abdominal pain, and signs of shock may appear.

Hepatitis

O Jaundice occurs late and is preceded by dark urine and clay-colored stools.
O Early findings include fatigue, nausea, vomiting, malaise, arthralgias, myalgias, headache, anorexia, photophobia, pharyngitis, cough, diarrhea or constipation, and low-grade fever.
O Findings during the icteric phase include weight loss, anorexia, right-upper-quadrant pain and tenderness, and an enlarged liver.

Pancreatitis (acute)

O Jaundice may occur.
O Primary symptom is usually severe epigastric pain that may radiate to the back and is relieved by lying with the knees flexed on the chest or sitting up and leaning forward.
O Other findings include nausea, persistent vomiting, Turner's or Cullen's sign, fever, and abdominal distention, rigidity, and tenderness.

Sickle cell anemia

O Jaundice occurs with impaired growth and development, increased susceptibility to infection, thrombotic complications, leg ulcers, swollen and painful joints, fever, chills, bone aches, and chest pain.

Other causes

Drugs

O Jaundice may occur with drugs that cause hepatic injury, such as acetaminophen, isoniazid, hormonal contraceptives, sulfonamides, mercaptopurine, erythromycin estolate, niacin, troleandomycin, androgenic steroids, 3-hydroxy-3-methylglutaryl coenzyme A (HMG-CoA) reductase inhibitors, phenothiazines, ethanol, methyldopa, rifampin, dilantin, phenylbutazone, and I.V. tetracycline.

Treatments

O Upper abdominal surgery may result in jaundice.
O Surgical shunts used to reduce portal hypertension may also produce jaundice.

Nursing considerations

O To decrease pruritus:
  – Frequently bathe the patient.
  – Apply an antipruritic lotion such as calamine.
  – Administer diphenhydramine or hydroxyzine.

Pediatric pointers

O Physiologic jaundice is common in neonates, developing 3 to 5 days after birth.

O In infants, obstructive jaundice usually results from congenital biliary atresia.

Geriatric pointers

O In patients older than age 60, jaundice is usually caused by cholestasis resulting from extrahepatic obstruction.

Patient teaching

O Teach the patient appropriate dietary changes he can make.
O Discuss ways to reduce pruritus.

Jaw pain

Overview

- May arise from the maxilla, mandible, or temporomandibular joint (TMJ)
- Usually results from disorders of the teeth, soft tissue, or glands of the mouth or throat or from local trauma or infection
- May develop gradually or abruptly
- May signal a life-threatening disorder

Emergency actions

Sudden severe jaw pain, especially when associated with chest pain, shortness of breath, or arm pain, may signal a myocardial infarction. Perform an electrocardiogram and obtain blood samples for cardiac enzyme levels. Administer oxygen, morphine sulfate, and a vasodilator as indicated.

Assessment

History

- Determine the onset, character, intensity, and frequency of jaw pain.
- Ask whether the jaw pain radiates to other areas.
- Ask about recent trauma, surgery, or procedures.
- Inquire about associated signs and symptoms, such as joint or chest pain, dyspnea, palpitations, fatigue, headache, malaise, anorexia, weight loss, intermittent claudication, diplopia, and hearing loss.
- Ask about aggravating or alleviating factors.

Physical assessment

- Inspect the painful area for redness; palpate for edema or warmth.
- Look for facial asymmetry.
- Check the TMJs, noting crepitus and ability to open the mouth.
- Palpate the parotid area for pain and swelling.
- Inspect and palpate the oral cavity for lesions, elevation of the tongue, or masses.

Medical causes

Angina pectoris

- Jaw and left arm pain may radiate from the substernal area.
- May be triggered by exertion, emotional stress, or ingestion of a heavy meal and subsides with rest or administration of nitroglycerin.
- Accompanying findings include shortness of breath, nausea, vomiting, tachycardia, dizziness, diaphoresis, and palpitations.

Arthritis

- With osteoarthritis, aching jaw pain increases with activity and may be accompanied by crepitus, enlarged joints with restricted range of motion, and stiffness on awakening that improves with activity.
- Rheumatoid arthritis causes symmetrical pain in all joints, including the jaw.
- Other findings of rheumatoid arthritis include tender, swollen joints with limited range of motion that are stiff after inactivity; myalgia; fatigue, weight loss; malaise; anorexia; lymphadenopathy; mild fever; painless, movable nodules on the elbows, knees, and knuckles; joint deformities and crepitus; and multiple systemic complications.

Head and neck cancer

- Jaw pain has an insidious onset.
- Other findings include a history of leukoplakia ulcers on the mucous membranes; palpable masses in the jaw, mouth, and neck; dysphagia; bloody discharge; drooling; lymphadenopathy; and trismus.

Hypocalcemic tetany

- Painful muscle contractions of the jaw and mouth occur with paresthesia and carpopedal spasms.
- Other findings include weakness, fatigue, palpitations, hyperreflexia, positive Chvostek's and Trousseau's signs, muscle twitching, choreiform movements, muscle cramps and, with severe hypocalcemia, laryngospasm with stridor, cyanosis, seizures, and arrhythmias.

Ludwig's angina

- Severe jaw pain in the mandibular area occurs with tongue elevation, sublingual edema, fever, and drooling.
- Progressive disease produces dysphagia, dysphonia, stridor, and dyspnea.

Myocardial infarction

- A life-threatening disorder — crushing substernal pain may radiate to the lower jaw, left arm, neck, back, or shoulder blades.
- Other findings include pallor, clammy skin, dyspnea, excessive diaphoresis, nausea, vomiting, anxiety, restlessness, a feeling of impending doom, low-grade fever, decreased or increased blood pressure, arrhythmias, an atrial gallop, new murmurs, and crackles.

Osteomyelitis

- Aching jaw pain may occur along with warmth, swelling, tenderness, erythema, and restricted jaw movement.
- Tachycardia, sudden fever, nausea, and malaise may occur with acute osteomyelitis.

Sinusitis

- Maxillary sinusitis produces intense boring pain in the maxilla and cheek that may radiate to the eye

along with a feeling of fullness, increased pain on percussion of the first and second molars and, in those with nasal obstruction, the loss of the sense of smell.
○ Sphenoid sinusitis produces chronic pain at the mandibular ramus and vertex of the head and in the temporal area.
○ Other features of both types of sinusitis include fever, halitosis, headache, malaise, cough, sore throat, and fever.

Suppurative parotitis

○ Onset of jaw pain, high fever, and chills is abrupt.
○ Other findings include erythema and edema of the overlying skin; a tender, swollen gland; and pus at the second molar.

Temporal arteritis

○ Sharp jaw pain occurs after chewing or talking.
○ Other findings include low-grade fever; generalized muscle pain; malaise; fatigue; anorexia; weight loss; throbbing, unilateral headache in the frontotemporal regions; swollen, nodular, tender and, possibly, pulseless temporal arteries; erythema of the overlying skin.

Temporomandibular joint disorders

○ Jaw pain at the TMJ; spasm and pain of the masticating muscle; clicking, popping, or crepitus of the TMJ; and restricted jaw movement may occur.
○ Other findings include localized pain that may radiate to other head and neck areas, teeth clenching, bruxism, ear pain, headache, deviation of the jaw to the affected side upon opening the mouth, and jaw subluxation or dislocation, especially after yawning.

Trauma

○ Jaw pain may occur with swelling and decreased jaw mobility.
○ Other findings include hypotension, tachycardia, lacerations, ecchymoses, hematomas, blurred vision, and rhinorrhea or otorrhea.

Trigeminal neuralgia

○ Paroxysmal attacks of intense unilateral jaw pain (stopping at the facial midline) or rapid-fire shooting sensations in one division of the trigeminal nerve (usually the mandibular or maxillary division) occur.
○ Pain is felt mainly over the lips and chin and in the teeth; mouth and nose areas may be hypersensitive; and corneal reflexes are diminished or absent (if the ophthalmic branch is involved).

Other causes

Drugs

○ Some drugs, such as phenothiazines, affect the extrapyramidal tract, causing dyskinesias; other cause tetany of the jaw from hypocalcemia.

Nursing considerations

○ If pain is severe, withhold food, liquids, and oral medications until diagnosis is confirmed.
○ Administer an analgesic.
○ Apply an ice pack if the jaw is swollen.
○ Discourage the patient from talking or moving the jaw.

Pediatric pointers

○ Mumps causes unilateral or bilateral swelling from the lower mandible to the zygomatic arch.
○ Parotiditis due to cystic fibrosis causes jaw pain.
○ When trauma causes jaw pain in children, always consider the possibility of abuse.

Patient teaching

○ Explain the disorder and treatments the patient needs.
○ Teach the patient the proper way to insert mouth splints.
○ Discuss ways to reduce stress.
○ Explain the identification and avoidance of triggers.

Jugular vein distention

Overview

- Abnormal fullness and height of pulse waves in internal or external jugular veins
- Involves a pulse wave height greater than 1¼" to 1½" (3 to 4 cm) above the angle of Louis with the patient in a supine position and his head elevated 45 degrees (See *Evaluating jugular vein distention.*)
- Reflects increased venous pressure in the right side of the heart, which in turn, indicates increased central venous pressure
- Occurs in cardiovascular disorders

Emergency actions

If you detect jugular vein distention in a patient with pale, clammy skin who suddenly appears anxious and dyspneic, take his blood pressure. If you note hypotension and paradoxical pulse, suspect cardiac tamponade. Elevate the foot of the bed 20 to 30 degrees, give supplemental oxygen, and monitor cardiac status and rhythm, oxygen saturation, and mental status. Start an I.V. line for medication administration and keep cardiopulmonary resuscitation equipment close by. Assemble equipment for emergency pericardiocentesis.

Assessment

History

- Find out about recent weight gain or swelling.
- Inquire about associated chest pain, shortness of breath, paroxysmal nocturnal dyspnea, anorexia, nausea, or vomiting.
- Obtain a medical history, including cancer or cardiac, pulmonary, hepatic, or renal disease.
- Obtain a drug history, noting use of diuretics.
- Inquire about diet history, especially sodium intake.

Assessment tip
Evaluating jugular vein distention

With the patient in a supine position, elevate the head of the bed 45 to 90 degrees. (In the normal patient, veins distend only when the patient lies flat.)

Next, locate the angle of Louis (sternal notch)—the reference point for measuring venous pressure. To do so, palpate the clavicles where they join the sternum (the suprasternal notch). Place your first two fingers on the suprasternal notch. Then, without lifting them from the skin, slide them down the sternum until you feel a bony protuberance—this is the angle of Louis.

Find the internal jugular vein (which indicates venous pressure more reliably than the external jugular vein). Shine a flashlight across the patient's neck to create shadows that highlight his venous pulse. Be sure to distinguish jugular vein pulsations from carotid artery pulsations. One way to do this is to palpate the vessel: Arterial pulsations continue, whereas venous pulsations disappear with light finger pressure. Also, venous pulsations increase or decrease with changes in body position; arterial pulsations remain constant.

Next, locate the highest point along the vein where you can see pulsations. Using a centimeter ruler, measure the distance between that high point and the sternal notch. Record this finding as well as the angle at which the patient was lying. A finding greater than 1¼" to 1½" (3 to 4 cm) above the sternal notch, with the head of the bed at a 45-degree angle, indicates jugular vein distention.

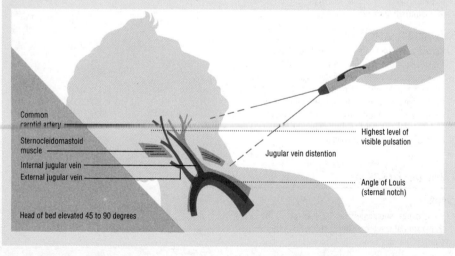

Common carotid artery

Sternocleidomastoid muscle

Internal jugular vein

External jugular vein

Head of bed elevated 45 to 90 degrees

Highest level of visible pulsation

Jugular vein distention

Angle of Louis (sternal notch)

Physical assessment

○ Check vital signs.
○ Inspect and palpate for edema.
○ Weigh the patient and compare weight to his baseline.
○ Auscultate lungs for crackles and heart for gallops, pericardial friction rub, and muffled heart sounds.
○ Inspect abdomen for distention.
○ Palpate and percuss for an enlarged liver.

Medical causes

Cardiac tamponade

○ A life-threatening condition — jugular vein distention occurs with anxiety, restlessness, cyanosis, chest pain, dyspnea, hypotension, and clammy skin.
○ Other features include tachycardia, tachypnea, muffled heart sounds, a pericardial friction rub, weak or absent peripheral pulses that decrease during inspiration (pulsus paradoxus), and hepatomegaly.

Heart failure

○ Right-sided heart failure commonly causes jugular vein distention, weakness, cyanosis, dependent edema, steady weight gain, confusion, and hepatomegaly.
○ Other findings of right-sided failure include nausea, vomiting, abdominal discomfort, anorexia, and ascites (a late sign).
○ Jugular vein distention is a late sign in left-sided heart failure.
○ Other findings of left-sided failure include fatigue, dyspnea, orthopnea, paroxysmal nocturnal dyspnea, tachypnea, tachycardia, crackles, a ventricular gallop, and arrhythmias.

Hypervolemia

○ Jugular vein distention occurs along with rapid weight gain, elevated blood pressure, bounding pulse, peripheral edema, dyspnea, and crackles.

Pericarditis (chronic constrictive)

○ Jugular vein distention is a progressive sign and more prominent on inspiration (known as Kussmaul's sign).
○ Other findings include chest pain, dependent edema, hepatomegaly, ascites, and pericardial friction rub.

Superior vena cava obstruction

○ Jugular vein distention may occur along with facial, neck, and upper arm edema.

Nursing considerations

○ If the patient has cardiac tamponade, prepare him for pericardiocentesis.
○ Restrict fluids and monitor intake and output.
○ Insert an indwelling urinary catheter if necessary.
○ If the patient has heart failure, administer a diuretic.

○ Routinely change the patient's position to avoid skin breakdown from peripheral edema.
○ Prepare the patient for central venous or pulmonary artery catheter insertion.

Pediatric pointers

○ Jugular vein distention is difficult to evaluate in infants, toddlers, and children because of their short, thick necks.

Patient teaching

○ Explain foods or drinks the patient should avoid.
○ Teach the patient to perform daily weight monitoring.
○ Explain what weight gain he should report.
○ Explain the importance of scheduled rest periods and help him plan for them.

Kernig's sign

Overview

○ Indicates meningeal irritation, herniated disk, or spinal tumor
○ Elicits resistance and hamstring muscle pain when the knee attempts to extend while the hip and knee are flexed 90 degrees (see *Eliciting Kernig's sign*)

Assessment

History

○ Ask about back pain that radiates to the legs, numbness, tingling, or weakness.
○ Inquire about a history of cancer or back injury.

Physical assessment

○ Assess motor function by inspecting the muscles and testing muscle tone and strength.
○ Perform cerebellar testing.
○ Assess sensory function by checking the patient's sensitivity to pain, light touch, vibration, position, and discrimination.

Medical causes

Lumbosacral herniated disk

○ Positive Kernig's sign may be elicited.

○ Sciatic pain on the affected side or both sides is an early finding.

Meningitis

○ Positive Kernig's sign usually occurs early, along with fever and, possibly, chills.

Spinal cord tumor

○ Kernig's sign can be occasionally elicited.
○ Earliest symptom of spinal cord tumor is pain felt locally or along the spinal nerve, commonly in the leg.

Subarachnoid hemorrhage

○ Kernig's sign and Brudzinski's sign can be elicited within minutes after the initial bleeding. (See *When Kernig's sign signals CNS crisis.*)

Nursing considerations

○ Closely monitor vital signs, intracranial pressure (ICP), and cardiopulmonary and neurologic status.
○ Ensure bed rest, quiet, and minimal stress.
○ For those with subarachnoid hemorrhage, darken the room and elevate the head of the bed at least 30 degrees to reduce ICP.
○ If the patient has a herniated disk or spinal tumor, he may require pelvic traction.

Pediatric pointers

○ Kernig's sign is considered ominous in children because of their greater potential for rapid deterioration.

Assessment tip
Eliciting Kernig's sign

To elicit Kernig's sign, place the patient in a supine position. Flex the leg at the hip and knee, as shown below. Then try to extend the leg while you keep the hip flexed. If the patient has pain and, possibly, a spasm in the hamstring muscle and resists further extension, you can assume that meningeal irritation has occurred.

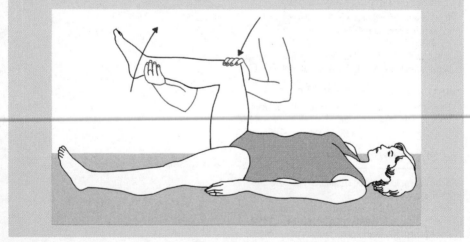

Because Kernig's sign may signal meningitis or subarachnoid hemorrhage — both life-threatening central nervous system (CNS) disorders — take the patient's vital signs immediately to obtain baseline information. Then test for Brudzinski's sign to obtain further evidence of meningeal irritation. Next, ask the patient or his family to describe the onset of illness. Typically, the progressive onset of headache, fever, nuchal rigidity, and confusion suggests meningitis. (The sudden onset of a severe headache, nuchal rigidity, photophobia and, possibly, loss of consciousness usually indicates subarachnoid hemorrhage.)

Meningitis
If a diagnosis of meningitis is suspected, ask about recent infections, especially tooth abscesses. Ask about exposure to infected people or to places where meningitis is endemic. Meningitis is usually a complication of another bacterial infection; draw blood for culture studies to determine the causative organism. If a tumor or abscess can be ruled out, prepare the patient for a lumbar puncture. Find out if the patient has a history of I.V. drug abuse, an open-head injury, or endocarditis. Insert an I.V. line and immediately begin giving an antibiotic.

Subarachnoid hemorrhage
If subarachnoid hemorrhage is the suspected diagnosis, ask about a history of hypertension, cerebral aneurysm, head trauma, or arteriovenous malformation. Also ask about sudden withdrawal of an antihypertensive.

Check the patient's pupils for dilation, and assess him for signs of increasing intracranial pressure, such as bradycardia, increased systolic blood pressure, and widened pulse pressure. Insert an I.V. line and administer supplemental oxygen.

Patient teaching
○ Teach the patient the signs and symptoms of meningitis.
○ Discuss ways to prevent meningitis.
○ Explain the activities that a patient with a herniated disk should avoid.
○ Teach the patient how to apply his back brace or cervical collar as needed.

Leg pain

Overview

○ May be gradual or sudden, localized or affecting the entire leg
○ May feel dull, burning, sharp, shooting, or tingling

⚡ Emergency actions

If the patient has acute leg pain and a history of trauma, quickly take his vital signs and determine the leg's neurovascular status.

Observe the leg's position and check for swelling, gross deformities, or abnormal rotation. Check distal pulses and note skin color and temperature. A pale, cool, and pulseless leg may indicate impaired circulation, which may require emergency surgery.

Assessment

History

○ Ask about the onset and description of pain.
○ Inquire about the use of assistive devices.
○ Obtain a medical history, including injury, surgery, or joint, vascular, or back problems.
○ Obtain a drug history.

Physical assessment

○ Observe the leg while the patient walks (if possible), stands, and sits.
○ If the leg isn't fractured, test hip and knee range of motion (ROM).
○ Check reflexes in the legs.
○ Compare both legs for symmetry, movement, and active ROM.
○ Assess sensation and strength.
○ If the leg is immobilized, check distal circulation, sensation, and mobility; stretch the toes to elicit associated pain.

Medical causes

Bone cancer

○ First, continuous deep or boring pain that worsens at night
○ Later, skin breakdown, impaired circulation, cachexia, fever, and impaired mobility

Compartment syndrome

○ Progressive, intense lower leg pain increases with passive muscle stretching is a major sign of this limb-threatening disorder.
○ Pain typically worsens despite analgesia.
○ Other findings include muscle weakness and paresthesia, but normal distal circulation.

Fracture

○ Severe, acute leg pain accompanies swelling and ecchymosis.
○ Other findings include deformity, muscle spasms, bony crepitation, paresthesia, absent pulse, mottled cyanosis, cool skin, and pain with movement.

Infection

○ Local leg pain occurs with erythema, swelling, streaking, and warmth.
○ Other features include fever, tachycardia, and loss of function of the affected limb.

Occlusive vascular disease

○ Continuous cramping pain may worsen with walking.
○ Other signs and symptoms include pain at night, cold feet, cold intolerance, numbness, tingling, ankle and lower leg edema, decreased or absent pulses, and increased capillary refill time.

Sciatica

○ Shooting, aching, or tingling pain radiates down the back of the leg.
○ Typically, activity exacerbates the pain and rest relieves it.

Strain or sprain

○ Acute strain causes sharp, transient pain and rapid swelling, followed by leg tenderness and ecchymosis.
○ Chronic strain produces stiffness, soreness, generalized leg tenderness, and pain on passive or active motion.
○ A sprain causes local pain, especially during joint movement; ecchymosis; local swelling; and loss of mobility.

Thrombophlebitis

○ Discomfort ranges from calf tenderness to severe pain and swelling, warmth, and heaviness.
○ Other features include fever, chills, malaise, muscle cramps, a positive Homans' sign, and superficial veins that are engorged, sensitive to pressure, and hard, thready, and cordlike.

Varicose veins

○ Nocturnal cramping; heaviness; diffuse, dull aching after prolonged standing or walking; and aching during menses occur.
○ Other findings include palpable nodules, orthostatic edema, and stasis pigmentation of the calves and ankles.

Venous stasis ulcers

○ Localized pain and bleeding occur.
○ Mottled, bluish pigmentation is characteristic, and local edema may occur.

Nursing considerations

- Check distal pulses and evaluate the legs for temperature, color, and sensation.
- Monitor thigh and calf circumference.
- Give an anticoagulant and antibiotic as needed.
- Use sandbags to immobilize the leg; apply ice and, if needed, skeletal traction.

Pediatric pointers

- Common causes of leg pain in children include fracture, osteomyelitis, and bone cancer.
- If parents fail to give adequate explanation for leg fracture, consider child abuse.

Patient teaching

- Explain the use of anti-inflammatory drugs, ROM exercises, and assistive devices.
- Discuss lifestyle changes the patient should make.
- Teach appropriate positioning to enhance blood flow and venous return.
- Discuss the need for physical therapy, as appropriate.

Level of consciousness, decreased

Overview

- Ranges from lethargy to stupor to coma
- Involves cerebral disturbance on both sides or disturbance in the reticular activating system
- May signal a life-threatening disorder
- Can deteriorate suddenly or gradually and can remain altered temporarily or permanently
- Can be indicated by a change in mental status — the most sensitive indicator of decreased level of consciousness (LOC)

Emergency actions

After evaluating the patient's airway, breathing, and circulation, use the Glasgow Coma Scale to determine LOC and to obtain baseline data. (See Using the Glasgow Coma Scale.)

Insert an artificial airway, elevate the head of the bed 30 degrees and, if spinal cord injury has been ruled out, turn the patient's head to the side. Prepare to suction the patient if needed. He may require hyperventilation to reduce carbon dioxide levels and decrease intracranial pressure (ICP). Then determine the rate, rhythm, and depth of spontaneous respirations. Support breathing with a handheld resuscitation bag if needed.

If Glasgow Coma Scale score is 7 or lower, intubation and resuscitation may be needed. Continue to monitor vital signs, looking for signs of increasing ICP, such as bradycardia and widening pulse pressure. When airway, breathing, and circulation are stabilized, perform a neurologic examination.

Assessment

History

- Ask family about headaches, dizziness, nausea, vision or hearing disturbances, weakness, and fatigue.
- Determine whether the family has noticed any changes in behavior, personality, memory, or temperament.
- Obtain a medical history, including neurologic disease or cancer and recent trauma or infection.
- Obtain a history of drug and alcohol use.

Physical assessment

- Perform a complete neurologic examination.
- Perform a physical assessment.

Medical causes

Adrenal crisis

- Decreased LOC, ranging from lethargy to coma, may develop within 12 hours of onset.
- Early signs and symptoms include progressive weakness, irritability, anorexia, headache, nausea, vomiting, diarrhea, abdominal pain, and fever.
- Later findings include hypotension; rapid, thready pulse; oliguria; cool, clammy skin; and flaccid extremities.

Brain abscess

- Decreased LOC varies from drowsiness to deep stupor.
- Intractable headache, nausea, vomiting, and seizures occur.
- Early signs and symptoms include constant intractable headache, nausea, vomiting, and seizures.
- Later findings include ocular disturbances and signs of infection.
- Other features include personality changes, confusion, abnormal behavior, dizziness, facial weakness, aphasia, ataxia, tremor, and hemiparesis.

Brain tumor

- LOC decreases slowly, from lethargy to coma.
- Apathy, behavior changes, memory loss, decreased attention span, morning headache, dizziness, aphasia, seizures, vision loss, ataxia, and sensorimotor disturbances may occur.
- In later stages findings include, papilledema, vomiting, bradycardia, and widening pulse pressure.
- In the final stages, findings include decorticate or decerebrate posture.

Cerebral aneurysm (ruptured)

- Somnolence, confusion and, at times, stupor characterize moderate bleeding.
- Deep coma occurs with severe bleeding, which can be fatal.
- Onset is usually abrupt with sudden, severe headache, nausea, and vomiting.
- Nuchal rigidity, back and leg pain, fever, restlessness, irritability, seizures, and blurred vision point to meningeal irritation.
- Other findings include hemiparesis, hemisensory defects, dysphagia, and visual defects.

Cerebral contusion

- Unconscious patients may have dilated, nonreactive pupils and decorticate or decerebrate posture.
- Conscious patients may be drowsy, confused, disoriented, agitated, or violent.
- Other signs and symptoms include blurred or double vision, fever, headache, pallor, diaphoresis, seizures, impaired mental status, slight hemiparesis, tachycardia, altered respirations, aphasia, and hemiparesis.

The Glasgow Coma Scale provides an easy way to describe a patient's mental status and to detect and interpret changes.
To use the Glasgow Coma Scale, test the patient's ability to respond to verbal, motor, and sensory stimulation. The scoring system doesn't determine exact level of consciousness, but it does provide an easy way to describe the patient's basic condition and helps to detect and interpret changes from baseline findings. A decreased reaction score in one or more categories may signal an impending neurologic crisis. A score of 7 or lower indicates severe neurologic damage.

Test	Reaction	Score
Eyes	Open spontaneously	4
	Open to verbal command	3
	Open to pain	2
	No response	1
Best motor response	Obeys verbal command	6
	Localizes painful stimulus	5
	Flexion — withdrawal	4
	Flexion — abnormal (decorticate rigidity)	3
	Extension (decerebrate rigidity)	2
	No response	1
Best verbal response	Oriented and converses	5
	Disoriented and converses	4
	Inappropriate words	3
	Incomprehensible sounds	2
	No response	1
Total		3 to 15

Diabetic ketoacidosis
○ Decrease in LOC is rapid and ranges from lethargy to coma.
○ Polydipsia, polyphagia, and polyuria precede decreased LOC.
○ Associated features include weakness, anorexia, abdominal pain, nausea, vomiting, orthostatic hypotension, fruity breath odor, Kussmaul's respirations, warm and dry skin, and a rapid, thready pulse.

Encephalitis
○ Decreased LOC may range from lethargy to coma within 48 hours of onset.
○ Other possible signs and symptoms include abrupt onset of fever, headache, nuchal rigidity, nausea, vomiting, irritability, personality changes, seizures, aphasia, ataxia, hemiparesis, nystagmus, photophobia, myoclonus, and cranial nerve palsies.

Encephalopathy
○ With hepatic encephalopathy, decreased LOC ranges from slight personality changes to coma depending on the stage.
○ With hypertensive encephalopathy, LOC progressively decreases from lethargy to stupor to coma.
○ With hypoglycemic encephalopathy, LOC rapidly deteriorates from lethargy to coma.

○ Hypoxic encephalopathy produces a sudden or gradual decrease in LOC, leading to coma and brain death.
○ With uremic encephalopathy, LOC decreases gradually from lethargy to coma.

Epidural hemorrhage (acute)
○ Momentary loss of consciousness is sometimes followed by a lucid interval.
○ Other signs and symptoms while the patient is lucid include severe headache, nausea, vomiting, and bladder distention.
○ Rapid deterioration in consciousness follows, possibly leading to coma.
○ Other findings include irregular respirations, seizures, decreased and bounding pulse, increased pulse pressure, hypertension, fixed and dilated pupils, unilateral hemiparesis or hemiplegia, decerebrate posture, and Babinski's reflex.

Heatstroke
○ As body temperature increases, LOC gradually decreases from lethargy to coma.
○ Early signs and symptoms include irritability, anxiety, severe headache, malaise, tachycardia, tachypnea, orthostatic hypotension, muscle cramps, rigidity, and syncope.

○ At the onset, skin is hot, flushed, and diaphoretic with blotchy cyanosis; when body temperature exceeds 105° F (40.5° C), skin becomes hot, flushed, and anhidrotic.

Hypernatremia

○ LOC deteriorates from lethargy to coma.
○ The patient is irritable and exhibits twitches that progress to seizures.
○ Other signs and symptoms include nausea, malaise, fever, thirst, flushed skin, dry mucous membranes, and a weak, thready pulse.

Hyperosmolar hyperglycemic nonketotic syndrome

○ LOC decreases rapidly from lethargy to coma.
○ Early findings include polyuria, polydipsia, weight loss, and weakness.
○ Later findings include hypotension, poor skin turgor, dry skin and mucous membranes, tachycardia, tachypnea, oliguria, and seizures.

Hypokalemia

○ LOC gradually decreases to lethargy.
○ Other signs and symptoms include confusion, nausea, vomiting, diarrhea, polyuria, weakness, decreased reflexes, malaise, dizziness, hypotension, arrhythmias, and abnormal electrocardiogram results.

Hyponatremia

○ Decreased LOC occurs in late stages.
○ Early nausea and malaise may progress to behavior changes, confusion, lethargy, incoordination and, eventually, seizures and coma.

Hypothermia

○ When severe, LOC decreases from lethargy to coma.
○ Mild to moderate cases produce memory loss, slurred speech, shivering, weakness, fatigue, and apathy.
○ Other early findings include ataxia, muscle stiffness, hyperactive deep tendon reflexes (DTRs), diuresis, tachycardia, bradypnea, decreased blood pressure, and cold, pale skin.
○ Later findings include muscle rigidity, decreased reflexes, peripheral cyanosis, bradycardia, arrhythmias, severe hypotension, shallow respirations, oliguria and, possibly, cardiopulmonary arrest.

Intracerebral hemorrhage

○ A life-threatening disorder — rapid, steady loss of consciousness occurs within hours and is accompanied by severe headache, dizziness, nausea, and vomiting.
○ Associated features include increased blood pressure, irregular respirations, Babinski's reflex, seizures, aphasia, decreased sensations, hemiplegia, decorticate or decerebrate posture, and dilated pupils.

Meningitis

○ Confusion and irritability occur; stupor, coma, and seizures may occur in severe cases.
○ Other findings include fever, chills, severe headache, nuchal rigidity, hyperreflexia, Kernig's and Brudzinski's signs, ocular palsies, photophobia, facial weakness, hearing loss, and opisthotonos.

Myxedema crisis

○ Decline in LOC may be swift.
○ Other findings include severe hypothermia, hypoventilation, hypotension, bradycardia, hypoactive reflexes, periorbital and peripheral edema, impaired hearing and balance, and seizures.

Pontine hemorrhage

○ A sudden, rapid decrease in LOC to the point of coma occurs within minutes.
○ Death occurs within hours.
○ Other findings include total paralysis, decerebrate posture, Babinski's reflex, absent doll's eye sign, and bilateral miosis.

Seizure disorders

○ A complex partial seizure causes decreased LOC, manifested as a blank stare, purposeless behavior, and unintelligible speech; an aura may precede the seizure; several minutes of mental confusion may follow the seizure.
○ An absence seizure involves a brief change in LOC, indicated by blinking or eye rolling, blank stare, and slight mouth movements.
○ A generalized tonic-clonic seizure typically begins with a loud cry and sudden loss of consciousness; consciousness returns after the seizure but the patient remains confused and may fall into deep sleep.
○ An atonic seizure produces sudden unconsciousness for a few seconds.
○ Status epilepticus, a life-threatening condition, involves rapidly recurring seizures.

Shock

○ Decreased LOC occurs late.
○ Other findings include confusion, anxiety, restlessness, hypotension, tachycardia, weak pulse with narrowing pulse pressure, dyspnea, oliguria, and cool, clammy skin.

Stroke

○ In thrombotic stroke, LOC changes may be abrupt or take several minutes, hours, or days.
○ Embolic stroke occurs suddenly and deficits peak immediately.
○ In hemorrhagic stroke, deficits develop over minutes or hours.
○ Other findings of stroke include disorientation, intellectual deficits, personality changes, emotional lability, dysarthria, dysphagia, ataxia, aphasia, agnosia, unilateral sensorimotor loss, vision disturbances, incontinence, and seizures.

Subdural hematoma (chronic)

○ LOC deteriorates slowly.
○ Other signs and symptoms include confusion, decreased ability to concentrate, personality changes, headache, light-headedness, seizures, and a dilated ipsilateral pupil with ptosis.

Subdural hemorrhage (acute)

○ A life-threatening condition — agitation and confusion are followed by progressively decreasing LOC from somnolence to coma.
○ Other features include headache, fever, unilateral pupil dilation, decreased pulse and respiratory rates, widening pulse pressure, seizures, hemiparesis, and Babinski's reflex.

Thyroid storm

○ LOC decreases suddenly and can progress to coma.
○ Irritability, restlessness, confusion, and psychotic behavior precede the deterioration.
○ Other findings include tremors, weakness, vision disturbances, tachycardia, arrhythmias, angina, acute respiratory distress, vomiting, diarrhea, and fever.

Transient ischemic attack

○ LOC decreases abruptly (with varying severity) and gradually returns to normal within 24 hours.
○ Other signs and symptoms include vision loss, nystagmus, aphasia, dizziness, dysarthria, unilateral hemiparesis or hemiplegia, tinnitus, paresthesia, dysphagia, and uncoordinated gait.

West Nile encephalitis

○ Stupor, disorientation, and coma occur with severe infection.
○ Other findings of severe infection include high fever, headache, neck stiffness, tremors, occasional seizures, and paralysis; rarely, death can occur.
○ Skin rash and lymphadenopathy may develop.

Other causes

Alcohol

○ Alcohol causes varying degrees of sedation, irritability, and incoordination; intoxication causes stupor.

Drugs

○ Overdose of barbiturates, other central nervous system depressants, or aspirin can cause sedation and other degrees of decreased LOC.

Poisoning

○ Toxins, such as lead, carbon monoxide, and snake venom, can cause varying degrees of decreased LOC.

Nursing considerations

○ Reassess LOC and neurologic status at least hourly.
○ Monitor ICP and intake and output.
○ Ensure airway patency and proper nutrition.
○ Keep the patient on bed rest with the side rails up.
○ Maintain seizure precautions.
○ Keep the head of the bed elevated to at least 30 degrees.
○ Don't give an opioid or a sedative.

Pediatric pointers

○ The primary cause of decreased LOC in children is head trauma.
○ Other causes include poisoning, hydrocephalus, meningitis, or brain abscess following an ear or a respiratory infection.

Patient teaching

○ Explain the treatments and procedures the patient needs.
○ Teach safety and seizure precautions.
○ Provide referrals to sources of support.
○ Discuss quality-of-life issues.

Lymphadenopathy

Overview

- Refers to enlargement of one or more lymph nodes
- May be generalized or localized
- Are cause for concern if more than ⅜″ (1 cm) in diameter

Assessment

History

- Ask about the onset, location, and description of swelling.
- Find out about recent infections or health problems.
- Ask about previous biopsies and personal or family history of cancer.

Physical assessment

- Note the size of any palpable lymph nodes and whether they're fixed or mobile, tender or nontender, and erythematous.
- Note the texture of palpable nodes.
- If lymph nodes are erythematous, check the area drained by that part of the lymph system for signs of infection.
- Palpate and percuss the spleen.

Medical causes

Acquired immunodeficiency syndrome

- Lymphadenopathy occurs with fatigue, night sweats, afternoon fevers, diarrhea, weight loss, and cough with several concurrent infections.

Anthrax (cutaneous)

- Lymphadenopathy, malaise, headache, and fever may develop.
- A small, elevated itchy lesion resembling an insect bite may progress into a painless, necrotic-centered ulcer.

Chronic fatigue syndrome

- Lymphadenopathy may occur with incapacitating fatigue, sore throat, low-grade fevers, myalgia, cognitive dysfunction, and sleep disturbances.
- Other signs and symptoms include arthralgia with arthritis, headache, and memory deficits.

Cytomegalovirus infection

- Generalized lymphadenopathy is accompanied by fever, malaise, and hepatosplenomegaly.
- Other features include a pruritic rash of small, erythematous macules that progresses to papules and then to vesicles.

Hodgkin's disease

- Extent of lymphadenopathy reflects stage of malignancy.
- Early findings include pruritus, fatigue, weakness, night sweats, malaise, weight loss, and fever.

Leukemia

- In acute lymphocytic leukemia, generalized lymphadenopathy is accompanied by fatigue, malaise, pallor, prolonged bleeding time, swollen gums, weight loss, bone or joint pain, hepatosplenomegaly, and low fever.
- In chronic lymphocytic leukemia, generalized lymphadenopathy appears early along with fatigue, malaise, and fever.
- Late findings of the chronic disorder include hepatosplenomegaly, severe fatigue, weight loss, bone tenderness, edema, pallor, dyspnea, tachycardia, palpitations, bleeding, anemia, and macular or nodular lesions.

Lyme disease

- As disease progresses, lymphadenopathy, constant malaise and fatigue, and intermittent headache, fever, chills, and aches develop.
- Arthralgia and, eventually, neurologic and cardiac abnormalities may develop.

Mononucleosis (infectious)

- Painful lymphadenopathy involves cervical, axillary, and inguinal nodes.
- Prodromal symptoms of headache, malaise, and fatigue appear 3 to 5 days before the appearance of the classic triad of lymphadenopathy, sore throat, temperature fluctuations with an evening peak.
- Other findings include hepatosplenomegaly, stomatitis, exudative tonsillitis, or pharyngitis.

Non-Hodgkin's lymphoma

- Painless enlargement of one or more peripheral lymph nodes is the most common sign.
- Generalized lymphadenopathy characterizes stage IV.
- Other features include dyspnea, cough, hepatosplenomegaly, fever, night sweats, fatigue, malaise, and weight loss.

Rheumatoid arthritis

- Lymphadenopathy is an early, nonspecific finding.
- Other signs and symptoms include fatigue, malaise, low fever, weight loss, and vague arthralgia and myalgia.
- Later findings include joint tenderness, swelling, and warmth; joint stiffness after inactivity; subcutaneous nodules on the elbows; joint deformity; muscle weakness; and muscle atrophy.

Sarcoidosis

- Generalized hilar and right paratracheal forms of lymphadenopathy with splenomegaly are common.

○ Initial signs and symptoms include arthralgia, fatigue, malaise, weight loss, and pulmonary symptoms.
○ Other signs and symptoms vary and may include breathlessness, cough, substernal chest pain, arrhythmias, muscle weakness and pain, phalangeal and nasal mucosal lesions, subcutaneous skin nodules, eye pain, photophobia, nonreactive pupils, seizures, and cranial or peripheral nerve palsies.

Syphilis
○ Localized lymphadenopathy occurs with painless canker that develops at site of sexual exposure.
○ In the second stage, generalized lymphadenopathy occurs along with a macular, papular, pustular, or nodular rash on the arms, trunk, palms (a diagnostic sign), soles, face, and scalp.
○ Other signs and symptoms include headache, malaise, anorexia, weight loss, nausea, vomiting, sore throat, and low fever.

Systemic lupus erythematosus
○ Generalized lymphadenopathy accompanies butterfly rash (hallmark sign), photosensitivity, Raynaud's phenomenon, and joint pain and stiffness.
○ Other signs and symptoms include pleuritic chest pain, cough, fever, anorexia, and weight loss.

Tuberculous lymphadenitis
○ Lymphadenopathy may be generalized or restricted to superficial lymph nodes.
○ Lymph nodes may become fluctuant and drain to surrounding tissue.
○ Other signs and symptoms include fever, chills, weakness, and fatigue.

Other causes

Drugs
○ Phenytoin may cause generalized lymphadenopathy.

Immunizations
○ Typhoid vaccination may cause generalized lymphadenopathy.

Nursing considerations

○ If the patient is uncomfortable, provide an antipyretic, a tepid sponge bath, or a hypothermia blanket.
○ If diagnostic tests reveal infection, check your facility's policy regarding infection control.

Pediatric pointers
○ Infection is the most common cause of lymphadenopathy in children.
○ If the child has a history of febrile seizures, provide an antipyretic.

Patient teaching
○ Teach the patient ways to prevent infection.
○ Explain the signs and symptoms of infection the patient should report.
○ Explain the reasons for isolation (as needed).
○ Stress the importance of a healthy diet and rest.

McBurney's sign

Overview

- Tenderness elicited by palpating the right-lower-quadrant over McBurney's point (see *Eliciting McBurney's sign*)
- Indicator of localized peritoneal inflammation in acute appendicitis

Assessment

History

- Ask about the onset, location, and description of abdominal pain.
- Determine what aggravates and alleviates the tenderness.
- Find out about other signs and symptoms, such as vomiting and a low-grade fever.

Physical assessment

- Before eliciting McBurney's sign, inspect the abdomen for distention, auscultate for hypoactive or absent bowel sounds, and test for tympany.
- Lightly palpate the abdomen to detect tenderness, rigidity, guarding, or pain.
- Observe the patient's facial expression for signs of pain.

Medical causes

Appendicitis

- McBurney's sign appears within the first 2 hours after the onset of appendicitis, after initial pain in the epigastric and periumbilical area shifts to the right lower quadrant.
- Persistent pain increases with walking or coughing.
- Nausea and vomiting occur at onset.
- Boardlike abdominal rigidity and rebound tenderness that worsen as the condition progresses accompany cutaneous hyperalgia, fever, constipation or diarrhea, tachycardia, retractive respirations, anorexia, and moderate malaise.
- Rupture causes sudden end to pain and the development of signs and symptoms of peritonitis.

Nursing considerations

- Make sure the patient receives nothing by mouth.
- Prepare the patient for appendectomy.
- Avoid administration of a cathartic or enema, which may cause the appendix to rupture.

Pediatric pointers

- McBurney's sign is also elicited in children with appendicitis.

Geriatric pointers

- In elderly patients, McBurney's sign may be decreased or absent.

Assessment tip
Eliciting McBurney's sign

To elicit McBurney's sign, help the patient into a supine position with his knees slightly flexed and his abdominal muscles relaxed. Palpate deeply and slowly in the right lower quadrant over McBurney's point— located about 2″ (5 cm) from the right anterior superior spine of the ilium, on a line between the spine and the umbilicus. Point pain and tenderness, a positive McBurney's sign, indicates appendicitis.

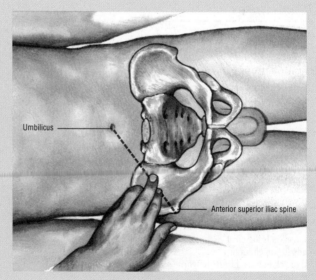

Umbilicus

Anterior superior iliac spine

Patient teaching

○ Explain which postoperative signs and symptoms the patient should report.
○ Instruct the patient on wound care.
○ Explain the needed activity restrictions.

McMurray's sign

Overview

- A palpable, audible click or pop elicited by rotating the tibia on the femur (see *Eliciting McMurray's sign*)
- An indicator of medial meniscal injury
- Don't elicit the sign in a patient with suspected fractures of the tibial plateau or femoral condyles

Assessment

History

- Ask about the onset and description of acute knee pain.
- Find out what aggravates and alleviates the pain.
- Obtain a medical history, including previous knee surgery, prosthetic replacement, and joint problems such as arthritis.

Physical assessment

- Assess the leg's range of motion (ROM), both passive and with resistance.

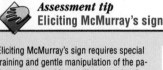

Assessment tip
Eliciting McMurray's sign

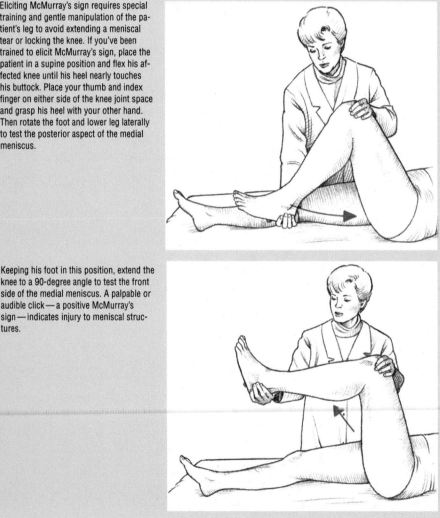

Eliciting McMurray's sign requires special training and gentle manipulation of the patient's leg to avoid extending a meniscal tear or locking the knee. If you've been trained to elicit McMurray's sign, place the patient in a supine position and flex his affected knee until his heel nearly touches his buttock. Place your thumb and index finger on either side of the knee joint space and grasp his heel with your other hand. Then rotate the foot and lower leg laterally to test the posterior aspect of the medial meniscus.

Keeping his foot in this position, extend the knee to a 90-degree angle to test the front side of the medial meniscus. A palpable or audible click—a positive McMurray's sign—indicates injury to meniscal structures.

○ Check for cruciate ligament stability by noting anterior or posterior movement of the tibia on the femur (drawer sign).
○ Measure the quadriceps muscles in both legs for symmetry.

Medical causes

Meniscal tear

○ McMurray's sign is usually elicited.
○ Other signs and symptoms include acute knee pain at the medical or lateral joint line, quadriceps weakening and atrophy, and decreased ROM or locking of the knee joint.

Nursing considerations

○ If trauma is the cause of the knee pain and the presence of McMurray's sign, prepare the patient for aspiration of the joint.
○ Immobilize and apply ice to the knee.
○ Apply a cast or knee immobilizer.

Pediatric pointers

○ McMurray's sign in adolescents is usually elicited in meniscal tears caused by sports injury.
○ It may also be elicited in children with congenital discoid meniscus.

Patient teaching

○ Explain the purpose of elevating the affected leg.
○ Teach knee exercises.
○ Explain the proper use of assistive devices the patient needs.
○ Explain the proper use of analgesics and anti-inflammatory drugs.
○ Discuss lifestyle changes the patient should make.

Melena

Overview

- Passage of black, tarry stools containing digested blood (see *Comparing melena to hematochezia*)
- Commonly indicates upper GI bleeding
- When severe, can signal acute bleeding and life-threatening hypovolemic shock

⭐ ***Emergency actions***

If the patient has severe melena, take orthostatic vital signs and look for other signs of hypovolemic shock. Insert a large-bore I.V. line to administer replacement fluids and allow blood transfusion. Obtain hematocrit, prothrombin time, International Normalized Ratio, and partial thromboplastin time. Place the patient flat with his head turned to the side and his feet elevated. Administer supplemental oxygen as needed.

Assessment

History

- Ask about the onset of melena.
- Determine the frequency and quantity of bowel movements.
- Ask about hematemesis or hematochezia.
- Find out about the use of anti-inflammatory drugs, alcohol, other GI irritants, or iron supplements.
- Obtain a drug history, noting the use of warfarin and other anticoagulants.

Physical assessment

- Inspect the mouth and nasopharynx for bleeding.
- Auscultate, percuss, and palpate the abdomen.
- Perform a cardiovascular assessment to detect signs and symptoms of shock.

Medical causes

Colon cancer

- Early right-sided tumor growth may cause melena and abdominal aching, pressure, or cramps.
- As right-sided colon cancer progresses, findings include weakness, fatigue, anemia, diarrhea or obstipation, anorexia, weight loss, vomiting, and signs and symptoms of obstruction.
- With left-sided tumor growth, melena is rare until late in the disease.
- Early signs and symptoms of left-sided colon cancer include rectal bleeding with intermittent abdominal fullness or cramping and rectal pressure.
- As left-sided colon cancer progresses obstipation, diarrhea, pencil-shaped stools may develop.

Esophageal cancer

- Melena is a late sign along with painful dysphagia, anorexia, and regurgitation.
- Earlier signs and symptoms include painless dysphagia, rapid weight loss, steady chest pain with substernal fullness, nausea, vomiting, and hematemesis.

Esophageal varices (ruptured)

- A life-threatening disorder — melena, hematochezia, and hematemesis may occur.
- Melena is preceded by signs of shock.
- Agitation or confusion signal developing hepatic encephalopathy.

Gastric cancer

- Melena and altered bowel habits may occur late.
- Common signs and symptoms include insidious onset of upper abdominal or retrosternal discomfort and chronic dyspepsia unrelieved by antacids and exacerbated by food.
- Other signs and symptoms include anorexia, nausea, hematemesis, pallor, fatigue, weight loss, and a feeling of abdominal fullness.

Gastritis

- Melena and hematemesis are common.
- Other features include mild epigastric or abdominal discomfort that's made worse by eating; belching; nausea; vomiting; and malaise.

Mallory-Weiss syndrome

- Massive bleeding from the upper GI tract is characteristic.
- Melena and hematemesis follow vomiting.
- Epigastric or back pain and signs and symptoms of shock may occur.

Mesenteric vascular occlusion

- Slight melena occurs with 2 to 3 days of persistent, mild abdominal pain.
- Later, abdominal pain becomes severe and may be accompanied by tenderness, distention, guarding, and rigidity.
- Anorexia, vomiting, fever, and profound shock may develop.

Peptic ulcer

- Melena may signal life-threatening hemorrhage.
- Other signs and symptoms include decreased appetite; nausea; vomiting; hematemesis; hematochezia; left epigastric pain that's gnawing, burning, or sharp; and signs and symptoms of shock.

Small-bowel tumors

- Tumors may bleed and produce melena.
- Other signs and symptoms include abdominal pain, distention, and increasing frequency and rising pitch of bowel sounds.

With GI bleeding, the site, amount, and rate of blood flow through the GI tract determine if a patient will develop melena (black, tarry stools) or hematochezia (bright red, bloody stools). Usually, melena indicates upper GI bleeding, and hematochezia indicates lower GI bleeding. However, with some disorders, melena may alternate with hematochezia. This chart helps differentiate these two commonly related signs.

Sign	*Sites*	*Characteristics*
Melena	Esophagus, stomach, duodenum; rarely, jejunum, ileum, ascending colon.	Black, loose, tarry stools. Delayed or minimal passage of blood through GI tract.
Hematochezia	Usually affecting the colon or lower; rapid hemorrhage of 1 L or more is associated with esophageal, stomach, or duodenal bleeding.	Bright red or dark, mahogany-colored stools; pure blood; blood mixed with formed stool; or bloody diarrhea. Reflects lower GI bleeding or rapid blood loss and passage of undigested blood through GI tract.

Thrombocytopenia

○ Melena or hematochezia may accompany other manifestations of bleeding tendency.
○ Malaise, fatigue, weakness, and lethargy are typical.

Other causes

Drug and alcohol

○ Aspirin, other nonsteroidal anti-inflammatory drugs (NSAIDs), or alcohol can cause melena.

Nursing considerations

○ Monitor vital signs and look closely for signs of hypovolemic shock.
○ Encourage bed rest.
○ Keep the perianal area clean and dry to prevent skin irritation and breakdown.
○ A nasogastric tube may be needed to drain gastric contents and for decompression.
○ Give blood transfusions according to hematocrit.

Pediatric pointers

○ Neonates may experience melena neonatorum from extravasation of blood into the alimentary canal.
○ In older children, melena usually results from peptic ulcer, gastritis, or Meckel's diverticulum.

Geriatric pointers

○ Patients with recurrent intermittent GI bleeding without a clear cause should be considered for angiography or an exploratory laparotomy.

Patient teaching

○ Explain the changes in bowel elimination that the patient needs to report.
○ Stress the importance of undergoing colorectal cancer screening.
○ Explain to the patient the need to avoid aspirin, other NSAIDs, and alcohol.

Mouth lesions

Overview

- Include ulcers (most common), cysts, firm nodules, hemorrhagic lesions, papules, vesicles, bullae, and erythematous lesions
- May occur anywhere on the lips, cheeks, hard and soft palate, salivary glands, tongue, gingivae, or mucous membranes (see *Common mouth lesions*)

Assessment

History

- Ask about the onset of lesions.
- Find out about pain, odor, drainage, or skin lesions.
- Obtain a drug history, including drug allergies and antibiotic use.
- Obtain a medical history, including malignancies, sexually transmitted diseases, I.V. drug use, recent infection, or trauma.
- Ask about dental history and oral hygiene habits.

Physical assessment

- Note lesion sites and character.
- Examine the lips for color and texture.
- Inspect and palpate the buccal mucosa and tongue for color, texture, contour, and lesions.
- Examine the oropharynx.
- Inspect the teeth and gums.
- Palpate the neck for adenopathy.

Medical causes

Acquired immunodeficiency syndrome

- Oral lesions may be an early sign of immunosuppression.
- Kaposi's sarcoma may appear on the hard palate as a flat or raised lesion, ranging in color from red to blue to purple; lesion may ulcerate and become painful.

Candidiasis

- Soft, elevated plaques usually develop on the buccal mucosa and tongue.
- In acute atrophic form, lesions are red and painful.
- In chronic hyperplastic form, lesions are white and firm.

Discoid lupus erythematosus

- Erythematous areas with white spots and radiating white striae appear on the tongue, buccal mucosa, and palate.
- Other findings include skin lesions on the face, enlarged hair follicles filled with scale, and alopecia.

Erythema multiforme

- Onset of vesicles and bullae on the lips and buccal mucosa is sudden.
- Erythematous macules and papules may form symmetrically on the hands, arms, feet, face, and neck, and, possibly, in the eyes and on genitalia.
- Other signs and symptoms include lymphadenopathy, fever, malaise, cough, throat and chest pain, vomiting, diarrhea, myalgia, arthralgia, fingernail loss, blindness, hematuria, and signs of renal failure.

Gingivitis (acute necrotizing ulcerative)

- Sudden occurrence of gingival ulcers that are covered with a grayish white pseudomembrane
- Tender or painful gingivae, intermittent gingival bleeding, halitosis, enlarged cervical lymph nodes, and fever

Gonorrhea

- Painful lip ulcerations may occur, along with rough, reddened, bleeding gingivae and a swollen, ulcerated tongue.
- Men may develop dysuria, purulent urethral discharge, and a reddened, edematous urinary meatus.
- Women may be asymptomatic or develop inflammation and a greenish yellow cervical discharge.

Herpes simplex 1

- Small, irritating vesicles develop on the oral mucosa following a brief period of prodromal tingling, itching, fever, and pharyngitis.
- Vesicles form on an erythematous base and then rupture, leaving a painful ulcer, followed by a yellowish crust.
- Other findings include submaxillary lymphadenopathy, increased salivation, halitosis, anorexia, and keratoconjunctivitis.

Herpes zoster

- Painful vesicles develop on the buccal mucosa, tongue, uvula, pharynx, and larynx.
- Small, red nodules erupt on one side of the thorax or up and down the arms and legs and rapidly become vesicles filled with clear fluid or pus; vesicles dry and form scabs about 10 days after the eruption.
- Other signs and symptoms include fever, malaise, pruritus, paresthesia or hyperesthesia, and tenderness along the course of the involved sensory nerve.

Leukoplakia, erythroplakia

- Leukoplakia is a white lesion that can't be removed by rubbing the mucosal surface.
- Erythroplakia is red and edematous and has a velvety surface.

Lichen planus

- White or gray, velvety, threadlike papules develop on the buccal mucosa or the tongue.
- Violet papules with white lines or spots then erupt on the genitalia, lower back, ankles, and anterior

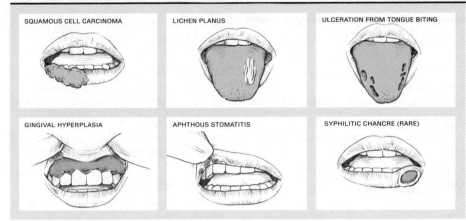

SQUAMOUS CELL CARCINOMA   LICHEN PLANUS   ULCERATION FROM TONGUE BITING

GINGIVAL HYPERPLASIA   APHTHOUS STOMATITIS   SYPHILITIC CHANCRE (RARE)

lower legs along with pruritus, nails with longitudinal ridges, and alopecia.

Squamous cell carcinoma

○ A painless ulcer with an elevated, indurated border most commonly appears on the lower lip.

Stomatitis (aphthous)

○ In the minor form, one or more erosions covered by a gray membrane and surrounded by a red halo appear on the mucosa.
○ In the major form, large, painful ulcers occur on the lips, cheek, tongue, and soft palate.

Syphilis

○ Primary syphilis typically produces a solitary painless, red ulcer (chancre) on the lip or in the mouth; ulcers appears as a crater with undulated, raised edges and a shiny center; lip chancre may develop a crust.
○ In the secondary stage, multiple painless ulcers covered by grayish plaque erupt in the mouth; a macular, papular, pustular, or nodular rash appears on the arms, trunk, palms, soles, face and scalp.
○ Other signs and symptoms in the secondary stage include lymphadenopathy, headache, malaise, anorexia, weight loss, nausea, vomiting, sore throat, low fever, metrorrhagia, and postcoital bleeding.
○ At the tertiary stage, chronic, painless, superficial nodules or deep granulomatous lesions develop on skin and mucous membranes, especially the tongue and palate.

Systemic lupus erythematosus

○ Oral lesions appear as erythematous areas from edema, petechiae, and superficial ulcers with a red halo and tendency to bleed.
○ Primary findings include nondeforming arthritis, butterfly rash across the nose and cheeks, and photosensitivity.

Other causes

Drugs

○ Chemotherapeutic drugs produce stomatitis.
○ Allergic reactions to penicillin, sulfonamides, gold, quinine, streptomycin, phenytoin, aspirin, and barbiturates can also cause oral lesions.
○ Inhaled steroids used for pulmonary disorders can also lead to oral lesions.

Treatments

○ Radiation therapy may cause oral lesions.

Nursing considerations

○ Provide a topical anesthetic such as lidocaine.
○ Provide oral hygiene.

Pediatric pointers

○ Causes of mouth ulcers in children include chickenpox, measles, scarlet fever, diphtheria, and hand-foot-and-mouth disease.
○ In neonates, mouth ulcers can result from candidiasis or congenital syphilis.

Geriatric pointers

○ Ill-fitting dentures can cause irritation, leading to inflammation and ulcers.

Patient teaching

○ Explain irritants to avoid.
○ Teach the patient proper mouth care and oral hygiene.
○ Explain the signs and symptoms the patient should report.

Murmurs

Overview

- Auscultatory sounds heard within the heart chambers or major arteries
- Classified by their timing and duration in the cardiac cycle, auscultatory location, loudness, configuration, pitch, and quality (see *Classifying murmurs*)
- Reflect accelerated, forward, or backward blood flow or decreased blood viscosity

✦ Emergency actions

In patients with bacterial endocarditis, new murmurs with crackles, distended jugular veins, orthopnea, and dyspnea may signal heart failure. In patients with acute myocardial infarction, a loud decrescendo holosystolic murmur at the apex that radiates to the axilla and left sternal border or throughout the chest is significant, particularly with a widely split S_2 and an atrial gallop. This murmur, with signs of acute pulmonary edema, usually indicates acute mitral insufficiency from the rupture of the chordae tendineae — a medical emergency.

Assessment

History

- Ask whether the murmur is new or existing.
- Find out about other symptoms, including palpitations, dizziness, syncope, chest pain, dyspnea, and fatigue.
- Obtain a medical history, including rheumatic fever, recent dental work, heart disease, or heart surgery.

Physical assessment

- Auscultate the heart and determine the type of murmur.
- Note the presence of cardiac arrhythmias, jugular vein distention, dyspnea, orthopnea, and crackles.
- Palpate the liver for enlargement or tenderness.

Medical causes

Aortic insufficiency

- In acute form, a soft, short diastolic murmur is heard over the left sternal border that is best heard with the patient leaning forward and at the end of a forced held expiration.
- Other acute findings include tachycardia, dyspnea, jugular vein distention, crackles, increased fatigue, and pale, cool extremities.
- In chronic form, a high-pitched, blowing, decrescendo diastolic murmur is heard over the second or third right intercostal space or the left sternal border; an Austin Flint murmur — a rumbling, mid-to-

late diastolic murmur best heard at the apex — may also occur.
- Other chronic signs and symptoms include palpitations, tachycardia, angina, increased fatigue, dyspnea, orthopnea, and crackles.

Aortic stenosis

- Murmur is systolic, harsh and grating, medium-pitched, crescendo-decrescendo, and heard loudest over the second right intercostal space with the patient leaning forward.
- Other features include dizziness, syncope, dyspnea on exertion, paroxysmal nocturnal dyspnea, fatigue, and angina.

Cardiomyopathy (hypertrophic)

- A harsh, late systolic murmur commonly accompanies an audible S_3 or S_4.
- Murmur decreases with squatting and increases with sitting down.
- Other signs and symptoms include dyspnea, chest pain, palpitations, dizziness, and syncope.

Mitral insufficiency

- Acute form produces medium-pitched blowing, early systolic or holosystolic decrescendo murmur at apex, along with a widely split S_2 and, commonly, S_4.
- Other acute findings include tachycardia and signs of acute pulmonary edema.
- Chronic form produces high-pitched, blowing, holosystolic plateau murmur that's loudest at apex and may radiate to axilla or back.
- Other chronic signs and symptoms include fatigue, dyspnea, and palpitations.

Mitral prolapse

- Midsystolic to late-systolic click with high-pitched late-systolic crescendo murmur occurs, best heard at the apex.
- Other signs and symptoms include cardiac awareness, migraine headaches, dizziness, weakness, syncope, palpitations, chest pain, dyspnea, severe episodic fatigue, mood swings, and anxiety.

Mitral stenosis

- Murmur is soft, low-pitched, rumbling, crescendo-decrescendo, and diastolic; is accompanied by a loud S_1 or opening snap; and best heard with the patient lying on his left side.
- With severe stenosis, murmur of mitral insufficiency may also be heard.
- Other findings include hemoptysis, exertional dyspnea, fatigue, and signs of acute pulmonary edema.

Papillary muscle rupture

- A life-threatening disorder — loud holosystolic murmur can be auscultated at apex.
- Other findings include severe dyspnea, chest pain, syncope, hemoptysis, tachycardia, and hypotension.

Rheumatic fever with pericarditis

○ A systolic murmur of mitral insufficiency, midsystolic murmur from swelling of the leaflet of the mitral valve, and a diastolic murmur of aortic insufficiency are common.
○ A pericardial friction rub along with murmurs and gallops is heard best with the patient leaning forward during forced expiration.
○ Other signs and symptoms include fever, joint and sternal pain, edema, and tachypnea.

Tricuspid insufficiency

○ Soft, high-pitched, holosystolic blowing murmur increases with inspiration and decreases with exhalation and Valsalva's maneuver, best heard over the lower left sternal border and the xiphoid area.
○ Late findings include exertional dyspnea, orthopnea, jugular vein distention, ascites, peripheral cyanosis and edema, muscle wasting, fatigue, weakness, and syncope.

Tricuspid stenosis

○ A diastolic murmur similar to that of mitral stenosis, but louder with inspiration and decreased with exhalation and Valsalva's maneuver, is produced.
○ Other findings include fatigue, syncope, peripheral edema, jugular vein distention, ascites, hepatomegaly, and dyspnea.

Other causes

Treatments

○ Prosthetic valve replacement may cause variable murmurs.

Nursing considerations

○ Give an antibiotic and an anticoagulant if needed.

Pediatric pointers

○ Innocent murmurs are commonly heard in young children.
○ Pathognomonic heart murmurs in infants and young children usually result from congenital heart disease.
○ Other murmurs can be acquired, as with rheumatic heart disease.

Teaching points

○ Explain the use of prophylactic antibiotics.
○ Explain the signs and symptoms the patient should report.

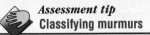

Assessment tip
Classifying murmurs

After you've auscultated a murmur, determine its timing in the cardiac cycle, location, loudness, configuration, pitch, and quality. Identifying these qualities will help you establish the type of murmur your patient has.

Timing can be characterized as systolic (between S_1 and S_2), holosystolic (continuous throughout systole), diastolic (between S_2 and S_1), or continuous throughout systole and diastole; systolic and diastolic murmurs can be further characterized as early, middle, or late.

Location refers to the area of maximum loudness, such as the apex, the lower left sternal border, or an intercostal space.

Loudness is graded on a scale of 1 to 6. A grade 1 murmur is very faint, detected only after careful auscultation. A grade 2 murmur is a soft, evident murmur. Murmurs considered to be grade 3 are moderately loud. A grade 4 murmur is a loud murmur with a possible intermittent thrill. Grade 5 murmurs are loud and associated with a palpable precordial thrill. Grade 6 murmurs are loud and, like grade 5 murmurs, are associated with a thrill. A grade 6 murmur is audible even when the stethoscope is lifted from the thoracic wall.

Configuration, or shape, refers to the nature of loudness—crescendo (grows louder), decrescendo (grows softer), crescendo-decrescendo (first rises, then falls), decrescendo-crescendo (first falls, then rises), plateau (even intensity), or variable (uneven intensity).

Pitch may be high or low.

Quality may be described as harsh, rumbling, blowing, scratching, buzzing, musical, or squeaking.

Muscle atrophy

Overview

○ Results from denervation or prolonged muscle disuse
○ Causes loss of motion or power

Assessment

History

○ Ask about the onset and progression of muscle atrophy.
○ Inquire about other signs and symptoms, such as weakness, pain, loss of sensation, and recent weight loss.
○ Obtain a medical history, including musculoskeletal or neurologic disorders, including trauma, and endocrine and metabolic disorders.
○ Ask about the use of drugs, particularly steroids.
○ Find out about alcohol use.

Physical assessment

○ Check all muscle groups for size, tonicity, and strength.
○ Measure the circumference of all limbs.
○ Check for muscle contractures in all limbs by fully extending joints and noting any pain resistance.
○ Palpate peripheral pulses for quality and rate.
○ Assess sensory function in and around the atrophied area.
○ Test deep tendon reflexes (DTRs).

Medical causes

Amyotrophic lateral sclerosis

○ Muscle weakness and atrophy that begins in one hand, spreads to the arm, and then develops in the other hand and arm are initial symptoms.
○ Eventually, weakness and atrophy spread to the trunk, neck, tongue, larynx, pharynx, and legs; progressive respiratory muscle weakness leads to respiratory insufficiency.
○ Other signs and symptoms include muscle flaccidity, fasciculations, hyperactive DTRs, slight leg muscle spasticity, dysphagia, impaired speech, excessive drooling, and depression.

Burns

○ Limited muscle movements from fibrous scar tissue, pain, and loss of serum proteins lead to atrophy.

Compartment syndrome and Volkmann's ischemic contracture

○ Muscle atrophy is a late sign along with contractures, paralysis, and loss of pulses.

○ Earlier signs and symptoms include severe pain that increases with passive muscle movement, weakness, and paresthesia.

Herniated disk

○ Muscle weakness, disuse, and, ultimately, atrophy develop.
○ Severe lower back pain, possibly radiating to the buttocks, legs, and feet is the primary symptom.
○ Other findings include muscle spasm, diminished reflexes, and sensory changes.

Hypercortisolism

○ Limb weakness and eventually atrophy occur.
○ Other cushingoid features include buffalo hump, moon face, truncal obesity, purple striae, thin skin, acne, easy bruising, poor wound healing, elevated blood pressure, fatigue, hyperpigmentation, and diaphoresis.
○ Men may develop impotence; women may develop hirsutism and menstrual irregularities.

Hypothyroidism

○ Reversible weakness and atrophy of proximal limb muscles may occur.
○ Other findings include muscle cramps and stiffness, cold intolerance; weight gain despite anorexia; mental dullness; dry, pale, cool, doughy skin; puffy face, hands, and feet; and bradycardia.

Meniscal tear

○ Quadriceps muscle atrophy is a classic sign.

Multiple sclerosis

○ Arm and leg atrophy, spasticity, and contractures result.
○ Other findings include diplopia, blurred vision, nystagmus, hyperactive DTRs, sensory loss or paresthesia, dysarthria, dysphagia, incoordination, ataxic gait, intention tremors, emotional lability, impotence, and urinary dysfunction.

Osteoarthritis

○ Atrophy proximal to involved joints eventually occurs.
○ Other late features include Heberden's nodes, Bouchard's nodes, crepitus and fluid accumulation, and contractures.

Parkinson's disease

○ Muscle rigidity, weakness, and disuse produces muscle atrophy.
○ Other findings include resting tremors, bradykinesia, a propulsive gait, a high-pitched and monotone voice, masklike facies, drooling, dysphagia, dysarthria, and oculogyric crisis or blepharospasm.

Peripheral nerve trauma

○ Muscle weakness and atrophy develop.

○ Other findings include paresthesia or sensory loss, pain, loss of reflexes supplied by the damaged nerve and, possibly, paralysis.

Peripheral neuropathy

○ Muscle weakness progresses slowly to flaccid paralysis and eventually to atrophy.
○ Other signs and symptoms include loss of vibration sense; paresthesia, hyperesthesia, or anesthesia in the hands and feet; mild to sharp, burning pain; anhidrosis; glossy red skin; and diminished or absent DTRs.

Protein deficiency

○ Muscle weakness and atrophy develop if the deficiency is chronic.
○ Other features include chronic fatigue, apathy, anorexia, dry skin, peripheral edema, and dull, sparse, dry hair.

Radiculopathy

○ Muscle atrophy and weakness develop along with paralysis, severe pain and, at times, loss of feeling in the areas supplied by the affected nerve.

Rheumatoid arthritis

○ Muscle atrophy occurs in the late stages.
○ Other late findings include deformities, crepitation with joint rotation, and multiple systemic complications.

Spinal cord injury

○ Muscle weakness and flaccid, then spastic, paralysis eventually lead to atrophy.
○ Other findings depend on the level of injury but may include respiratory insufficiency or paralysis, sensory losses, bowel and bladder dysfunction, hyperactive DTRs, positive Babinski's reflex, sexual dysfunction, and anhidrosis.

Stroke

○ Muscle weakness and eventually atrophy of the arms, legs, face, and tongue occurs.
○ Other findings vary but may include dysarthria, aphasia, ataxia, apraxia, agnosia, visual disturbances, altered level of consciousness, personality changes, bowel and bladder dysfunction, seizures, and ipsilateral paresthesia or sensory loss.

Thyrotoxicosis

○ Insidious, generalized muscle weakness and atrophy are produced.
○ Other signs and symptoms include extreme anxiety, fatigue, heat intolerance, diaphoresis, tremors, tachycardia, palpitations, ventricular or atrial gallop, dyspnea, weight loss, an enlarged thyroid gland, and exophthalmos.

Other causes

Drugs

○ Prolonged steroid therapy interferes with muscle metabolism and leads to atrophy.

Treatments

○ Prolonged immobilization from bed rest, casts, splints, or traction may cause muscle weakness and atrophy.

Nursing considerations

○ Encourage frequent, active or passive range-of-motion exercises.
○ Apply splints or braces, if needed.
○ If you find resistance to full extension during exercise, consult the physical therapist.
○ Use heat, drugs, or relaxation techniques to relax resistant muscles.

Pediatric pointers

○ In young children, profound muscle weakness and atrophy can result from muscular dystrophy.
○ Muscle atrophy may also result from cerebral palsy and poliomyelitis, and from paralysis from meningocele and myelomeningocele.

Patient teaching

○ Show the patient how to use assistive devices as needed.
○ Emphasize safety measures the patient should adopt.
○ Teach the patient an exercise regimen to follow.

Muscle spasms

Overview

○ Involve strong, painful contractions of the muscle
○ Most commonly occur in the calf and foot

⚡ Emergency actions

If the patient complains of frequent or unrelieved spasms in many muscles with paresthesia in his hands and feet, quickly attempt to elicit Chvostek's and Trousseau's signs. If these signs are present, suspect hypocalcemia. Evaluate respiratory function, watching for the development of laryngospasm. Provide supplemental oxygen as needed and anticipate intubation and mechanical ventilation. Insert an I.V. line for administration of a calcium supplement. Monitor cardiac status and begin resuscitation if needed.

Assessment

History

○ Ask about the onset and description of spasms.
○ Find out what causes, aggravates, or alleviates the spasms.
○ Inquire about weakness, sensory loss, or paresthesia.
○ Obtain a drug and diet history.
○ Ask about recent vomiting or diarrhea.

Physical assessment

○ Check muscle strength and tone.
○ Check all major muscle groups and note whether movements precipitate spasms.
○ Palpate peripheral pulses for presence and quality.
○ Examine limbs for color, capillary refill, edema, and temperature changes.
○ Test reflexes and sensory function in all limbs.

Medical causes

Amyotrophic lateral sclerosis

○ Muscle spasms may accompany progressive muscle weakness and atrophy that typically begin in one hand, spread to the arm, and then spread to the other hand and arm.
○ Eventually, muscle weakness and atrophy affect the trunk, neck, tongue, larynx, pharynx, and legs.
○ Other signs and symptoms include respiratory insufficiency, muscle spasticity, coarse fasciculations, hyperactive deep tendon reflexes (DTRs), dysphagia, impaired speech, excessive drooling, and depression.

Arterial occlusive disease

○ Spasms and intermittent claudication occur in the leg.
○ Other findings include loss of peripheral pulses; pallor or cyanosis; decreased sensation; hair loss; dry or scaling skin; edema; and ulcerations.

Cholera

○ Muscle spasms, severe water and electrolyte loss, thirst, weakness, decreased skin turgor, tachycardia, and hypotension occur along with abrupt watery diarrhea and vomiting.

Dehydration

○ Limb and abdominal cramps and muscle twitching may occur.
○ Other signs and symptoms include a slight fever, decreased skin turgor, dry mucous membranes, tachycardia, orthostatic hypotension, muscle twitching, seizures, nausea, vomiting, and oliguria.

Fracture

○ Localized spasms and pain are mild if fracture is nondisplaced; intense if severely displaced.
○ Other features include swelling, limited mobility, and bony crepitation.

Hypocalcemia

○ Tetany is the classic feature.
○ Other findings include Chvostek's and Trousseau's signs; paresthesia of the lips, fingers, and toes; choreiform movements; hyperactive DTRs; fatigue; palpitations; and arrhythmias.

Hypothyroidism

○ Spasms and stiffness occur with leg muscle hypertrophy or proximal limb weakness and atrophy.
○ Other findings include forgetfulness and mental instability; fatigue; cold intolerance; dry, pale, cool, doughy skin; puffy face, hands, and feet; periorbital edema; dry, sparse, brittle hair; bradycardia; and weight gain despite anorexia.

Muscle trauma

○ Excessive muscle strain may cause mild to severe spasms.
○ The injured area may be painful, swollen, reddened, and warm.

Respiratory alkalosis

○ Acute onset of muscle spasms may be accompanied by twitching and weakness, carpopedal spasms, circumoral and peripheral paresthesia, vertigo, syncope, pallor, and anxiety.
○ Cardiac arrhythmias may occur with severe alkalosis.

Spinal injury or disease

○ Resulting muscle spasms worsen with movement.

Other causes

Drugs

○ Corticosteroids, diuretics, and estrogens may result in spasms.

Nursing considerations

○ Help alleviate spasms by slowly stretching the affected muscle in the direction opposite the contraction.
○ If needed, give a mild analgesic.

Pediatric pointers

○ Muscle spasms may indicate hypoparathyroidism, osteomalacia, rickets or, rarely, congenital torticollis.

Patient teaching

○ Explain immobilization and wrapping the injured area.
○ Discuss pain relief measures.
○ Help the patient learn to use assistive devices as needed.

Muscle spasticity

Overview

- The state of excessive muscle tone manifested by increased resistance to stretching and heightened reflexes
- Also known as *muscle hypertonicity*
- Caused by an upper-motor-neuron lesion, spasticity usually occurs in the arms and leg muscles (see *How spasticity develops*)

⭐ Emergency actions

In a patient with a recent skin puncture or laceration, generalized spasticity and trismus indicate tetanus; if you suspect tetanus, look for signs of respiratory distress. Provide ventilatory support if needed and monitor the patient closely.

Assessment

History

- Ask about the onset, duration, and progression of spasticity.
- Ask about how the spasticity started and what aggravates it.
- Find out about other muscular changes or other symptoms.
- Obtain a medical history, including a history of trauma or degenerative or vascular disease.

Physical assessment

- Take vital signs.
- Perform a neurologic assessment.
- Test reflexes and evaluate motor and sensory function in all limbs.
- Evaluate muscles for wasting and contractures.

Medical causes

Amyotrophic lateral sclerosis

- Spasticity, spasms, coarse fasciculations, hyperactive deep tendon reflexes (DTRs), and a positive Babinski's sign result.
- Earlier findings include progressive muscle weakness and flaccidity that typically begin in the hands and arms and eventually spread to the trunk, neck, larynx, pharynx, and legs.
- Other signs and symptoms include respiratory insufficiency, dysphagia, dysarthria, excessive drooling, and depression.

Epidural hemorrhage

- Limb spasticity is a late and ominous sign.
- Other findings include a momentary loss of consciousness after head trauma, followed by a lucid interval and then a rapid deterioration in level of consciousness (LOC).
- Other findings include hemiparesis or hemiplegia; seizures; fixed, dilated pupils; high fever; decreased and bounding pulse; widened pulse pressure; elevated blood pressure; irregular respiratory pattern; a positive Babinski's sign; and decerebrate posture.

How spasticity develops

Motor activity is controlled by pyramidal and extrapyramidal tracts that originate in the motor cortex, basal ganglia, brain stem, and spinal cord. Nerve fibers from the various tracts converge and synapse at the anterior horn in the spinal cord. Together, they maintain segmental muscle tone by modulating the stretch reflex arc. This arc, shown in simplified form, is basically a negative feedback loop in which muscle stretch (stimulation) causes reflexive contraction (inhibition), thus maintaining muscle length and tone.

Damage to certain tracts results in the loss of inhibition and disruption of the stretch reflex arc. Uninhibited muscle stretch produces exaggerated, uncontrolled muscle activity, accentuating the reflex arc and eventually resulting in spasticity.

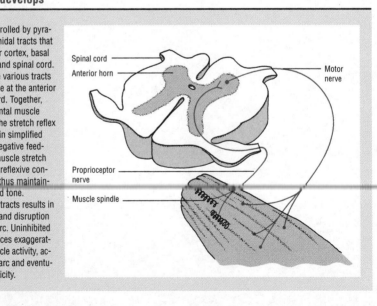

Spinal cord

Anterior horn

Motor nerve

Proprioceptor nerve

Muscle spindle

Multiple sclerosis

○ Muscle spasticity, hyperreflexia, and contractures may eventually develop.
○ Progressive weakness and atrophy occur early.
○ Other findings include diplopia, blurring or loss of vision, nystagmus, sensory loss or paresthesia, dysarthria, dysphagia, incoordination, ataxic gait, intention tremors, emotional lability, impotence, and urinary dysfunction.

Spinal cord injury

○ Spastic paralysis in the affected limbs follows initial flaccid paralysis.
○ Spasticity and muscle atrophy increase for up to 2 years after the injury, then gradually regress to flaccidity.
○ Other findings vary with the level of the injury and may include respiratory insufficiency or paralysis, sensory losses, bowel and bladder dysfunction, hyperactive DTRs, positive Babinski's sign, anhidrosis, and bradycardia.

Stroke

○ Spastic paralysis may develop on the affected side following the acute stage.
○ Other findings vary and may include dysarthria, aphasia, ataxia, apraxia, agnosia, ipsilateral paresthesia or sensory loss, visual disturbance, altered LOC, personality changes, emotional lability, bowel and bladder dysfunction, and seizures.

Nursing considerations

○ Give drugs for pain and an antispasmodic.
○ Passive range-of-motion exercises, splinting, traction, and application of heat may help relieve spasms and prevent contractures.
○ Maintain a calm, quiet environment, and encourage bed rest.
○ In cases of prolonged, uncontrollable spasticity, nerve blocks or surgical transection may be needed.

Pediatric pointers

○ In children, muscle spasticity may be a sign of cerebral palsy.

Patient teaching

○ Teach the patient to use assistive devices, as needed.
○ Discuss ways of maintaining independence.

Muscle weakness

Overview

○ Detected by observing and measuring the strength of an individual muscle or muscle group

Assessment

History

○ Determine the onset and location of weakness.
○ Ask what aggravates the weakness.
○ Find out about other symptoms, including muscle or joint pain, altered sensory function, and fatigue.
○ Obtain a medical history, including hyperthyroidism, musculoskeletal or neurologic problems, recent trauma, and family history of chronic muscle weakness.
○ Obtain an alcohol and drug history.

Physical assessment

○ Test major muscles on both sides. (See *Testing muscle strength*, pages 260 and 261.)
○ Test for range of motion (ROM) at all major joints.
○ Test sensory function in the involved areas.
○ Test deep tendon reflexes (DTRs) on both sides.

Medical causes

Amyotrophic lateral sclerosis

○ Muscle weakness and atrophy in one hand rapidly spread to the arm and then to the other hand and arm.
○ Eventually, weakness and atrophy spread to the trunk, neck, tongue, larynx, pharynx, and legs.
○ Respiratory insufficiency results from progressive respiratory muscle weakness.

Brain tumor

○ Weakness varies with the tumor's location and size.
○ Other findings include headache, vomiting, diplopia, decreased visual acuity, decreased level of consciousness (LOC), pupillary changes, decreased motor strength, hemiparesis, hemiplegia, diminished sensations, ataxia, seizures, and behavioral changes.

Guillain-Barré syndrome

○ Rapidly progressive, symmetrical weakness and pain ascends from the feet to the arms and facial nerves; may progress to motor paralysis and respiratory failure.
○ Other findings include sensory loss or paresthesia, muscle flaccidity, loss of DTRs, tachycardia or bradycardia, fluctuating hypertension and orthostatic hypotension, diaphoresis, bowel and bladder incontinence, facial diplegia, dysphagia, dysarthria, and hypernasality.

Head trauma

○ Varying degrees of muscle weakness occur.
○ Other findings include decreased LOC, otorrhea or rhinorrhea, raccoon eyes and Battle's sign, sensory disturbances, and signs of increased intracranial pressure.

Herniated disk

○ Muscle weakness, disuse and, ultimately, atrophy occurs.
○ Severe lower back pain, possibly radiating to the buttocks, legs, and feet — usually on one side — is the primary symptom.
○ Diminished reflexes and sensory changes may occur.

Hodgkin's disease

○ Muscle weakness may accompany painless, progressive lymphadenopathy.
○ Other signs and symptoms include paresthesia, fatigue, persistent fever, night sweats, and weight loss.

Hypercortisolism

○ Limb weakness and atrophy occur.
○ Other cushingoid features include buffalo hump, moon face, truncal obesity, purple striae, thin skin, acne, elevated blood pressure, fatigue, hyperpigmentation, easy bruising, poor wound healing, and diaphoresis.
○ Impotence may occur in males; hirsutism and menstrual irregularities may occur in females.

Hypothyroidism

○ Reversible weakness and atrophy of proximal limb muscles may occur.
○ Other findings include muscle cramps; cold intolerance; weight gain despite anorexia; mental dullness; dry, pale doughy skin; puffy face, hands, and feet; impaired hearing and balance; and bradycardia.

Multiple sclerosis

○ Muscle weakness in one or more limbs may progress to atrophy, spasticity, and contractures.
○ Other findings include diplopia, blurred vision, vision loss, nystagmus, hyperactive DTRs, sensory loss or paresthesia, dysarthria, dysphagia, incoordination, ataxic gait, intention tremors, emotional lability, and urinary dysfunction.

Myasthenia gravis

○ Gradually progressive skeletal muscle weakness and fatigue are the principal symptoms.
○ Early signs include weak eye closure, ptosis, diplopia, a masklike facies, difficulty chewing and swallowing, nasal regurgitation of fluid with hypernasality, and a hanging jaw and bobbing head.
○ Respiratory failure may eventually occur.

Osteoarthritis

○ Progressive muscle disuse and weakness lead to atrophy.

- Other signs and symptoms include crepitation; enlarged edematous joints; Heberden's nodes; increased pain in damp, cold weather; joint stiffness; limited ROM; pain relieved by resting joints; and smooth, taut, shiny skin.

Paget's disease
- Muscle weakness, paralysis, paresthesia, and pain may develop.
- Bowed tibias, frequent fractures, and kyphosis may also develop.

Parkinson's disease
- Muscle weakness accompanies rigidity.
- Other findings include a pill-rolling tremor in one hand, propulsive gait, dysarthria, bradykinesia, drooling, dysphagia, a masklike facies, and a high-pitched, monotonous voice.

Peripheral nerve trauma
- Muscle weakness and atrophy are accompanied by paresthesia, pain, and loss of reflexes supplied by damaged nerve.

Peripheral neuropathy
- Muscle weakness progresses slowly to flaccid paralysis.
- Other signs and symptoms include loss of vibration sense; paresthesia, hyperesthesia, or anesthesia in the hands and feet; hypoactive or absent DTRs; mild to sharp burning pain; anhidrosis; and glossy red skin.

Potassium imbalance
- With hypokalemia, temporary muscle weakness occurs; may be accompanied by nausea, vomiting, diarrhea, decreased mentation, leg cramps, diminished reflexes, malaise, polyuria, dizziness, hypotension, and arrhythmias.
- With hyperkalemia, weakness may progress to flaccid paralysis accompanied by irritability, confusion, hyperreflexia, paresthesia or anesthesia, oliguria, anorexia, nausea, diarrhea, abdominal cramps, tachycardia or bradycardia, and arrhythmias.

Rhabdomyolysis
- Muscle weakness or pain occurs with fever, nausea, vomiting, malaise, dark urine, and signs of acute renal failure.

Rheumatoid arthritis
- Symmetric muscle weakness may accompany increased warmth, swelling, and tenderness in involved joints; pain; and stiffness.

Seizure disorder
- Temporary generalized muscle weakness may occur after generalized tonic-clonic seizure; aura may precede the seizure.

- Other postictal signs and symptoms include headache, muscle soreness, and profound fatigue.

Spinal trauma and disease
- Severe muscle weakness, leading to flaccidity or spasticity and, eventually, paralysis, occurs.

Stroke
- Weakness may progress to hemiplegia and atrophy.
- Other findings include dysarthria, aphasia, ataxia, apraxia, agnosia, ipsilateral paresthesia or sensory loss, visual disturbance, altered LOC, personality changes, bowel and bladder dysfunction, headache, and seizures.

Thyrotoxicosis
- Insidious, generalized muscle weakness and atrophy may occur.
- Other findings include anxiety, fatigue, heat intolerance, diaphoresis, tremors, tachycardia, palpitations, ventricular or atrial gallop, dyspnea, weight loss, enlarged thyroid gland, exophthalmos, and warm, flushed skin.

Other causes

Drugs
- Aminoglycoside antibiotics may worsen weakness in patients with myasthenia gravis.
- Generalized muscle weakness can result from prolonged corticosteroid use, digoxin, and excessive doses of dantrolene.

Immobility
- Immobilization, prolonged bed rest, or inactivity can lead to muscle weakness in the involved extremity.

Nursing considerations

- Provide assistive devices as needed.
- Protect the patient from injury.
- If sensory loss occurs, guard against pressure ulcer formation and thermal injury.
- With chronic weakness, provide ROM exercises or splint the limbs as needed.
- Allow for adequate rest periods.
- Give drugs for pain as needed.

Pediatric pointers
- Muscular dystrophy is a major cause of muscle weakness in children.

Patient teaching
- Teach the patient how to use assistive devices as needed.
- Explain the importance of frequent position changes and rest periods.

Obtain an overall picture of your patient's motor function by testing strength in 10 selected muscle groups. Ask the patient to attempt normal range-of-motion movements against your resistance. If the muscle group is weak, change the amount of resistance as needed to permit accurate assessment. If needed, position the patient so his limbs don't have to resist gravity, and repeat the test.

Arm muscles

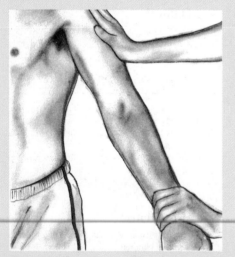

Biceps. With your hand on the patient's hand, have him flex his forearm against your resistance. Watch for biceps contraction.

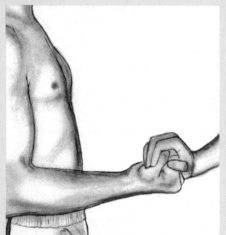

Deltoid. With the patient's arm fully extended, place one hand over his deltoid muscle and the other on his wrist. Ask him to abduct his arm to a horizontal position against your resistance; as he does so, palpate for deltoid contraction.

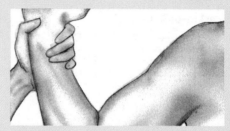

Triceps. Have the patient abduct and hold his arm midway between flexion and extension. Hold and support his arm at the wrist and ask him to extend it against your resistance. Watch for triceps contraction.

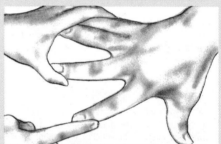

Dorsal interossei. Have the patient extend and spread his fingers and tell him to try to resist your attempt to squeeze them together.

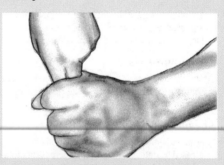

Forearm and hand (grip). Have the patient grasp your middle and index fingers and squeeze as hard as he can. To prevent pain or injury to the examiner, the examiner should cross his fingers.

Rate muscle strength on a scale from 0 to 5:
0 = Total paralysis
1 = Visible or palpable contraction, but no movement
2 = Full muscle movement with force of gravity eliminated
3 = Full muscle movement against gravity, but no movement against resistance
4 = Full muscle movement against gravity; partial movement against resistance
5 = Full muscle movement against both gravity and resistance — normal strength.

Leg muscles

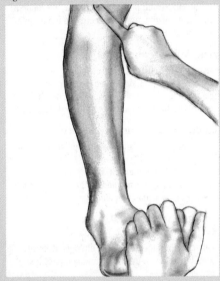

Anterior tibial. With the patient's leg extended, place your hand on his foot and ask him to dorsiflex his ankle against your resistance. Palpate for anterior tibial contraction.

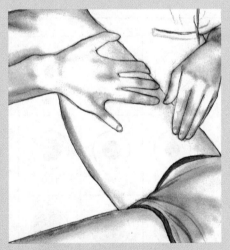

Psoas. While you support his leg, have the patient raise his knee and then flex his hip against your resistance. Watch for psoas contraction.

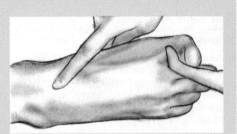

Extensor hallucis longus. With your finger on the patient's great toe, have him dorsiflex the toe against your resistance. Palpate for extensor hallucis contraction.

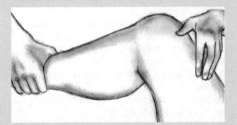

Quadriceps. Have the patient bend his knee slightly while you support his lower leg. Then ask him to extend the knee against your resistance; as he's doing so, palpate for quadriceps contraction.

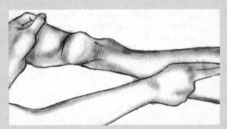

Gastrocnemius. With the patient on his side, support his foot and ask him to plantarflex his ankle against your resistance. Palpate for gastrocnemius contraction.

Mydriasis

Overview

- Pupillary dilation caused by contraction of the dilator of the iris
- May be a normal response to stimuli or drugs

Assessment

History

- Ask about other eye problems, such as pain, blurring, diplopia, or visual field defects.
- Obtain a health history, focusing on eye or head trauma, glaucoma and other ocular problems, and neurologic and vascular disorders.
- Obtain a complete drug history.

Physical assessment

- Inspect and compare the pupils' size, color, and shape. (See *Grading pupil size*.)
- Test each pupil for light reflex, consensual response, and accommodation.
- Perform a swinging flashlight test to evaluate a decreased response to direct light coupled with a normal consensual response.
- Check eyes for ptosis, swelling, and ecchymosis.
- Test visual acuity in both eyes with and without correction.
- Evaluate extraocular muscle function by checking the six cardinal fields of gaze.

Medical causes

Aortic arch syndrome

- Mydriasis in both eyes occurs late.
- Other ocular findings include visual blurring, transient vision loss, and diplopia.
- Other signs and symptoms include dizziness and syncope; neck, shoulder, and chest pain; bruits; loss of radial and carotid pulses; paresthesia; intermittent claudication; and, possibly, decreased blood pressure in the arms.

Carotid artery aneurysm

- Mydriasis in one eye may be accompanied by bitemporal hemianopsia, decreased visual acuity, hemiplegia, decreased level of consciousness, headache, aphasia, behavioral changes, and hypoesthesia.

Glaucoma (acute angle-closure)

- Moderate mydriasis and loss of pupillary reflex occur with excruciating pain, redness, decreased visual acuity, visual blurring, halo vision, conjunctival injection, a cloudy cornea and, in 2 to 5 days without treatment, permanent blindness.

Oculomotor nerve palsy

- Mydriasis in one eye is commonly the first sign.
- Other findings include ptosis, diplopia, decreased pupillary reflexes, exotropia, and complete loss of accommodation.

 Assessment tip
Grading pupil size

To ensure accurate evaluation of pupillary size, compare your patient's pupils to the scale shown at right. Keep in mind that maximum constriction may be less than 1 mm and maximum dilation greater than 9 mm.

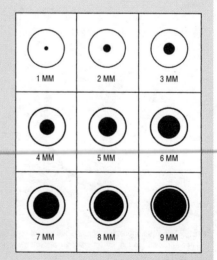

Traumatic iridoplegia

○ Mydriasis and loss of pupillary reflex caused by paralysis of sphincter of iris is usually transient.
○ Other findings include a quivering iris, ecchymosis, pain, and swelling.

Other causes

Drugs

○ Mydriasis can be caused by anesthesia induction, anticholinergics, antihistamines, sympathomimetics, barbiturates (overdose), estrogens, and tricyclic antidepressants.
○ Topical mydriatic drugs and cycloplegics are given for their mydriatic effect.

Surgery

○ Traumatic mydriasis commonly results from ocular surgery.

Nursing considerations

Pediatric pointers

○ Mydriasis occurs in children as a result of ocular trauma, drugs, Adie's syndrome and, most commonly, increased intracranial pressure.

Patient teaching

○ Discuss the effects of mydriatic drugs and reducing their adverse effects.

Myoclonus

Overview

- Involves sudden, shocklike contractions of the muscles
- May be isolated or repetitive, rhythmic or arrhythmic, symmetrical or asymmetrical, synchronous or asynchronous, generalized or focal
- May be triggered by certain stimuli

✦ Emergency actions

Check for seizure activity. Take vital signs to rule out arrhythmias or a blocked airway. If the patient has a seizure, gently help him lie down. Place a pillow or a rolled-up towel under the head to prevent concussion. Loosen any constrictive clothing, especially around the neck, and turn the head to one side to prevent airway occlusion or aspiration of secretions.

Assessment

History

- Ask about the frequency, severity, location, and circumstances of myoclonus.
- Determine whether the patient has had previous seizures.
- Find out what causes the patient's myoclonus.

Physical assessment

- Evaluate level of consciousness (LOC) and mental condition.
- Check for muscle rigidity and wasting.
- Test for deep tendon reflexes (DTRs).
- Complete neurologic and musculoskeletal assessments.

Medical causes

Alzheimer's disease

- Generalized myoclonus may occur in advanced stages.
- Other late findings include mild choreoathetoid movements, muscle rigidity, bowel and bladder incontinence, delusions, and hallucinations.

Creutzfeldt-Jakob disease

- Diffuse myoclonic jerks are initially random; they gradually become rhythmic and symmetrical in response to sensory stimuli.
- Other effects include ataxia, aphasia, hearing loss, muscle rigidity and wasting, fasciculations, hemiplegia, vision disturbances and, possibly, blindness.

Encephalitis (viral)

- Myoclonus is intermittent.
- Other findings vary but may include rapidly decreasing LOC, fever, headache, irritability, nuchal rigidity, vomiting, seizures, aphasia, ataxia, hemiparesis, facial muscle weakness, nystagmus, ocular palsies, and dysphagia.

Encephalopathy

- In hepatic encephalopathy, myoclonic jerks are produced in association with asterixis and focal or generalized seizures.
- In hypoxic encephalopathy, generalized myoclonus or seizures occur almost immediately after restoration of cardiopulmonary function.
- In uremic encephalopathy, myoclonic jerks and seizures are common.

Epilepsy

- With idiopathic epilepsy, localized myoclonus usually occurs singly or in short bursts in an arm or leg upon awakening.
- With myoclonic epilepsy, myoclonus is initially infrequent and localized but becomes more frequent and generalized over a period of months.

Other causes

Drug withdrawal

- Myoclonus may be seen in patients with alcohol, opioid, or sedative withdrawal or alcohol withdrawal delirium.

Poisoning

- Acute intoxication with methyl bromide, bismuth, or strychnine may produce an acute onset of myoclonus and confusion.

Nursing considerations

- If myoclonus is progressive, take seizure precautions.
- Keep an oral airway and suction equipment at the bedside.
- Pad the bed's side rails and remove potentially harmful objects.
- Remain with the patient while he walks.
- Give drugs that suppress myoclonus as needed.

Pediatric pointers

- Myoclonus may result from subacute sclerosing panencephalitis, severe meningitis, progressive poliodystrophy, childhood myoclonic epilepsy, and encephalopathies.

Patient teaching

○ Talk with the patient about taking safety measures and seizure precautions.
○ Refer the patient to social service or community resources as needed.

Nasal obstruction

Overview

- Typically benign, but may cause discomfort or voice changes or alter sense of taste and smell

Assessment

History

- Ask about the onset, duration, frequency, and description of obstruction.
- Inquire about associated drainage, sinus pain, or headaches.
- Take a drug and alcohol history.
- Find out about previous trauma or surgery.
- Ask about recent travel.

Physical assessment

- Assess airflow and the condition of the turbinates and nasal septum.
- Evaluate the orbits for any evidence of decreased vision, excess tearing, or abnormal appearance of the eye.
- Palpate over the frontal and maxillary sinuses for tenderness.
- Examine the ears for effusions.
- Inspect the oral cavity, pharynx, nasopharynx, and larynx.
- Palpate the neck for adenopathy.

Medical causes

Basilar skull fracture

- Cerebrospinal fluid rhinorrhea may develop.
- Other findings include epistaxis, otorrhea, and a bulging tympanic membrane from blood or fluid.
- Fracture may also cause headache, facial paralysis, nausea, vomiting, impaired eye movement, ocular deviation, vision and hearing loss, depressed level of consciousness, Battle's sign, and raccoon eyes.

Common cold

- Watery discharge, sneezing, and nasal obstruction occur.
- Related signs and symptoms include sinus pain, reduced sense of taste and smell, sore throat, malaise, myalgia, arthralgia, and mild headache.

Hypothyroidism

- Nasal obstruction may occur.
- Other signs and symptoms include fatigue, weight gain despite anorexia, cold intolerance, facial edema, impaired memory, brittle hair, thick skin and tongue, bradycardia, and a hoarse voice.

Nasal deformities

- A deviated nasal septum may cause nasal obstruction.
- A perforated nasal septum may cause a sensation of nasal congestion due to altered airflow.

Nasal fracture

- Mucosal swelling, epistaxis, abscess, or a septal deviation caused by trauma results in nasal obstruction.
- Other findings include periorbital ecchymoses and edema, nasal deformity and pain, and crepitation of the nasal bones.

Nasal polyps

- Nasal obstruction, anosmia, and clear, watery drainage develop.
- Translucent, pear-shaped polyps occur.

Nasal tumors

- Nasal obstruction, rhinorrhea, epistaxis, pain, foul discharge, and cheek swelling may occur.

Nasopharyngeal tumors

- Nasal obstruction, rhinorrhea, epistaxis, otitis media, and nasal speech may occur.
- Neck mass or conductive hearing loss may be the first sign of cancer of the nasopharynx.

Pregnancy

- Vascular engorgement of the mucosa results in obstruction.
- Other findings include clear or blood-tinged drainage, sneezing, and edematous and bluish turbinates.

Rhinitis

- Allergic rhinitis produces watery discharge and nasal obstruction as well as sneezing, increased lacrimation, decreased sense of smell, postnasal drip, and itching of the eyes, nose, and ears.
- Vasomotor rhinitis produces a profuse watery nasal discharge in addition to nasal obstruction, sneezing, postnasal drip, and swollen turbinates.
- Atrophic rhinitis produces chronic and continuous nasal obstruction along with intermittent, foul-smelling, purulent drainage.

Sinusitis

- Acute sinusitis produces marked nasal obstruction along with fever, severe pain over the involved sinuses, and thick, purulent drainage.
- Chronic sinusitis produces persistent or recurrent nasal obstruction as well as thick, intermittently purulent rhinorrhea and discomfort over the involved sinuses.

Wegener's granulomatosis

- Besides nasal obstruction, other nasal findings include crusting, epistaxis, mucopurulent discharge, and cartilaginous necrosis of the septum and bridge of the nose.

Other causes

Drugs
○ Topical nasal vasoconstrictors may cause rebound rhinorrhea and nasal obstruction.
○ Antihypertensives may cause nasal congestion.

Surgery
○ Nasal obstruction may occur after sinus or cranial surgery or even after rhinoplasty.

Nursing considerations

○ Promote fluid intake to thin secretions, as needed.
○ Give an antihistamine, a decongestant, an analgesic, or an antipyretic.

Pediatric pointers
○ Acute nasal obstruction in children commonly results from the common cold; chronic obstruction typically results from large adenoids.
○ In neonates, choanal atresia is the most common congenital cause of nasal obstruction.
○ Cystic fibrosis may cause nasal polyps, resulting in obstruction.

Patient teaching
○ Teach the patient proper use of nasal vasoconstrictor sprays.
○ Explain activity restrictions to a patient requiring surgery.

Nausea

Overview

- A sensation of profound revulsion to food or of impending vomiting

Assessment

History

- Ask about the onset and description of nausea.
- Determine aggravating or alleviating factors.
- Obtain a medical history, including GI, endocrine, and metabolic disorders; cancer; and infections.
- Ask about vomiting, abdominal pain, and changes in bowel habits.
- Ask about the possibility of pregnancy.

Physical assessment

- Inspect the skin for jaundice, bruises, and spider angiomas; assess skin turgor.
- Inspect for abdominal distention.
- Auscultate for bowel sounds and bruits.
- Palpate for abdominal rigidity and tenderness and test for rebound tenderness.
- Palpate and percuss the liver.

Medical causes

Anthrax (GI)

- Initial signs and symptoms include nausea, vomiting, loss of appetite, and fever which may progress to abdominal pain, severe bloody diarrhea, and hematemesis.

Appendicitis

- A brief period of nausea may accompany onset of abdominal pain.
- Other findings include abdominal rigidity and tenderness, cutaneous hyperalgesia, fever, constipation or diarrhea, tachycardia, anorexia, and malaise.

Cholecystitis (acute)

- Nausea typically follows severe right-upper-quadrant pain that may radiate to the back or shoulders, commonly after meals.
- Associated findings include vomiting, flatulence, abdominal tenderness, rigidity and distention, fever with chills, diaphoresis, and a positive Murphy's sign.

Cholelithiasis

- Nausea accompanies severe right-upper-quadrant or epigastric pain.

- Other signs and symptoms include vomiting, abdominal tenderness and guarding, flatulence, belching, epigastric burning, tachycardia, restlessness and, with occlusion of the common bile duct, jaundice, clay-colored stools, fever, chills, and a positive Murphy's sign.

Cirrhosis

- Nausea, vomiting, anorexia, abdominal pain, and constipation or diarrhea occur.
- As the disease progresses, jaundice and hepatomegaly may occur with abdominal distention, spider angiomas, fetor hepaticus, enlarged superficial abdominal veins, and mental changes.

Diverticulitis

- Nausea, intermittent crampy abdominal pain, constipation or diarrhea, low-grade fever and, in many cases, a palpable, fixed mass occur.
- Other findings include anorexia, bloody stools, and flatulence.

Electrolyte imbalances

- Nausea and vomiting occur with cardiac arrhythmias, tremors or seizures, anorexia, malaise, and weakness.

Escherichia coli 0157:H7

- Nausea, watery or bloody diarrhea, vomiting, fever, and abdominal cramps occur.

Gastritis

- Nausea is common, especially after ingestion of alcohol, aspirin, spicy foods, or caffeine.
- Vomiting, epigastric pain, belching, and malaise may occur.

Gastroenteritis

- Nausea, vomiting, diarrhea, and abdominal cramping occur.
- Fever, malaise, hyperactive bowel sounds, abdominal pain and tenderness, and signs of dehydration and electrolyte imbalance may occur.

Hepatitis

- Nausea is an early symptom.
- Vomiting, fatigue, myalgia, arthralgia, headache, anorexia, photophobia, pharyngitis, cough, and fever also occur early in the preicteric phase.

Hyperemesis gravidarum

- Unremitting nausea and vomiting persist beyond the first trimester of pregnancy.
- Other signs and symptoms include weight loss, signs of dehydration, headache, and delirium.

Inflammatory bowel disease

- Nausea, vomiting, abdominal pain, and anorexia may occur, but the most common sign is recurrent diarrhea with blood, pus, and mucus.

Intestinal obstruction

○ Nausea, vomiting, constipation, and abdominal pain occur.
○ Other findings include abdominal distention and tenderness, visible peristaltic waves, and hyperactive (in partial obstruction) or hypoactive or absent bowel sounds (in complete obstruction).

Irritable bowel syndrome

○ Nausea, dyspepsia, and abdominal distention may result.
○ Other signs and symptoms include lower abdominal pain and tenderness relieved by defecation, diurnal diarrhea alternating with constipation or normal bowel function, small stools with visible mucus, and a feeling of incomplete evacuation.

Labyrinthitis

○ Nausea and vomiting occur with vertigo, progressive hearing loss, nystagmus, and tinnitus.

Lactose intolerance

○ Nausea, diarrhea, cramps, bloating, and gas occur after eating dairy products.

Ménière's disease

○ Sudden, brief, recurrent attacks of nausea, vomiting, vertigo, tinnitus, nystagmus and, eventually, hearing loss occur.

Metabolic acidosis

○ Nausea, vomiting, anorexia, diarrhea, Kussmaul's respirations, and decreased level of consciousness may develop.

Migraine headache

○ Nausea and vomiting may occur along with photophobia, light flashes, increased sensitivity to noise, light-headedness, partial vision loss, and paresthesia of the lips, face, and hands.

Motion sickness

○ Nausea and vomiting occur along with possible headache, dizziness, fatigue, diaphoresis, hypersalivation, and dyspnea.

Myocardial infarction

○ Nausea and vomiting may occur but the cardinal symptom is severe substernal chest pain that may radiate to the left arm, jaw, or neck.
○ Other findings include dyspnea, pallor, clammy skin, diaphoresis, altered blood pressure, and arrhythmias.

Pancreatitis (acute)

○ Nausea, usually followed by vomiting, is an early symptom.
○ Other signs and symptoms include severe pain upper abdominal pain that may radiate to the back; abdom-

inal tenderness and rigidity; anorexia; diminished bowel sounds; and fever.

Peptic ulcer

○ Nausea and vomiting follow attacks of sharp or gnawing, burning epigastric pain when the stomach is empty or after ingesting alcohol, caffeine, or aspirin.

Peritonitis

○ Nausea and vomiting accompany acute abdominal pain.
○ Other findings include fever; chills; tachycardia; hypoactive or absent bowel sounds; abdominal rigidity, and tenderness; diaphoresis; hypotension; and shallow respirations.

Rhabdomyolysis

○ Nausea, vomiting, fever, malaise, and dark urine are common.
○ Tenderness, swelling, and muscle weakness may develop.

Thyrotoxicosis

○ Nausea and vomiting may accompany severe anxiety, heat intolerance, diaphoresis, diarrhea, tremor, tachycardia, and palpitations.
○ Other signs include exophthalmos, ventricular or atrial gallop, and an enlarged thyroid gland.

Other causes

Drugs

○ Antineoplastics, opiates, ferrous sulfate, levodopa, oral potassium chloride replacements, estrogens, sulfasalazine, antibiotics, quinidine, anesthetics, digoxin, theophylline overdose, and nonsteroidal anti-inflammatory drugs

Radiation and surgery

○ Radiation therapy can cause nausea and vomiting.
○ Postoperative nausea and vomiting is common.

Nursing considerations

○ Provide measures to ease the patient's nausea.
○ Evaluate fluid, electrolyte, and acid-base balance.
○ Elevate the patient's head or position him on his side.
○ Be prepared to insert a nasogastric tube if needed.

Patient teaching

○ Discuss what aggravates nausea and how to avoid it.

Neck pain

Overview

- May originate from any neck structure
- May be referred from other areas of the body

★ Emergency actions

If the patient's neck pain results from trauma, first immobilize the cervical spine, preferably with a long backboard and Philadelphia collar. Take vital signs and perform a quick neurologic examination. Give oxygen as needed. Intubation or tracheostomy and mechanical ventilation may be necessary. Ask how the injury occurred. Examine the neck for abrasions, swelling, lacerations, erythema, and ecchymoses.

Assessment

History

- Find out about the onset and description of pain.
- Ask about alleviating, aggravating, or precipitating factors.
- Find about associated symptoms such as headache.
- Obtain a medical and drug history.

Physical assessment

- Inspect the neck, shoulders, and cervical spine for swelling, masses, erythema, and ecchymoses.
- Assess active range of motion (ROM) in the neck and note any pain.
- Examine posture.
- Test and compare bilateral muscle strength.
- Check sensation in the arms.
- Assess hand grasp and arm reflexes.
- If the patient's condition permits, test for Brudzinski's and Kernig's signs.
- Palpate the cervical lymph nodes for enlargement

Medical causes

Cervical extension injury

- Anterior pain usually diminishes within several days after injury.
- Posterior pain persists and may even intensify.
- Other signs and symptoms include tenderness, swelling and nuchal rigidity, arm or back pain, occipital headache, muscle spasms, visual blurring, and unilateral miosis on the affected side.

Cervical spine fracture

- Severe neck pain may occur with intense occipital headache, quadriplegia, deformity, and respiratory paralysis.

Cervical spine tumor

- Metastatic tumors typically produce persistent neck pain; primary tumors cause mild to severe pain along a specific nerve root.
- Other findings may include paresthesia, arm and leg weakness that progresses to atrophy and paralysis, and bowel and bladder incontinence.

Cervical spondylosis

- Posterior neck pain that may radiate is aggravated by and restricts movement.
- Accompanying findings include paresthesia, weakness, and stiffness.

Cervical stenosis

- Neck and arm pain, paresthesia, muscle weakness or paralysis, gait and balance problems, and decreased ROM may occur.

Herniated cervical disk

- Variable neck pain that's referred along a specific dermatome is aggravated by and restricts movement.
- Paresthesia and other sensory disturbances and arm weakness may also occur.

Hodgkin's disease

- Generalized pain may eventually affect the neck.
- Lymphadenopathy, the classic sign, may accompany paresthesia, muscle weakness, fever, fatigue, weight loss, malaise, and hepatomegaly.

Laryngeal cancer

- Neck pain radiating to the ear is a late sign.
- Other findings include dysphagia, dyspnea, hemoptysis, stridor, hoarseness, and cervical lymphadenopathy.

Lymphadenitis

- Enlarged and inflamed cervical lymph nodes cause acute pain.
- Fever, chills, and malaise may also occur.

Meningitis

- Neck pain may accompany nuchal rigidity.
- Related signs and symptoms include fever, headache, photophobia, positive Brudzinski's and Kernig's signs, and decreased level of consciousness (LOC).

Neck sprain

- Pain, slight swelling, stiffness, and restricted ROM result.
- Ligament rupture causes pain, marked swelling, ecchymosis, muscle spasms, and nuchal rigidity with head tilt.

Paget's disease

- Cervical vertebrae deformity may produce severe neck pain, paresthesia, and arm weakness as the disease progresses.

A lightweight, molded polyethylene collar designed to hold the neck straight with the chin slightly elevated and tucked in, the Philadelphia cervical collar immobilizes the cervical spine, decreases muscle spasms, and relieves some pain. It also prevents further injury and promotes healing. When applying the collar, fit it snugly around the patient's neck and attach the Velcro fasteners or buckles at the back. Check the patient's airway and his neurovascular status to ensure that the collar isn't too tight. Also, make sure that the collar isn't placed too high in front, which can hyperextend the neck. In a patient with a neck sprain, hyperextension may cause the ligaments to heal in a shortened position; in a patient with a cervical spine fracture, it could cause serious neurologic damage.

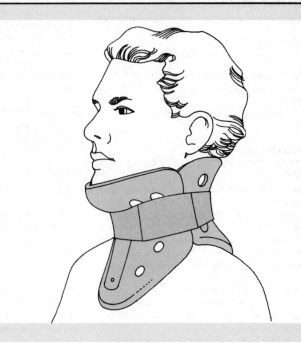

Rheumatoid arthritis

○ Moderate to severe pain may radiate along a specific nerve root.
○ Other features include increased stiff joints, paresthesia, muscle weakness, low-grade fever, anorexia, malaise, fatigue, neck deformity, and warmth, swelling, and tenderness in involved joints.

Spinous process fracture

○ Fracture near the cervicothoracic junction produces acute pain that radiates to shoulders.
○ Other findings include swelling, tenderness, restricted ROM, muscle spasm, and deformity.

Subarachnoid hemorrhage

○ A life-threatening condition — moderate to severe neck pain and rigidity, headache, and decreased LOC may occur.
○ Kernig's and Brudzinski's signs are present.

Torticollis

○ Severe neck pain accompanies recurrent unilateral stiffness and muscle spasms.
○ Stiffness of the neck muscles is followed by a momentary twitching or contraction that pulls the head to the affected side.

Tracheal trauma

○ Neck pain and respiratory difficulty occur.

○ Torn tracheal mucosa produces mild to moderate pain and may result in airway occlusion, hemoptysis, hoarseness, and dysphagia.

Nursing considerations

○ Give an anti-inflammatory and an analgesic as needed.
○ Apply cervical collar, as appropriate. (See *Applying a Philadelphia collar.*)
○ Neck trauma may not initially produce a lot of pain; immobilization is necessary until significant injury is ruled out.

Pediatric pointers

○ The most common causes of neck pain in children are meningitis and trauma.

Patient teaching

○ Explain any activities the patient needs to limit.
○ Teach the patient to apply the cervical collar, if needed.
○ Provide reinforcement for exercises the patient needs to do.

Nipple discharge

Overview

○ Characterized as intermittent or constant, as unilateral or bilateral, and by color, consistency, and composition
○ Is relatively common in parous women

Assessment

History

○ Ask about the onset, duration, and description of discharge.
○ Inquire about associated pain, tenderness, itching, warmth, and changes in breast or nipple contour.
○ Ask about use of herbs; some have estrogenic effects and cause nipple discharge as an adverse effect.
○ Determine the onset, location, size, and consistency of any breast lumps.
○ Find out about the use of hormones.
○ Obtain a complete gynecologic and obstetric history.
○ Determine the patient's normal menstrual cycle and date of last menses.
○ Ask about breast swelling and tenderness, bloating, irritability, headaches, abdominal cramping, nausea, or diarrhea related to menses.
○ Assess her risk factors for breast cancer.

Physical assessment

○ Characterize the discharge. (See *Eliciting nipple discharge.*)
○ Examine the nipples and breasts with the patient in four positions.
○ Check for nipple deviation, flattening, retraction, redness, asymmetry, thickening, excoriation, erosion, or cracking.
○ Inspect the breasts for asymmetry, irregular contours, dimpling, erythema, and peau d'orange.
○ With the patient in a supine position, palpate breasts and axillae for lumps.
○ Note the size, location, delineation, consistency, and mobility of any lumps.

Medical causes

Breast abscess

○ A thick, purulent discharge may be produced from a cracked nipple or an infected duct.
○ Other findings include abrupt onset of high fever with chills; breast pain, tenderness, and erythema; a palpable soft nodule or generalized induration; and nipple retraction.

Breast cancer

○ Bloody, watery, or purulent discharge may emit from a normal-appearing nipple.
○ Characteristic findings include a hard, irregular, fixed lump; erythema; dimpling; peau d'orange; changes in contour; nipple deviation, flattening, or retraction; axillary lymphadenopathy; and breast pain.

Choriocarcinoma

○ A white or grayish milky discharge may occur with persistent uterine bleeding and bogginess and vaginal masses.

Herpes zoster

○ Bilateral, spontaneous, intermittent galactorrhea may occur.
○ Other characteristic findings include shooting or burning pain, eruption of small red nodules or vesicles on the thorax and possibly the arms and legs, headache, fever, malaise, and pruritus, paresthesia, or hyperesthesia in affected areas.

Intraductal papilloma

○ Discharge is unilateral serous, serosanguineous, or bloody from only one duct.
○ Subareolar nodules, breast pain, and tenderness may occur.

Mammary duct ectasia

○ A thick, sticky, grayish discharge from multiple ducts may be the first sign; discharge may be bilateral and is usually spontaneous.
○ Other findings include a rubbery, poorly delineated lump beneath the areola, with a blue-green discoloration of the overlying skin; nipple retraction; and redness, swelling, tenderness, and burning pain in the areola and nipple.

Paget's disease

○ Serous or bloody unilateral discharge emits from denuded skin on the nipple, which is red, intensely itchy and, possibly, eroded or excoriated.

Prolactin-secreting pituitary tumor

○ Bilateral galactorrhea may occur.
○ Other findings include amenorrhea, infertility, decreased libido, vaginal secretions, headaches, and blindness.

Proliferative (fibrocystic) breast disease

○ Bilateral clear, milky, or straw-colored discharge occurs.
○ Multiple round, soft, tender, mobile nodules are palpable on both breasts in the upper outer quadrants.
○ Nodule size, tenderness, and discharge increase during the luteal phase of the menstrual cycle.

If your patient has a history or evidence of nipple discharge, you can attempt to elicit it during your examination. Help the patient into a supine position, and gently squeeze the nipple between your thumb and index finger (as shown top right); note any discharge through the nipple. Then place your fingers on the areola, as shown below right, and palpate the entire areolar surface, watching for any discharge through areolar ducts.

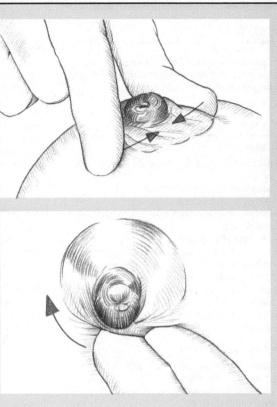

Trauma

○ Bilateral galactorrhea can result from trauma to the breasts.
○ Other findings vary with the cause and severity of trauma but may include chest pain, dyspnea, bruising, flail chest, cardiac tamponade, pulmonary artery tears, ventricular rupture, shock, and bronchial, tracheal, or esophageal tears.

Other causes

Drugs

○ Antihypertensive drugs, cimetidine, hormonal contraceptives, metoclopramide, psychotropic agents, or verapamil may cause galactorrhea.

Surgery

○ Chest wall surgery may stimulate thoracic nerves, causing intermittent bilateral galactorrhea.

Nursing considerations

○ Clearly explain the nature and origin of the discharge.
○ Apply a breast binder.

Pediatric pointers

○ Nipple discharge in children and adolescents is rare.
○ Infants may produce a milky discharge between 3 days and 2 weeks after birth due to maternal hormonal influences.

Geriatric pointers

○ In postmenopausal women, breast changes are considered malignant until proven otherwise.

Patient teaching

○ Explain the importance of being aware of discharge characteristics.
○ Explain when to seek medical attention.
○ Discuss the importance of breast self-examinations, medical appointments, and mammograms.

Nocturia

Overview

- Excessive urination of 500 ml or more at night
- The patient may awaken one or more times during the night to empty his bladder

Assessment

History

- Ask about the onset, frequency, and pattern of nocturia.
- Inquire about precipitating factors.
- Determine the volume voided.
- Find out about associated color, odor, or consistency changes of urine.
- Note the pattern of fluid intake.
- Review associated pain, burning, difficulty urinating, and costovertebral angle (CVA) tenderness.
- Obtain a medical history, including a personal or family history of renal or urinary tract disorders or endocrine and metabolic diseases.
- Obtain a drug history, noting use of diuretics, a cardiac glycoside, or an antihypertensive.

Physical assessment

- Palpate and percuss the kidneys, CVA, and bladder.
- Inspect the urinary meatus.
- Inspect urine specimen for color, odor, and presence of sediment.

Medical causes

Benign prostatic hyperplasia

- Nocturia occurs possibly with frequency, hesitation, incontinence, reduced force and caliber of the urine stream, hematuria, lower abdominal fullness, perineal pain, and constipation.
- Palpation reveals an enlarged prostate.

Bladder neoplasm

- Nocturia, a late sign, involves frequent voiding of small to moderate amounts of urine.
- Characteristic signs and symptoms include hematuria, bladder distention, urinary frequency and urgency, dysuria, pyuria, vomiting, diarrhea, insomnia, and bladder, rectal, flank, back, or leg pain.

Cystitis

- Nocturia is marked by frequent, small voidings and accompanied by dysuria and tenesmus in all form of cystitis.
- In bacterial cystitis, findings include urinary urgency; hematuria; fatigue; suprapubic, perineal, flank, and lower back pain; and, occasionally, low-grade fever.
- In chronic interstitial cystitis, Hunner's ulcers and gross hematuria may occur.
- In viral cystitis, urinary urgency, hematuria, and fever may develop.

Diabetes insipidus

- Nocturia occurs early and involves periodic voiding of moderate to large amounts of urine.
- Polydipsia and dehydration may also develop.

Diabetes mellitus

- Nocturia, an early sign, involves frequent, large voidings.
- Associated findings include daytime polyuria, polydipsia, polyphagia, frequent urinary tract infections, recurrent yeast infections, vaginitis, weakness, fatigue, weight loss, and signs of dehydration.

Hypercalcemic nephropathy

- Nocturia involves the periodic voiding of moderate to large amounts of urine.
- Daytime polyuria, polydipsia and, occasionally, hematuria and pyuria occur.

Hypokalemic nephropathy

- Nocturia involves the periodic voiding of moderate to large amounts of urine.
- Other findings include polydipsia, daytime polyuria, muscle weakness or paralysis, hypoactive bowel sounds, and increased susceptibility to pyelonephritis.

Prostate cancer

- Nocturia occurs late and is characterized by infrequent voidings of moderate amounts of urine.
- Other characteristics include dysuria, difficulty initiating a urine stream, interrupted urine stream, bladder distention, urinary frequency, weight loss, pallor, weakness, perineal pain, constipation, and a hard, irregularly shaped, nodular prostate on palpation.

Pyelonephritis (acute)

- Nocturia is common and involves infrequent voiding of moderate amounts of urine; urine may appear cloudy.
- Other findings include a high, sustained fever with chills, fatigue, flank pain, CVA tenderness, weakness, dysuria, hematuria, urinary frequency and urgency, and tenesmus.
- Occasionally, anorexia, nausea, vomiting, diarrhea, and hypoactive bowel sounds occur.

Renal failure (chronic)

- Nocturia involving infrequent voiding of moderate amounts of urine occurs relatively early; oliguria or anuria may develop.
- Other signs and symptoms include fatigue, ammonia breath odor, Kussmaul's respirations, peripheral edema, elevated blood pressure, decreased level of consciousness, confusion, emotional lability, muscle

twitching, anorexia, metallic mouth taste, constipation or diarrhea, petechiae, ecchymoses, pruritus, yellow- or bronze-tinged skin, nausea, and vomiting.

Other causes

Drugs
○ Drugs that mobilize edematous fluid or produce diuresis may cause nocturia.

Nursing considerations

○ Maintain fluid balance.
○ Monitor vital signs, intake and output, and daily weight.
○ Document frequency of nocturia, amount, and specific gravity.
○ Plan administration of a diuretic for daytime hours, if possible.
○ Plan rest periods to compensate for sleep lost.

Pediatric pointers
○ With the exception of prostate disorders, causes of nocturia are generally the same for children and adults.

Geriatric pointers
○ Postmenopausal women have decreased bladder elasticity, but urine output remains constant, resulting in nocturia.

Patient teaching
○ Explain the importance of reducing fluid intake and voiding before bedtime.

Nystagmus

Overview

- Involuntary oscillations of one or both eyeballs
- May be pendular (equal in rate in both directions) or jerk (fast and then slow) (see *Assessing nystagmus*)
- May be rhythmic and may be horizontal, vertical, rotary, or mixed
- May be transient or sustained, and occur spontaneously or on deviation or fixation of the eyes
- Results from pathology in the visual perceptual area, vestibular system, cerebellum, or brain stem

Assessment

History

- Ask about the onset, duration, and description of nystagmus.
- Inquire about recent infection of the ear or respiratory tract.
- Note a history of head trauma or cancer.
- Find out about associated vertigo, dizziness, tinnitus, nausea or vomiting, numbness, weakness, bladder dysfunction, and fever.

Physical assessment

- Evaluate level of consciousness (LOC) and vital signs.
- Be alert for signs of increased intracranial pressure (ICP), such as pupillary changes, drowsiness, elevated systolic pressure, and altered respirations.
- Test extraocular muscle function.
- Note when nystagmus occurs as well as its velocity and direction.
- Test reflexes.
- Evaluate motor and sensory function.
- Test the cranial nerves.

Medical causes

Encephalitis

- Jerk nystagmus is typically accompanied by altered LOC ranging from lethargy to coma.
- It may be preceded by sudden onset of fever, headache, and vomiting.
- Other findings include nuchal rigidity, seizures, aphasia, ataxia, photophobia, and cranial nerve palsies.

Head trauma

- Brain stem injury may cause horizontal jerk nystagmus.
- Other findings include pupillary changes, altered respiratory pattern, coma, and decerebrate posture.

Labyrinthitis (acute)

- Sudden onset of jerk nystagmus is accompanied by dizziness, vertigo, tinnitus, nausea, and vomiting.
- Fast component of the nystagmus is toward the unaffected ear.
- Gradual sensorineural hearing loss may occur.

Ménière's disease

- Acute attacks of jerk nystagmus, severe nausea, dizziness, vertigo, progressive hearing loss, and tinnitus occur.
- Direction of jerk nystagmus varies from one attack to the next.

Multiple sclerosis

- Jerk or pendular nystagmus may occur intermittently.
- It may be preceded by diplopia, blurred vision, and paresthesia.
- Other findings include muscle weakness or paralysis, spasticity, hyperreflexia, intention tremor, gait ataxia, dysphagia, dysarthria, impotence, constipation, emotional instability, and urinary frequency, urgency, and incontinence.

Stroke

- A stroke involving the posterior inferior cerebellar artery may cause sudden horizontal or vertical jerk nystagmus that may be gaze dependent.
- Other findings include dysphagia, dysarthria, loss of pain and temperature sensation in the ipsilateral face and contralateral trunk and limbs, ipsilateral Horner's syndrome, cerebellar signs, and signs of increased ICP.

Other causes

Drugs and alcohol

- Jerk nystagmus may result from alcohol intoxication and barbiturate, phenytoin, or carbamazepine toxicity.

Nursing considerations

- Provide for the patient's safety.

Pediatric pointers

- In children, pendular nystagmus may be idiopathic, or it may result from early impaired vision associated with certain disorders.

Patient teaching

- Instruct the patient about safety measures.
- Caution the patient about the importance of avoiding sudden position changes.

Assessment tip
Assessing nystagmus

The various types of jerk and pendular nystagmus are illustrated here.

Jerk nystagmus
Convergence-retraction nystagmus refers to the irregular jerking of the eyes back into the orbit during upward gaze. It can indicate midbrain tegmental damage.

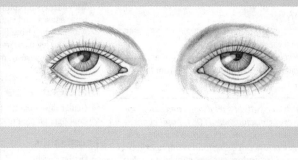

Downbeat nystagmus refers to the irregular downward jerking of the eyes during downward gaze. It can signal lower medullary damage.

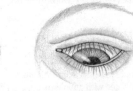

Vestibular nystagmus, the horizontal or rotary movement of the eyes, suggests vestibular disease or cochlear dysfunction.

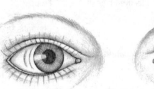

Pendular nystagmus
Horizontal, or pendular, nystagmus refers to oscillations of equal velocity around a center point. It can indicate congenital loss of visual acuity or multiple sclerosis.

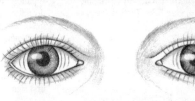

Vertical, or seesaw, nystagmus is the rapid, seesaw movement of the eyes: One eye appears to rise while the other appears to fall. It suggests an optic chiasm lesion.

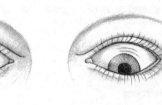

Ocular deviation

Overview

- Abnormal eye movement
- May be conjugate (both eyes move together) or disconjugate (one eye moves separately from the other)

Emergency actions

Take the patient's vital signs and assess for altered level of consciousness (LOC), pupil changes, motor or sensory dysfunction, and severe headache. If possible, ask him about behavioral changes or recent head trauma. Respiratory support may be necessary.

Assessment

History

- Find out the duration of ocular deviation.
- Ask if it's associated with double vision, eye pain, headache, motor or sensory changes, or fever.
- Obtain a medical history, including hypertension, diabetes, allergies, and thyroid, neurologic, muscular disorders, and ocular history (such as eye or head trauma or surgery).

Physical assessment

- Perform a complete neurologic assessment, including a complete eye assessment.
- Observe for partial or complete ptosis.
- Observe for spontaneous head tilts or turns that compensate for ocular deviation.
- Check for eye redness or periorbital edema.
- Assess visual acuity.
- Evaluate extraocular muscle function by testing the six cardinal positions of gaze. (See *Testing the six cardinal positions of gaze.*)

Medical causes

Brain tumor

- Ocular deviation depends on the site and extent of the tumor.
- Other signs and symptoms include headaches that are most severe in the morning, behavioral changes, memory loss, dizziness, confusion, vision loss, motor and sensory dysfunction, aphasia, signs of hormonal imbalance, and slowly deteriorating LOC from lethargy to coma.
- Late signs include papilledema, vomiting, increased systolic pressure, widening pulse pressure, and decorticate posture.

Cerebral aneurysm

- Typically, ocular deviation and diplopia are the first signs.

- Ptosis, a dilated pupil on the affected side, and a severe headache (on one side, usually in the front) are other major signs and symptoms.
- With aneurysm rupture, abrupt intensification of pain, nausea, and vomiting occur.
- With bleeding from the site, meningeal irritation, back and leg pain, fever, irritability, seizures, blurred vision, hemiparesis, dysphagia, and visual defects may develop.

Diabetes mellitus

- Ocular deviation, ptosis, and the sudden onset of diplopia and pain occur.

Encephalitis

- Ocular deviation and diplopia may occur.
- Fever, headache, and vomiting are followed by signs of meningeal irritation and neuronal damage.
- Rapid deterioration of LOC may occur within 24 to 48 hours.

Head trauma

- The nature of ocular deviation depends on the site and extent of head trauma.
- Visible soft-tissue injury, bony deformity, facial edema, and clear or bloody otorrhea or rhinorrhea may be present.
- Other signs and symptoms include blurred vision, diplopia, nystagmus, behavioral changes, headache, motor and sensory dysfunction, signs of increased ICP, and a decreased LOC that may progress to coma.

Multiple sclerosis

- Ocular deviation may be an early sign.
- Diplopia, blurred vision, and sensory dysfunction occur.
- Other signs and symptoms include nystagmus, constipation, muscle weakness, paralysis, spasticity, hyperreflexia, intention tremor, gait ataxia, dysphagia, dysarthria, impotence, emotional lability, and urinary frequency, urgency, and incontinence.

Myasthenia gravis

- Ocular deviation may accompany the more common first signs of diplopia and ptosis.
- May affect only the eye muscles or progress to other muscle groups, causing altered facial expression, difficulty chewing, dysphagia, weakened voice, impaired fine hand movements, and respiratory distress.

Ophthalmoplegic migraine

- Ocular deviation and diplopia persist for days after the pain subsides.
- Other findings include headache on one side with possible ptosis on the same side; temporary hemiplegia; irritability, depression, or slight confusion; and sensory deficits.

To perform an assessment of extraocular muscle function, sit directly in front of the patient and ask her to remain still while you hold a cylindrical object, such as a penlight, directly in front of and about 18″ (46 cm) away from her nose. Ask the patient to hold her head still and to watch the object as you move it clockwise through each of the six cardinal positions, returning the object to midpoint after each movement. (Three positions are shown here: left lateral, left superior, and left inferior.)

The ocular muscles must work with the muscles producing the opposite movement. Normally, when one muscle contracts, its opposite relaxes to produce a smooth motion.

Throughout the test, the patient's eyes should remain parallel as they move. Note any abnormal findings, such as nystagmus or the deviation of one eye away from the object.

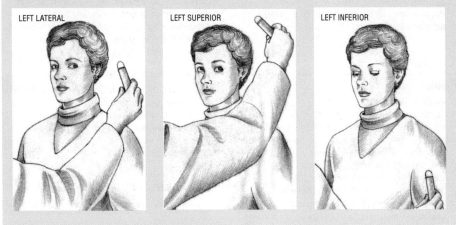

LEFT LATERAL   LEFT SUPERIOR   LEFT INFERIOR

Orbital blowout fracture

○ Limited extraocular movement and ocular deviation may occur.
○ Typically, upward gaze is absent.
○ Other signs and symptoms include pain, diplopia, nausea, periorbital edema, ecchymosis, and a globe that may be displaced downward and inward.

Orbital tumor

○ Ocular deviation occurs as the tumor gradually enlarges.
○ Other findings include an edematous eyelid, proptosis, diplopia, and blurred vision.

Stroke

○ Ocular deviation depends on the site and extent of the stroke.
○ Other findings vary and may include altered LOC, contralateral hemiplegia and sensory loss, dysarthria, dysphagia, homonymous hemianopsia, blurred vision, and diplopia.
○ Additional findings include urine retention or incontinence or both, constipation, behavioral changes, headache, vomiting, and seizures.

Thyrotoxicosis

○ Exophthalmos occurs, which causes limited extraocular movement and ocular deviation.

○ Usually, the upward gaze weakens first, followed by diplopia.
○ Other findings include lid retraction, a wide-eyed staring gaze, excessive tearing, edematous eyelids and, sometimes, inability to close the eyes.
○ Main findings include tachycardia, palpitations, weight loss despite increased appetite, diarrhea, tremors, an enlarged thyroid gland, dyspnea, nervousness, diaphoresis, heat intolerance, and an atrial or ventricular gallop.

Nursing considerations

○ If you suspect an acute neurologic disorder, monitor vital signs and neurologic status.

Pediatric pointers

○ In children, the most common cause of ocular deviation is nonparalytic strabismus.

Patient teaching

○ Explain the disorder and its treatment.
○ Explain changes in LOC that need to be reported.
○ Provide information about maintaining a safe environment.
○ Teach ways of reducing environmental stress.

Oligomenorrhea

Overview

- Abnormally infrequent menstrual bleeding (three to six menstrual cycles per year)
- Common in infertile, early postmenarchal, and perimenopausal women
- May develop gradually or may follow a period of gradually lengthening cycles
- May alternate with normal menses or progress to secondary amenorrhea

Assessment

History

- Ask the patient's age.
- Obtain a menstrual history, including age at menarche and characteristics and duration of bleeding.
- Ask about ovulatory bleeding.
- Note hormonal contraceptive use.
- Note previous gynecologic disorders.
- Ask about problems with breast-feeding.
- Determine weight gain or loss and exercise patterns.
- Find out about excessive thirst, frequent urination, fatigue, jitteriness, palpitations, headache, dizziness, and impaired peripheral vision.
- Obtain a drug history.

Physical assessment

- Take vital signs and weigh the patient.
- Inspect for increased facial hair growth, sparse body hair, male distribution of fat and muscle, acne, and clitoral enlargement.
- Note if the skin is abnormally dry or moist; check hair texture.
- Look for signs of psychological or physical stress.
- Rule out pregnancy.

Medical causes

Adrenal hyperplasia

- Oligomenorrhea may occur with signs of androgen excess, such as clitoral enlargement, deepening voice, acne, and male distribution of hair, fat, and muscle mass.

Anorexia nervosa

- Sporadic oligomenorrhea or amenorrhea may occur along with a morbid fear of being fat and a weight loss of more than 20% of the patient's ideal body weight.
- Other findings include dramatic skeletal muscle atrophy and loss of fatty tissue; dry or sparse scalp hair; lanugo on the face and body; constipation; decreased libido; and blotchy or sallow, dry skin.

Diabetes mellitus

- Oligomenorrhea may be an early sign; in juvenile-onset diabetes, the patient may never have had normal menses.
- Other findings include excessive hunger, polydipsia, polyuria, polyphagia, weakness, fatigue, dry mucous membranes, poor skin turgor, irritability, emotional lability, and weight loss.

Hypothyroidism

- Oligomenorrhea
- Fatigue; cold intolerance; dry, flaky, inelastic skin; constipation; puffy face, hands, and feet; bradycardia; decreased mental acuity; hoarseness; periorbital edema; ptosis; dry, sparse hair; thick, brittle nails; and unexplained weight gain

Polycystic ovary disease

- Oligomenorrhea, amenorrhea, menometrorrhagia, or irregular menses may occur.
- Infertility, anovulation, and enlarged, palpable ovaries are common.
- Other findings include male distribution of body hair and muscle mass, facial hair growth, acne, and obesity.

Prolactin-secreting pituitary tumor

- Oligomenorrhea or amenorrhea may be the first sign.
- Accompanying signs and symptoms include galactorrhea, infertility, loss of libido, and sparse pubic hair.
- Headache and visual field disturbances signal tumor expansion.

Thyrotoxicosis

- Oligomenorrhea may occur with reduced fertility.

Other causes

Drugs

- Drugs that increase androgen level — such as corticosteroids, corticotropin, anabolic steroids, danazol, and injectable and implantable contraceptives — may cause oligomenorrhea.
- Other drugs that may cause oligomenorrhea include phenothiazine derivatives, amphetamines, and antihypertensives.

Nursing considerations

- Prepare the patient for diagnostic tests.

Pediatric pointers

- Oligomenorrhea in teenagers is associated with immature hormonal function.
- Prolonged oligomenorrhea may signal congenital adrenal hyperplasia or Turner's syndrome.

Geriatric pointers

○ Oligomenorrhea in perimenopausal woman usually indicates impending onset of menopause.

Patient teaching

○ Teach the patient techniques of recording basal body temperature.
○ Explain the use of a home ovulation test.
○ Provide information about the use of contraceptives.

Oliguria

Overview

- Defined as urine output of less than 400 ml/24 hours
- Major sign of renal and urinary tract disorders
- Typically occurs abruptly and may herald serious, possibly life-threatening, hemodynamic instability

Assessment

History

- Ask about usual voiding patterns and the onset and description of oliguria.
- Find out about pain or burning on urination, fever, loss of appetite, thirst, dyspnea, chest pain, or recent weight gain or loss.
- Record the patient's daily fluid intake.
- Obtain a medical history, including renal, urinary tract, or cardiovascular disorders; recent traumatic injury or surgery with significant blood loss; and recent transfusions.
- Ask about use of alcohol.
- Obtain a drug history.
- Note exposure to nephrotoxic agents, such as heavy metals, organic solvents, anesthetics, or radiographic contrast media.

Physical assessment

- Take vital signs and weigh the patient.
- Palpate the kidneys for tenderness and enlargement.
- Percuss for costovertebral angle (CVA) tenderness.
- Inspect the flanks for edema or erythema.
- Auscultate the heart and lungs for abnormal sounds and the flank area for bruits.
- Assess for edema or signs of dehydration.
- Obtain a urine specimen, and inspect it for abnormal color, odor, or sediment; measure its specific gravity.

Medical causes

Acute tubular necrosis

- Oliguria, an early sign, may occur abruptly (in shock) or gradually (in nephrotoxicity) and persists for about 2 weeks, followed by polyuria.
- Other findings include signs of hyperkalemia, uremia, and heart failure.

Calculi

- Oliguria or anuria may result.
- Excruciating pain radiates from the CVA to the flank, the suprapubic region, and the external genitalia.
- Other signs and symptoms include urinary frequency and urgency, dysuria, hematuria or pyuria, nausea,

vomiting, hypoactive bowel sounds, abdominal distention and, possibly, fever and chills.

Glomerulonephritis (acute)

- Oliguria or anuria
- Mild fever, fatigue, gross hematuria, proteinuria, generalized edema, elevated blood pressure, headache, nausea, vomiting, flank and abdominal pain, and signs of pulmonary congestion

Heart failure

- In left-sided heart failure, oliguria
- Dyspnea, fatigue, weakness, peripheral edema, distended neck veins, tachycardia, tachypnea, crackles, and a dry or productive cough
- In advanced failure, orthopnea, cyanosis, clubbing, ventricular gallop, diastolic hypertension, cardiomegaly, and hemoptysis

Hypovolemia

- Oliguria may occur.
- Other signs and symptoms include orthostatic hypotension, apathy, lethargy, fatigue, muscle weakness, anorexia, nausea, thirst, dizziness, sunken eyeballs, poor skin turgor, and dry mucous membranes.

Pyelonephritis (acute)

- Oliguria, high fever with chills, fatigue, flank pain, CVA tenderness, weakness, nocturia, dysuria, hematuria, urinary frequency and urgency, and tenesmus occur.
- Anorexia, nausea, diarrhea, and vomiting may also develop.

Renal artery occlusion (bilateral)

- Oliguria or, more commonly, anuria may accompany severe, constant upper abdominal and flank pain, nausea and vomiting, hypoactive bowel sounds, fever, and diastolic hypertension.

Renal failure (chronic)

- Oliguria is a major sign of end-stage chronic renal failure.
- Other signs and symptoms include fatigue, weakness, irritability, uremic fetor, ecchymoses, petechiae, peripheral edema, elevated blood pressure, confusion, emotional lability, drowsiness, coarse muscle twitching, muscle cramps, peripheral neuropathies, anorexia, metallic taste in the mouth, nausea, vomiting, constipation or diarrhea, stomatitis, pruritus, pallor, and yellow- or bronze-tinged skin.
- Eventually, seizures, coma, and uremic frost develop.

Renal vein occlusion (bilateral)

- Occasionally, oliguria occurs with acute low back and flank pain, CVA tenderness, fever, pallor, hematuria, enlarged and palpable kidneys, edema and, possibly, signs of uremia.

Sepsis

○ Oliguria, fever, chills, restlessness, confusion, diaphoresis, anorexia, vomiting, diarrhea, pallor, hypotension, and tachycardia occur.
○ Signs of local infection may be produced.

Toxemia of pregnancy

○ Oliguria may be accompanied by elevated blood pressure, dizziness, diplopia, blurred vision, nausea and vomiting, irritability, and frontal headache.
○ Oliguria is preceded by generalized edema and sudden weight gain of more than 3 lb (1.4 kg) per week during the second trimester or more than 1 lb (0.5 kg) per week during the third trimester.
○ If the condition progresses to eclampsia, seizures and coma may occur.

Urethral stricture

○ Oliguria is accompanied by chronic urethral discharge, urinary frequency and urgency, dysuria, pyuria, and diminished urine stream.

Other causes

Diagnostic studies

○ Radiographic studies that use contract media may cause nephrotoxicity and oliguria.

Drugs

○ Oliguria may result from drugs that cause decreased renal perfusion (diuretics), nephrotoxicity (most notably aminoglycosides and chemotherapeutics), urine retention (adrenergics and anticholinergics), or urinary obstruction associated with precipitation of urinary crystals (sulfonamides and acyclovir).

Nursing considerations

○ Monitor vital signs, intake and output, and daily weight.
○ Restrict fluids to 600 ml to 1 L more than the urinary output for the previous day, if indicated.
○ Provide diet low in sodium, potassium, and protein.

Pediatric pointers

○ In a neonate, oliguria may result from edema or dehydration, congenital heart disease, respiratory distress syndrome, sepsis, congenital hydronephrosis, acute tubular necrosis, and renal vein thrombosis.
○ Causes of oliguria in children ages 1 to 5 include hemolytic-uremic syndrome and acute poststreptococcal glomerulonephritis.

Geriatric pointers

○ In elderly patients, oliguria may result from an underlying disorder, overall poor muscle tone because of inactivity, poor fluid intake, and infrequent voiding attempts.

Patient teaching

○ Explain fluid and dietary restrictions the patient needs.

Orthopnea

Overview

- Refers to difficulty breathing in a supine position
- Is a common symptom of cardiopulmonary disorders that produce dyspnea
- Results from increased hydrostatic pressure in the pulmonary vasculature related to being in the supine position
- May be reported that the patient can't catch his breath when lying down or that he sleeps in a reclining chair or propped up by pillows
- May be classified as two- or three-pillow orthopnea

Assessment

History

- Ask about the onset and description of orthopnea.
- Note how many pillows are used for sleeping.
- Obtain a medical history, including history of cardiopulmonary disorders, such as myocardial infarction, rheumatic heart disease, heart failure, valvular disease, asthma, emphysema, or chronic bronchitis.
- Find out about smoking and alcohol habits.
- Inquire about associated cough, dyspnea, fatigue, weakness, loss of appetite, or chest pain.
- Obtain a drug history.

Physical assessment

- Take vital signs.
- Check for other signs of increased respiratory effort, such as accessory muscle use, shallow respirations, and tachypnea.
- Note barrel chest.
- Inspect skin for pallor or cyanosis, and inspect the fingers for clubbing.
- Observe and palpate for edema.
- Check jugular vein distention.
- Auscultate the lungs and heart.
- Monitor oxygen saturation.

Medical causes

Chronic obstructive pulmonary disease

- Orthopnea and other dyspneic complaints are accompanied by accessory muscle use, tachypnea, tachycardia, and paradoxical pulse.
- Other findings include diminished breath sounds, rhonchi, crackles, and wheezing on auscultation; dry or productive cough with copious sputum; anorexia; weight loss; and edema.
- Barrel chest, cyanosis, and clubbing are late signs.

Left-sided heart failure

- If heart failure is acute, orthopnea may begin suddenly; if chronic, it may be constant.
- Early findings include progressively severe dyspnea, Cheyne-Stokes respirations, paroxysmal nocturnal dyspnea, fatigue, weakness, a cough that may occasionally produce clear or blood-tinged sputum, tachycardia, tachypnea, and crackles.
- Late findings include cyanosis, clubbing, ventricular gallop, and hemoptysis.

Mediastinal tumor

- Orthopnea is an early sign, but many patients are asymptomatic until the tumor enlarges.
- Other signs and symptoms as the tumor enlarges include retrosternal chest pain, dry cough, hoarseness, dysphagia, stertorous respirations, palpitations, cyanosis, suprasternal retractions on inspiration, tracheal deviation, dilated jugular and superficial chest veins, and edema of the face, neck, and arms.

Valvular heart disease

- Orthopnea may result from valvular heart disease.
- Signs and symptoms may vary according to valve involved.
  - Signs and symptoms of aortic insufficiency include fatigue, dyspnea, palpitations, dizziness, and angina. With heart failure, orthopnea, paroxysmal nocturnal dyspnea, and cough may also occur.
  - Signs and symptoms of aortic stenosis include syncope, angina, and dyspnea on exertion. With left-sided heart failure, orthopnea may also occur.
  - Signs and symptoms of mitral insufficiency include fatigue, dyspnea, palpitations, angina, and orthopnea.
  - Signs and symptoms of mitral stenosis include fatigue, weakness, dyspnea on exertion, nocturnal dyspnea, palpitations, and orthopnea.

Nursing considerations

- Place the patient in semi-Fowler's or high Fowler's position.
- Alternatively, have the patient lean over a bedside table with his chest forward.
- If needed, administer oxygen via nasal cannula.
- To reduce lung fluid, give a diuretic.
- Monitor intake and output.
- For the patient with left-sided heart failure, give angiotensin-converting enzyme inhibitors.
- Insert a central venous line or pulmonary artery catheter, as needed.

Pediatric pointers

- Common causes of orthopnea in children include heart failure, croup syndrome, cystic fibrosis, and asthma.

○ Sleeping in an infant seat may improve symptoms for a young child.

Geriatric pointers

○ If the patient is using more than one pillow in bed, consider a noncardiogenic pulmonary cause.

Patient teaching

○ Explain the signs and symptoms the patient should report.
○ Explain dietary and fluid restrictions the patient needs.
○ Discuss daily weight measurement.

Orthostatic hypotension

Overview

- A blood pressure drop of 15 to 20 mm Hg or more (with or without an increase in the heart rate of at least 20 beats/minute) upon rising from a supine to a sitting or standing position
- Also called *postural hypotension*
- Failure of compensatory vasomotor responses to adjust to position changes
- Light-headedness, syncope, or blurred vision

Emergency actions

Check for tachycardia, altered level of consciousness (LOC), and pale, clammy skin. If present, suspect hypovolemic shock. Insert a large-bore I.V. line for fluid or blood replacement. Take vital signs frequently and monitor the patient's intake and output.

Assessment

History

- Ask about dizziness, weakness, or fainting when standing.
- Inquire about fatigue, orthopnea, nausea, headache, abdominal or chest discomfort, and GI bleeding.
- Obtain a drug history.

Physical assessment

- Check skin turgor.
- Palpate peripheral pulses.
- Auscultate the heart and lungs.
- Test muscle strength and observe gait for unsteadiness.

Medical causes

Adrenal insufficiency

- Orthostatic hypotension may be accompanied by fatigue, muscle weakness, poor coordination, anorexia, nausea, vomiting, fasting hypoglycemia, weight loss, irritability, abdominal pain, hyperpigmentation, and a weak, irregular pulse.
- Other signs and symptoms include diarrhea, constipation, decreased libido, amenorrhea, syncope, and enhanced taste, smell, and hearing.

Amyloidosis

- Orthostatic hypotension is common.
- Other signs and symptoms vary widely and include angina, tachycardia, dyspnea, orthopnea, fatigue, and cough.

Diabetic autonomic neuropathy

- Orthostatic hypotension, syncope, dysphagia, constipation or diarrhea, painless bladder distention with overflow incontinence, impotence, and retrograde ejaculation

Hyperaldosteronism

- Orthostatic hypotension with sustained elevated blood pressure occurs.
- Other findings include muscle weakness, intermittent flaccid paralysis, fatigue, headache, paresthesia, vision disturbance, nocturia, polydipsia, personality changes and, possibly, tetany.

Hyponatremia

- Orthostatic hypotension with headache, profound thirst, nausea, vomiting, muscle twitching and weakness, fatigue, oliguria or anuria, tachycardia, abdominal cramps, irritability, seizures, decreased LOC, and cold clammy skin
- If severe, cyanosis, thready pulse, and eventually vasomotor collapse

Hypovolemia

- Orthostatic hypotension with apathy, fatigue, muscle weakness, anorexia, nausea, and profound thirst.
- Other signs and symptoms include dizziness, oliguria, sunken eyeballs, poor skin turgor, and dry mucous membranes.

Other causes

Drugs

- Antihypertensives, diuretics in large doses, levodopa, monoamine oxidase inhibitors, morphine, nitrates, phenothiazines, spinal anesthesia, and tricyclic antidepressants may cause orthostatic hypotension.

Treatments

- Orthostatic hypotension is common with prolonged bed rest.
- Sympathectomy may cause orthostatic hypotension by disrupting normal vasoconstrictive mechanisms.

Nursing considerations

- Elevate the head of the bed, and help the patient to a sitting position with his feet dangling over the side of the bed; if tolerated, have him sit in a chair briefly.
- Evaluate the need for assistive devices.
- Monitor intake and output and weigh the patient daily.
- Help the patient with walking.

Pediatric pointers

- The causes of orthostatic hypotension in children may be the same as those in adults.

Geriatric pointers

○ Elderly patients commonly experience autonomic dysfunction, which can show up as orthostatic hypotension.
○ Postprandial hypotension may occur 45 to 60 minutes after a meal.

Patient teaching

○ Explain the importance of avoiding volume depletion.
○ Explain how to change position gradually.

Otorrhea

Overview

○ Drainage from the ear
○ May be bloody, purulent, clear, or serosanguineous

Assessment

History

○ Ask about the onset and description of drainage.
○ Find out about pain, tenderness, vertigo, or tinnitus.
○ Obtain a medical history, including recent upper respiratory infection or head trauma, and history of cancer, dermatitis, or immunosuppressant therapy.

Physical assessment

○ Inspect the external ear, and apply pressure on the tragus and mastoid area to elicit tenderness; then insert an otoscope.
○ Observe for edema, erythema, crusts, or polyps.
○ Inspect the tympanic membrane, note color changes, perforation, absence of the normal light reflex, or a bulging membrane.
○ Test hearing acuity and perform Weber's and Rinne tests.
○ Palpate the neck and preauricular, parotid, and postauricular areas for lymphadenopathy.
○ Test the function of cranial nerves VII, IX, X, and XI.

Medical causes

Allergy

○ Tympanic membrane perforation may cause clear or cloudy otorrhea, rhinorrhea, and itchy, watery eyes.
○ Other signs and symptoms include nasal congestion and an itchy nose and throat.

Assessment tip
Examining a child's ear

To examine a child's ear safely and accurately, restrain the child by having him sit on a parent's lap with the ear to be examined facing you. Have him put one arm around the parent's waist and the other down at his side, and then ask the parent to hold the child in place. Alternatively, if you are alone with the child, ask him to lie on his abdomen with his arms at his sides and his head turned so the affected ear faces the ceiling. Bend over him, restraining his upper body with your elbows and upper arms.

Aural polyps

○ Foul, purulent, and possibly blood-streaked discharge
○ Partial hearing loss

Basilar skull fracture

○ Otorrhea may be clear and watery and show a positive reaction on glucose test, or it may be bloody.
○ Other signs and symptoms include hearing loss, cerebrospinal fluid or bloody rhinorrhea, periorbital raccoon eyes, mastoid ecchymosis (Battle's sign), cranial nerve palsies, decreased level of consciousness, and headache.

Dermatitis of the external ear canal

○ With contact dermatitis, vesicles produce clear, watery otorrhea with edema and erythema of the external ear canal.
○ Infectious eczematoid dermatitis causes purulent otorrhea with erythema and crusting of the external ear canal.
○ With seborrheic dermatitis, otorrhea has greasy scales and flakes.

Mastoiditis

○ Thick, purulent, yellow otorrhea becomes increasingly profuse.
○ Main findings include low-grade fever and dull aching and tenderness in the mastoid area.
○ Conductive hearing loss may develop.

Myringitis (infectious)

○ Small, reddened, blood-filled blebs or blisters rupture, causing serosanguineous otorrhea.
○ Other findings include severe ear pain and tenderness over the mastoid process.
○ In the chronic form, purulent otorrhea, pruritus, and gradual hearing loss occur.

Otitis externa

○ Acute form usually causes purulent, yellow, sticky, foul-smelling otorrhea.
○ Associated acute signs and symptoms include edema, erythema, pain, and itching of the auricle and external ear; severe tenderness with movement of the mastoid, tragus, mouth, or jaw; tenderness and swelling of surrounding nodes; partial conductive hearing loss; and low-grade fever and headache ipsilateral to the affected ear.
○ Chronic form usually causes scanty, intermittent otorrhea that may be serous or purulent as well as edema and slight erythema.

Otitis media

○ With acute otitis media, rupture of the tympanic membrane produces bloody, purulent otorrhea and conductive hearing loss that worsens over several hours.

- With acute suppurative otitis media, otorrhea may accompany signs and symptoms of upper respiratory infection, dizziness, fever, nausea, and vomiting.
- Chronic otitis media causes intermittent, purulent, foul-smelling otorrhea; gradual conductive hearing loss; pain; nausea; and vertigo.

Trauma
- Bloody otorrhea may result.
- Otorrhea may be accompanied by partial hearing loss.

Tumor
- A benign tumor of the jugular glomus may cause bloody otorrhea.
- Other signs and symptoms of this benign disorder include throbbing discomfort, tinnitus that resembles the sound of the patient's heartbeat, progressive stuffiness of the affected ear, vertigo, conductive hearing loss and, possibly, a reddened mass behind the tympanic membrane.
- Squamous cell carcinoma of the external ear causes purulent otorrhea with itching; deep, boring pain; hearing loss; and, in late stages, facial paralysis.
- In squamous cell carcinoma of the middle ear, blood-tinged otorrhea occurs early accompanied by hearing loss of the affected side; pain and facial paralysis are late signs.

Nursing considerations

- Apply warm, moist compresses, heating pads, or hot water bottles to the ears.
- Use cotton wicks to clean the ear or to apply topical drugs.
- Keep eardrops at room temperature; instillation of cold eardrops may cause vertigo.
- If the patient has impaired hearing, make sure he understands what's explained to him.

Pediatric pointers
- Perforation of the tympanic membrane from otitis media is the most common cause of otorrhea in infants and young children.
- Children may insert foreign bodies into their ears, resulting in infection, pain, and purulent discharge.
- Because the auditory canal of a child lies horizontal, the pinna must be pulled downward and backward to examine the ear. (See *Examining a child's ear.*)

Patient teaching
- Instruct the patient on safe ways to blow his nose and clean his ears.
- Stress the use of earplugs when swimming.
- Explain the signs and symptoms the patient needs to report.

Pallor

Overview

- Refers to abnormal paleness or loss of skin color
- Develops suddenly or gradually
- Can be difficult to detect in darker-skinned patients because black skin may be ashen grey and brown skin may be yellowish brown.
- Can be generalized or localized
- Is caused chiefly by anemia (see *How pallor develops*)

⭐ Emergency actions

If generalized pallor develops suddenly, look for signs of shock and prepare to rapidly infuse fluids or blood. Keep emergency resuscitation equipment nearby.

Assessment

History

- Obtain a medical history, including anemia, renal failure, heart failure, or diabetes.
- Ask about diet, especially intake of green vegetables.
- Ask about the onset and description of the pallor.
- Explore what aggravates and alleviates the pallor.
- Inquire about dizziness, fainting, orthostasis, weakness, fatigue, dyspnea, chest pain, palpitations, menstrual irregularities, or loss of libido.

Physical assessment

- Assess vital signs, checking for orthostatic hypotension.
- Auscultate the heart for heart murmurs or gallops.
- Auscultate the lungs for crackles.
- Check skin temperature.
- Note skin ulceration.
- Palpate peripheral pulses.

Medical causes

Anemia

- Pallor begins gradually; skin is gray or sallow.
- Other findings include fatigue, dyspnea, tachycardia, bounding pulse, atrial gallop, systolic bruit over the carotid arteries and, possibly, crackles and bleeding tendencies.

Arterial occlusion (acute)

- Pallor begins abruptly in the extremity with occlusion.
- Line of demarcation separates cool, pale, cyanotic, and mottled skin from normal skin.

How pallor develops

Pallor may result from decreased peripheral oxyhemoglobin or decreased total oxyhemoglobin. The flowchart below illustrates the progression to pallor.

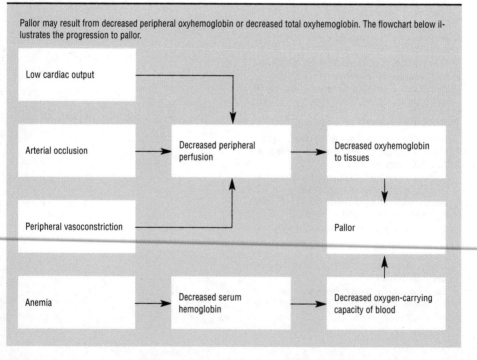

○ Other findings include severe pain, intense intermittent claudication, paresthesia, paresis in the affected extremity, and absent pulses below the occlusion.

Arterial occlusive disease (chronic)

○ Pallor is specific to an extremity.
○ Pallor develops gradually and is aggravated by elevating the extremity.
○ Other findings include intermittent claudication, weakness, cool skin, diminished pulses in the extremity and, possibly, ulceration and gangrene.

Cardiac arrhythmias

○ Acute pallor may occur with an irregular, rapid, or slow pulse; dizziness; weakness and fatigue; hypotension; confusion; palpitations; diaphoresis; oliguria; and, possibly, loss of consciousness.

Frostbite

○ Pallor is localized to the frostbitten area, which feels cold, waxy and, possibly, hard; sensation may be absent.
○ Skin turns purplish blue as skin thaws; if frostbite is severe, blistering and gangrene may follow.

Orthostatic hypotension

○ Pallor occurs abruptly on rising from a recumbent position along with a drop in blood pressure, tachycardia, and dizziness.
○ Loss of consciousness is possible.

Raynaud's disease

○ Upon exposure to cold or stress, the fingers abruptly turn pale (a classic sign), then cyanotic.
○ With rewarming, fingers become red and paresthetic.
○ With chronic disease, ulceration may occur.

Shock

○ In hypovolemic and cardiogenic shock, acute pallor occurs early with restlessness, thirst, tachycardia, tachypnea, and cool, clammy skin.
○ As shock progresses, skin becomes increasingly clammy, pulse becomes more rapid and thready, and hypotension develops with narrowing pulse pressure.
○ Other findings include oliguria, subnormal body temperature, and decreased level of consciousness (LOC).

Vasopressor syncope

○ Sudden pallor immediately precedes or accompanies loss of consciousness.
○ These fainting spells may be triggered by emotional stress or pain and usually last for a few seconds or minutes.
○ Before loss of consciousness, diaphoresis, nausea, yawning, hyperpnea, weakness, confusion, tachycardia, and dim vision may occur followed by bradycardia, hypotension, a few clonic jerks, and dilated pupils.

Nursing considerations

○ Administer blood and fluids as well as a diuretic, cardiotonic, and an antiarrhythmic, as needed.
○ Frequently monitor vital signs, intake and output, electrocardiogram, and hemodynamic status.

Pediatric pointers

○ Pallor in children can also stem from a congenital heart defect or chronic lung disease.

Patient teaching

○ For anemia, explain the importance of an iron-rich diet and rest.
○ For frostbite and Raynaud's disease, discuss cold-protection measures.
○ For orthostatic hypotension, explain the need to rise slowly.

Palpitations

Overview

- Conscious awareness of one's own heartbeat
- Usually felt over the precordium or in the throat or neck
- May be regular or irregular, fast or slow, paroxysmal or sustained
- May be described as pounding, jumping, turning, fluttering, flopping, or as skipping a beat

Emergency actions

Ask the patient about dizziness or shortness of breath. Then inspect for pale, cool, clammy skin. Take vital signs, noting hypotension and irregular or abnormal pulse. If these signs are present, suspect cardiac arrhythmia. Begin cardiac monitoring and, if needed, deliver electroshock therapy. Start an I.V. line to administer an antiarrhythmic, if needed.

Assessment

History

- Ask about the onset and description of palpitations.
- Inquire about aggravating and alleviating factors.
- Note associated signs and symptoms, such as dizziness, syncope, weakness, fatigue, angina, and pale, cool skin.
- Obtain a medical history, including cardiovascular or pulmonary disorder, or hypoglycemia.
- Obtain a drug history, including recently prescribed digoxin.
- Ask about caffeine, tobacco, and alcohol use.

Physical assessment

- Perform a complete cardiac and pulmonary assessment.
- Auscultate heart for gallops and murmurs.
- Auscultate lungs for abnormal breath sounds.

Medical causes

Anemia

- Palpitations occur, especially on exertion, with pallor, fatigue, and dyspnea.
- Other findings include systolic ejection murmur, bounding pulse, tachycardia, crackles, an atrial gallop, and a systolic bruit over the carotid arteries.

Anxiety attack (acute)

- Palpitations may be accompanied by diaphoresis, facial flushing, trembling, and an impending sense of doom.
- Hyperventilation may lead to dizziness, weakness, and syncope.

- Other findings include tachycardia, precordial pain, shortness of breath, restlessness, and insomnia.

Cardiac arrhythmias

- Paroxysmal or sustained palpitations may be accompanied by dizziness, weakness, and fatigue.
- Other findings include an irregular, rapid, or slow pulse rate; decreased blood pressure; confusion; pallor; chest pain; syncope; oliguria; and diaphoresis.

Hypertension

- Sustained palpitations may occur alone or with headache, dizziness, tinnitus, and fatigue.
- Blood pressure typically exceeds 140/90 mm Hg.
- Nausea, vomiting, seizures, and decreased level of consciousness (LOC) may also occur.

Hypocalcemia

- Palpitations occur with weakness and fatigue.
- Paresthesia progresses to muscle tension and carpopedal spasms.
- Related findings include muscle twitching, hyperactive deep tendon reflexes, chorea, and positive Chvostek's and Trousseau's signs.

Hypoglycemia

- Sustained palpitations occur with fatigue, irritability, hunger, cold sweats, tremors, tachycardia, anxiety, and headache.
- Eventually, blurred or double vision, muscle weakness, hemiplegia, and altered LOC develop.

Mitral prolapse

- Paroxysmal palpitations accompany sharp, stabbing, or aching precordial pain and midsystolic click, followed by an apical systolic murmur.
- Other findings include dyspnea, dizziness, severe fatigue, migraine headache, anxiety, paroxysmal tachycardia, crackles, and peripheral edema.

Mitral stenosis

- Early on, sustained palpitations accompany exertional dyspnea and fatigue.
- Loud S_1 or opening snap and a rumbling diastolic murmur at the apex are heard on auscultation.
- Other findings include an atrial gallop and, with advanced disease, orthopnea, dyspnea at rest, paroxysmal nocturnal dyspnea, peripheral edema, jugular vein distention, ascites, hepatomegaly, and atrial fibrillation.

Pheochromocytoma

- Paroxysmal palpitations occur with dramatically elevated blood pressure (the main sign).
- Other findings include tachycardia, headache, chest or abdominal pain, diaphoresis, warm and pale or flushed skin, paresthesia, tremors, insomnia, nausea, vomiting, and anxiety.

Thyrotoxicosis

○ Sustained palpitations may be accompanied by tachycardia, dyspnea, diarrhea, nervousness, tremors, diaphoresis, heat intolerance, weight loss despite increased appetite, atrial or ventricular gallop and, possibly, exophthalmos.

Other causes

Drugs

○ Drugs, such as digoxin, sympathomimetics, ganglionic blockers, beta blockers, calcium channel blockers, atropine, and minoxidil, that precipitate cardiac arrhythmias or increase cardiac output may cause palpitations.

Exercise

○ Exercise can cause palpitations.

Nursing considerations

○ Monitor for signs of reduced cardiac output and cardiac arrhythmias.
○ Prepare for procedures such as cardioversion.
○ Provide supplemental oxygen.
○ Provide for rest periods.

Pediatric pointers

○ Palpitations commonly result from fever and congenital heart defects.

Patient teaching

○ Explain diagnostic tests the patient needs.
○ Teach the patient how to reduce anxiety.

Papular rash

Overview

- Consists of small, raised, circumscribed papules
- May erupt anywhere on the body in various configurations
- May be acute or chronic (see *Recognizing common skin lesions*)

Assessment

History

- Ask about onset, course of rash, and characteristics, such as itching, burning, or tenderness.
- Inquire about fever, headache, and GI distress.
- Obtain a medical history, including allergies, previous rashes and skin disorders, infections, childhood diseases, sexual history, sexually transmitted diseases, cancers, and exposure to chemicals and pesticides.

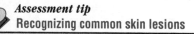

Assessment tip
Recognizing common skin lesions

Use the illustrations below to help you identify common skin lesions. Remember to keep a centimeter ruler handy to measure the size of the lesion accurately.

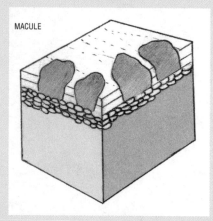

MACULE

A small (usually less than 1 cm in diameter), flat blemish or discoloration that can be brown, tan, red, or white and has the same texture as the surrounding skin

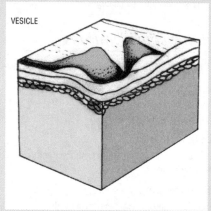

VESICLE

A small (less than 0.5 cm in diameter), thin-walled, raised blister containing clear, serous, purulent, or bloody fluid

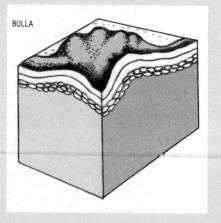

BULLA

A raised, thin-walled blister greater than 0.5 cm in diameter that contains clear or serous fluid

PUSTULE

A circumscribed, pus- or lymph-filled, elevated lesion that varies in diameter; may be firm or soft and white or yellow

○ Obtain a drug history.
○ Ask about recent insect or rodent bite or exposure to infectious disease.

Physical assessment

○ Note the color, configuration, and location of rash.
○ Perform a whole-body examination of skin, hair, and nails.

Medical causes

Acne vulgaris

○ Inflamed papules, pustules, nodules, or cysts appear on the face, shoulders, chest, and back.
○ Lesions may be painful and pruritic.

Anthrax (cutaneous)

○ Initially appears as a small, painless, pruritic macular or papular lesion.
○ A vesicle develops within 2 days and then evolves into a painless ulcer with a black, necrotic center.

WHEAL

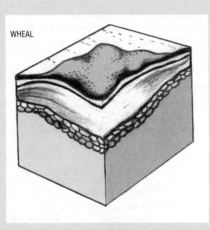

A slightly raised, firm lesion of variable size and shape that's surrounded by edema (skin may be red or pale)

PAPULE

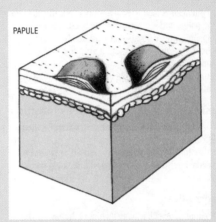

A small, solid, raised lesion less than 1 cm in diameter with red to purple skin discoloration

NODULE

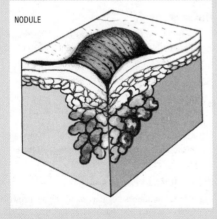

A small, firm, circumscribed, elevated lesion 1 to 2 cm in diameter with possible skin discoloration

TUMOR

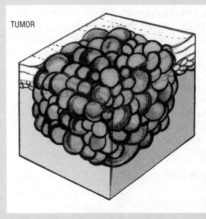

A solid, raised mass usually larger than 2 cm in diameter with possible skin discoloration

○ Lymphadenopathy, malaise, headache, and fever may develop.

Dermatitis (perioral)

○ Tiny, discrete, erythematous papules and pustules that may be pruritic and painful appear on the nasolabial fold, chin, and upper lip area.

Erythema migrans

○ Papular or macular rash starts as a single lesion and spreads at margins while clearing centrally.
○ Commonly appears of the thighs, trunk, or upper arms.
○ Accompanying findings include fever, chills, headache, malaise, nausea, vomiting, fatigue, backache, knee pain, and stiff neck.

Gonococcemia

○ Erythematous macular rash erupts sporadically on the palms and soles and rapidly becomes maculopapular, vesiculopustular, and hemorrhagic.
○ Mature lesion is raised with a gray, necrotic center, surrounded by erythema, and heals in 3 to 4 days.
○ Eruptions may be accompanied by fever and joint pain.

Human immunodeficiency virus infection

○ A generalized maculopapular rash occurs with acute infection.
○ Other findings include fever, malaise, sore throat, headache, lymphadenopathy, and hepatosplenomegaly.

Insect bites

○ A papular, macular, or petechial rash may be accompanied by fever, myalgia, headache, lymphadenopathy, nausea, and vomiting.

Kaposi's sarcoma

○ Purple or blue papules or macules of vascular origin appear on the skin, mucous membrane, and viscera.
○ Lesions decrease in size with firm pressure and then return to their original size within 10 to 15 seconds.
○ Lesions may become scaly and may ulcerate with bleeding.

Lichen amyloidosis

○ Discrete, firm, hemispherical, pruritic papules appear on the anterior tibiae, feet, and thighs.
○ Papules may be brown or yellow and smooth or scaly.

Lichen planus

○ White lines or spots mark discrete, flat, angular or polygonal, violet papules.
○ Papules may be linear or may coalesce into plaques and usually appear on the lumbar region, genitalia, ankles, anterior tibiae, and wrists.

○ Rash usually develops first on the buccal mucosa as a lacy network of white or gray threadlike papules or plaques.
○ Other findings include pruritus, distorted fingernails, and atrophic alopecia.

Mononucleosis (infectious)

○ A maculopapular rash that resembles rubella is an early sign.
○ Headache, malaise, and fatigue typically precede the rash.
○ Other findings include sore throat, cervical lymphadenopathy, hepatosplenomegaly, and fluctuating temperature with an evening peak of 101° to 102° F (38.3° to 38.9° C).

Pityriasis rosea

○ Initially, an erythematous, slightly raised, oval lesion appears anywhere on the body.
○ Later, yellow to tan or erythematous patches with scaly edges appear on the trunk, arms, and legs; commonly erupting along body cleavage lines in a pine tree-shaped pattern.

Polymorphic light eruption

○ Papular, vesicular, or nodular rash appears on sun-exposed areas.
○ Other symptoms include pruritus, headache, and malaise.

Psoriasis

○ Initially, small, erythematous pruritic and, sometimes, painful papules appear on the scalp, chest, elbows, knees, back, buttocks, and genitalia.
○ Eventually, papules enlarge and coalesce, forming elevated, red, scaly plaques covered by characteristic silver scales.
○ Other findings include pitted fingernails and arthralgia.

Rosacea

○ Persistent erythema, telangiectasia, and recurrent eruption of papules and pustules on the forehead, malar areas, nose, and chin occur.

Sarcoidosis

○ Small, erythematous or yellow-brown papules appear around the eyes and mouth and on the nose, nasal mucosa, and upper back.
○ Other findings include dyspnea with a nonproductive cough, fatigue, arthralgia, weight loss, lymphadenopathy, vision loss, and dysphagia.

Seborrheic keratosis

○ Benign skin tumors begin as small, yellow-brown papules on the chest, back, or abdomen, eventually enlarging and becoming deeply pigmented.

Smallpox

○ Maculopapular rash develops on the oral mucosa, pharynx, face, and forearms and then spreads to the trunk and legs.
○ Within 2 days, rash becomes vesicular, and, later, round, firm pustules develop that are deeply embedded in the skin.
○ After 8 to 9 days, pustules form a crust; later the scab separates from the skin, leaving a pitted scar.
○ Initial findings include high fever, malaise, prostration, severe headache, backache, and abdominal pain.

Syphilis

○ A discrete, reddish brown, mucocutaneous rash and general lymphadenopathy herald the onset of secondary syphilis.
○ Rash may be papular, macular, pustular, or nodular and erupts between rolls of fat on the trunk and proximally on the arms, palms, soles, face, and scalp.
○ Other findings include headache, malaise, anorexia, weight loss, nausea, vomiting, sore throat, low-grade fever, temporary alopecia, and brittle, pitted nails.

Systemic lupus erythematosus

○ A characteristic butterfly-shaped rash of erythematous maculopapules or discoid plaques in a malar distribution across the nose and cheeks
○ Photosensitivity, nondeforming arthritis, patchy alopecia, mucous membrane ulceration, fever, chills, lymphadenopathy, anorexia, weight loss, abdominal pain, diarrhea or constipation, dyspnea, hematuria, headache, and irritability

Other causes

Drugs

○ Antibiotics, benzodiazepines, lithium, phenylbutazone, gold salts, allopurinol, isoniazid, and salicylates may cause transient maculopapular rashes, usually on the trunk.

Nursing considerations

○ Apply cool compresses or an antipruritic lotion.
○ Administer an antihistamine for allergic reactions and an antibiotic for infection.

Pediatric pointers

○ Common causes of papular rashes in children are infectious diseases, scabies, insect bites, allergies, drug reactions, and miliaria.

Geriatric pointers

○ An erythematous area, sometimes with firm papules, may be the first sign of a pressure ulcer.

Patient teaching

○ Teach the paient appropriate skin care measures.
○ Explain ways to reduce itching.
○ Discuss signs and symptoms the patient needs to report.

Paradoxical pulse

Overview

- Refers to decline in blood pressure of more than 10 mm Hg during inspiration (see *Detecting and measuring paradoxical pulse*)
- May cause peripheral pulses to weaken or disappear if it falls more than 20 mm Hg
- Results from an exaggerated inspirational increase in negative intrathoracic pressure
- May signal cardiac tamponade

> **Emergency actions**
>
> *Quickly take the patient's other vital signs. Check for additional signs and symptoms of cardiac tamponade, such as dyspnea, tachypnea, diaphoresis, jugular vein distention, tachycardia, narrowed pulse pressure, and hypotension. Emergency pericardiocentesis to aspirate blood or fluid from the pericardial sac may be needed. Evaluate the effectiveness of pericardiocentesis by measuring the degree of paradoxical pulse; it should decrease after aspiration.*

Assessment

History

- Ask about a history of chronic cardiac or pulmonary disease.
- Ask about other signs and symptoms, such as a cough or chest pain.

Assessment tip
Detecting and measuring paradoxical pulse

To accurately detect and measure paradoxical pulse, use a sphygmomanometer or an intra-arterial monitoring device. Inflate the blood pressure cuff 10 to 20 mm Hg beyond the peak systolic pressure. Then deflate the cuff at a rate of 2 mm Hg/second until you hear the first Korotkoff sound during expiration. Note the systolic pressure. As you continue to slowly deflate the cuff, observe the patient's respiratory pattern. If a paradoxical pulse is present, the Korotkoff sounds will disappear with inspiration and return with expiration. Continue to deflate the cuff until you hear Korotkoff sounds during both inspiration and expiration, and again note the systolic pressure. Subtract this reading from the first one to determine the degree of pulsus paradoxus. A difference of more than 10 mm Hg is abnormal.

You can also detect paradoxical pulse by palpating the radial pulse over several cycles of slow inspiration and expiration. Marked pulse diminution during inspiration indicates a paradoxical pulse.

Physical assessment

- Auscultate for abnormal breath sounds.
- Complete cardiac and pulmonary assessments.

Medical causes

Cardiac tamponade

- Paradoxical pulse is common.
- When severe, the classic findings of hypotension, diminished or muffled heart sounds, and jugular vein distention occur.
- Related findings include chest pain, pericardial rub, narrowed pulse pressure, anxiety, restlessness, clammy skin, hepatomegaly, dyspnea, tachypnea, and cyanosis.
- If cardiac tamponade develops gradually, paradoxical pulse may be accompanied by weakness, anorexia, and weight loss.

Chronic obstructive pulmonary disease

- Paradoxical pulse results from wide fluctuations in intrathoracic pressure.
- Other findings include dyspnea, tachypnea, wheezing, cough, accessory muscle use, barrel chest, clubbing, rhonchi, crackles, cyanosis, edema, and labored, pursed-lip breathing.

Pericarditis (chronic constrictive)

- Paradoxical pulse may occur.
- Other findings include pericardial rub, chest pain, exertional dyspnea, orthopnea, hepatomegaly, ascites, peripheral edema, and Kussmaul's sign.

Pulmonary embolism (massive)

- Paradoxical pulse results from decreased left ventricular filling and stroke volume.
- Other findings include severe apprehension, dyspnea, tachypnea, pleuritic chest pain, cyanosis, and jugular vein distention.
- With circulatory collapse, hypotension, and a weak, rapid pulse occur.
- With pulmonary infarction, hemoptysis, decreased breath sounds, and a pleural rub may develop.

Right ventricular infarction

- Paradoxical pulse may occur with elevated jugular venous or central venous pressure.
- Related findings include those of myocardial infarction and right-sided heart failure.

Nursing considerations

- Monitor vital signs and frequently check the degree of pulsus paradoxus.
- Perform vigorous respiratory treatment.

Pediatric pointers

○ Paradoxical pulse commonly occurs in children with chronic pulmonary disease, especially during an acute asthma attack.

○ A paradoxical pulse above 20 mm Hg is a reliable indicator of cardiac tamponade.

Patient teaching

○ Teach the patient with chronic obstructive pulmonary disease how to care for himself.

Paralysis

Overview

- Refers to total loss of voluntary motor function from severe cortical or pyramidal tract damage
- Can be local or widespread, symmetrical or asymmetrical, transient or permanent, and spastic or flaccid
- Classified as paraplegia, quadriplegia, or hemiplegia

⭐ Emergency actions

If paralysis develops suddenly, suspect trauma or acute vascular insult. Immobilize the patient's spine, determine level of consciousness (LOC), take vital signs, and assess for signs of increasing intracranial pressure (ICP). Elevate the patient's head 30 degrees, if possible, to reduce ICP. Evaluate respiratory status, administer oxygen, and provide intubation and mechanical ventilation, as needed.

Assessment

History

- Determine the onset (and preceding events), duration, intensity, and progression of paralysis.
- Obtain a medical history, including neurologic or neuromuscular disease, recent infectious illness, sexually transmitted disease, cancer, recent injury, or recent immunizations.
- Find out about fever, headache, vision disturbances, dysphagia, nausea and vomiting, bowel or bladder dysfunction, muscle pain or weakness, and fatigue.

Physical assessment

- Perform a complete neurologic examination.
- Test cranial nerve, motor and sensory function, and deep tendon reflexes (DTRs).
- Assess strength in all major muscle groups, noting any muscle atrophy.

Medical causes

Amyotrophic lateral sclerosis

- A life-threatening disorder — spastic or flaccid paralysis occurs in the major muscle groups and progresses to total paralysis.
- Early findings include progressive muscle weakness, fasciculations, hyperreflexia, and muscle atrophy.
- Later, respiratory distress, dysarthria, drooling, choking, and difficulty chewing occur.

Bell's palsy

- Transient paralysis in muscles on one side of the face
- Increased tearing, drooling, inability to close eyelid, and a diminished or absent corneal reflex

Brain tumor

- If a tumor affects the motor cortex of the frontal lobe, contralateral hemiparesis progresses to hemiplegia.
- Early findings include frontal headache and behavioral changes.
- Later findings include seizures, aphasia, and signs of increased ICP.

Conversion disorder

- Loss of voluntary movement can affect any muscle group and has no obvious physical cause.
- Paralysis appears and disappears unpredictably.

Encephalitis

- Variable paralysis develops in the late stages.
- Earlier findings include rapidly deteriorating LOC, fever, headache, photophobia, vomiting, signs of meningeal irritation, aphasia, ataxia, nystagmus, ocular palsies, myoclonus, and seizures.

Guillain-Barré syndrome

- A rapidly developing, reversible paralysis begins as leg muscle weakness and ascends symmetrically; respiratory muscle paralysis may be life-threatening.

Head trauma

- Sudden paralysis may occur; location and extent vary, depending on the injury.
- Other findings include decreased LOC, sensory disturbances, headache, blurred or double vision, nausea, vomiting, and focal neurologic disturbances.

Migraine headache

- Hemiparesis, scotomas, paresthesia, confusion, dizziness, photophobia, and other transient symptoms may precede the onset of a throbbing unilateral headache and may persist after it subsides.

Multiple sclerosis

- Paralysis waxes and wanes until the later stages, when it may become permanent; it ranges from monoplegia to quadriplegia.
- Late findings vary and may include muscle weakness and spasticity, hyperreflexia, intention tremor, gait ataxia, dysphagia, dysarthria, impotence, constipation, and urinary frequency, urgency, and incontinence.

Myasthenia gravis

- Muscle weakness and fatigue produce paralysis of certain muscle groups.
- Paralysis is usually transient in early stages but becomes more persistent as the disease progresses.
- Other findings include ptosis, diplopia, lack of facial mobility, dysphagia, dyspnea, and shallow respirations.

Neurosyphilis

○ Irreversible hemiplegia may occur in the late stages, accompanied by dementia, cranial nerve palsies, meningitis, personality changes, tremors, and abnormal reflexes.

Parkinson's disease

○ Extreme rigidity can progress to paralysis, particularly in the extremities.
○ Tremors, bradykinesia, and "lead-pipe" or "cogwheel" rigidity are the classic signs.

Peripheral nerve trauma

○ Loss of motor and sensory function in the innervated area may occur.
○ Muscles become flaccid and atrophied, and reflexes are lost.

Peripheral neuropathy

○ Muscle weakness may lead to flaccid paralysis and atrophy.
○ Related findings include paresthesia, loss of vibration sensation, hypoactive or absent DTRs, neuralgia, and skin changes.

Rabies

○ Progressive flaccid paralysis, vascular collapse, coma, and death within 2 weeks of contact with an infected animal
○ Early symptoms: fever; headache; hyperesthesia; photophobia; and excessive salivation, lacrimation, and perspiration
○ Within 2 to 10 days, agitation, cranial nerve dysfunction, cyclic respirations, high fever, urine retention, drooling, and hydrophobia

Seizure disorders

○ Transient local paralysis from focal seizures, which may be preceded by an aura

Spinal cord injury

○ Complete spinal cord transection results in permanent spastic paralysis below the level of the injury; reflexes may return after spinal shock resolves.
○ Partial transection causes variable paralysis and paresthesia.

Spinal cord tumor

○ Paresis, pain, paresthesia, and variable sensory loss may occur.
○ Condition may progress to spastic paralysis with hyperactive DTRs and bladder and bowel incontinence.

Stroke

○ Contralateral paresis or paralysis can result if the motor cortex is involved.
○ Other findings include headache, vomiting, seizures, decreased LOC, dysphagia, ataxia, contralateral paresthesia or sensory loss, apraxia, aphasia, vision disturbances, and bowel and bladder dysfunction.

Subarachnoid hemorrhage

○ Sudden paralysis (temporary or permanent) may occur.
○ Other findings include severe headache, mydriasis, photophobia, aphasia, decreased LOC, nuchal rigidity, vomiting, and seizures.

Thoracic aortic aneurysm

○ Sudden transient paralysis
○ Prominent symptoms: severe chest pain radiating to the neck, shoulders, back, and abdomen and a sensation of tearing in the thorax
○ Other findings: diaphoresis, dyspnea, tachycardia, cyanosis, diastolic heart murmur, and abrupt loss of radial and femoral pulses or wide variations in pulses and blood pressure between the arms and legs

Transient ischemic attack

○ Transient paresis or paralysis on one side with paresthesia, blurred or double vision, dizziness, aphasia, dysarthria, and decreased LOC

West Nile encephalitis

○ Paralysis may occur in more severe infections, accompanied by fever, neck stiffness, decreased LOC, seizures, headache, rash, and lymphadenopathy.

Other causes

Drugs

○ Neuromuscular blockers produce paralysis.
○ Electroconvulsive therapy can produce acute, but transient, paralysis.

Nursing considerations

○ Change the patient's position frequently and provide skin care to prevent breakdown.
○ Administer frequent chest physiotherapy.
○ Perform passive range-of-motion exercises to maintain muscle tone.
○ Apply splints to prevent contractures.
○ Use footboards or other devices to prevent footdrop.
○ Arrange for physical, speech, and occupational therapy, as appropriate.

Pediatric pointers

○ Children may develop paralysis from hereditary or congenital disorders.

Patient teaching

○ Provide referrals to social and psychological services.

Paresthesia

Overview

- Refers to abnormal sensation or combination of sensations — commonly described as numbness, prickling, or tingling — along peripheral nerve pathways
- May develop suddenly or gradually and may be transient or permanent

Assessment

History

- Ask about the onset and nature of abnormal sensations.
- Inquire about other findings, such as sensory loss and paresis.
- Find out about recent traumatic injury, surgery, or invasive procedure.
- Take a medical history, including neurologic, cardiovascular, metabolic, renal and chronic inflammatory disorders.

Physical assessment

- Assess level of consciousness (LOC) and cranial nerve function.
- Test muscle strength and deep tendon reflexes (DTRs) in affected limbs.
- Evaluate light touch, pain, temperature, vibration, and position sensation.
- Note skin color and temperature, and palpate pulses.

Medical causes

Arterial occlusion (acute)

- Sudden paresthesia and coldness in one or both legs with a saddle embolus
- Paresis, intermittent claudication, aching pain at rest, and absent pulses below the occlusion

Arteriosclerosis obliterans

- Paresthesia may occur in the affected leg, along with intermittent claudication, pallor, paresis, coldness, and diminished or absent popliteal and pedal pulses.

Arthritis

- If the cervical spine is affected, paresthesias may occur in the neck, shoulders, and arms.
- If the lumbar spine is affected, paresthesias may occur in the legs and feet.

Brain tumor

- Progressive contralateral paresthesia may occur with tumors of the sensory cortex.

- Agnosia, apraxia, agraphia, homonymous hemianopsia, and loss of proprioception may also occur.

Buerger's disease

- Feet become cold, cyanotic, and numb after exposure to cold; later they redden, become hot, and tingle.
- Other findings include intermittent claudication, weak peripheral pulses, migratory superficial thrombophlebitis and, later, ulceration, muscle atrophy, and gangrene.

Diabetes mellitus

- Paresthesia and a burning sensation in the hands and legs
- Other findings: anosmia, fatigue, polyuria, polydipsia, weight loss, and polyphagia.

Guillain-Barré syndrome

- Transient paresthesia may precede muscle weakness, which usually begins in the legs and ascends to the arms and facial nerves.
- Other findings include dysarthria, dysphagia, nasal speech, orthostatic hypotension, bladder and bowel incontinence, diaphoresis, tachycardia and, possibly, life-threatening respiratory muscle paralysis.

Head trauma

- Paresthesia with a concussion or contusion
- Variable paresis or paralysis, decreased LOC, headache, blurred or double vision, nausea, vomiting, dizziness, and seizures.

Heavy metal or solvent poisoning

- Acute or gradual paresthesia
- Mental status changes, tremors, weakness, seizures, and GI distress.

Herniated disk

- Paresthesia may occur along with severe pain, muscle spasms, and weakness.

Herpes zoster

- Paresthesia occurs early in the dermatome supplied by affected spinal nerve.
- Within several days, a pruritic, erythematous, vesicular rash associated with sharp, shooting, or burning pain occurs in the affected dermatome.

Hyperventilation syndrome

- Transient paresthesia in hands, feet, and perioral area
- Agitation, vertigo, syncope, pallor, muscle twitching and weakness, carpopedal spasm and arrhythmias

Hypocalcemia

- Asymmetrical paresthesia in fingers, toes, and circumoral area

○ Muscle weakness, twitching or cramps; palpitations; hyperactive DTRs; carpopedal spasm; and positive Chvostek's and Trousseau's sign

Migraine headache

○ Paresthesia in hands, face, and perioral area may signal an impending migraine headache.
○ Other early findings include scotomas, hemiparesis, confusion, dizziness, and photophobia.

Multiple sclerosis

○ An early symptom, paresthesia commonly waxes and wanes until the later stages when it becomes permanent.
○ Other findings include muscle weakness, spasticity, and hyperreflexia.

Peripheral nerve trauma

○ Paresthesia and dysesthesia in the area supplied by the affected nerve
○ Flaccid paralysis or paresis, hyporeflexia, and sensory loss

Peripheral neuropathy

○ Progressive paresthesia in all extremities
○ Muscle weakness that may progress to flaccid paralysis and atrophy, loss of vibration sensation, diminished or absent DTRs, and cutaneous changes

Rabies

○ Paresthesia, coldness, and itching at site of an animal bite in the early stage

Raynaud's disease

○ Exposure to cold or stress turns fingers pale, cold, and cyanotic; with rewarming, they become red, throbbing, aching, swollen, and paresthetic.

Seizure disorders

○ Paresthesia of the lips, fingers, and toes results from seizures originating in the parietal lobe.
○ Paresthesia may act as auras that precede tonic-clonic seizures.

Spinal cord injury

○ Paresthesia may occur in partial spinal cord transection, after spinal shock resolves, at or below the level of the lesion.
○ Sensory and motor loss varies.

Spinal cord tumors

○ Paresthesia, paresis, pain, and sensory loss occur.
○ Eventually, paresis may cause spastic paralysis with hyperactive DTRs and, possibly, bladder and bowel incontinence.

Stroke

○ Although contralateral paresthesia may occur, sensory loss is more common.

○ Associated findings vary and may include contralateral hemiplegia, decreased LOC, and homonymous hemianopsia.

Systemic lupus erythematosus

○ Paresthesia may occur, but primary findings include nondeforming arthritis, photosensitivity, and a butterfly-shaped rash across the nose and cheeks.

Thoracic outlet syndrome

○ Paresthesia occurs suddenly when the affected arm is raised and abducted.
○ Arm becomes pale and cool, with diminished pulses.

Transient ischemic attack

○ Abrupt paresthesia limited to an isolated body part
○ Decreased LOC, dizziness, unilateral vision loss, nystagmus, aphasia, dysarthria, tinnitus, facial weakness, dysphagia, and ataxic gait

Vitamin B deficiency

○ Paresthesia and weakness in the arms and legs
○ Burning leg pain, hypoactive DTRs, variable sensory loss, changes in mental status, and impaired vision

Other causes

Drugs

○ Phenytoin, chemotherapeutics, D-penicillamine, isoniazid, nitrofurantoin, chloroquine, and parenteral gold therapy may produce transient paresthesia.

Radiation therapy

○ Long-term radiation therapy may cause peripheral nerve damage, resulting in paresthesia.

Nursing considerations

○ Monitor neurologic status.
○ Help the patient perform daily activities as needed.
○ If sensory deficits are present, protect the patient from injury.

Pediatric pointers

○ Children usually can't describe this symptom.
○ Hereditary polyneuropathies are first recognized in childhood.

Patient teaching

○ Discuss safety measures.
○ Tell the patient which signs and symptoms to report.

Peau d'orange

Overview

- Edematous thickening and pitting of breast skin resembling an orange peel (See *Recognizing peau d'orange.*)
- Usually a late sign of breast cancer

Assessment

History

- Ask when peau d'orange was first noticed.
- Inquire about lumps, pain, or other breast changes.
- Find out about associated malaise, achiness, and weight loss.
- Take a lactation history.
- Obtain a history of previous breast or axillary surgery.

Physical assessment

- Estimate extent of peau d'orange.
- Check for breast erythema and induration.
- Assess nipples for discharge, deviation, retraction, dimpling, and cracking.
- Palpate peau d'orange for warmth or induration.
- Palpate the rest of the breast for lumps.
- Palpate axillary lymph nodes, noting enlargement.
- Take the patient's temperature.

Medical causes

Breast abscess

- Peau d'orange with malaise, breast tenderness and erythema, and a sudden fever with shaking chills.
- Purulent discharge from a cracked nipple and possibly a mass.

Breast cancer

- Peau d'orange usually begins in the dependent part of the breast or the areola.
- Palpation typically reveals a firm, immobile mass that adheres to the skin above the area of peau d'orange .
- Other findings may include changes in breast contour, size, or symmetry; nipples may reveal deviation, erosion, retraction, and a thin and watery, bloody, or purulent discharge.

Erysipelas

- A well-demarcated, erythematous, elevated area, typically with a peau d'orange texture
- Pain, warmth, fever, and fatigue

Graves' disease

- Raised, thickened, hyperpigmented, peau d'orange areas that join together
- Weight loss, palpitations, anxiety, heat intolerance, tremor, and amenorrhea

Assessment tip
Recognizing peau d'orange

In peau d'orange, the skin appears to be pitted (as shown at right). This condition usually indicates late-stage breast cancer.

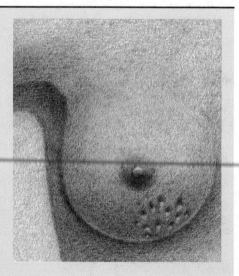

Nursing considerations

○ After cancer is ruled out, treat the underlying disorder.
○ Provide emotional support.

Patient teaching

○ Explain diagnostic tests the patient needs.
○ Teach the patient how to do monthly breast self-examinations.
○ Discuss signs and symptoms the patient needs to report.

Pericardial rub

Overview

- The scratching, grating, or crunching sound made when two inflamed layers of the pericardium slide over each other
- Three types: presystolic, systolic, and diastolic (see *Understanding pericardial rubs*)
- Ranges from faint to loud
- Best heard along the lower left sternal border during deep inspiration

History

- Take a medical history, noting cardiac dysfunction, myocardial infarction, cardiac surgery, pericarditis, rheumatoid arthritis, chronic renal failure, infection, or systemic lupus erythematosus.
- Obtain a description of any chest pain, including character, location, and aggravating and alleviating factors.

Physical assessment

- Take vital signs, noting hypotension, tachycardia, irregular pulse, tachypnea, and fever.
- Inspect for jugular vein distention, edema, ascites, and hepatomegaly.
- Auscultate heart sounds; to listen for a pericardial friction rub, have the patient sit upright, lean forward and exhale. (See *Pericardial rub or murmur?*)
- Auscultate the lungs for crackles. (*See Comparing auscultation findings.*)

Medical causes

Pericarditis

- Pericardial rub, the classic sign of acute pericarditis, is accompanied by sharp precordial or retrosternal pain that radiates to the left shoulder, neck, and back.
- Pain worsens with deep breathing, coughing, and lying flat.

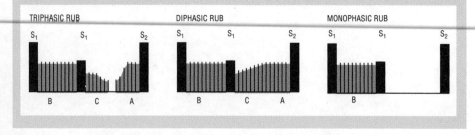

Assessment tip
Understanding pericardial rubs

The complete, or classic, pericardial rub is triphasic. Its three sound components are linked to phases of the cardiac cycle. The *presystolic* component (A) reflects atrial systole and precedes the first heart sound (S_1). The *systolic* component (B) — usually the loudest — reflects ventricular systole and occurs between the S_1 and the second heart sound (S_2). The early *diastolic* component (C) reflects ventricular diastole and follows the S_2.

Sometimes, the early diastolic component merges with the presystolic component, producing a diphasic to-and-fro sound on auscultation. In other patients, auscultation may detect only one component — a monophasic rub, typically during ventricular systole.

TRIPHASIC RUB   DIPHASIC RUB   MONOPHASIC RUB

S_1 S_1 S_2 S_1 S_1 S_2 S_1 S_1 S_2

B   C   A   B   C   A   B

During auscultation, you may detect a pleural friction rub, crackles, or a pericardial friction rub—three abnormal sounds that are commonly confused. Use this chart to help clarify auscultation findings.

Finding	Cause	Quality	Location	Timing
Pleural rub	Inflamed visceral and parietal pleural surfaces rub against each other.	Loud and grating, creaking, or squeaking	Best heard over the low axilla or the anterior, lateral, or posterior base of the lung	Occurs in late inspiration and early expiration but ceases when the patient holds his breath; persists during coughing
Crackles	Air suddenly enters fluid-filled airways.	Nonmusical clicking or rattling	Best heard at less distended and more dependent areas of the lungs, usually at the bases	Occurs chiefly during inspiration
Pericardial rub	Inflamed layers of the pericardium rub against each other.	Hard and grating, scratching, or crunching	Best heard along the lower left sternal border	Occurs in relation to heartbeat; most noticeable during deep inspiration and continues even when the patient holds his breath

○ Pain lessens when the patient sits up and leans forward.

○ Other findings of the acute condition include fever, dyspnea, tachycardia, and arrhythmias.

○ In the chronic condition, a pericardial rub develops gradually and may be accompanied by peripheral edema, ascites, Kussmaul's sign, hepatomegaly, dyspnea, orthopnea, paradoxical pulse, and chest pain.

Other causes

Drugs

○ Procainamide and chemotherapeutics can cause pericarditis.

Nursing considerations

○ Monitor the patient's cardiovascular status.

○ If the pericardial rub disappears, look for signs of cardiac tamponade; if the signs develop, prepare the patient for pericardiocentesis.

○ Ensure that the patient gets adequate rest.

○ Give an anti-inflammatory, antiarrhythmic, diuretic, or antimicrobial to treat the underlying cause.

○ Anticipate pericardiectomy to promote cardiac filling and contraction.

Pediatric pointers

○ A pericardial rub may develop with bacterial pericarditis, a life-threatening condition that usually occurs before age 6.

○ A pericardial rub may occur after surgery to correct congenital cardiac anomalies.

Patient teaching

○ Explain the underlying disorder and its treatments.

○ Explain what the patient can do to minimize his symptoms.

Peristaltic waves, visible

Overview

- Occur when peristalsis increases in strength and frequency as the intestine contracts to force its contents past an obstruction
- Usually, peristaltic waves aren't visible; if they are, they consist of waves that appear suddenly and vanish quickly
- Best detected by stooping at the patient's side and inspecting abdominal contour while he's in a supine position

Assessment

History

- Obtain a medical history, including a history of pyloric ulcer, stomach cancer, chronic gastritis, intestinal obstruction, intestinal tumors or polyps, gallstones, chronic constipation, and hernia.
- Ask about recent abdominal surgery.
- Take a drug history.
- Find out about related signs and symptoms, such as abdominal pain, nausea, and vomiting.
- Obtain a description of the vomitus, including consistency, amount, and color.

Physical assessment

- Inspect the abdomen for distention, surgical scars, adhesions, or visible bowel loops.
- Auscultate for bowel sounds.
- Roll the patient from side to side and then auscultate for succussion splash, which is a splashing sound in the stomach from retained secretions caused by pyloric obstruction.
- Percuss for tympany. (See *Performing an abdominal assessment.*)

Assessment tip
Performing an abdominal assessment

When performing an abdominal assessment, use this sequence:
1. Inspection
2. Auscultation
3. Percussion
4. Palpation
   Palpating or percussing the abdomen before you auscultate can change the character of the patient's bowel sounds, resulting in an inaccurate assessment.

- Palpate abdomen for rigidity and tenderness.
- Check skin and mucous membranes for dryness and poor skin turgor.
- Take vital signs, noting tachycardia and hypotension.

Medical causes

Large-bowel obstruction

- Visible peristaltic waves in the upper abdomen are an early sign.
- Obstipation (severe constipation) may be the earliest sign.
- Other characteristic findings include nausea, colicky abdominal pain, abdominal distention, and hyperactive bowel sounds.

Pyloric obstruction

- Peristaltic waves may be detected in a swollen epigastrium or in the left upper quadrant, usually beginning near the left rib margin and rolling from left to right.
- Auscultation reveals a loud succussion splash.
- Related findings include vague epigastric discomfort or colicky pain after eating; nausea; vomiting; anorexia; and weight loss.

Small-bowel obstruction

- Peristaltic waves rolling across the upper abdomen and intermittent, cramping, periumbilical pain are early signs along with hyperactive bowel sounds and slight abdominal distention.
- Other findings include nausea; vomiting of bilious or, later, fecal material; and constipation.
- With partial obstruction, diarrhea may occur.

Nursing considerations

- Withhold food and fluids.
- If obstruction is confirmed, perform nasogastric suctioning to decompress the stomach and small bowel.
- Provide frequent oral hygiene.
- Monitor for dehydration.
- Frequently monitor vital signs and intake and output.

Pediatric pointers

- In infants, visible peristaltic waves may indicate pyloric stenosis.
- In small children, peristaltic waves may be visible normally or may indicate bowel obstruction.

Geriatric pointers

- In elderly patients, always check for fecal impaction, which is common in this age-group.

○ Obtain a detailed drug history; antidepressants and antipsychotics can predispose to constipation and bowel obstruction.

Patient teaching
○ Discuss diet and fluid requirements.
○ Encourage the use of stool softeners and increased intake of high-fiber foods for patients with chronic constipation.

Photophobia

Overview

- Refers to abnormal sensitivity to light
- Commonly indicates increased eye sensitivity without any underlying pathology
- May indicate a systemic disorder, an ocular disorder or trauma, or the use of certain drugs

Assessment

History

- Ask about the onset and severity of photophobia.
- Inquire about recent eye trauma, chemical splash, or exposure to rays of a sun lamp.
- Obtain a description of the location, duration, intensity, and characteristics of any pain or discomfort.
- Find out about vision changes or increased tearing.

Physical assessment

- Take vital signs.
- Assess neurologic status.
- Assess visual activity, unless the cause is a chemical burn.
- Inspect the eyes' external structures.
- Examine the conjunctivae and sclera, noting their color.
- Characterize the amount and consistency of any discharge.
- Check pupillary reaction to light.
- Evaluate extraocular muscle function by testing the six cardinal positions of gaze.
- Test visual acuity.

Medical causes

Burns

- With a chemical burn, photophobia and eye pain may be accompanied by erythema and blistering on the face and lids, miosis, diffuse conjunctival injection, blurred vision, inability to keep the eyes open, and corneal changes.
- With ultraviolet radiation burn, photophobia occurs with moderate to severe eye pain.

Conjunctivitis

- Photophobia occurs when conjunctivitis affects the cornea.
- Other common findings include conjunctival injection, increased tearing, a foreign-body sensation, a feeing of fullness around the eyes, and eye pain, burning, and itching.
- Allergic conjunctivitis causes stringy eye discharge and milky red injection.
- Bacterial conjunctivitis causes brilliant red conjunctiva with copious, mucopurulent, flaky eye discharge.
- Fungal conjunctivitis produces a thick, purulent discharge; extreme redness; and crusting, sticky eyelids.
- Viral conjunctivitis causes copious tearing with little discharge and enlarged preauricular nodes.

Corneal abrasion

- Photophobia is usually accompanied by excessive tearing, conjunctival injection, visible corneal damage, blurred vision, eye pain, and foreign-body sensation in the eye.

Corneal foreign body

- Photophobia may occur with miosis, intense eye pain, foreign-body sensation, slightly impaired vision, conjunctival injection, and profuse tearing.

Corneal ulcer

- Severe photophobia and eye pain are aggravated by blinking.
- Impaired visual acuity, blurring, eye discharge, conjunctival injection, and sticky eyelids may also occur.
- A bacterial ulcer may also cause an irregularly shaped corneal ulcer and pupillary constriction.
- A fungal ulcer may be surrounded by progressively clearer rings.

Dry eye syndrome

- Photophobia may occur, but eye pain, conjunctival injection, a foreign-body sensation, itching, excessive mucus secretion and, possibly, decreased tearing and difficulty moving the eyelids are more common symptoms.

Iritis (acute)

- Severe photophobia occurs, along with conjunctival injection, moderate to severe eye pain, and blurred vision.
- Pupil may be constricted and respond poorly to light.

Keratitis (interstitial)

- Photophobia occurs along with eye pain, blurred vision, dramatic conjunctival injection, and grayish pink corneas.

Meningitis (acute bacterial)

- Photophobia occurs with such signs as nuchal rigidity, hyperreflexia, Brudzinski's and Kernig's signs, fever, chills, and opisthotonos.
- Related findings include headache, vomiting, ocular palsies, facial weakness, pupillary abnormalities, hearing loss, seizures, and altered level of consciousness.

Migraine headache

- Photophobia and noise sensitivity are prominent features.

○ Other findings include fatigue, blurred vision, nausea, and vomiting.

Scleritis

○ Photophobia occurs along with severe eye pain, conjunctival injection, a bluish purple sclera, and profuse tearing.

Uveitis

○ Photophobia results from both anterior and posterior uveitis.
○ Anterior uveitis also produces moderate to severe eye pain, severe conjunctival injection, and a small, nonreactive pupil.
○ Posterior uveitis develops slowly, causing visual floaters, eye pain, pupil distortion, conjunctival injection, and blurred vision.

Other causes

Drugs

○ Mydriatics, amphetamines, cocaine, and ophthalmic antifungals can cause photophobia.

Nursing considerations

○ Darken the room and tell the patient to close his eyes.
○ Administer corticosteroids and antibiotic drops or ointment.
○ If the underlying disorder can be identified, begin treatment for it.
○ Saline drops or other lubricating ointment can soothe dry eyes and improve photophobia.

Pediatric pointers

○ Suspect photophobia in a child who squints, rubs his eyes frequently, or wears sunglasses indoors and outside.
○ Congenital disorders such as albinism and childhood diseases, such as measles and rubella, can cause photophobia.

Patient teaching

○ Teach the patient ways to increase comfort.
○ Explain diagnostic tests the patient needs.

Pleural rub

Overview

- Loud, coarse, grating, creaking, or squeaking sound that may be auscultated during late inspiration or early expiration
- Indicative of inflammation of the visceral and parietal pleural lining
- Heard best over the low axilla or the anterior, lateral, or posterior bases of the lungs fields with the patient upright

> ### Emergency actions
>
> *Quickly look for signs of respiratory distress. Check for hypotension, tachycardia, and decreased level of consciousness. If you see signs of distress, open and maintain an airway. Endotracheal intubation and supplemental oxygen may be necessary. Insert a large-bore I.V. line to deliver drugs and fluids. Elevate the patient's head 30 degrees. Monitor cardiac status constantly, and check vital signs frequently.*

Assessment

History

- Obtain a description of chest pain, including onset, location, severity, duration, radiation, and aggravating and alleviating factors.
- Take a medical history, including rheumatoid arthritis, a respiratory or cardiovascular disorder, recent trauma, asbestos exposure, and radiation therapy.
- Ask about smoking history.

Physical assessment

- Auscultate the lungs with the patient sitting upright and breathing deeply and slowly through the mouth.
- Determine whether the rub is in one lung or both.
- Listen for absent or diminished breath sounds.
- Palpate for decreased chest motion and percuss for flatness or dullness.
- Observe for clubbing and pedal edema.

Medical causes

Asbestosis

- Pleural rub, exertional dyspnea, cough, chest pain, and crackles may occur.
- As the disease advances, clubbing and dyspnea develop.

Lung cancer

- A pleural rub may be heard in the area of the lung that's affected by the cancer.

- Other findings include a cough (possibly with hemoptysis), dyspnea, chest pain, weight loss, anorexia, fatigue, clubbing, fever, and wheezing.

Pleurisy

- A pleural rub occurs early.
- The main symptom is sudden, intense, unilateral chest pain in the lower and lateral parts of the chest; deep breathing, coughing, and thoracic movements aggravate the pain.
- Other findings include decreased breath sounds, inspiratory crackles, dyspnea, tachypnea, tachycardia, cyanosis, fever, and fatigue.

Pneumonia (bacterial)

- A pleural rub after a dry, painful, hacking, productive cough
- Shaking chills, high fever, headache, dyspnea, pleuritic chest pain, tachypnea, tachycardia, grunting respirations, nasal flaring, dullness to percussion, decreased breath sounds, and cyanosis

Pulmonary embolism

- A pleural rub may occur over the affected area of the lung.
- The first symptom is usually sudden dyspnea, which may be accompanied by angina or unilateral pleuritic chest pain.
- Other findings include a nonproductive cough or a cough that produces blood-tinged sputum, tachycardia, tachypnea, low-grade fever, restlessness, and diaphoresis.

Rheumatoid arthritis

- A unilateral pleural rub may occur.
- Typical early findings include fatigue, persistent low-grade fever, weight loss, and vague arthralgia and myalgia.
- Later findings include warm, swollen, painful joints; joint stiffness after activity; subcutaneous nodules on the elbows; joint deformity; and muscle weakness and atrophy.

Systemic lupus erythematosus

- A pleural rub — accompanied by hemoptysis, dyspnea, pleuritic chest pain, and crackles — may occur with pulmonary involvement.
- More characteristic effects include a butterfly-shaped rash, nondeforming joint pain and stiffness, and photosensitivity.
- Fever, anorexia, weight loss, and lymphadenopathy may also occur.

Tuberculosis (pulmonary)

- A pleural rub may occur over the affected part of the lung.
- Early findings include weight loss, night sweats, low-grade fever in the afternoon, malaise, dyspnea, anorexia, and easy fatigability.

- Disease progression produces pleuritic chest pain, fine crackles over the upper lobes, and a productive cough with blood-streaked sputum.
- Advanced findings include chest wall retraction, tracheal deviation, and dullness to percussion.

Other causes

Treatments

- Thoracic surgery and radiation therapy can cause pleural rub.

Nursing considerations

- Monitor the patient's respiratory status and vital signs.
- If the patient has a persistent dry, hacking cough that tires him, give an antitussive.
- Administer oxygen and an antibiotic.

Pediatric pointers

- Auscultate for a pleural rub in a child who has grunting respirations, reports chest pain, or protects his chest.
- A pleural rub in a child is usually an early sign of pleurisy.

Geriatric pointers

- Pleuritic chest pain may mimic cardiac chest pain.

Patient teaching

- Prepare the patient for diagnostic tests.
- Discuss pain relief measures.
- Explain signs and symptoms the patient needs to report.

Polydipsia

Overview

○ Refers to excessive thirst
○ May reflect decreased fluid intake, increased urine output, or excessive loss of water and salt

Assessment

History

○ Determine the patient's average fluid intake and output.
○ Obtain a description of his urinary patterns.
○ Take a personal or family history of diabetes or kidney disease.
○ Take a drug history.
○ Ask about recent weight loss.

Physical assessment

○ Obtain the patient's blood pressure and pulse when he's in supine and standing positions.
○ Check for signs of dehydration.

Medical causes

Diabetes insipidus

○ Polydipsia, excessive voiding of dilute urine, and nocturia occur.
○ Fatigue and signs of dehydration occur in severe cases.

Diabetes mellitus

○ Polydipsia is a classic finding.
○ Polyuria, polyphagia, nocturia, and signs of dehydration may also occur.

Hypercalcemia

○ In later stages, polydipsia occurs with polyuria, nocturia, constipation, paresthesia and, occasionally, hematuria and pyuria.
○ If hypercalcemia is severe, vomiting, decreased level of consciousness, and renal failure develop.

Hypokalemia

○ Polydipsia, polyuria, and nocturia may develop.
○ Other related signs and symptoms include muscle weakness or paralysis, fatigue, decreased bowel sounds, hypoactive deep tendon reflexes, and arrhythmias.

Psychogenic polydipsia

○ This psychiatric condition causes polydipsia in the absence of a physiologic stimulus to drink.
○ No apparent reason for excessive thirst or fluid intake exists.
○ The condition may be well-tolerated if water intoxication and hyponatremia don't occur
○ Related findings include confusion, headache, irritability, weight gain, elevated blood pressure, stupor, and coma.

Renal disorders (chronic)

○ Polydipsia and polyuria signal kidney damage.
○ Other related findings include nocturia, weakness, elevated blood pressure, pallor and, in later stages, oliguria.

Sickle cell anemia

○ Polydipsia and polyuria occur as nephropathy develops.
○ Other related signs and symptoms include abdominal pain and cramps, arthralgia and, occasionally, lower extremity skin ulcers and such bone deformities as kyphosis.

Thyrotoxicosis

○ Polydipsia may occur infrequently with this disorder.
○ Characteristic findings include tachycardia, palpitations, weight loss despite increased appetite, diarrhea, tremors, nervousness, heat intolerance, and enlarged thyroid.

Other causes

Drugs

○ Diuretics and demeclocycline may produce polydipsia.
○ Phenothiazines and anticholinergics can cause dry mouth, making the patient so thirsty that he drinks compulsively.

Nursing considerations

○ Record total intake and output.
○ Weigh the patient at the same time each day using the same scale.
○ Check blood pressure and pulse in supine and standing positions.
○ Give the patient ample liquids.

Pediatric pointers

○ In children, polydipsia usually stems from diabetes insipidus or diabetes mellitus.
○ Psychogenic polydipsia in children may reflect emotional difficulties.

Patient teaching

○ Explain the underlying disorder and treatment the patient needs.
○ Teach the patient about diet, exercise, and home blood glucose monitoring.
○ Stress the importance of reporting significant weight gain or loss.

Polyphagia

Overview

○ Refers to voracious or excessive eating
○ Can be persistent or intermittent, resulting from endocrine and psychological disorders as well as the use of certain drugs

Assessment

History

○ Ask about food intake during previous 24 hours, noting frequency of meals and amounts of types of foods eaten.
○ Note recent changes in food habits.
○ Inquire about the pattern of overeating.
○ Ask about any conditions triggering overeating, such as stress, depression, or menstruation.
○ Ask the patient about vomiting or headache after overeating.
○ Explore other relevant signs and symptoms, such as a recent gain or loss of weight; feeling tired, nervous, or excitable; and heat intolerance, dizziness, palpitations, diarrhea, or increased thirst or urination.
○ Obtain a complete drug history, including the use of laxatives or enemas.

Physical assessment

○ Weigh the patient and observe him when you tell him his current weight.
○ Inspect the patient's skin to detect dryness or poor turgor.
○ Palpate for thyroid enlargement.

Medical causes

Anxiety

○ Polyphagia may result from mild to moderate anxiety or emotional stress.
○ Mild anxiety may produce restlessness, sleeplessness, irritability, repetitive questioning, and constant seeking of attention and reassurance.
○ Moderate anxiety may produce selective inattention and difficulty concentrating.
○ Other effects of anxiety include muscle tension, diaphoresis, GI distress, palpitations, tachycardia, and urinary and sexual dysfunction.

Bulimia

○ Polyphagia alternates with self-induced vomiting, fasting, or diarrhea.
○ Bulimia most commonly occurs in women ages 18 to 29.

○ The patient typically weighs less than normal but has a morbid fear of obesity, is depressed, has low self-esteem, and conceals her overeating.

Diabetes mellitus

○ Polyphagia occurs with weight loss, polydipsia, and polyuria.
○ Other characteristic signs and symptoms include nocturia, weakness, fatigue, and signs of dehydration, such as dry mucous membranes and poor skin turgor.

Migraine headache

○ Polyphagia sometimes precedes a migraine headache.
○ The patient may experience changes in appetite and food cravings.
○ Other early signs and symptoms include fatigue, nausea, vomiting, light and noise sensitivity, and a visual aura.

Premenstrual syndrome

○ Appetite changes, such as food cravings and binges, may occur.
○ Other findings include abdominal bloating, depression, insomnia, headache, paresthesia, diarrhea or constipation, edema and temporary weight gain, palpitations, back pain, breast swelling and tenderness, oliguria, and easy bruising.

Thyrotoxicosis

○ Despite constant polyphagia, weight loss occurs.
○ Other characteristic signs and symptoms include weakness, nervousness, diarrhea, tremors, thin and brittle hair and nails, diaphoresis, dyspnea, palpitations, tachycardia, heat intolerance, exophthalmos, atrial or ventricular gallop, and an enlarged thyroid.

Other causes

Drugs

○ Corticosteroids and cyproheptadine may increase appetite, causing weight gain.

Nursing considerations

○ Monitor the patient's eating habits.
○ Weigh the patient once or twice per week.
○ Refer the patient to a registered dietitian for nutritional counseling, if needed.
○ Provide emotional support.

Pediatric pointers

○ In children, polyphagia commonly results from juvenile diabetes.

- In infants ages 6 to 18 months, polyphagia can result from a malabsorptive disorder.
- Polyphagia may also occur in a child experiencing a growth spurt.

Patient teaching

- Refer the patient for nutritional counseling.
- Provide referral for personal or family counseling.
- Provide emotional support and help the patient to understand the disease process.

Polyuria

Overview

○ Daily production and excretion of more than 3 L of urine

Assessment

History

○ Explore the frequency and pattern of polyuria.
○ Ask for a description of patterns and amounts of daily fluid intake.
○ Inquire about fatigue, increased thirst, or weight loss.
○ Obtain a medical history of visual deficits, headaches, head trauma, urinary tract obstruction, diabetes mellitus, renal disorder, chronic hypokalemia or hypercalcemia, or psychiatric disorder.
○ Take a drug history.

Physical assessment

○ Take vital signs, noting increased body temperature, tachycardia, and orthostatic hypotension.
○ Inspect for signs of dehydration.
○ Perform a neurologic assessment, noting any change in level of consciousness.
○ Palpate the bladder and inspect the urethral meatus.
○ Obtain a urine specimen and check specific gravity.

Medical causes

Acute tubular necrosis

○ During the diuretic phase, urine output of more than 8 L/day gradually subsides after about 1 week.
○ Urine specific gravity (1.101 or less) increases as polyuria subsides.
○ Related findings include weight loss, decreasing edema, and nocturia.

Diabetes insipidus

○ Polyuria of about 5 L/day occurs, with urine specific gravity of 1.005 or less.
○ Accompanying findings include polydipsia, nocturia, fatigue, and signs of dehydration.

Diabetes mellitus

○ Polyuria is seldom more than 5 L/day, and urine specific gravity is typically more than 1.020.
○ Other findings include polydipsia, polyphagia, weight loss, frequent urinary tract infections and yeast vaginitis, fatigue, signs of dehydration, and nocturia.

Glomerulonephritis (chronic)

○ Polyuria gradually progresses to oliguria.

○ Urine output is usually less than 4 L/day; specific gravity is about 1.010.
○ Related GI findings include anorexia, nausea, and vomiting.
○ Other findings include drowsiness, fatigue, edema, headache, elevated blood pressure, dyspnea, nocturia, hematuria, frothy or malodorous urine, and proteinuria.

Hypercalcemia

○ Polyuria of more than 5 L/day with a urine specific gravity of about 1.010
○ Polydipsia, nocturia, constipation, paresthesia, and, occasionally, hematuria, and pyuria
○ With severe hypercalcemia, anorexia, vomiting, stupor progressing to coma, and renal failure

Hypokalemia

○ Prolonged potassium depletion causes polyuria of less than 5 L/day with a urine specific gravity of about 1.010.
○ Other findings include polydipsia, circumoral and foot paresthesia, hypoactive deep tendon reflexes, fatigue, hypoactive bowel sounds, nocturia, arrhythmias, and muscle cramping, weakness, or paralysis.

Postobstructive uropathy

○ After resolution of a urinary tract obstruction, polyuria — usually more than 5 L/day with a urine specific gravity of less than 1.010 — occurs for up to several days before gradually subsiding.
○ Other findings include bladder distention, edema, nocturia, and weight loss.

Pyelonephritis

○ Polyuria of less than 5 L/day with a low but variable urine specific gravity occurs in acute disease.
○ Other findings of the acute condition include persistent high fever, flank pain, hematuria, costovertebral angle tenderness, chills, weakness, dysuria, urinary frequency and urgency, tenesmus, and nocturia.
○ Chronic pyelonephritis produces polyuria of less than 5 L/day that declines as renal function worsens; urine specific gravity is usually about 1.010 but may be higher if proteinuria is present.
○ Other effects of the chronic condition include irritability, paresthesia, fatigue, nausea, vomiting, diarrhea, drowsiness, anorexia, pyuria and, in late stages, elevated blood pressure.

Sickle cell anemia

○ Polyuria occurs with a urinary output of less than 5 L/day with a specific gravity of about 1.020.
○ Additional findings include polydipsia, fatigue, abdominal cramps, arthralgia, priapism and, occasionally, leg ulcers and bony deformities.

Other causes

Diagnostic tests

○ Radiographic tests that use contrast media may cause transient polyuria.

Drugs

○ Diuretics produce polyuria.
○ Cardiotonics, vitamin D, demeclocycline, phenytoin, lithium, methoxyflurane, and propoxyphene can also produce polyuria.

Nursing considerations

○ Record intake and output, and weigh the patient daily.
○ Monitor vital signs.
○ Encourage fluid intake to maintain adequate fluid balance.

Pediatric pointers

○ The major causes of polyuria in children are congenital nephrogenic diabetes insipidus, medullary cystic disease, polycystic renal disease, and distal renal tubular acidosis.
○ Because a child's fluid balance is more delicate than an adult's, check urine's specific gravity at each voiding and be alert for signs of dehydration.

Geriatric pointers

○ Chronic pyelonephritis is commonly associated with an underlying disorder.

Patient teaching

○ Explain the facts about underlying disorder.
○ Explain fluid replacement.
○ Instruct the patient on weight monitoring.
○ Explain the signs and symptoms of dehydration the patient needs to report.

Pruritus

Overview

- Unpleasant itching sensation that provokes scratching to gain relief
- Exacerbated by increased skin temperature, poor skin turgor, local vasodilation, dermatoses, and stress

Assessment

History

- Ask about the onset, frequency, duration, and intensity of pruritus.
- Determine location, whether it's localized or generalized, and what aggravates and alleviates it.
- Ask about contact with irritants.
- Obtain a description of skin care practices.
- Take a drug history.
- Obtain a medical history.
- Find out about recent travel and pets in the home.

Physical assessment

- Observe for signs of scratching, such as excoriation, purpura, scabs, scars, or lichenification.
- Look for primary lesions to help confirm dermatoses.

Medical causes

Anemia (iron deficiency)

- Pruritus occasionally occurs.
- Late findings include exertional dyspnea, fatigue, listlessness, pallor, irritability, headache, tachycardia, poor muscle tone and, possibly, murmurs.
- Chronic anemia causes spoon-shaped (koilonychias) and brittle nails (cheilosis), cracked mouth corners, a smooth tongue (glossitis), and dysphagia.

Anthrax (cutaneous)

- Early infection causes small, painless or pruritic, macular or papular lesion resembling an insect bite.
- In 1 or 2 days, lesion develops into a vesicular lesion and then a painless ulcer with a black, necrotic center.
- Other findings include lymphadenopathy, malaise, headache, or fever.

Conjunctivitis

- All forms cause eye itching, burning, and pain along with photophobia, conjunctival injection, a foreign-body sensation, and excessive tearing.

Dermatitis

- Pruritus may be accompanied by a skin lesion.

- Atopic dermatitis begins with intense, severe pruritus and an erythematous rash on dry skin at flexion points.
- In chronic atopic dermatitis, lesions may progress to dry, scaly skin with white dermatographism, blanching, and lichenification.
- In contact dermatitis, itchy, small vesicles may ooze and scale and are surrounded by redness; localized edema may occur with a severe reaction.
- Dermatitis herpetiformis initially causes intense pruritus; 8 to 12 hours later, symmetrically distributed lesions form on the buttocks, shoulders, elbows, and knees.

Enterobiasis

- Intense perianal pruritus occurs, especially at night.
- Other findings include irritability, scratching, skin irritation and, sometimes, vaginitis.

Hemorrhoids

- Anal pruritus, rectal pain, and constipation may occur.

Hepatobiliary disease

- Pruritus, commonly accompanied by jaundice, may be generalized or localized to the palms and soles.
- Other findings include right-upper-quadrant pain, clay-colored stools, chills, fever, flatus, belching, a bloated feeling, epigastric burning, and bitter fluid regurgitation.
- Later findings include mental changes, ascites, bleeding tendencies, spider angiomas, palmar erythema, dry skin, fetor hepaticus, enlarged superficial abdominal veins, bilateral gynecomastia, and hepatomegaly.

Herpes zoster

- Within 4 days of fever and malaise, pruritus, paresthesia or hyperesthesia, and severe, deep pain develop in a dermatome distribution.
- Up to 2 weeks after initial symptoms, red, nodular skin eruptions appear on the painful areas and become vesicular; about 10 days later, vesicles rupture and form scabs.

Hodgkin's disease

- Severe, unexplained itching occasionally occurs.
- Early findings include persistent fever, night sweats, fatigue, weight loss, malaise, and painless lymph node swelling.
- Later findings include hepatomegaly, splenomegaly, dyspnea, dysphagia, dry cough, hyperpigmentation, jaundice, and pallor.

Lichen simplex chronicus

- Localized pruritus and a circumscribed scaling patch with sharp margins develop.
- Later, skin thickens and papules form.

Pediculosis

○ Pruritus in the area of infestation is a prominent symptom of infestation.

○ Pediculosis capitis may cause scalp excoriation from scratching; foul-smelling, lusterless, matted hair; occipital and cervical lymphadenopathy; and oval, gray-white nits on hair shafts.

○ Pediculosis corporis initially causes red papules, which become urticarial from scratching; later, rashes or wheals may develop.

○ Pediculosis pubis is marked by nits or adult lice and erythematous, itching papules in pubic hair or hair around the anus, abdomen, or thighs.

Pityriasis rosea

○ Pruritus that's aggravated by a hot bath or shower occasionally occurs.

○ An erythematous herald patch forms and progresses to scaly, yellow, erythematous patches that erupt on the trunk or extremities and persist for 2 to 6 weeks.

Polycythemia vera

○ Pruritus is generalized or localized to the head, neck, face, and extremities; hot baths and showers typically aggravate it.

○ A deep purplish red develops on the oral mucosa, gingivae, and tongue.

○ Related findings include headache, dizziness, fatigue, dyspnea, paresthesia, impaired mentation, tinnitus, double or blurred vision, scotoma, hypotension, intermittent claudication, urticaria, ruddy cyanosis, hepatosplenomegaly, and ecchymosis.

Psoriasis

○ Pruritus and pain commonly occur.

○ Small erythematous papules enlarge or coalesce to form red, elevated plaques with silver scales on the scalp, chest, elbows, knees, back, buttocks, and genitals.

Renal failure (chronic)

○ Pruritus may develop gradually or suddenly.

○ Other findings include ammonia breath odor, oliguria or anuria, fatigue, decreased mental acuity, muscle twitching and cramps, anorexia, nausea, vomiting, peripheral neuropathies, and coma.

Scabies

○ Localized pruritus that awakens the patient typically occurs.

○ Threadlike lesions appear with a swollen nodule or red papule.

Thyrotoxicosis

○ Generalized pruritus may precede or accompany the characteristic findings of tachycardia, palpitations, weight loss despite increased appetite, tremors, diarrhea, an enlarged thyroid, dyspnea, nervousness, diaphoresis, heat intolerance and, possibly, exophthalmos.

Tinea pedis

○ Severe foot pruritus typically occurs with scales and blisters between the toes and a dry, scaly squamous inflammation on the sole.

Urticaria

○ Extreme pruritus and stinging occur as transient erythematous or whitish wheals form on the skin or mucous membranes.

Vaginitis

○ Localized pruritus commonly occurs with foul-smelling vaginal discharge that may be purulent, white or gray, and curdlike.

○ Perineal pain and urinary symptoms may occur.

Other causes

Drug hypersensitivity

○ When mild and localized, an allergic reaction to drugs such as penicillin and sulfonamides can cause pruritus, erythema, urticaria, and edema.

Nursing considerations

○ Administer a topical or oral corticosteroid, an antihistamine, or a tranquilizer.

Pediatric pointers

○ Many adult disorders also cause pruritus in children, but they may affect different parts of the body.

○ Such childhood diseases as measles and chickenpox can also cause pruritus.

Patient teaching

○ Teach the patient ways to control pruritus.

Psychotic behavior

Overview

- Inability or unwillingness to recognize and acknowledge reality and to relate to others
- May begin suddenly or insidiously
- May progress from vague complaints of fatigue, insomnia, or headache to withdrawal, social isolation, and preoccupation with certain issues resulting from gross impairment in functioning
- *Delusions* are persistent beliefs that have no basis in reality or in the patient's knowledge or experience
- *Illusions* are misinterpretations of external sensory stimuli
- *Bizarre language* reflects a communication disruption
- *Perseveration* is a persistent verbal or motor response

Assessment

History

- Obtain a description of problem and any precipitating circumstances.
- Take a drug history.
- Find out about the use of alcohol or illicit drugs.
- Obtain the family's description of the patient's relationships, communication patterns, and role.
- Take a family history of psychiatric or emotional illness.

Physical assessment

- Assess the patient's appearance, behavior, mood, thought, coping mechanisms, and potential for self-destructive behavior.
- Watch for cognitive, linguistic, or perceptual abnormalities.
- Look for unusual gestures, posture, gait, tone of voice, and mannerisms.
- Determine whether the patient is responding to stimuli.

Medical causes

Organic disorders

- Psychotic behavior can result from alcohol withdrawal syndrome, cocaine or amphetamine intoxication, cerebral hypoxia, and nutritional disorders.
- Endocrine disorders such as adrenal dysfunction and severe infections such as encephalitis can also cause psychotic behavior.
- Neurologic causes include Alzheimer's disease and other dementias.

Psychiatric disorders

- Psychotic behavior usually occurs with bipolar disorder, personality disorder, schizophrenia, and some pervasive developmental disorders.

Other causes

Drugs

- Albuterol, alprazolam, amantadine, anticholinergics, asparaginase, atropine, bromocriptine, cimetidine, clonidine, corticotropin, cortisone, cycloserine, dapsone, diazepam, digoxin, disopyramide, disulfiram, indomethacin, lidocaine, methyldopa, prednisone, propranolol, thyroid hormones, and vincristine
- Almost any drug can provoke psychotic behavior as a rare, severe adverse or idiosyncratic reaction.

Nursing considerations

- Continuously evaluate the patient's orientation to reality.

Controlling psychotic behavior

A patient who displays psychotic behavior may be terrified and unable to differentiate between himself and his environment. To control his behavior and to prevent injury to the patient, staff, and others, follow these guidelines:

- Remove potentially dangerous objects, such as belts or metal utensils, from the patient's environment.
- Help the patient discern what's real and unreal in an honest and genuine way.
- Be straightforward, concise, and nonthreatening when speaking to the patient. Discuss simple, concrete subjects, and avoid theories or philosophical issues.
- Positively reinforce the patient's perceptions of reality, and correct his misperceptions in a matter-of-fact way.
- *Never* argue with the patient, but also don't support his misperceptions.
- If the patient is frightened, stay with him.
- Touch the patient to provide reassurance *only* if you've done this before and know that it's safe.
- Move the patient to a safer, less-stimulating environment.
- Provide one-on-one care if the patient's behavior is extremely bizarre, disturbing to other patients, or dangerous to himself.
- Give drugs, as appropriate.

- Call the patient by his preferred name, tell him your name, describe where he is, and use clocks and calendars to help develop a conception of reality.
- Administer antipsychotics or other drugs, as needed.
- Monitor the patient's eating and elimination habits.
- Prepare the patient for transfer to a mental health center, if needed. (See *Controlling psychotic behavior*.)

Pediatric pointers

- In children, psychotic behavior may result from early infantile autism, symbiotic infantile psychosis, or childhood schizophrenia.
- An adolescent patient who exhibits psychotic behavior may have a history of several days' drug use or lack of sleep or food.

Patient teaching

- Explain the importance of structured activities.

Ptosis

Overview

- Refers to excessive drooping of one or both upper eyelids
- Can be constant, progressive, or intermittent
- Can be congenital or acquired

Assessment

History

- Ask about the onset of ptosis and whether the condition has worsened or improved.
- Find out about recent traumatic eye injury.
- Inquire about eye pain or headache.
- Determine whether the patient has experienced vision changes.
- Take a drug history, noting especially the use of a chemotherapeutic drug.

Physical assessment

- Assess the degree of ptosis.
- Check for eyelid edema, exophthalmos, and conjunctival injection.
- Evaluate extraocular muscle function.
- Examine pupil size, color, shape, and reaction to light.
- Test visual acuity.

Medical causes

Alcoholism

- Ptosis as well as complications such as severe weight loss, jaundice, ascites, and mental disturbances, can result from long-term alcohol abuse.

Botulism

- Cranial nerve dysfunction causes ptosis, dysarthria, dysphagia, and diplopia.
- Other findings include dry mouth, sore throat, weakness, vomiting, diarrhea, hyporeflexia, and dyspnea.

Cerebral aneurysm

- Sudden ptosis, diplopia, a dilated pupil, and inability to rotate the eye can occur.
- Ruptured aneurysm, a life-threatening condition, produces sudden severe headache, nausea, vomiting, and decreased level of consciousness (LOC).
- Other findings include nuchal rigidity, back and leg pain, fever, restlessness, irritability, seizures, blurred vision, hemiparesis, sensory deficits, dysphagia, and visual defects.

Hemangioma

- Ptosis may occur along with exophthalmos, limited extraocular movement, swollen periorbital tissue, and blurred vision.

Levator muscle maldevelopment

- Ptosis results from isolated dystrophy of the levator muscle.
- Lid lag on downgaze is an important clue to diagnosis.

Myasthenia gravis

- Gradual ptosis in both eyes is commonly the first sign.
- Ptosis is accompanied by weak eye closure and diplopia.
- Other findings include muscle weakness and fatigue, masklike facies, difficulty chewing or swallowing, dyspnea, cyanosis and, possibly, paralysis.

Myotonic dystrophy

- Mild to severe ptosis in both eyes may occur.
- Distinctive cataracts with iridescent dots in the cortex, miosis, diplopia, decreased tearing, and muscular and testicular atrophy may occur.

Ocular muscle dystrophy

- Ptosis progresses slowly to complete closure of the eyelids.
- Other findings include progressive external ophthalmoplegia and muscle weakness and atrophy of the upper face, neck, trunk, and limbs.

Ocular trauma

- Mild to severe ptosis can result from trauma to the nerve or muscles that control the eyelids.
- Eye pain, lid swelling, ecchymosis, and decreased visual acuity may occur.

Parinaud's syndrome

- Ptosis, enophthalmos, nystagmus, lid retraction, dilated pupils with absent or poor light response, and papilledema occur.
- Ocular muscles fail to move voluntarily.

Subdural hematoma (chronic)

- Ptosis may be a late sign, along with one dilation of one pupil and sluggishness.
- Headache, behavioral changes, and decreased LOC commonly occur.

Other causes

Drugs

- Vinca alkaloids can produce ptosis.

Lead poisoning

- With lead poisoning, ptosis develops over 3 to 6 months; other findings include anorexia, nausea, vomiting, diarrhea, colicky abdominal pain, a lead line in the gums, decreased LOC, tachycardia, hypotension, irritability, and peripheral nerve weakness.

Nursing considerations

○ Orient the patient with decreased visual acuity to his surroundings.
○ Provide special spectacle frames that suspend the eyelid by traction with a wire crutch.

Pediatric pointers

○ In congenital ptosis, ptosis is unilateral, constant, and accompanied by lagophthalmos, which causes the infant to sleep with his eyes open.

Patient teaching

○ Discuss self-esteem issues.
○ Prepare the patient for the diagnostic tests he needs.
○ Prepare the patient for surgery, if needed.

Pulse, absent or weak

Overview

- When generalized, indicates a life-threatening condition, such as shock or arrhythmia (see *Managing an absent or weak pulse*, pages 328 and 329.)
- When localized, may indicate acute arterial occlusion

Assessment

History

- Review the medical history, including heart disease.
- Take a drug history.
- Question him about associated signs and symptoms, such as chest pain or dyspnea.

Physical assessment

- Palpate the remaining arterial pulses for comparison. (See *Evaluating peripheral pulses*.)
- Check other vital signs.
- Evaluate cardiopulmonary status.

Assessment tip
Evaluating peripheral pulses

The rate, amplitude, and symmetry of peripheral pulses provide important clues to cardiac function and the quality of peripheral perfusion. To gather these clues, palpate peripheral pulses lightly with the pads of your index, middle, and ring fingers, as space permits.

Rate
Count all pulses for at least 30 seconds (60 seconds when recording vital signs). The normal rate is between 60 and 100 beats/minute.

Amplitude
Palpate the blood vessel during ventricular systole. Describe pulse amplitude by using a scale such as the one here:
 4+ = bounding
 3+ = increased
 2+ = normal
 1+ = weak, thready
 0 = absent.
Use a stick figure to easily document the location and amplitude of all pulses.

Symmetry
Simultaneously palpate pulses (except for the carotid pulse) on both sides of the patient's body, and note any inequality. Always assess peripheral pulses methodically, moving from the arms to the legs.

Medical causes

Aortic aneurysm (dissecting)

- Weak or absent arterial pulses occur distal to the affected area when circulation to the innominate, left common carotid, subclavian, or femoral artery is affected.
- Tearing pain develops suddenly in the chest and neck and may radiate to the back and abdomen.
- Other findings include syncope, loss of consciousness, weakness or transient paralysis of the legs or arms, diastolic murmur of aortic insufficiency, hypotension, and mottled skin below the waist.

Aortic stenosis

- The carotid pulse is weak.
- Paroxysmal or exertional dyspnea, chest pain, and syncope are common.
- Other findings include an atrial gallop, a harsh systolic ejection murmur, crackles, palpitations, fatigue, and narrowed pulse pressure.

Arterial occlusion

- With acute occlusion, arterial pulses far from the obstruction are weak and then absent.
- Affected limb has severe pain, varying degrees of paralysis, intermittent claudication, and paresthesia; is cool, pale, and cyanotic, with increased capillary refill time; and has a line of color and temperature demarcation at the level of obstruction.
- With chronic occlusion, pulses in the affected limb weaken gradually.

Cardiac arrhythmias

- Generalized weak pulses may accompany cool, clammy skin.
- Other findings include hypotension, chest pain, dyspnea, dizziness, and decreased level of consciousness (LOC).

Cardiac tamponade

- In this life-threatening condition, a weak, rapid pulse accompanies these classic findings: paradoxical pulse, jugular vein distention, hypotension, and muffled heart sounds.
- Other findings include paradoxical pulse, jugular vein distention, hypotension, muffled heart sounds, narrowed pulse pressure, pericardial friction rub, hepatomegaly, anxiety, restlessness, cyanosis, chest pain, dyspnea, tachypnea, and cold, clammy skin.

Coarctation of the aorta

- Bounding pulses occur in the arms and neck, with decreased pulsations and systolic pulse pressure in the lower extremities.
- Auscultation may reveal a systolic ejection click accompanied by a systolic ejection murmur.

Peripheral vascular disease

- A weakening and loss of peripheral pulses occurs.

- Aching pain occurs distal to the occlusion that worsens with exercise and abates with rest.
- Other findings include cool skin, decreased hair growth in the affected limb, and impotence with an occlusion of the descending aorta or femoral areas.

Pulmonary embolism

- A generalized weak, rapid pulse occurs.
- Other features include an abrupt onset of chest pain, tachycardia, apprehension, syncope, diaphoresis, and cyanosis.
- Acute respiratory findings include tachypnea, dyspnea, decreased breath sounds, crackles, a pleural friction rub, and a cough, possibly with blood-tinged sputum.

Shock

- With *anaphylactic shock,* pulses become rapid and weak and then uniformly absent within seconds or minutes after exposure to an allergen.
- With *cardiogenic shock,* peripheral pulses are absent and central pulses are weak, depending on the degree of vascular collapse.
- With *hypovolemic shock,* all peripheral pulses become weak and then uniformly absent, depending on the severity of hypovolemia.
- With *septic shock,* all pulses in the extremities first become weak and then become absent.

Thoracic outlet syndrome

- Gradual or abrupt weakness or loss of pulses in arms occurs.
- Pulse changes commonly occur after the patient works with his hands above his shoulders, lifts a weight, or abducts his arm.
- Other findings include paresthesia and pain along the ulnar distribution of the arm that resolves when the arm returns to a neutral position.

Other causes

Treatments

- Localized absent pulse may occur away from the arteriovenous shunts used for dialysis.

Nursing considerations

- Monitor vital signs.
- Measure daily weight, intake and output, and central venous pressure.

Pediatric pointers

- Radial, dorsal pedal, and posterior tibial pulses aren't easily palpable in infants and small children.
- In children and young adults, weak or absent pulses in the legs may indicate coarctation of the aorta.

Patient teaching

- Teach the techniques for checking pulse.
- Explain the signs and symptoms the patient needs to report.
- Discuss foods and fluids the patient should avoid.
- Emphasize avoidance of activities that reduce circulation.

An absent or weak pulse can result from any one of several life-threatening disorders. Your evaluation and interventions will vary, depending on whether the weak or absent pulse is generalized or localized to one extremity. They'll also depend on associated signs and symptoms. Use the flowchart below to help you establish priorities for successfully managing this emergency.

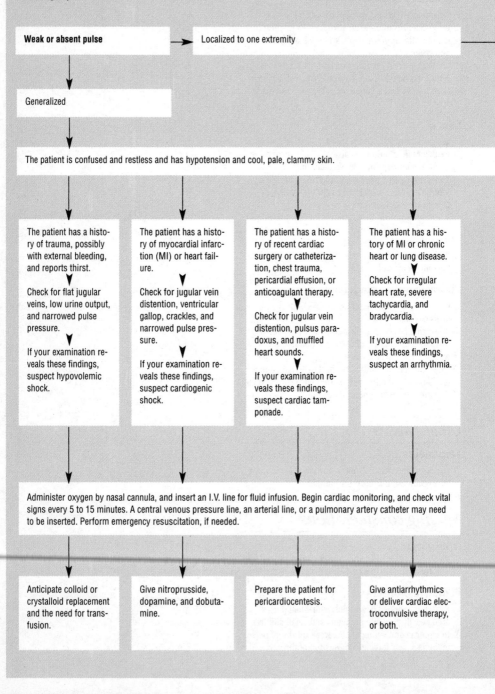

Weak or absent pulse → Localized to one extremity

Generalized

The patient is confused and restless and has hypotension and cool, pale, clammy skin.

The patient has a history of trauma, possibly with external bleeding, and reports thirst.

Check for flat jugular veins, low urine output, and narrowed pulse pressure.

If your examination reveals these findings, suspect hypovolemic shock.

The patient has a history of myocardial infarction (MI) or heart failure.

Check for jugular vein distention, ventricular gallop, crackles, and narrowed pulse pressure.

If your examination reveals these findings, suspect cardiogenic shock.

The patient has a history of recent cardiac surgery or catheterization, chest trauma, pericardial effusion, or anticoagulant therapy.

Check for jugular vein distention, pulsus paradoxus, and muffled heart sounds.

If your examination reveals these findings, suspect cardiac tamponade.

The patient has a history of MI or chronic heart or lung disease.

Check for irregular heart rate, severe tachycardia, and bradycardia.

If your examination reveals these findings, suspect an arrhythmia.

Administer oxygen by nasal cannula, and insert an I.V. line for fluid infusion. Begin cardiac monitoring, and check vital signs every 5 to 15 minutes. A central venous pressure line, an arterial line, or a pulmonary artery catheter may need to be inserted. Perform emergency resuscitation, if needed.

Anticipate colloid or crystalloid replacement and the need for transfusion.

Give nitroprusside, dopamine, and dobutamine.

Prepare the patient for pericardiocentesis.

Give antiarrhythmics or deliver cardiac electroconvulsive therapy, or both.

Examine the affected extremity for cool, mottled skin and pain.

If your examination reveals these findings, suspect arterial occlusive disease.

Prepare the patient for diagnostic tests to confirm or rule out arterial occlusion, such as arteriography, aortography, or Doppler ultrasonography. Don't elevate the affected extremity. Start an I.V. line in an unaffected arm or leg, and administer heparin or thrombotic, as needed. Anticipate preparing the patient for emergency embolectomy or peripheral angioplasty.

The patient has a history of trauma, congenital heart disease, or hypertension and reports severe, tearing chest pain.

Check for pulse quality and blood pressure variation between upper and lower extremities.

If your examination reveals these findings, suspect dissecting aortic aneurysm or aortic coarctation.

The patient has a history of severe infection—commonly gram-negative, urinary, or respiratory tract infection.

Check for fever, chills, and widened pulse pressure.

If your examination reveals these findings, suspect septic shock.

The patient has a history of an insect sting, drug ingestion, or exposure to another possible allergen.

Check for urticaria, wheezing or stridor, and dyspnea.

If your examination reveals these findings, suspect anaphylactic shock.

The patient has a history of venous stasis or deep vein thrombosis and reports sharp, substernal chest pain.

Check for dyspnea, crackles, pleural friction rub, and hemoptysis.

If your examination reveals these findings, suspect pulmonary embolism.

Administer oxygen by nasal cannula and insert an I.V. line for fluid infusion. Begin cardiac monitoring, and check vital signs every 5 to 15 minutes. A central venous pressure line, an arterial line, or a pulmonary artery catheter may need to be inserted. Give emergency resuscitation, if needed.

Prepare the patient for surgery and give an antihypertensive or nitroprusside.

Give antibiotics and vasopressors.

Emergency endotracheal intubation or cricothyrotomy and administration of epinephrine may be needed.

Endotracheal intubation and anticoagulant or thrombolytic therapy may be needed.

Pulse, bounding

Overview

○ Bounding pulse is produced by large waves of pressure as blood ejects from the left ventricle with each contraction
○ Bounding pulse is characterized by regular, recurrent expansion and contraction of the arterial walls
○ Pulse is strong and easily palpable
○ Pulse may be visible over superficial peripheral arteries
○ Pulse isn't obliterated by the pressure of palpation

Assessment

History

○ Ask about weakness, fatigue, shortness of breath, or other health changes.

Assessment tip
Assessing peripheral pulse sites

You can assess your patient's pulse rate, rhythm and amplitude at several sites, including those shown in the illustration below.

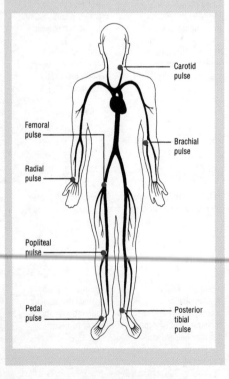

Carotid pulse

Femoral pulse

Brachial pulse

Radial pulse

Popliteal pulse

Pedal pulse

Posterior tibial pulse

○ Take a medical history, noting hyperthyroidism, anemia, or a cardiovascular disorder.
○ Ask about alcohol use.

Physical assessment

○ Check vital signs.
○ Auscultate heart and lungs for abnormal sounds, rates, or rhythms.
○ Complete the cardiovascular assessment. (See *Assessing peripheral pulse sites*.)

Medical causes

Alcoholism (acute)

○ A rapid, bounding pulse and flushed face result from vasodilation.
○ An odor of alcohol on the breath and an ataxic gait are common.
○ Other findings include hypothermia, bradypnea, labored and loud respirations, nausea, vomiting, diuresis, decreased level of consciousness, and seizures.

Anemia

○ Bounding pulse may be accompanied by systolic ejection murmur, tachycardia, an atrial gallop, a ventricular gallop, and a systolic bruit over the carotid artery.
○ Other findings include fatigue, pallor, dyspnea and, possibly, bleeding tendencies.

Aortic insufficiency

○ Bounding pulse is characterized by rapid, forceful expansion of the arterial pulse followed by rapid contraction.
○ Widened pulse pressure also occurs.
○ Other relevant signs and symptoms include weakness, severe dyspnea, hypotension, ventricular gallop, tachycardia, pallor, chest pain, strong and abrupt carotid pulsations, *pulsus biferiens,* an early systolic murmur, a murmur hard over the femoral artery during systole and diastole, a high-pitched diastolic murmur that starts with the second heart sound, and an apical diastolic rumble (Austin Flint murmur).
○ With chronic aortic insufficiency, most patients are asymptomatic until age 40 or 50 when exertional dyspnea, increased fatigue, orthopnea, paroxysmal nocturnal dyspnea, angina, and syncope may develop.

Febrile disorder

○ Bounding pulse may occur with fever.
○ Accompanying findings reflect the underlying disorder and may include fatigue, chills, malaise, anorexia, tachycardia, tachypnea, and diaphoresis.

Thyrotoxicosis

○ A rapid, full, bounding pulse occurs.
○ Other relevant signs and symptoms include tachycardia, palpitations, an atrial or ventricular gallop, weight loss despite increased appetite, diarrhea, an enlarged thyroid, dyspnea, tremors, nervousness, chest pain, exophthalmos, heat intolerance, signs of cardiovascular collapse, and warm, moist, and diaphoretic skin.

Nursing considerations

○ If bounding pulse is accompanied by rapid or irregular heartbeat, connect the patient to a cardiac monitor for further evaluation.
○ Provide for rest periods to reduce metabolic demands.
○ Administer iron supplements, if indicated.
○ Monitor intake and output.
○ Weigh the patient daily.
○ Restrict fluids, as necessary.

Pediatric pointers

○ A bounding pulse can be normal in infants or children.
○ It can also result from patent ductus arteriosus if the left-to-right shunt is large.

Patient teaching

○ Discuss diet modifications and fluid restrictions the patient needs.
○ Stress the need for rest periods.
○ Emphasize the importance of avoiding alcohol, and refer the patient to Alcoholics Anonymous.
○ Explain signs and symptoms he needs to report.

Pulse pressure, narrowed

Overview

○ Refers to the difference between systolic and diastolic blood pressures of less than 30 mm Hg
○ Occurs when peripheral vascular resistance increases, cardiac output declines, or intravascular volume markedly decreases (see *Understanding pulse pressure changes*)
○ Is usually a late sign

Assessment

History

○ Ask about specific cardiac symptoms, such as chest pain, dizziness, or syncope.

○ Obtain a medical history.
○ Assess risk factors for heart disease.

Physical assessment

○ Check for signs of heart failure, such as hypotension, tachycardia, dyspnea, jugular vein distention, pulmonary crackles, and decreased urine output.
○ Check for changes in skin temperature or color.
○ Palpate peripheral pulses, noting their strength.
○ Evaluate level of consciousness (LOC).
○ Auscultate for heart murmurs.

Medical causes

Aortic stenosis

○ Narrowed pulse pressure occurs late in significant stenosis.
○ Other findings include atrial or ventricular gallop, chest pain, angina, crackles, fatigue, dyspnea, paroxysmal nocturnal dyspnea, syncope, and a harsh, systolic ejection murmur.

Understanding pulse pressure changes

The amount of blood that the ventricles eject into the arteries with each beat—known as *stroke volume*—and the arteries' *peripheral resistance* to blood flow affect pulse pressure and systolic and diastolic blood pressures. For example, pulse pressure narrows when systolic pressure falls (lower right), diastolic pressure rises (upper left), or both. These changes reflect decreased stroke volume, increased peripheral resistance, or both.

Pulse pressure widens when systolic pressure rises (upper right), diastolic pressure falls (lower left), or both. These changes reflect increased stroke volume, decreased peripheral resistance, or both.

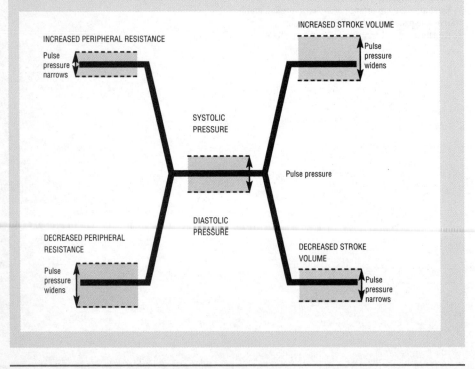

Cardiac tamponade

○ A life-threatening disorder — pulse pressure narrows by 10 to 20 mm Hg.
○ Paradoxical pulse, jugular vein distention, hypotension, and muffled heart sounds are classic.
○ Other findings include anxiety, restlessness, cyanosis, clammy skin, chest pain, dyspnea, tachypnea, decreased LOC, pericardial rub, hepatomegaly, and a weak, rapid pulse.

Heart failure

○ Narrowed pulse pressure occurs relatively late.
○ Tachypnea, palpitations, dependent edema, steady weight gain despite nausea and anorexia, chest tightness, hypotension, diaphoresis, pallor, a ventricular gallop, inspiratory crackles, oliguria and, possibly, a tender palpable liver may also occur.
○ Later, hemoptysis, cyanosis, marked hepatomegaly, and marked pitting edema may occur.

Shock

○ Narrowed pulse pressure occurs late.
○ Peripheral pulses first become weak and then uniformly absent in anaphylactic, hypovolemic, and septic shock.
○ In cardiogenic shock, peripheral pulses are absent and central pulses are weak.
○ Anaphylactic shock may result in hypotension, anxiety, restlessness, feelings of doom, intense itching, urticaria, dyspnea, stridor, hoarseness, chest or throat tightness, skin flushing, and seizures.
○ Cardiogenic shock may produce hypotension, tachycardia, tachypnea, cyanosis, oliguria, restlessness, confusion, obtundation, and cold, pale, clammy skin.
○ Deepening hypovolemia shock leads to hypotension, oliguria, confusion, decreased LOC and, possibly, hypothermia.
○ As septic shock progresses, the patient exhibits thirst, anxiety, restlessness, confusion, hypotension, cool and cyanotic extremities, cold and clammy skin and, eventually, severe hypotension, oliguria or anuria, respiratory failure, and coma.

○ Stress the importance of rest periods to reduce fatigue.

Nursing considerations

○ Monitor closely for changes in pulse rate or quality and for hypotension.
○ Assess for changes in LOC.

Pediatric pointers

○ In children, narrowed pulse pressure can result from congenital aortic stenosis as well as from the disorders that affect adults.

Patient teaching

○ Explain the disorder and its treatments.
○ Explain foods and fluids the patient should avoid.

Pulse pressure, widened

Overview

- Systolic pressure is more than 50 mm Hg higher than diastolic pressure
- Widened pulse pressure commonly occurs as a physiologic response to fever, hot weather, exercise, anxiety, anemia, or pregnancy

✷ Emergency actions

If the patient's level of consciousness (LOC) is decreased and you suspect his widened pulse pressure comes from increased intracranial pressure (ICP), check his vital signs and oxygen saturation. Maintain a patent airway. Provide supplemental oxygen and ventilatory support to keep the patient's partial pressure of arterial oxygen above 90 mm Hg or his oxygen saturation above 95%. Give osmotic diuretics such as mannitol by I.V. infusion to decrease ICP. Insert an indwelling urinary catheter; monitor intake and output during mannitol therapy. Start ICP monitoring. Administer analgesics as ordered. Hyperventilation therapy to decrease the patient's partial pressure of arterial carbon dioxide and to treat ICP remains controversial but may be needed for short intervals when ICP and neurologic deterioration increase. Perform a neurologic examination. Use the Glasgow Coma Scale to evaluate LOC. Check cranial nerve function—especially cranial nerves III, IV, and VI—and assess pupillary reactions, reflexes, and muscle tone. Continue ICP monitoring. Check for edema and auscultate for murmurs.

Assessment

History

- Obtain a medical history, including family's history.
- Take a drug history.
- Ask about such associated signs and symptoms as chest pain, shortness of breath, weakness, fatigue, or syncope.

Physical assessment

- Assess for signs and symptoms of heart failure, such as crackles, dyspnea, and jugular vein distention.
- Check for changes in skin temperature and color and strength of peripheral pulses.
- Evaluate LOC.
- Auscultate the heart for murmurs.
- Check for peripheral edema.

Medical causes

Aortic insufficiency

- Pulse pressure widens progressively as the valve deteriorates.
- Other relevant signs and symptoms include a bounding pulse, an atrial or ventricular gallop, chest pain, palpitations, pallor, pulsus biferiens, signs of heart failure (crackles, dyspnea, jugular vein distention), heart murmurs such as an early diastolic murmur and an apical diastolic rumble (Austin Flint murmur), and strong, abrupt carotid pulsations.

Arteriosclerosis

- Pulse pressure widens following moderate hypertension.
- Other findings include signs of vascular insufficiency, such as claudication, angina, and speech and vision disturbances.

Febrile disorders

- Fever can cause widened pulse pressure.
- Other symptoms vary by the underlying disorder but may include fatigue, chills, malaise, anorexia, tachycardia, tachypnea, and diaphoresis.

Increased ICP

- A life-threatening condition—widening pulse pressure is an intermediate to late sign of increased ICP.
- Decreased LOC is the earliest and most sensitive indicator of increased ICP.
- Cushing's triad—bradycardia, hypertension, and respiratory pattern changes—is characteristic of increasing ICP.
- Other findings include headache, vomiting, impaired or unequal motor movement, vision disturbances, and pupillary changes.

Nursing considerations

- If the patient displays increased ICP, continually reevaluate his neurologic status.
- Be alert for restlessness, confusion, unresponsiveness, or decreased LOC.
- Watch for subtle changes in condition.

Pediatric pointers

- Widened pulse pressure is an intermediate to late sign of increased ICP.
- Widened pulse pressure can occur with patent ductus arteriosus (PDA) but may not be evident at birth; the older child with PDA experiences exertional dyspnea, with pulse pressure that widens even further on exertion.

Geriatric pointers

○ Widened pulse pressure is a more reliable predictor of cardiovascular events in elderly patients than increased systolic and diastolic blood pressure.

Patient teaching

○ Explain needed dietary modifications, such as restricting sodium and saturated fats.
○ Stress the importance of planning rest periods.
○ If the patient has decreased LOC, discuss specific safety measures.

Pulse rhythm, abnormal

Overview

○ Refers to irregular expansion and contraction of peripheral arterial walls
○ May be persistent or sporadic, rhythmic or arrhythmic
○ Reflects an underlying cardiac arrhythmia (see *Abnormal pulse rhythm: A clue to cardiac arrhythmias*)

★ Emergency actions

Quickly look for signs of reduced cardiac output, such as decreased level of consciousness (LOC), hypotension, or dizziness. Promptly obtain an electrocardiogram (ECG) and possibly a chest X-ray, and begin cardiac monitoring. Insert an I.V. line for administration of emergency cardiac drugs, and give oxygen by nasal cannula or mask. Closely monitor vital signs, pulse quality, and cardiac rhythm. Keep emergency intubation, cardioversion, and suction equipment handy.

Assessment

History
○ Ask about the onset, quality, quantity, location, and radiation of pain.
○ Obtain a medical history, including heart disease and treatment for arrhythmias.
○ Take a drug history and check compliance.
○ Ask about caffeine or alcohol intake.

Physical assessment
○ Check apical and peripheral arterial pulses; check for a pulse deficit.
○ Auscultate heart sounds for abnormalities.
○ Count the apical beat for 60 seconds, noting the frequency of skipped peripheral beats.

Medical causes

Cardiac arrhythmias
○ An abnormal pulse rhythm may be the only sign; pulse may be weak, rapid, or slow.
○ Palpitations, a fluttering heartbeat, or weak and skipped beats may be reported by the patient.
○ Dull chest pain or discomfort and hypotension may occur.
○ Other findings include decreased urine output, dyspnea, tachypnea, pallor, and diaphoresis.
○ Neurologic findings include confusion, dizziness, light-headedness, decreased LOC and, sometimes, seizures.

Nursing considerations

○ Sedate the patient for cardioversion therapy if needed.
○ Prepare the patient for transfer to a cardiac or intensive care unit.
○ Check vital signs frequently to detect bradycardia, tachycardia, hypertension, or hypotension, tachypnea, or dyspnea.
○ Collect blood samples for serum electrolyte, cardiac enzyme, and drug level studies.
○ Obtain a 12-lead ECG and compare with previous tracings.

Pediatric pointers
○ Arrhythmias also produce pulse rhythm abnormalities in children.

Patient teaching
○ Tell the patient to keep a diary of activities and symptoms.
○ Educate the patient on the importance of avoiding tobacco and caffeine.
○ Discuss strategies to improve medication compliance.
○ Instruct the patient on taking his pulse rate.
○ Explain the signs and symptoms he needs to report.

An abnormal pulse rhythm may be your only clue that the patient has a cardiac arrhythmia, but this sign doesn't help you pinpoint the specific type of arrhythmia. For that, you need a cardiac monitor or an electrocardiogram (ECG) machine. The ECG strips below show some common cardiac arrhythmias that can cause abnormal pulse rhythms.

Arrhythmia	*Pulse rhythm and rate*	*Results*
Sinus arrhythmia	Irregular rhythm; fast, slow, or normal rate	• Reflex vagal tone inhibition (heart rate increases with inspiration and decreases with expiration) related to normal respiratory cycle • May result from drugs, as in digoxin toxicity • Occurs most often in children and young adults
Premature atrial contractions (PACs)	Irregular rhythm during PACs; fast, slow, or normal rate	• Occasional PACs may be normal • Isolated PACs may indicate atrial irritation—for example, from anxiety or excessive caffeine intake; increasing PACs may herald other arrhythmias • May result from heart failure, chronic obstructive pulmonary disease (COPD), or use of cardiac glycosides, aminophylline, or an adrenergic
Paroxysmal atrial tachycardia	Regular rhythm with abrupt onset and termination of arrhythmia; heart rate exceeding 140 beats/minute	• May occur in otherwise normal, healthy people who are experiencing physical or psychological stress, hypoxia, or digoxin toxicity; who use marijuana; or who consume excessive amounts of caffeine or other stimulants • May precipitate angina or heart failure
Atrial fibrillation	Irregular rhythm; atrial rate exceeding 400 beats/minute; ventricular rate varies	• May result from heart failure, COPD, hypertension, sepsis, pulmonary embolus, mitral valve disease, atrial irritation, postcoronary bypass, or valve replacement surgery • Preload inconsistent because atria don't contract; cardiac output changes with each beat; emboli may also result
Second-degree atrioventricular heart block, type I (Wenckebach)	Irregular ventricular rhythm; fast, slow or normal rate	• Commonly transient; may progress to complete heart block • May result from inferior wall myocardial infarction, digoxin or quinidine toxicity, vagal stimulation, electrolyte imbalance, or arteriosclerotic heart disease
Premature ventricular contractions (multifocal)	Usually irregular rhythm with a long pause after the premature beat; fast, slow, or normal rate	• Arise from different ventricular sites or from the same site with changing patterns of conduction • May result from caffeine or stress, alcohol ingestion, myocardial ischemia or infarction, myocardial irritation by pacemaker electrodes, hypocalcemia, hypercalcemia digoxin toxicity, or exercise

Pulsus biferiens

Overview

○ Refers to hyperdynamic, double-beating pulse characterized by two systolic peaks separated by midsystolic dip
○ Typically has a taller or more forceful first peak
○ Occurs when a large volume of blood is rapidly ejected from the left ventricle
○ Can be palpated in the peripheral arteries or observed on an arterial pressure wave recording (see *Comparing arterial pressure waves*)

Assessment

History

○ Take a medical history, including cardiac disorders.
○ Take a drug history.
○ Ask about associated signs and symptoms, such as dyspnea, chest pain, or fatigue.
○ Ask about the onset of symptoms and aggravating or alleviating factors.

Physical assessment

○ Take vital signs.
○ Auscultate for abnormal heart or breath sounds.
○ Assess peripheral pulses. (See *Detecting pulsus biferiens.*)
○ Complete the cardiopulmonary assessment.

Assessment tip
Comparing arterial pressure waves

The waveforms shown here help differentiate a normal arterial pulse from pulsus alternans, pulsus biferiens, and paradoxical pulse.

NORMAL ARTERIAL PULSE

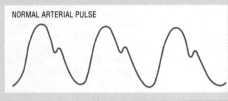

The percussion wave in a *normal arterial pulse* reflects ejection of blood into the aorta (early systole). The tidal wave is the peak of the pulse wave (later systole), and the dicrotic notch marks the beginning of diastole.

PULSUS ALTERNANS

Pulsus alternans is a beat-to-beat alternation in pulse size and intensity. Although the rhythm of pulsus alternans is regular, the volume varies. If you take the blood pressure of a patient with this abnormality, you'll first hear a loud Korotkoff sound and then a soft sound, continually alternating. Pulsus alternans commonly accompanies states of poor contractility that occur with left-sided heart failure.

PULSUS BIFERIENS

Pulsus biferiens is a double-beating pulse with two systolic peaks. The first beat reflects pulse pressure; the second, reverberation from the periphery. Pulsus biferiens commonly occurs with aortic insufficiency (aortic stenosis, aortic regurgitation), hypertrophic cardiomyopathy, or high cardiac output states.

PULSUS PARADOXUS

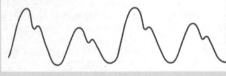

Inspiration Expiration Inspiration

Paradoxical pulse is an exaggerated decline in blood pressure during inspiration, resulting from an increase in negative intrathoracic pressure. A paradoxical pulse that exceeds 10 mm Hg is considered abnormal and may result from cardiac tamponade, constrictive pericarditis, or severe lung disease.

To detect pulsus biferiens, lightly palpate the carotid, brachial, radial, or femoral artery. (The pulse is easiest to palpate in the carotid artery.) At the same time, listen to the patient's heart sounds to determine if the two palpable peaks occur during systole. If they do, you'll feel the double pulse between the first and second heart sounds.

Medical causes

Aortic insufficiency

○ Aortic insufficiency is the most common organic cause of biferiens pulse.
○ Other findings include exertional dyspnea, fatigue, orthopnea, paroxysmal nocturnal dyspnea, ventricular gallop, tachycardia, chest pain, palpitations, pallor, strong and abrupt carotid pulsations, widened pulse pressure, and one or more murmurs, especially an apical diastolic rumble (Austin Flint murmur).

Aortic stenosis with aortic insufficiency

○ Pulse rate rises slowly and the second wave of the double beat is the more forceful one.
○ Dyspnea and fatigue are common.

High cardiac output states

○ Pulsus biferiens commonly occurs with high cardiac output states, such as anemia, thyrotoxicosis, fever, and exercise.
○ Other findings vary with the underlying disorder and may include tachycardia, a cervical venous hum, and widened pulse pressure.

Hypertrophic obstructive cardiomyopathy

○ Pulsus biferiens occurs with the pulse rising rapidly and the first wave being the more forceful one.
○ Other findings include a systolic murmur, dyspnea, angina, fatigue, and syncope.

Nursing considerations

○ Prepare the patient for diagnostic tests.
○ Schedule regular rest periods.
○ Monitor intake and output and daily weight.

Pediatric pointers

○ Pulsus biferiens may be palpated in children with a large patent ductus arteriosus as well as those with congenital aortic stenosis and insufficiency.

Patient teaching

○ Explain the facts about the disorder and its treatment.
○ Explain signs and symptoms of heart failure to report.
○ Discuss the planning of rest periods.

Pupils, nonreactive

Overview

○ Refers to failure of pupils to constrict in response to light or dilate when light is removed (see *Assessing pupillary reaction*)
○ May signal a life-threatening emergency or brain death
○ Can occur with optic drug use

Emergency actions

If the patient is unconscious and develops nonreactive pupils, quickly take his vital signs. Look for decerebrate or decorticate posture, bradycardia, elevated systolic blood pressure, and widened pulse pressure. One dilated, nonreactive pupil may be an early sign of uncal brain herniation. Emergency surgery to decrease intracranial pressure (ICP) may be necessary. Insert an I.V. line to administer a diuretic, an osmotic agent, or a corticosteroid to treat increased ICP. The patient may need controlled hyperventilation.

Assessment

History

○ Ask about the use of eyedrops and when they were last instilled.
○ Ask about pain and its location, intensity, and duration.

Physical assessment

○ Check visual acuity in both eyes.
○ Test the pupillary reaction to accommodation.
○ Examine the cornea and iris for abnormalities.
○ Measure intraocular pressure (IOP).
○ Perform ophthalmoscopic and slit-lamp examinations.
○ Cover the affected eye with a protective metal shield.

Assessment tip
Assessing pupillary reaction

To evaluate pupillary reaction to light, first test the patient's direct light reflex. Darken the room and cover one of the patient's eyes while you hold open the opposite eyelid. Using a bright penlight, bring the light toward the patient from the side and shine it directly into his opened eye. If normal, the pupil will promptly constrict. Next, test the consensual light reflex. Hold the patient's eyelids open and shine the light into one eye while watching the pupil of the opposite eye. If normal, both pupils will promptly constrict. Repeat both procedures in the opposite eye.

Medical causes

Botulism

○ Nonreactive pupils and mydriasis in both eyes usually appear 12 to 36 hours after ingestion of tainted food.
○ Other early findings include blurred vision, diplopia, ptosis, strabismus, extraocular muscle palsies, anorexia, nausea, vomiting, diarrhea, and dry mouth.
○ Vertigo, deafness, hoarseness, nasal voice, dysarthria, and dysphagia follow.
○ Progressive muscle weakness and absent deep tendon reflexes evolve over 2 to 4 days, resulting in severe constipation and paralysis of respiratory muscles with respiratory distress.

Encephalitis

○ Initially sluggish pupils become dilated and nonreactive.
○ Decreased accommodation and other symptoms of cranial nerve palsies develop.
○ A decreased level of consciousness, high fever, headache, vomiting, and nuchal rigidity occur within 48 hours.
○ Aphasia, ataxia, nystagmus, hemiparesis, and photophobia may occur with seizures.

Glaucoma (acute angle-closure)

○ Moderately dilated, nonreactive pupil occurs in the affected eye in this ophthalmic emergency.
○ Sudden blurred vision, followed by excruciating pain in and around the affected eye occurs.
○ Other findings include seeing halos around white lights at night, conjunctival injection, corneal clouding, and decreased visual acuity.
○ Nausea and vomiting occur with severely elevated IOP.

Ocular trauma

○ A transient or permanent nonreactive, dilated pupil may result from severe damage to the iris or optic nerve.
○ Eye pain, eye edema, and ecchymoses may occur.
○ A V-shaped notch in the pupillary rim, indicating a tear in the iris sphincter muscle may be seen on slit-lamp examination.

Oculomotor nerve palsy

○ A dilated, nonreactive pupil and loss of the accommodation reaction is the first sign.
○ May signal life-threatening brain herniation.

Uveitis

○ In anterior uveitis, a small, nonreactive pupil appears suddenly and is accompanied by severe eye pain, conjunctival injection, and photophobia.
○ With posterior uveitis, similar features develop insidiously, along with blurred vision and distorted pupil shape.

Wernicke's disease
○ Nonreactive pupils occur late in disease.
○ Initial findings include an intention tremor accompanied by a sluggish pupillary reaction.
○ Other ocular findings include diplopia, gaze paralysis, nystagmus, ptosis, decreased visual acuity, and conjunctival injection.
○ Orthostatic hypotension, tachycardia, ataxia, apathy, and confusion may also occur.

Other causes

Drugs
○ Instillation of a topical mydriatic or cycloplegic may induce a temporarily nonreactive pupil in the affected eye.
○ Opiates cause pinpoint pupils with a minimal light response that can be seen only with a magnifying glass.
○ Atropine poisoning produces widely dilated, nonreactive pupils.

Nursing considerations

○ If the patient is conscious, monitor his pupillary light reflex.
○ If the patient is unconsciousness, close his eyes to prevent corneal exposure.

Pediatric pointers
○ The most common cause of nonreactive pupils in children is oculomotor nerve palsy from increased ICP.

Patient teaching
○ Teach proper methods for instilling eye drops.
○ Explain methods of reducing photophobia.
○ Stress the importance of follow-up care to check IOP.

Pupils, sluggish

Overview

- Refers to abnormally slow pupillary response to light
- Can occur in one pupil or both; a normal pupillary reaction always occurs in bilaterally
- Indicates dysfunction of cranial nerves II and III, which mediate the light reflex
- Accompanies degenerative disease of the central nervous system and diabetic neuropathy

Assessment

History

- Obtain a medical history.
- Find out about the use of eyedrops and when they were used last.
- Ask about pain and other ocular symptoms.

Physical assessment

- Test visual acuity.
- Assess pupillary reaction to accommodation.
- Examine the cornea and iris for irregularities, scars, and foreign bodies.
- Measure intraocular pressure (IOP).

Medical causes

Adie's syndrome

- Sluggish pupillary response with abrupt onset of mydriasis, progressing to a nonreactive pupil
- Other findings: blurred vision, and hypoactive for absent deep tendon reflexes in the arms and legs

Diabetic neuropathy

- Sluggish pupillary response with long-standing disease.
- Other findings: orthostatic hypotension, syncope, dysphagia, episodic constipation or diarrhea, painless bladder distention with overflow incontinence, retrograde ejaculation, and impotence.

Encephalitis

- Sluggish response in both pupils is an initial symptom.
- Later, dilated, nonreactive pupils, decreased accommodation, and other cranial nerve palsies may occur.
- Other findings include decreased level of consciousness, headache, high fever, vomiting, nuchal rigidity, aphasia, ataxia, nystagmus, hemiparesis, photophobia, and seizures.

Herpes zoster

- A sluggish pupillary response may occur if nasociliary nerve is affected.
- Examination of the conjunctive reveals follicles.
- Other ocular findings include a serous discharge, absence of tears, ptosis, and extraocular muscle palsy.

Iritis (acute)

- A sluggish pupillary response and conjunctival injection occur in the affected eye.
- The pupil may remain constricted; pupil will be irregularly shaped if posterior synechiae have formed.
- Sudden onset of eye pain, photophobia, and blurred vision may also occur.

Multiple sclerosis

- Small, irregularly shaped pupils that react better to accommodation than to light.
- Ptosis, nystagmus, diplopia, and blurred vision.
- Early, vision problems and sensory impairment.
- Later, muscle weakness and paralysis; intention tremor, spasticity, hyperreflexia, and gait ataxia; dysphagia and dysarthria; constipation; urinary urgency, frequency, and incontinence; impotence; and emotional instability.

Myotonic dystrophy

- Sluggish pupillary reaction with lid lag, ptosis, miosis and, possibly, diplopia
- Decreased visual acuity from cataract formation; muscle weakness and atrophy; and testicular atrophy

Tertiary syphilis

- Sluggish pupillary reaction in the late stage of neurosyphilis
- Marked weakness of extraocular muscles, visual field defects, and decreased visual acuity

Wernicke's disease

- Early, an intention tremor with a sluggish pupillary reaction; later, pupils may be nonreactive
- Diplopia, gaze paralysis, nystagmus, ptosis, decreased visual acuity, and conjunctival injection
- Possible orthostatic hypotension, tachycardia, ataxia, apathy, and confusion

Nursing considerations

- A sluggish pupillary reaction isn't diagnostically significant.
- Treat the underlying disorder.
- If vision is affected, provide for the patient's safety.
- Monitor for eye pain and changes in vision.

Pediatric pointers

- Children experience sluggish pupillary reactions for the same reasons as adults.

Geriatric pointers

○ A sluggish pupillary response may occur normally in elderly people, whose pupils become smaller and less responsive with age.

Patient teaching

○ Stress the importance of regular ophthalmologic examinations.
○ Explain the facts about the disease.
○ Explain ways of reducing photophobia.
○ Teach the patient self-care for diabetes, if needed.

Purpura

Overview

- Extravasation of red blood cells from the blood vessels into the skin, subcutaneous tissue, or mucous membranes
- Involves easily visible purplish or brownish red discoloration
- Discoloration fails to blanch with pressure
- Purpuric lesions include petechiae, ecchymoses, and hematomas (see *Identifying purpuric lesions*)

History

- Ask about the onset and location of lesions.
- Take a drug and diet history.
- Find out about a personal or family history of bleeding disorders or easy bruising.
- Inquire about recent illnesses, trauma, and transfusions.
- Ask about other signs, such as epistaxis, bleeding gums, hematuria, hematochezia, fever, and heavy menstrual flow.

Physical assessment

- Inspect the entire skin surface and mucous membranes to determine the type, size, location, distribution, and severity of purpuric lesions.

Medical causes

Cholesterol emboli

- Purpura typically occurs in the lower extremities of patients with atherosclerotic vascular disease, after anticoagulation therapy or an invasive arterial procedure.
- Other findings include livedo reticularis, cyanosis, gangrene, nodules, and ulceration of the skin.

Disseminated intravascular coagulation

- Purpura occurs in different degrees.
- Cutaneous oozing, hematemesis, or bleeding from incision or needle insertion sites may occur.
- Other findings include acrocyanosis, nausea, dyspnea, seizures, oliguria, and severe muscle, back, and abdominal pain.

Dysproteinemias

- Petechiae and ecchymoses occur along with bleeding tendencies in multiple myeloma and cryoglobulinemia.
- Hyperglobulinemia typically begins insidiously with occasional outbreaks of purpura over the lower legs and feet.

Fat emboli

- Petechiae occur on the upper body a few days after a major injury.
- Other findings include fever, tachycardia, tachypnea, blood-tinged sputum, cyanosis, anxiety, altered level of consciousness, seizures, coma, or rash.

Idiopathic thrombocytopenic purpura

- Scattered petechiae on the distal arms and legs are an early sign.
- Deep-lying ecchymoses may also occur.
- Other findings include epistaxis, easy bruising, hematuria, hematemesis, and menorrhagia.

Leukemia

- Widespread, persistent petechiae appear on the skin, mucous membranes, retina, and serosal surfaces.
- Other findings include fever, abdominal or bone pain, lymphadenopathy, splenomegaly, swollen and bleeding gums, epistaxis, and other bleeding tendencies.

Liver disease

- Purpura, particularly ecchymoses, and other bleeding tendencies may occur.

Meningococcemia

- Cutaneous and oropharyngeal petechiae and purpura are initially discrete but become confluent, developing into hemorrhagic bullae and ulcerations.
- Sudden, severe infection results in extensive purpura and ecchymosis with irregular borders, most notably on the extremities.
- Other findings include spiking fevers, chills, myalgia, and arthralgia progressing to headache, neck stiffness, and nuchal rigidity.

Myeloproliferative disorders

- Hemorrhage accompanied by ecchymoses and ruddy cyanosis can occur.
- The oral mucosa takes on a deep purplish red hue, and slight trauma causes swollen gums to bleed.
- Other findings include pruritus, urticaria, lethargy, fatigue, weight loss, headache, dizziness, vertigo, dyspnea, paresthesia, visual alterations, intermittent claudication, hypertension, hepatosplenomegaly, and impaired mentation.

Nutritional deficiencies

- With vitamin C deficiency, purpura patches join together to form ecchymoses on the inner thighs and lower buttocks.
- With vitamin K deficiency, abnormal bleeding tendencies, such as ecchymosis, gum bleeding, epistaxis, and hematuria.
- With vitamin B_{12} and folic acid deficiencies, varying degrees of purpura.

Rocky Mountain spotted fever

○ Initial skin lesions are small pink macules that evolve into blatant petechiae and palpable purpura; palms and soles are particularly affected.

○ Fever, severe headache, myalgia, photophobia, nausea, and vomiting; later, shock and death

Septicemia

○ Purpura, especially petechiae

○ Fever, chills, headache, tachycardia, lethargy, diaphoresis, anorexia, and signs of specific infection

Systemic lupus erythematosus

○ Purpura may occur with other cutaneous findings.

○ Characteristic butterfly-shaped rash appears in the disorder's acute phase.

○ Common findings include nondeforming joint pain and stiffness, Raynaud's phenomenon, seizures, psychotic behavior, photosensitivity, fever, anorexia, weight loss, and lymphadenopathy.

Trauma

○ Local or widespread purpura

Other causes

Procedures and diagnostic tests

○ Invasive diagnostic tests may produce local ecchymoses and hematomas.

○ Procedures that disrupt circulation, coagulation, or platelet activity or production can cause purpura.

Drugs

○ Anticoagulants

Nursing considerations

○ Apply pressure and cold compresses to hematomas for the first 24 hours to reduce bleeding; then apply hot compresses to speed absorption of blood.

Pediatric pointers

○ Neonates commonly exhibit petechiae, particularly on the head, neck, and shoulders, after vertex deliveries.

○ The most common type of purpura in children is allergic purpura.

○ When assessing a child with purpura, be alert for signs of possible child abuse.

Geriatric pointers

○ Purpura can be a consequence of aging.

○ Chronic stasis produces dusky reddish purpura on the legs after prolonged standing.

Patient teaching

○ Explain treating the underlying disease.

○ Discuss the avoidance of fade creams.

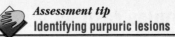

Assessment tip
Identifying purpuric lesions

Purpuric lesions fall into three categories: petechiae, ecchymoses, and hematomas. Use the illustrations below to help you accurately identify purpuric lesions in your patients.

Petechiae

Petechiae are painless, round, pinpoint lesions, 1 to 3 mm in diameter. Caused by extravasation of red blood cells into cutaneous tissue, these red or brown lesions usually arise on dependent portions of the body. They appear and fade in crops and can group to form ecchymoses.

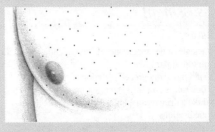

Ecchymoses

Ecchymoses, another form of blood extravasation, are larger than petechiae. These purple, blue, or yellow-green bruises vary in size and shape and can arise anywhere on the body as a result of trauma. Ecchymoses usually appear on the arms and legs of patients with bleeding disorders.

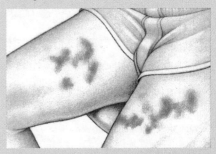

Hematomas

Hematomas are palpable ecchymoses that are painful and swollen. Usually the result of trauma, superficial hematomas are red, whereas deep hematomas are blue. Hematomas commonly exceed 1 cm in diameter, but their size varies widely.

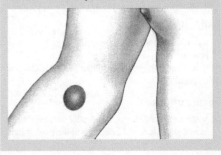

Pustular rash

Overview

○ Rash is made up of crops of pustules — visible collections of pus within or beneath the epidermis, commonly in a hair follicles or sweat pores.
○ Pustules vary greatly in size and shape.
○ Rash can be generalized or localized to the hair follicles or sweat glands.

Assessment

History

○ Ask about the appearance, location, and onset of the first pustular lesion.
○ Find out about preceding lesions.
○ Determine how the lesions spread.
○ Take a drug history, including the use of topical medications.
○ Ask about a family history of skin disorders.

Physical assessment

○ Assess entire skin surface, noting if it's dry, oily, or moist.
○ Record the exact location and distribution of skin lesions, noting color, shape, and size.

Medical causes

Acne vulgaris

○ Pustules accompany papules, nodules, cysts, and open and closed comedones.
○ Lesions commonly appear on the face, shoulders, back, and chest.
○ Other findings include pain on pressure, pruritus, burning and, if chronic, scars.

Blastomycosis

○ Small, painless, nonpruritic macules or papules can enlarge to well-circumscribed, verrucous, crusted, or ulcerated lesions edged by pustules.
○ Other findings include pleuritic chest pain and a dry, hacking or productive cough with occasional hemoptysis.

Folliculitis

○ Individual pustules each pierced by a hair
○ Pruritus
○ If the condition progresses, hard painful nodules of furunculosis

Furunculosis

○ Acute, deep-seated, red, hot, tender abscess evolves from a staphylococcal folliculitis at the base of hair follicles.

○ Most commonly occur in areas prone to repeated infection, such as the face, neck, forearms, groin, axillae, buttocks, and legs.
○ Pustules remain tense for 2 to 4 days and then become fluctuant.
○ With rupture, pus and necrotic material are discharged, pain subsides, but erythema and edema may persist.

Gonococcemia

○ A rash of scanty, pinpoint erythematous macules rapidly becomes vesiculopustular, maculopapular and, frequently, hemorrhagic.
○ Mature lesions are elevated, with dirty gray necrotic centers and surrounding erythema.
○ Rash occurs on palms and soles, usually during the first day that other signs and symptoms, such as fever and joint pain, occur.
○ Rash disappears after 3 or 4 days but may recur with each episode of fever.

Impetigo contagiosa

○ Vesicles form and break, and a crust forms from the exudate: a thick, yellow crust in streptococcal impetigo and a thin, clear crust in staphylococcal impetigo.
○ Painless itching occurs in both forms.

Nummular or annular dermatitis

○ Numerous coinlike or ringed pustular lesions appear, usually on the extensor surfaces of the extremities, posterior trunk, buttocks, and lower legs.
○ Lesions commonly ooze a purulent exudate, itch severely, and become crusted and scaly rapidly.

Pustular miliaria

○ Pustular lesions begin as tiny erythematous papulovesicles at sweat pores.
○ Diffuse erythema may radiate from the lesion.
○ Rash and associated burning and pruritus worsen with sweating.

Rosacea

○ Acute episodes of pustules, papules, and edema occur with telangiectasia.
○ Rosacea is characterized by persistent erythema.
○ It may begin as a flush covering the forehead, malar region, nose, and chin.
○ Intermittent episodes gradually become more persistent, and the skin develops varying degrees of erythema.

Scabies

○ Threadlike channels or burrows under skin characterize scabies; pustules, vesicles, and excoriations may also occur.
○ Lesions have a swollen nodule or red papule that contains the itch mite.

Smallpox

○ A maculopapular rash develops on the mucosa of the mouth, pharynx, face, and forearms and then spreads to the trunk and legs.
○ Initial findings include high fever, malaise, prostration, severe headache, and abdominal pain.
○ Within 2 days, the rash becomes vesicular and later, pustular.
○ Pustules are round, firm, and deeply embedded in the skin.
○ After 8 to 9 days the pustules form a crust, and later the scab separates from the skin, leaving a pitted scar.

Varicella zoster

○ Extremely painful and pruritic vesicles and pustules occur along a dermatome.
○ Chronic pain may persist for months.

Other causes

Drugs

○ Bromides and iodides commonly cause a pustular rash.
○ Corticotropin, corticosteroids, dactinomycin, trimethadione, lithium, phenytoin, phenobarbital, isoniazid, hormonal contraceptives, androgens, and anabolic steroids may also cause a pustular rash.

Nursing considerations

○ Until infection is ruled out, take wound and skin isolation precautions.
○ If the organism is infectious, don't allow any drainage to touch unaffected skin.

Pediatric pointers

○ Varicella, erythema toxicum neonatorum, candidiasis, impetigo, infantile acropustulosis, and acrodermatitis enteropathica may produce a pustular rash in children.

Patient teaching

○ Explain methods to prevent the spread of infection.
○ Provide emotional support.
○ Provide information about relieving pain and itching.

Pyrosis

Overview

- Substernal burning sensation that rises in the chest and may radiate to the neck or throat
- Also called *heartburn*
- Caused by reflux of gastric contents into the esophagus
- Commonly accompanied by regurgitation
- Usually develops after meals or when the patient lies down, bends over, lifts heavy objects, or exercises vigorously; improves when the patient sits upright or takes an antacid (see *How pyrosis occurs*)

Assessment

History

- Ask about a history of heartburn.
- Find out about factors that aggravate, alleviate, or trigger heartburn.
- Determine the location of pain and whether it radiates.
- Ask about other signs and symptoms, including regurgitation.

Physical assessment

- Perform an abdominal assessment.
- Examine the mouth and throat.

Medical causes

Esophageal cancer

- Painless dysphagia that progressively worsens is an early symptom.
- Regurgitation and aspiration commonly occur at night.
- Other findings include rapid weight loss, steady pain in the front and back of chest, hoarseness, sore throat, nausea, vomiting, and a feeling of substernal fullness.

Esophageal diverticula

- Pyrosis, regurgitation, and dysphagia may occur, although the disorder usually causes no symptoms.
- Other findings include chronic cough, halitosis, chest pain, a bad taste in the mouth, and a gurgling in the esophagus when liquids are swallowed.

Gastroesophageal reflux disease

- Pyrosis, which is typically severe, is the most common symptom.
- Pyrosis tends to be chronic, occurs 30 to 60 minutes after eating, and may be triggered by certain foods or beverages.

- Pyrosis worsens when the patient lies down or bends and abates when he sits upright or takes an antacid.
- Other findings include postural regurgitation, dysphagia, flatulent dyspepsia, and dull retrosternal pain that may radiate.

Hiatal hernia

- Eructation after eating, with heartburn, regurgitation of sour-tasting fluid, and abdominal distention.
- Dull substernal or epigastric pain, radiating to the shoulder.
- Dysphagia, nausea, weight loss, dyspnea, tachypnea, a cough, and halitosis.

Obesity

- Reflux and resulting pyrosis from increased intra-abdominal pressure.
- Hypertension, cardiovascular disease, diabetes mellitus, renal disease, gallbladder disease, and psychosocial difficulties.

Peptic ulcer disease

- Pyrosis and indigestion usually signal the start of a peptic ulcer attack.
- Gnawing, burning pain in the left epigastrium may occur 2 or 3 hours after eating or when the stomach is empty (usually at night) and is relieved by eating or taking an antacid or antisecretory.

Scleroderma

- Reflux with pyrosis from esophageal dysfunction.
- The sensation of food sticking behind the breastbone, odynophagia, bloating after meals, and weight loss.
- Abdominal distention, constipation or diarrhea, and malodorous floating stools.
- Early, blanching, pruritus, cyanosis, and stress- or cold-induced erythema of the fingers and toes.
- Later, finger and joint pain, stiffness, and swelling; skin thickening on the hands and forearms; masklike facies; and flexion contractures.
- With advanced disease, arrhythmias, dyspnea, cough, malignant hypertension, and signs of renal failure.

Other causes

Drugs

- Tolbutamide, aspirin, anticholinergics, and drugs that have anticholinergic effects may cause or aggravate pyrosis.

Lifestyle

- Large meals or pregnancy may cause or aggravate pyrosis.

Serving as a barrier to reflux, the lower esophageal sphincter (LES) normally relaxes only to allow food to pass from the esophagus into the stomach. However, hormonal fluctuations, mechanical stress, and the effects of certain foods and drugs can lower LES pressure. When LES pressure falls and intra-abdominal or intragastric pressure rises, the normally contracted LES relaxes inappropriately and allows reflux of gastric acid or bile secretions into the lower esophagus. There, the acids or secretions irritate and inflame the esophageal mucosa, producing pyrosis.

Persistent inflammation can cause LES pressure to decrease even more and may trigger a cycle of reflux and pyrosis.

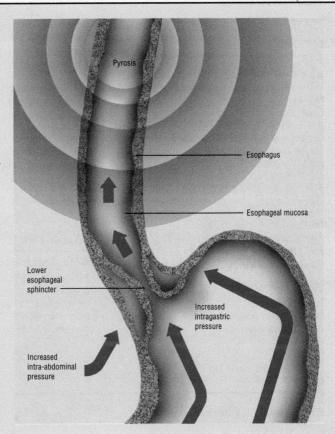

Nursing considerations

○ Prepare the patient for diagnostic tests.
○ Position the patient to alleviate pyrosis.
○ Give antacids, if needed.

Pediatric pointers

○ Help a child describe the sensation to aid differentiation between esophageal pain and pyrosis.

Geriatric pointers

○ Elderly patients with peptic ulcer disease commonly present with nonspecific abdominal discomfort or weight loss.
○ Elderly patients are at greater risk for complications from nonsteroidal anti-inflammatories.
○ Many develop pyrosis caused by intolerance to spicy foods.

Patient teaching

○ Discuss lifestyle changes, such as eating frequent, small meals and sitting upright for 2 hours after meals.

○ Explain dietary restrictions and guidelines the patient needs to use.
○ Explain measures to prevent increased intra-abdominal pressure.
○ Discuss the importance of stopping smoking and drugs that reduce sphincter control.

Raccoon eyes

Overview

○ Refers to periorbital ecchymoses that don't result from facial soft-tissue trauma (see *Recognizing raccoon eyes*)
○ Usually an indicator of basilar skull fracture
○ Develops when damage at the time of fracture tears the meninges and causes the venous sinuses to bleed into the arachnoid villi and the cranial sinuses
○ May be the only indicator of basilar skull fracture

Assessment

History
○ Find out when the head injury occurred and the nature of the injury.
○ Obtain a medical history.

Physical assessment
○ Take vital signs.
○ Evaluate level of consciousness (LOC) using the Glasgow Coma Scale.

○ Evaluate function of the cranial nerves, especially I (olfactory), III (oculomotor), IV (trochlear), VI (abducens), and VII (facial).
○ Assess for signs and symptoms of increased intracranial pressure.
○ Test visual acuity.
○ Assess gross hearing.
○ Note irregularities in the facial or skull bones.
○ Observe for swelling, localized pain, a Battle's sign, or lacerations of the face or scalp.
○ Check for ecchymoses over the mastoid bone.
○ Inspect for hemorrhage or cerebrospinal fluid (CSF) leakage from the nose or ears.
○ Test any drainage with a sterile gauze pad and note whether a halo sign is present, indicating CSF.
○ Use a glucose reagent strip to test any clear drainage for glucose.

Medical causes

Basilar skull fracture
○ Raccoon eyes are produced after head trauma that doesn't involve the orbital area.
○ Other findings vary with the fracture site and may include pharyngeal hemorrhage, epistaxis, rhinorrhea, otorrhea, and a bulging tympanic membrane from blood or CSF.

Assessment tip
Recognizing raccoon eyes

It's usually easy to differentiate "raccoon eyes" from the "black eye" associated with facial trauma. Raccoon eyes (shown at right) are always bilateral. They develop within 2 or 3 days of a closed-head injury that results in basilar skull fracture. In contrast, the periorbital ecchymosis that occurs with facial trauma can affect one eye or both. A black eye usually develops within hours of injury.

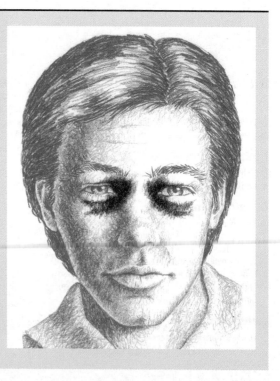

○ Additional findings include difficulty hearing, head-ache, nausea, vomiting, cranial nerve palsies, a positive Battle's sign, and altered LOC.

Other causes

Surgery
○ Raccoon eyes occurring after craniotomy may indicate a meningeal tear and bleeding into the sinuses.

Nursing considerations

○ Keep the patient on complete bedrest.
○ Perform frequent neurologic evaluations to reevaluate his LOC.
○ Check vital signs frequently; look for changes such as bradycardia, bradypnea, hypertension, and fever.
○ Instruct the patient not to blow his nose, cough vigorously, or strain to avoid worsening a dural tear.
○ If otorrhea or rhinorrhea is present, don't attempt to stop the flow; instead, place a sterile loose gauze pad under the nose or ear to absorb the drainage.
○ Monitor the amount of drainage and test it with a glucose reagent strip to confirm or rule out CSF.
○ To prevent further tearing of the mucous membranes and infection, never suction or pass a nasogastric tube through the patient's nose.
○ Observe for signs and symptoms of meningitis, such as fever and nuchal rigidity, and expect to administer a prophylactic antibiotic.
○ If the dural tear doesn't heal spontaneously, contrast cisternography may be performed to locate the tear, possibly followed by corrective surgery.

Pediatric pointers
○ Raccoon eyes in children are usually caused by a basilar skull fracture after a fall.

Patient teaching
○ Explain the signs and symptoms of neurologic deterioration to report.
○ Explain the activity limitations the patient needs.
○ Give the patient instructions for care of a scalp wound.

Rebound tenderness

Overview

- Refers to intense, elicited abdominal pain caused by rebound of the palpated tissues (see *Eliciting rebound tenderness*)
- Also called Blumberg's sign
- A reliable indicator of peritonitis or peritoneal inflammation
- May be localized, as in an abscess, or generalized, as in perforation of an intra-abdominal organ
- Occurs usually with abdominal pain, tenderness, and rigidity

Emergency actions

If you elicit rebound tenderness in a patient who's experiencing constant, severe abdominal pain, quickly take his vital signs. Insert a large-bore I.V. catheter and begin administering I.V. fluids. Insert an indwelling urinary catheter and monitor intake and output. Give supplemental oxygen as needed, and continue to monitor the patient for signs of shock, such as hypotension and tachycardia.

Assessment

History

- Ask about the event that led up to the tenderness.

Assessment tip
Eliciting rebound tenderness

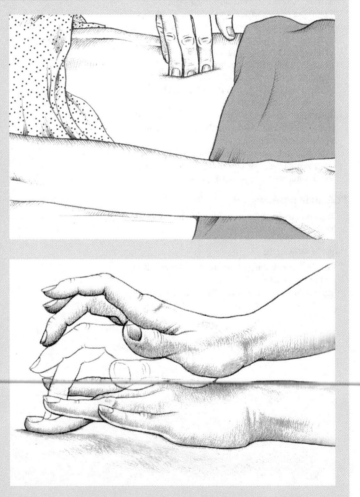

To elicit rebound tenderness, help the patient into a supine position, and push your fingers deeply and steadily into his abdomen (as shown). Quickly release the pressure. Pain that results from the rebound of palpated tissue (rebound tenderness) indicates peritoneal inflammation or peritonitis.

You can also elicit this symptom on a miniature scale by percussing the patient's abdomen lightly and indirectly (as shown). Better still, simply ask the patient to cough. This allows you to elicit rebound tenderness without having to touch the patient's abdomen and may also increase his cooperation because he won't associate exacerbation of his pain with your actions.

- Inquire about what aggravates and alleviates the tenderness.
- Find out about other signs and symptoms, such as nausea, vomiting, fever, or abdominal bloating or distention, or changes in bowel and bladder function.
- Take a medical history.

Physical assessment

- Inspect the abdomen for distention, visible peristaltic waves, and scars.
- Auscultate for bowel sounds and characterize their motility.
- Palpate for associated rigidity or guarding, starting with light palpation and, if needed, progressing to deep palpation.
- Percuss the abdomen noting any tympany.

Medical causes

Peritonitis

- A life-threatening disorder; rebound tenderness is accompanied by sudden and severe abdominal pain, which may be diffuse or localized.
- Pain may worsen with movement.
- Typical findings include weakness, pallor, excessive sweating, and cold skin.
- Other findings include hypoactive or absent bowel sounds, tachypnea, nausea, vomiting, positive psoas and obturator signs, high fever, and abdominal distention, rigidity, and guarding.
- Shoulder pain and hiccups suggest inflammation of the diaphragmatic peritoneum.

Nursing considerations

- Promote comfort by helping the patient flex his knees or assume a semi-Fowler's position.
- An analgesic may mask other symptoms.
- Give an antiemetic and antipyretic.
- Withhold oral drugs and fluids because of decreased intestinal motility and the probability that the patient may require surgery.
- Give an antibiotic.
- Inset a nasogastric tube, if needed.
- Give continuous parenteral fluid or nutrition.

Pediatric pointers

- Because eliciting rebound tenderness may be difficult in young children, look for such clues as an anguished facial expression or intensified crying.
- When eliciting this symptom, use assessment techniques that produce minimal tenderness.

Geriatric pointers

- May be diminished or absent in elderly patients.

Patient teaching

- Explain the signs and symptoms the patient needs to report immediately.
- Instruct the patient in postoperative care.

Rectal pain

Overview

- Discomfort arising in the anorectal area
- A common symptom of anorectal disorders
- May result from or be aggravated by diarrhea, constipation, or passage of stool
- May be aggravated by intense pruritus and continued scratching associated with drainage of mucus, blood, or feces that irritates the skin and nerve endings

Assessment

History

- Obtain a description of pain, including quality and intensity and what aggravates and alleviates the pain.
- Find out about other signs and symptoms, such as rectal bleeding, presence of mucus or pus, and constipation or diarrhea.
- Ask the date of last bowel movement.
- Obtain a dietary history.

Physical assessment

- Inspect the rectal area for bleeding, drainage, or protrusions.
- Check for inflammation and other lesions.
- Perform a rectal examination, if needed.
- Assess stool for occult blood.

Medical causes

Abscess

- A superficial abscess produces constant, throbbing, local pain that's exacerbated by sitting or walking.
- With a deep abscess, the pain may begin insidiously high in the rectum or even in the lower abdomen and be accompanied by an indurated anal mass, fever, malaise, anal swelling and inflammation, purulent drainage, and local tenderness.
- A prostatic abscess occasionally produces rectal pain and may be accompanied by urine frequency with retention, dysuria, and fever.

Anal fissure

- Sharp rectal pain occurs on defecation.
- A burning sensation and gnawing pain may continue up to 4 hours after defecation.
- Fear of provoking pain may lead to acute constipation.
- Other findings include anal pruritus and extreme tenderness, and the patient may report finding spots of blood on the toilet tissue after defecation.

Anorectal fistula

- Pain develops when a tract formed between the anal canal and skin temporarily seals.
- Other findings include pruritus and drainage of pus, mucus, blood and, occasionally, stool.

Cryptitis

- Dull anal pain or discomfort occurs with anal pruritus.
- Intense pain may occur when the anal sphincter contracts.

Hemorrhoids

- Rectal pain worsens during defecation and subsides after it.
- Usually, rectal pain is accompanied by severe itching.
- Fear of provoking pain may lead to constipation.
- With internal hemorrhoids, mild, intermittent bleeding characteristically occurs as spotting on toilet tissue or on the stool surface.

Proctalgia fugax

- Muscle spasms of the rectum and pelvic floor produce sudden episodes of severe rectal pain.
- The pain is sometimes associated with stress or anxiety and relieved by food and drink.
- The pain may awaken the patient.

Rectal cancer

- Rectal pain, bleeding, tenesmus, and a hard, nontender mass are typical findings in this rare form of cancer.

Other causes

Anal intercourse

- Shearing forces may cause inflammation or tearing of the mucous membranes and discomfort.

Nursing considerations

- Apply analgesic ointment or give suppositories.
- Give a stool softener, if needed.
- Apply cold compresses to help shrink protruding hemorrhoids, prevent thrombosis, and reduce pain.
- If the patient's condition permits, place him in Trendelenburg's position with his buttocks elevated to further relieve pain.
- Provide emotional support and privacy.

Pediatric pointers

- Observe any child with rectal pain for bleeding, drainage, and signs of infection.
- Acute anal fissure is a common cause of rectal pain and bleeding in children, whose fear of provoking the pain may lead to constipation.
- Infants who seem to have pain on defecation should be evaluated for congenital rectal anomalies.

○ Look for other indicators of sexual abuse in all children who complain of rectal pain.

Geriatric pointers

○ Perform a thorough evaluation because elderly patients typically underreport their symptoms and have an increased risk of neoplastic disorders.

Patient teaching

○ Instruct the patient on how to ease discomfort.
○ Discuss proper diet and fluid intake.
○ Discuss stool softeners.

Respirations, grunting

Overview

- A deep, low-pitched grunting sound at the end of each breath
- Occurs as the glottis closes
- Indicates intrathoracic disease with lower respiratory involvement
- May be soft and heard only on auscultation, or loud and clearly audible without a stethoscope
- Intensity of the grunting reflects the severity of the respiratory distress

★ Emergency actions

Quickly place the patient in a comfortable position and check for signs of respiratory distress. Monitor oxygen saturation and administer oxygen and drugs such as bronchodilators. Have emergency equipment available and intubate the patient if necessary. Obtain arterial blood gas (ABG) analysis to determine oxygenation.

Assessment

History

- Ask about the onset of grunting respirations.
- Find out the gestational age of an infant.
- Find out if anyone in the home has recently had an upper respiratory tract infection.
- Inquire about a personal history of frequent colds or upper respiratory tract infections.
- Ask about a history of respiratory syncytial virus.
- Note changes in activity level or feeding pattern.

Physical assessment

- Observe for use of accessory muscles and retractions during respiration.
- Check for cyanosis, diaphoresis, retractions, and edema.
- Auscultate the lungs, noting diminished or abnormal sounds.
- Characterize the color, amount, and consistency of any discharge or sputum.
- Note the characteristics of the cough, if any.

Medical causes

Asthma

- Grunting respirations may be apparent during severe attack.
- As the attack progresses, dyspnea, audible wheezing, chest tightness, and coughing occur.

Heart failure

- Grunting respirations accompany increasing pulmonary edema as a late sign of left-sided heart failure.
- Other findings include productive cough, crackles, and chest wall retractions.
- Cyanosis may also be evident, depending on the underlying congenital cardiac defect.

Pneumonia

- Grunting respirations accompany diminished breath sounds, scattered crackles, sibilant rhonchi, high fever, tachypnea, a productive cough, anorexia, and lethargy.
- As the disorder progresses, severe dyspnea, substernal and subcostal retractions, nasal flaring, cyanosis, and increasing lethargy may occur.
- GI signs, such as vomiting, diarrhea, and abdominal distention may also be seen.

Respiratory distress syndrome

- Initially, audible expiratory grunting occurs with intercostal, subcostal, or substernal retractions; tachycardia; and tachypnea.
- Later, as the infant tires, apnea or irregular respirations replace grunting.
- Cyanosis, frothy sputum, dramatic nasal flaring, lethargy, bradycardia, and hypotension characterize severe distress.

Nursing considerations

- Closely monitor the patient's condition.
- Keep emergency equipment nearby.
- Administer oxygen using an oxygen hood or tent.
- Continually monitor ABG levels and deliver the minimum amount of oxygen possible to avoid causing retinopathy of prematurity.
- Begin inhalation therapy with a bronchodilator.
- If the patient has pneumonia, give an I.V. antimicrobial.
- Perform chest physiotherapy.
- Provide emotional support to the patient and family.

Pediatric pointers

- Grunting respirations may be a chief sign of respiratory distress in infants and children. (See *Positioning an infant for chest physical therapy*.)

Patient teaching

- Explain the sights and sounds of intensive care.
- Teach techniques for home respiratory care and therapy.
- Give instructions on the proper use of prescribed drugs.
- Explain the signs and symptoms to report.

Positioning an infant for chest physical therapy

An infant with grunting respirations may need chest physical therapy to mobilize and drain excess lung secretions. Auscultate first to locate congested areas and determine the best drainage position. Then review the illustrations here, which show the various drainage positions and where to place your hands for percussion. When you percuss the infant, use the fingers of one hand. Vibrate these fingers and move them toward the infant's head to facilitate drainage.

Hold the infant upright and about 30 degrees forward to percuss and drain the apical segments of the upper lobes.

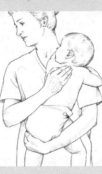

Place the infant in a supine position to percuss and drain the anterior segments of the upper lobes.

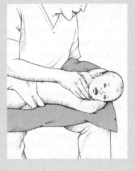

Use this position to percuss and drain the posterior segments of the upper lobes.

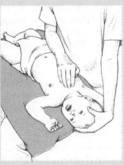

Hold the infant at a 45-degree angle on his side with his head down about 15 degrees to percuss and drain the right middle lobe.

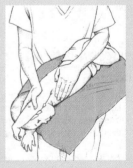

Place the infant in a supine position with his head 30 degrees lower than his feet to percuss and drain the anterior segments of the lower lobes.

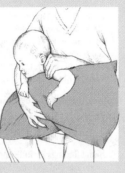

Place the infant in a prone position with his head down 30 degrees to percuss and drain the posterior basal segments of the lower lobes.

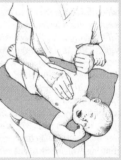

Place the infant on his side with his head down 30 degrees to percuss and drain the lateral basal segments of the lower lobes. Repeat this on the other side.

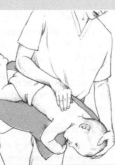

Use a prone position to percuss and drain the superior segments of the lower lobes.

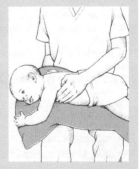

Respirations, shallow

Overview

- A diminished volume of air during inspiration
- Trigger accelerated respiratory rate as the patient attempts to obtain enough oxygen
- Lead to inadequate gas exchange as muscles tire and compensatory increase in respirations diminishes
- May develop suddenly or gradually and may last briefly or become chronic
- Are key signs of respiratory distress and neurologic deterioration

Emergency actions

Look for impending respiratory failure or arrest. Look for signs of airway obstruction. If the patient is choking, perform four back blows and four abdominal thrusts to try to expel the foreign object. If secretions occlude the patient's airway, use suction.

If the patient is also wheezing, check for stridor, nasal flaring, and the use of accessory muscles. Administer oxygen with a face mask or handheld resuscitation bag. Attempt to calm the patient.

If the patient loses consciousness, insert an artificial airway and prepare for endotracheal intubation and ventilatory support. Measure his tidal volume and minute volume with a Wright respirometer to determine the need for mechanical ventilation. (See Measuring lung volumes.) *Check arterial blood gas (ABG) levels, heart rate, blood pressure, and oxygen saturation.*

Assessment

History

- If the patient is not in severe respiratory distress, take a complete medical history, including chronic respiratory disorders or respiratory tract infection, neurologic or neuromuscular disease, surgery, and trauma.
- Ask if the patient has had a tetanus booster within the past 10 years.
- Ask about smoking history.
- Take a drug history and explore the possibility of drug abuse.
- Determine the onset and duration of shallow respirations.
- Ask about factors that exacerbate or relieve shallow respirations.
- Note any changes in appetite, weight, activity level, and behavior.

Physical assessment

- Evaluate the patient's level of consciousness (LOC) and his orientation to time, person, and place.
- Observe for spontaneous movements.
- Test muscle strength and deep tendon reflexes.
- Inspect the chest for deformities or abnormal movements.
- Inspect the extremities for cyanosis, edema, and digital clubbing.
- Palpate for expansion and diaphragmatic tactile fremitus.
- Percuss for hyperresonance or dullness.
- Auscultate for diminished, absent, or adventitious breath sounds and for abnormal or distant heart sounds.
- Examine the abdomen for distention, tenderness, or masses.

Medical causes

Acute respiratory distress syndrome

- A life-threatening disorder; rapid, shallow respirations and dyspnea appear initially, sometimes after the patient appears stable.
- Other findings include intercostal and suprasternal retractions, diaphoresis, rhonchi, crackles, restlessness, apprehension, decreased LOC, cyanosis, and tachycardia.

Amyotrophic lateral sclerosis

- Progressive degenerative respiratory muscle weakness leads to progressive shallow, ineffective respirations.
- Initial findings include upper extremity muscle weakness and wasting.
- Other findings include muscle cramps and atrophy, hyperreflexia, slight spasticity of the legs, coarse fasciculations of the affected muscle, impaired speech, and difficulty chewing and swallowing.

Asthma

- Rapid, shallow respirations result from bronchospasm and decreased alveolar gas exchange.
- Related respiratory findings include wheezing, rhonchi, a dry cough, dyspnea, prolonged expirations, intercostal and supraclavicular retractions on inspiration, nasal flaring, chest tightness, tachycardia, diaphoresis, and the use of accessory muscles.

Atelectasis

- Decreased lung expansion or pleuritic pain causes sudden onset of rapid, shallow respirations.
- Other findings include a dry cough, dyspnea, tachycardia, anxiety, cyanosis, diaphoresis, dullness to percussion, decreased breath sounds and vocal fremitus, inspiratory lag, and substernal or intercostal retractions.

Bronchiectasis

- Increased secretions obstruct airflow in the bronchi, leading to shallow respirations and a productive

Use a Wright respirometer to measure tidal volume (the amount of air inspired with each breath) and minute volume (the volume of air inspired in a minute—or tidal volume multiplied by respiratory rate). You can connect the respirometer to an intubated patient's airway using an endotracheal tube (shown here) or a tracheostomy tube. If the patient isn't intubated, connect the respirometer to a face mask, making sure the seal over the patient's mouth and nose is airtight.

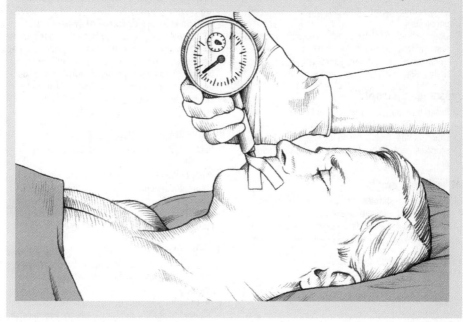

cough with copious, foul-smelling, mucopurulent sputum (a classic finding).
○ Other findings include hemoptysis, wheezing, rhonchi, coarse crackles during inspiration, and late-stage clubbing.

Chronic bronchitis

○ Shallow respirations result from chronic airway inflammation.
○ A nonproductive, hacking cough that later becomes productive is an early sign.
○ Other findings include prolonged expirations, wheezing, dyspnea, accessory muscle use, barrel chest, cyanosis, tachypnea, scattered rhonchi, coarse crackles, and late-stage clubbing.

Emphysema

○ Increased breathing effort causes muscle fatigue, leading to chronic shallow respirations.
○ Other findings include dyspnea, anorexia, malaise, tachypnea, diminished breath sounds, cyanosis, pursed-lip breathing, accessory muscle use, barrel chest, chronic productive cough, and late-stage clubbing.

Flail chest

○ Decreased air movement results in rapid, shallow respirations; paradoxical chest wall motion.
○ Other findings include tachycardia, hypotension, ecchymoses, cyanosis, and pain over the affected area.

Fractured ribs

○ Sharp, severe pain on inspiration may cause shallow respirations.
○ Other findings include dyspnea, cough, splinting, and tenderness and edema at the fracture site.

Guillain-Barré syndrome

○ Progressive ascending paralysis causes rapid or progressive onset of shallow respirations.
○ Muscle weakness begins in the lower limbs and extends to the face.
○ Other findings include paresthesia, dysarthria, diminished or absent corneal reflex, nasal speech, dysphagia, ipsilateral loss of facial muscle control, and flaccid paralysis.

Kyphoscoliosis

○ Skeletal cage distortion cause rapid, shallow respirations from reduced lung capacity.

- Accompanying features include back pain, fatigue, tracheal deviation, ineffective coughing, and dyspnea.

Multiple sclerosis

- Muscle weakness causes progressive shallow respirations.
- Early findings include diplopia, blurred vision, and paresthesia.
- Other possible findings include nystagmus, constipation, paralysis, spasticity, hyperreflexia, intention tremor, ataxic gait, dysphagia, dysarthria, urinary dysfunction, impotence, and emotional lability.

Muscular dystrophy

- Progressive thoracic deformity and muscle weakness cause shallow respirations to occur.
- Other findings include waddling gait, contractures, scoliosis, lordosis, and muscle atrophy or hypertrophy.

Myasthenia gravis

- Progressive respiratory muscle weakness leads to shallow respirations, dyspnea, and cyanosis.
- Other findings include fatigue, weak eye closure, ptosis, diplopia, and difficulty chewing and swallowing.

Obesity

- The work of breathing may cause shallow respirations.

Parkinson's disease

- Fatigue and weakness lead to progressive shallow respirations.
- Disorder slowly progresses to increased rigidity, masklike facies, stooped posture, shuffling gait, dysphagia, drooling, dysarthria, and pill-rolling tremor.

Pleural effusion

- Restricted lung expansion causes shallow respirations.
- Other findings include nonproductive cough, weight loss, dyspnea, pleural friction rub, tachycardia, tachypnea, decreased chest motion, decreased or absent breath sounds, and pleuritic chest pain.

Pneumonia

- Pulmonary consolidation results in rapid, shallow respirations.
- Accompanying findings include dyspnea, fever, shaking chills, chest pain, cough, tachycardia, decreased breath sounds, crackles, rhonchi, myalgia, fatigue, anorexia, headache, and cyanosis.

Pneumothorax

- Shallow respirations and dyspnea begin suddenly.
- Related findings include tachycardia, tachypnea, nonproductive cough, cyanosis, accessory muscle use, asymmetrical chest expansion, anxiety, restlessness, subcutaneous crepitation, diminished or absent breath sounds on the affected side, and sudden, sharp, severe chest pain that worsens with movement.

Pulmonary edema

- Pulmonary vascular congestion causes rapid, shallow respirations.
- Early findings include exertional dyspnea, paroxysmal nocturnal dyspnea, nonproductive cough, tachycardia, tachypnea, crackles, and a ventricular gallop.
- Severe pulmonary edema produces more rapid, labored respirations; widespread crackles; a productive cough with frothy, bloody sputum; worsening tachycardia; arrhythmias; cold, clammy skin; cyanosis; hypotension; and thready pulse.

Pulmonary embolism

- Rapid, shallow respirations and severe dyspnea begin suddenly.
- Other findings include tachycardia, tachypnea, a nonproductive cough or a productive cough with blood-tinged sputum, low-grade fever, restlessness, pleural friction rub, crackles, diffuse wheezing, chest pain, and signs of circulatory collapse.

Spinal cord injury

- Diaphragmatic breathing and shallow respirations may occur in injury to the C5 to C8 cervical vertebrae.
- Other findings include quadriplegia with flaccidity followed by spastic paralysis, areflexia, hypotension, sensory loss below the level of injury, and bowel and bladder incontinence.

Upper airway obstruction

- Partial airway obstruction causes acute shallow respirations with sudden gagging and dry, paroxysmal coughing; hoarseness; stridor; and tachycardia.
- Other findings include dyspnea, decreased breath sounds, wheezing, and cyanosis.

Other causes

Drugs

- Opioids, sedatives and hypnotics, tranquilizers, neuromuscular blockers, magnesium sulfate, and anesthetics can produce slow, shallow respirations.

Surgery

- After abdominal or chest surgery, pain from chest splinting and decreased chest wall motion may cause shallow respirations.

Nursing considerations

- Position the patient upright to ease his breathing.

○ Ensure adequate hydration and the use humidification as needed.
○ Give oxygen, a bronchodilator, a mucolytic, an expectorant, or an antibiotic.
○ Turn the patient frequently.
○ Monitor the patient for increasing lethargy, which may indicate rising carbon dioxide levels.

Pediatric pointers

○ In children, shallow respirations commonly indicate a life-threatening condition.
○ Airway obstruction can occur rapidly because of the narrow passageways; if it does, administer back blows or chest thrusts but not abdominal thrusts, which can damage internal organs.

Geriatric pointers

○ Stiffness or deformity of the chest wall may cause shallow respirations.

Patient teaching

○ Explain the importance of coughing and deep breathing.
○ Provide emotional support and teach the caregiver to do so as well.

Respirations, stertorous

Overview

- Are characterized by harsh, rattling, or snoring sound
- Result from the vibration of relaxed oropharyngeal structures during sleep or coma, causing partial airway obstruction
- Occurs normally in about 10% of the population, especially middle-age, obese men
- May be aggravated by the ingestion of alcohol or sedatives before bed and by sleeping in a supine position

✦ Emergency actions

Check the patient's mouth and throat for edema, redness, masses, or foreign objects. If edema is marked, take vital signs, including oxygen saturation levels. Observe for signs and symptoms of respiratory distress, such as dyspnea, tachypnea, using accessory muscles, intercostal muscle retractions, and cyanosis. Elevate the head of bed 30 degrees to help ease the patient's breathing and reduce edema. Then administer supplemental oxygen and intubate, perform a tracheostomy, or provide mechanical ventilation. Insert an I.V. line for fluid and drug access and begin cardiac monitoring.

Assessment

History

- Ask the patient's sleeping partner about his snoring habits.
- Ask about factors that decrease snoring.
- Inquire about sleeptalking and sleepwalking.
- Ask about signs of sleep deprivation, such as personality changes, headaches, daytime somnolence, or decreased mental acuity.

Physical assessment

- Perform a complete respiratory assessment.
- Examine the head, nose, and throat.
- If you detect stertorous respirations while the patient is sleeping, observe his breathing pattern for 3 to 4 minutes.
- Watch for periods of apnea and note their length.

Medical causes

Airway obstruction

- With partial obstruction, stertorous respirations may be accompanied by wheezing, dyspnea, tachypnea, intercostal retractions, and nasal flaring.

- In complete obstruction, the patient abruptly loses ability to talk and displays diaphoresis, tachycardia, and inspiratory chest movement but absent breath sounds; severe hypoxemia rapidly ensues, resulting in cyanosis, loss of consciousness, and cardiopulmonary collapse.

Obstructive sleep apnea

- Loud and disruptive snoring is a major characteristic, commonly affecting the obese.
- Snoring alternates with periods of sleep apnea, which usually end with loud gasping sounds.
- Alternating tachycardia and bradycardia, and hypertension may occur.
- Sleep disturbances such as somnambulism and talking during sleep may occur.
- Other relevant findings may include a generalized headache, feeling tired and unrefreshed, daytime sleepiness, depression, hostility, and decreased mental acuity.

Pickwickian syndrome

- Defined as a group of symptoms that primarily affect extremely obese patients.
- Obstructive sleep apnea with disruptive snoring and disturbed sleep at night results from excessive fatty tissue surrounding the chest muscles.
- Related signs and symptoms include excessive sleepiness during the day, shortness of breath, flushed face or bluish tinge to the face, elevated blood pressure, and enlarged liver.

Other causes

Procedures

- Endotracheal intubation, suction, or surgery may cause significant palatal or uvular edema, resulting in stertorous respirations.

Nursing considerations

- Give a corticosteroid or an antibiotic.
- To reduce palatal and uvular inflammation and edema, provide cool, humidified oxygen.
- Monitor the patient's respiratory status.

Pediatric pointers

- The most common cause of stertorous respirations is nasal or pharyngeal obstruction from tonsillar or adenoid hypertrophy or the presence of a foreign body.

Geriatric pointers

- Encourage the patient to seek treatment for sleep apnea or significant hypertrophy of tonsils or adenoids.

Patient teaching

○ Discuss the importance and methods of weight loss.
○ Explain the set-up and use of continuous or bilevel positive airway pressure device.
○ Teach the patient how to elevate his head while sleeping.
○ Provide information and recommend a smoking cessation program if the patient smokes.
○ Provide teaching on the use of a BiPAP or CPAP device for a patient with sleep apnea.

Retractions, costal and sternal

Overview

- Visible indentations of the soft tissue covering the chest wall
- Suprasternal, intercostal, subcostal, or substernal
- Classic sign of respiratory distress in infants and children

✦ Emergency actions

If you detect retractions in a child, check quickly for other signs of respiratory distress. Prepare the child for suctioning, insertion of an artificial airway, and administration of oxygen. Observe the depth and location of retractions. Also note the rate, depth, and quality of respirations. Look for accessory muscle use, nasal flaring during inspiration, or grunting during expiration. Note whether the child appears restless or lethargic. Auscultate the child's lungs to detect abnormal breath sounds. (See Observing retractions.*)*

Assessment

History

- Ask the parents about the child's medical and birth history.
- Ask about recent signs of upper respiratory infection.
- Determine the frequency of past respiratory problems during the past year.
- Inquire about recent exposure to cold, flu, or respiratory ailment.
- Find out about aspiration of food, liquid, or foreign body.
- Inquire about a personal or family history of allergies or asthma.

Physical assessment

- If the child isn't in severe distress, complete a cardiopulmonary assessment.
- Take the child's vital signs, including his temperature.

Medical causes

Asthma attack

- Intercostal and suprasternal retractions may accompany acute attack.
- Retractions are preceded by dyspnea, wheezing, a hacking cough, and pallor.
- Related findings include cyanosis or flushing, crackles, rhonchi, diaphoresis, tachycardia, tachypnea, a frightened, anxious expression and, with severe distress, nasal flaring.

Bronchiolitis

- Intercostal and subcostal retractions, nasal flaring, tachypnea, dyspnea, cough, restlessness, and a slight fever may occur, most commonly in children younger than age 2.

Croup (spasmodic)

- Attacks of a barking cough, hoarseness, dyspnea, and restlessness occur.
- As distress worsens, findings include suprasternal, substernal, and intercostal retractions; nasal flaring; tachycardia; cyanosis; and an anxious, frantic expression.

Epiglottiditis

- A life-threatening disorder; this infection may precipitate severe respiratory distress with suprasternal, substernal, and intercostal retractions.
- Early findings include sudden onset of a barking cough, stridor, and a high fever, sore throat, hoarseness, dysphagia, drooling, dyspnea, and restlessness.

Heart failure

- Intercostal and substernal retractions occur along with nasal flaring, progressive tachypnea, grunting respirations, edema, and cyanosis.
- Other findings include productive cough, crackles, jugular vein distention, tachycardia, right-upper-quadrant pain, anorexia, and fatigue.

Laryngotracheobronchitis (acute)

- Substernal and intercostal retractions follow low to moderate fever, runny nose, poor appetite, a barking cough, hoarseness, and inspiratory stridor.
- Other findings include tachycardia; shallow, rapid respirations; restlessness; irritability; and pale, cyanotic skin.

Pneumonia (bacterial)

- Subcostal and intercostal retractions follow signs and symptoms of acute infection.
- Other findings include nasal flaring, dyspnea, tachypnea, grunting respirations, cyanosis, a productive cough, and diminished breath sounds, crackles, and sibilant rhonchi over the affected lung.

Respiratory distress syndrome

- A life-threatening disorder; substernal and subcostal retractions are early signs.
- Other early findings include tachypnea, tachycardia, and expiratory grunting.
- As respiratory distress worsens, intercostal and suprasternal retractions occur, and apnea or irregular respirations replace grunting.
- Other findings include nasal flaring, cyanosis, lethargy, and eventual unresponsiveness, bradycardia, and hypotension.

When you observe retractions in infants and children, note their exact location—an important clue to the cause and severity of respiratory distress. For example, subcostal and substernal retractions usually result from lower respiratory tract disorders; suprasternal retractions, from upper respiratory tract disorders.

Mild intercostal retractions alone may be normal. However, intercostal retractions with subcostal and substernal retractions may indicate moderate respiratory distress. Deep suprasternal retractions typically indicate severe distress.

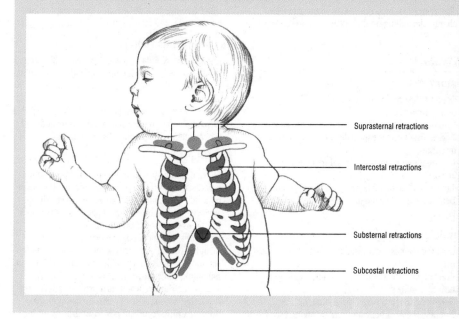

Suprasternal retractions

Intercostal retractions

Substernal retractions

Subcostal retractions

Nursing considerations

○ Monitor vital signs frequently.
○ Keep suction equipment and an airway at the bedside.
○ If the infant weighs less than 15 lb (6.8 kg), place him in an oxygen hood; if he weighs more, place him in a cool mist tent.
○ Perform chest physical therapy with postural drainage.
○ Give a bronchodilator and a steroid.

Pediatric pointers

○ When examining a child for retractions, know that crying may accentuate the contractions.

Geriatric pointers

○ Retractions are more difficult to assess in an older patient who's obese or who has chronic chest wall stiffness or deformity.

Patient teaching

○ Instruct the patient in how to take prescribed drugs properly at home.

○ Give instructions for providing a humidified environment.
○ Stress the importance of ensuring adequate hydration.

Rhinorrhea

Overview

- Free discharge of thin nasal mucus
- Self-limiting or chronic
- Clear, purulent, bloody, or serosanguineous discharge, depending on the cause

Assessment

History

- Obtain a description of the onset and characteristics of the rhinorrhea.
- Find out about aggravating and alleviating factors.
- Take a drug history, especially the use of nose drops or sprays.
- Inquire about exposure to nasal irritants at home or at work.
- Take a medical history, including seasonal allergies.
- Determine whether the patient recently had a head injury.

Physical assessment

- Examine the nose, checking airflow from each nostril.
- Evaluate the size, color, and condition of the turbinate mucosa.
- Note if the mucosa is red, pale, blue, or gray.
- Examine the area beneath each turbinate. (See *Using a nasal speculum*.)
- Palpate over the frontal, ethmoid, and maxillary sinuses for tenderness.
- Collect a small amount of drainage on a glucose reagent strip to differentiate nasal mucus from cerebrospinal fluid (CSF).
- Test for anosmia.

Medical causes

Basilar skull fracture

- Produces CSF rhinorrhea that increases when the head is lowered.
- Other findings include epistaxis, otorrhea, a bulging tympanic membrane, headache, facial paralysis, nausea, vomiting, impaired eye movement, ocular deviation, vision and hearing loss, depressed level of consciousness, Battle's sign, and raccoon eyes.

Common cold

- Initial watery nasal discharge may become thicker and mucopurulent.
- Related findings include sneezing, nasal congestion, a dry and hacking cough, sore throat, mouth breathing, and transient loss of smell and taste.

- Other findings include malaise, fatigue, myalgia, arthralgia, a slight headache, low-grade fever, dry lips, and a red upper lip and nose.

Headache (cluster)

- Rhinorrhea may accompany a cluster headache.
- Related ocular effects include miosis, ipsilateral tearing, conjunctival injection, and ptosis.
- Other findings include flushing, facial diaphoresis, bradycardia, and restlessness.

Nasal or sinus tumors

- Intermittent, bloody or serosanguineous discharge is produced, which may be purulent and foul-smelling.
- Nasal congestion, postnasal drip, and headache may also occur.
- A cheek mass or eye displacement, facial paresthesia or pain, and nasal obstruction may occur in the advanced stages of a paranasal sinus tumor.

Rhinitis

- Allergic rhinitis produces an episodic, profuse watery discharge with increased tearing; nasal congestion; itchy eyes, nose, and throat; postnasal drip; sneezing; mouth breathing; impaired sense of smell; frontal or temporal headache; pale, engorged turbinates; and pale, boggy mucosa.
- Atrophic rhinitis produces scanty, purulent, and foul-smelling nasal discharge with nasal obstruction and pale pink, shiny mucosa.
- Vasomotor rhinitis produces a profuse watery nasal discharge accompanied by chronic nasal obstruction, sneezing, recurrent postnasal drip, blue nasal mucosa, and pale, swollen turbinates.

Sinusitis

- With acute sinusitis, a thick and purulent nasal discharge leads to a purulent postnasal drip that results in throat pain and halitosis; accompanying features include nasal congestion, severe pain and tenderness over the involved sinuses, fever, headache, and malaise.
- With chronic sinusitis, the nasal discharge is scanty, thick, and intermittently purulent, with nasal congestion, discomfort or pressure over the involved sinuses, a chronic sore throat, and nasal polyps.

Wegener's granulomatosis

- Bloody, mucopurulent discharge is accompanied by conductive hearing loss, crusting, epistaxis, and tissue necrosis of the nose.

Other causes

Drugs

- Nasal sprays or nose drops containing vasoconstrictors that are used longer than 5 days may cause rebound rhinorrhea.

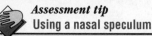
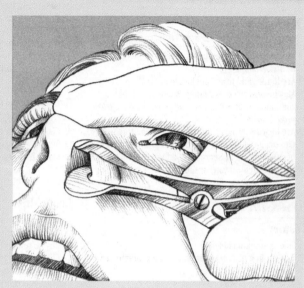

To visualize the interior of the nares, use a nasal speculum and a good light source, such as a penlight. Hold the speculum in the palm of one hand and the penlight in the other hand. Have the patient tilt the head back slightly and rest it against a wall or other firm support, if possible. Insert the speculum blades about ½″ (1.3 cm) into the nasal vestibule, as shown.

Place your index finger on the tip of the patient's nose for stability. Carefully open the speculum blades. Shine the light source in the direction of the nares. Now, inspect the nares, as shown. The mucosa should be deep pink. Note any discharge, masses, lesions, or mucosal swellings. Check the nasal septum for perforation, bleeding, or crusting. Bluish turbinates suggest allergy. A rounded, elongated projection suggests a polyp.

Surgery

○ Cerebrospinal rhinorrhea may occur after sinus or cranial surgery.

Nursing considerations

○ Give an antihistamine, a decongestant, an analgesic, or an antipyretic.
○ Encourage increased fluid intake to thin secretions.

Pediatric pointers

○ Rhinorrhea in children may stem from choanal atresia, allergic or chronic rhinitis, acute ethmoiditis, or congenital syphilis.
○ Assume that rhinitis and nasal obstruction in one nostril is caused by a foreign body in the nose until proven otherwise.

Geriatric pointers

○ Elderly patients may experience increased adverse reactions to drugs used to treat rhinorrhea, such as elevated blood pressure or confusion.

Patient teaching

○ Explain the proper use of nasal over-the-counter sprays.

Rhonchi

Overview

- Are continuous adventitious breath sounds detected by auscultation
- Are louder and lower-pitched than crackles
- May be described as rattling, sonorous, bubbling, rumbling, or musical (see *Comparing adventitious breath sounds*)
- Are heard over large airways such as the trachea
- Can occur when air flows through passages that have been narrowed by secretions, a tumor or foreign body, bronchospasm, or mucosal thickening

Assessment

History

- Take a smoking history.
- Ask about a history of asthma or other pulmonary disorder.
- Take a drug history.

Physical assessment

- Take vital signs, including oxygen saturation.
- Characterize the patient's respirations as rapid or slow, shallow or deep, and regular or irregular.
- Inspect the chest, noting the use of accessory muscles.
- Listen for audible wheezing or gurgling.
- Auscultate for other abnormal breath sounds and note location.
- Percuss the chest, and note frequency and productivity of cough.

Medical causes

Acute respiratory distress syndrome

- A life-threatening disorder; initial features include dyspnea, rhonchi, crackles, and rapid, shallow respirations.
- Intercostal and suprasternal retractions, diaphoresis, and fluid accumulation occur with developing hypoxemia.
- As hypoxemia worsens, findings include difficulty breathing, restlessness, apprehension, decreased level of consciousness, cyanosis, motor dysfunction, and tachycardia.

Aspiration of foreign body

- Inspiratory and expiratory rhonchi and wheezing occur because of increased secretions.
- Other findings include diminished breath sounds over the obstructed area, fever, pain, and cough.

Asthma

- An asthma attack can cause rhonchi, crackles and, commonly, wheezing.
- Other findings include apprehension, a dry cough that later becomes productive, prolonged expirations, accessory muscle use, nasal flaring, tachypnea, tachycardia, diaphoresis, flushing or cyanosis, and intercostal and supraclavicular retractions on inspiration.

Bronchiectasis

- Lower-lobe rhonchi and crackles occur.
- Classic sign is a cough that produces mucopurulent, foul-smelling sputum.
- Other findings include fever, weight loss, exertional dyspnea, fatigue, malaise, halitosis, weakness, and late-stage clubbing.

Bronchitis

- Sonorous rhonchi and wheezing occur in acute tracheobronchitis; other features include chills, sore throat, fever, muscle and back pain, substernal tightness, and a cough that becomes productive as secretions increase.
- Scattered rhonchi, coarse crackles, wheezing, high-pitched piping sounds, and prolonged expirations occur with chronic bronchitis; accompanying findings include exertional dyspnea, increased accessory muscle use, barrel chest, cyanosis, tachypnea, and late-stage clubbing.

Emphysema

- Sonorous rhonchi may occur, but faint, high-pitched wheezing is more typical.
- Other findings include weight loss, anorexia, malaise, barrel chest, peripheral cyanosis, exertional dyspnea, accessory muscle use on inspiration, tachypnea, grunting expirations, late-stage clubbing, and a mild, chronic, cough with scant sputum.

Pneumonia

- Bacterial pneumonias can cause rhonchi and a dry cough that later becomes productive.
- Related findings include shaking chills, high fever, myalgia, headache, pleuritic chest pain, tachypnea, tachycardia, dyspnea, cyanosis, diaphoresis, decreased breath sounds, and fine crackles.

Other causes

Diagnostic tests

- Pulmonary function tests or bronchoscopy can loosen secretions and mucus, causing rhonchi.

Respiratory therapy

- Respiratory therapy may produce rhonchi from loosened secretions and mucus.

The characteristics of discontinuous and continuous adventitious breath sounds are compared in the chart below. Note the timing of each sound during inspiration and expiration on the corresponding graphs.

Sound	*Characteristics*

DISCONTINUOUS SOUNDS

Fine crackles

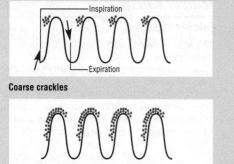

- Intermittent
- Nonmusical
- Soft
- High-pitched
- Short, cracking, popping
- Heard during inspiration (5 to 10 msec)

Coarse crackles

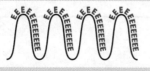

- Intermittent
- Nonmusical
- Loud
- Low-pitched
- Bubbling, gurgling
- Heard during early inspiration and possibly during expiration (20 to 30 msec)

CONTINUOUS SOUNDS

Wheezes

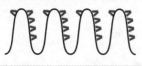

- Musical
- High-pitched
- Squeaking
- Mainly heard during expiration but may also occur during inspiration

Rhonchi

- Musical
- Low-pitched
- Snoring, moaning
- Heard during both inspiration and expiration, but are more prominent during expiration

Nursing considerations

- To ease breathing, place the patient in semi-Fowler's position.
- Give an antibiotic, a bronchodilator, and an expectorant.
- Provide humidification to thin secretions, relieve inflammation, and preventing drying.
- Promote coughing, deep breathing, and incentive spirometry.
- Provide pulmonary physiotherapy with postural drainage and percussion to loosen secretions.
- Use tracheal suctioning, if necessary, to clear secretions.

Pediatric pointers

- Rhonchi in children can result from bacterial pneumonia, cystic fibrosis, and croup syndrome.
- Because a respiratory tract disorder may begin abruptly and progress rapidly in an infant or a child, observe closely for signs of airway obstruction.

Patient teaching

- Explain deep-breathing and coughing techniques.
- Explain the need for increasing fluid intake.
- Discuss increasing activity levels.

Romberg's sign

Overview

- Refers to inability to maintain balance when standing erect with feet together and eyes closed (see *Assessing Romberg's sign*)
- Indicates a vestibular or proprioceptive disorder or a disorder of the spinal tracts when sign is positive
- May indicate cerebellar disorder

Assessment

History

- Obtain a medical history including previous neurologic symptoms and disorders.
- Ask about sensory changes and their onset.

Physical assessment

- Perform other neurologic screening tests, including proprioception.
- Test the patient's awareness of body part position.
- Test the patient's direction of movement.
- Test sensation and two-point discrimination in all dermatomes.
- Test and characterize the patient's deep tendon reflexes (DTRs).
- Test the patient's vibratory sense.
- Assess for hearing loss.
- Observe for nystagmus.

Medical causes

Multiple sclerosis

- A positive Romberg's sign may occur in multiple sclerosis.
- Early findings may include vision changes, diplopia, and paresthesia.
- Other findings include nystagmus, constipation, muscle weakness and spasticity, hyperreflexia, dysphagia, dysarthria, incontinence, urinary frequency and urgency, impotence, and emotional instability.

Assessment tip
Assessing Romberg's sign

Observe the patient's balance as he stands with his eyes open, feet together, and arms at his sides. Then ask him to close his eyes. Hold your arms out on either side of him to protect him if he sways. If he falls to one side, the result of the Romberg's test is positive.

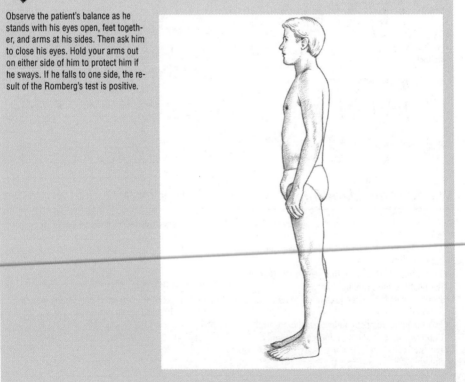

Peripheral nerve disease

○ Positive Romberg's sign may be accompanied by impotence, fatigue, and paresthesia, hyperesthesia, or anesthesia in the hands and feet.
○ Related findings include incoordination, ataxia, burning in the affected area, progressive muscle weakness and atrophy, hypoactive DTRs, and loss of vibration sense.

Pernicious anemia

○ A positive Romberg's sign and loss of proprioception in the lower limbs reflect peripheral nerve and spinal cord damage.
○ Gait changes (usually ataxia), muscle weakness, impaired coordination, paresthesia, and sensory loss may be present.
○ Other findings include a sore tongue, a positive Babinski's reflex, fatigue, blurred vision, diplopia, and light-headedness.

Spinal cerebellar degeneration

○ Positive Romberg's sign accompanies decreased visual acuity, fatigue, paresthesia, loss of vibration sense, incoordination, ataxic gait, hypoactive DTRs, and muscle weakness and atrophy.

Spinal cord disease

○ Positive Romberg's sign may accompany pain, fasciculations, muscle weakness and atrophy, and loss of sphincter tone, proprioception, and vibration sense.
○ DTRs may be hypoactive at the level of the lesion and hyperactive above it.

Vestibular disorders

○ Positive Romberg's sign may accompany vertigo, nystagmus, nausea, tinnitus, hearing loss, and vomiting.

Nursing considerations

○ Help the patient with ambulation.
○ Keep a night-light on and raise the side rails of the bed.

Pediatric pointers

○ Romberg's sign can't be tested until a child can stand without support and follow commands.
○ A positive sign in children commonly results from spinal cord disease.

Patient teaching

○ Provide instruction on safety measures to avoid injury.
○ Teach the patient the proper use of assistive devices.

Salivation, decreased

Overview

○ Diminished production or excretion of saliva
○ Also called *xerostomia*

Assessment

History

○ Ask about the onset and course of dry mouth.
○ Take a drug history.
○ Determine what aggravates or alleviates the condition.
○ Ask about burning or itching eyes and changes in sense of smell or taste.
○ Ask about recent dental or oral procedures.

Physical assessment

○ Inspect mouth for abnormalities.
○ Observe eyes for conjunctival irritation, matted lids, and corneal epithelial thickening.
○ Perform simple tests of smell and taste to detect impairment.
○ Check for enlarged parotid and submaxillary glands. (See *Examining salivary glands and ductal openings.*)
○ Palpate for tender or enlarged areas along the neck.

Assessment tip
Examining salivary glands and ductal openings

When a patient reports decreased salivation, assess the parotid and submaxillary glands for enlargement and the ductal openings for salivary flow.

To detect an enlarged parotid gland, ask the patient to clench his teeth, thereby tensing the masseter muscle. Then palpate the parotid duct (about 2″ [5 cm] long); you should be able to feel it against the tensed muscle, on the cheek just below the zygomatic arch. Next, check the ductal orifice, opposite the second molar. Using a gloved finger, palpate the orifice for enlargement, and observe for drainage.

Palpate the submaxillary gland. About the size of a walnut, this gland is located under the mandible, anterior to the angle of the jaw. Using a gloved finger, palpate the floor of the mouth for enlargement of the submaxillary ductal orifice.

Finally, test both ductal openings for salivary flow. Place cotton under the patient's tongue, have him sip pure lemon juice, and then remove the cotton and observe salivary flow from each opening. Document your findings.

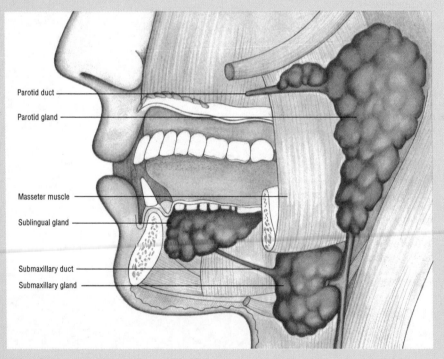

Medical causes

Dehydration
○ Decreased saliva production causes dry oral mucous membranes.
○ Other findings include decreased skin turgor, reduced urine output, hypotension, tachycardia, and a low-grade fever.

Facial nerve paralysis
○ Diminished saliva production, decreased sense of taste, and decreased facial muscle movement occur.
○ Affected side of the face may sag and appear mask-like.

Salivary duct obstruction
○ Reduced salivation with local pain and swelling of the face or neck.
○ Symptoms are most noticeable when eating or drinking.

Sjögren's syndrome
○ Diminished secretions from the lacrimal, parotid, and submaxillary glands produce the characteristic findings of decreased or absent salivation and dry eyes with a persistent burning, gritty sensation.
○ Dryness of the nose, respiratory tract, vagina, and skin may also occur.
○ Related oral findings include difficulty chewing, talking, and swallowing as well as ulcers and soreness of the lips and mucosa.
○ Other findings include parotid and submaxillary gland enlargement, nasal crusting, epistaxis, fatigue, lethargy, nonproductive cough, abdominal discomfort, and polyuria.
○ Signs and symptoms of rheumatoid arthritis and other connective tissue disorder may occur.

Other causes

Drugs
○ Anticholinergics, antihistamines, tricyclic antidepressants, phenothiazines, clonidine, and opioid analgesics can decrease salivation; this effect disappears after stopping therapy.

Radiation
○ Excessive irradiation of mouth or face from radiation therapy or dental X-rays may cause transient decreased salivation.

Nursing considerations
○ Allow extra time for speaking, eating, and swallowing.

Pediatric pointers
○ Mouth breathing and anticholinergics are causes of decreased salivation in children.

Patient teaching
○ Describe ways to relieve dry mouth.
○ Instruct the patient in proper oral hygiene and dental care.
○ Explain the proper use of pilocarpine.

Salivation, increased

Overview

- Also known as *polysialia* or *ptyalism*
- An uncommon symptom that results from GI disorders, systemic disorders, use of certain drugs, or exposure to certain toxins
- Saliva may also accumulate because of difficulty swallowing

Assessment

History

- Ask about fatigue, fever, headache, or sore throat.
- Inquire about recent exposure to toxins.
- Take a drug history, noting use of iodides, cholinergics, and miotics.
- Take a medical history.

Physical assessment

- Test for a gag reflex.
- Observe ability to swallow and chew.
- Note any drooling.
- Inspect the mouth for lesions; note their appearance.
- Palpate any mouth lesions and describe their appearance.
- Inspect the uvula, gingivae, and pharynx.
- Palpate lymph nodes, and determine if parotid glands are swollen or sore.

Medical causes

Bell's palsy

- Facial nerve paralysis causes an inability to control salivation or close the eye on the affected side.
- Affected side of the face sags and is expressionless, the nasolabial fold flattens, and the palpebral fissure (the distance between the upper and lower eyelids) widens.
- Other findings include diminished or absent corneal reflex and partial loss of taste or abnormal taste sensation.

Pregnancy

- In early months, increased salivation, nausea, gum swelling, and breast tenderness may occur.

Stomatitis

- Mucosal ulcers may be accompanied by moderately increased salivation, mouth pain, fever, and erythema.
- Spontaneous healing usually occurs in 7 to 10 days, but scarring and recurrence are possible.

Syphilis

- With secondary syphilis, mucosal ulcers cause increased salivation that may persist up to 1 year.
- Related findings include fever, malaise, headache, anorexia, weight loss, nausea, vomiting, sore throat, and lymphadenopathy.
- A symmetrical rash appears on the arms, trunk, palms, soles, face, and scalp.
- Condylomata develop in the genital and perianal areas.

Tuberculosis

- Certain forms may produce solitary, irregularly shaped mouth or tongue ulcers, covered with exudate, that cause increased salivation.
- Other findings include weight loss, anorexia, fever, fatigue, malaise, dyspnea, cough, night sweats (a common sign), and hemoptysis.

Other causes

Arsenic poisoning

- Common effects of arsenic poisoning are diarrhea, diffuse skin hyperpigmentation, and edema of the face, eyelids and ankles; increased salivation occurs infrequently.
- Other findings include garlicky breath odor, pruritus, headache, drowsiness, confusion, and weakness.

Drugs

- Increased salivation may occur with iodide toxicity, but the earliest symptoms are a brassy taste and a burning sensation in the mouth and throat; other findings include sneezing, irritated eyelids, and pain in the frontal sinus.
- Pilocarpine and other miotics used to treat glaucoma may be absorbed systemically, increasing salivation.
- Cholinergics, such as bethanechol and neostigmine, may cause increased salivation.

Mercury poisoning

- Stomatitis, characterized by increased salivation and a metallic taste, commonly occurs.
- Teeth may be loose with painful, swollen gums that are prone to bleeding.
- Blue line appears on the gingivae.
- Other findings include personality changes, memory loss, abdominal cramps, diarrhea, paresthesia, and tremors of the eyelids, lips, tongue, and fingers.

Nursing considerations

- Increased salivation doesn't require treatments beyond those needed to correct the underlying disorder.
- If the patient has difficulty swallowing, suction the mouth as needed.

Pediatric pointers

○ Increased salivation in children may stem from the same conditions that affect adults or from congenital esophageal atresia.

Geriatric pointers

○ Drooling is common in elderly the patients with Parkinson's disease.

Patient teaching

○ Instruct the patient in proper oral hygiene.
○ Emphasize the importance of obtaining proper dental care.

Scotoma

Overview

- Refers to an area of partial or complete blindness within an otherwise normal or slightly impaired visual field
- Usually located within the central 30-degree area of the normal visual field
- Ranges from absolute blindness to a barely detectable loss of visual acuity
- Classified as absolute, relative, or scintillating
- Can typically pinpoint the location in the visual field (see *Locating scotomas*)

Assessment

History

- Take a medical history, including eye disorders, vision problems, or chronic systemic disorders.
- Obtain a drug history.

Physical assessment

- Test visual acuity.
- Inspect pupils for size, equality, and reaction to light.
- Make sure an ophthalmoscopic examination is performed and intraocular pressure (IOP) is measured.
- Identify and characterize the scotoma using visual field tests.

Medical causes

Chorioretinitis

- A paracentral scotoma develops.

Assessment tip
Locating scotomas

Scotomas, or blind spots, are classified according to the affected area of the visual field. The normal scotoma — shown in the temporal region of the right eye — appears in black in all the illustrations.

The *normally present scotoma* represents the position of the optic nerve head in the visual field. It appears between 10 and 20 degrees on this chart of the normal visual field.

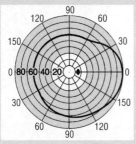

A *central scotoma* involves the point of central fixation. It's always associated with decreased visual acuity.

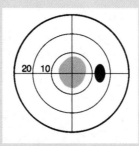

A *centrocecal scotoma* involves the point of central fixation and the area between the blind spot and the fixation point.

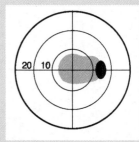

A *paracentral scotoma* affects an area of the visual field that is nasal or temporal to the point of central fixation.

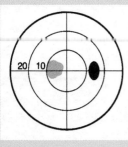

An *arcuate scotoma* arches around the fixation point, usually ending on the nasal side of the visual field.

An *annular scotoma* forms a circular defect around the fixation point. It's common with retinal pigmentary degeneration.

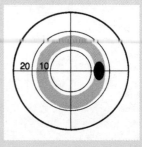

- Examination reveals clouding and cells in the vitreous, subretinal hemorrhage, and neovascularization.
- Photophobia with blurred vision may be present.

Glaucoma

- Prolonged elevation of IOP can cause an arcuate scotoma.
- Cupping of the optic disk, loss of peripheral vision, and reduced visual acuity occurs with poorly controlled glaucoma.
- Rainbow-colored halos may appear around lights.

Macular degeneration

- A central scotoma develops.
- Examination reveals changes in the macular area.
- Other findings include changes in visual acuity and color perception, and in perception of the size and shape of objects.

Migraine headache

- Transient scintillating scotomas, usually on one side, can occur during the aura.
- Other findings include paresthesia of the lips, face, or hands; slight confusion; dizziness; nausea and vomiting; and photophobia.

Optic neuritis

- A central, circular, or centrocecal scotoma with vision loss.
- In one or both eyes.
- Severe vision loss or blurring and pain, especially with eye movement.
- Hyperemia of the optic disk, retinal vein distention, blurred disk margins, and filling of the physiologic cup.

Retinitis pigmentosa

- Annular scotoma progresses concentrically until only tunnel vision remains.
- The earliest symptom — impaired night vision — appears during adolescence.
- Other findings include narrowing of the retinal blood vessels, pallor of the optic disk and, eventually, blindness.

- Explain the progression and complications of the disease.
- Explain which signs and symptoms the patient needs to report.
- Discuss which rehabilitation services are available.
- Discuss which assistive devices are available.
- Stress the importance of regular eye examinations.
- If the disorder involves the fovea centralis, explain the use of the Amsler grid.

Nursing considerations

- Provide safety measures.
- Give prescribed drugs.

Pediatric pointers

- In young children, visual field testing is difficult and requires patience; confrontation visual field testing is the method of choice.

Patient teaching

- Emphasize the importance of compliance with drug therapy.

Scrotal swelling

Overview

○ Occurs when a condition affecting the testicles, epididymis, or scrotal skin produces edema or a mass
○ Can be in one or both testicles and painful or painless

> ### ★ Emergency actions
>
> *If the patient also has severe pain, ask when the swelling began. Using a Doppler stethoscope, evaluate blood flow to the testicle. If it's decreased or absent, suspect testicular torsion and prepare the patient for surgery. Withhold food and fluids. Insert I.V. line and apply ice pack to the scrotum to reduce pain and swelling. An attempt may be made to untwist the cord manually, but even if this is successful, the patient may still require surgery for stabilization.*

Assessment

History

○ Ask about a history of injury to scrotum, urethral discharge, cloudy urine, increased urinary frequency, dysuria, sexually transmitted disease, prostate surgery, or prolonged catheterization.
○ Find out about recent illness, particularly mumps.
○ Obtain a history of sexual activity.
○ Ask which body positions alleviate or aggravate swelling.

Physical assessment

○ Take the vital signs, especially noting fever.
○ Palpate the abdomen for tenderness and swelling.
○ Examine the genital area.
○ Assess the scrotum with the patient in a supine position and then standing.
○ Check the testicles' position in the scrotum.
○ Palpate the scrotum for a cyst or lump, note tenderness or firmness.
○ Transilluminate the scrotum to distinguish a fluid-filled cyst from a solid mass.

Medical causes

Epididymal cysts

○ Painless scrotal swelling occurs.

Epididymitis

○ Inflammation, pain, extreme tenderness, and swelling develop in the groin and scrotum.
○ Other findings include high fever, malaise, urethral discharge and cloudy urine, lower abdominal pain on the affected side, and hot, red, dry, flaky and thin scrotal skin.

Hernia

○ Swelling and a soft or unusually firm scrotum are produced.
○ Nausea, anorexia, vomiting, and reduced bowel sounds may occur if the bowel is obstructed.

Hydrocele

○ Fluid accumulation produces gradual scrotal swelling that's usually painless.
○ The scrotum may be soft and cystic or firm and tense.
○ Palpation reveals a round, nontender scrotal mass.

Orchitis (acute)

○ Sudden painful swelling of one or both testicles occurs.
○ Related findings include hot, reddened scrotum; fever; chills; lower abdominal pain; nausea; vomiting; and extreme weakness.

Scrotal trauma

○ Scrotal swelling, bruising, and severe pain result.
○ The scrotum may appear dark blue.
○ Nausea, vomiting, and difficulty urinating may also occur.

Spermatocele

○ Moveable, painless cystic mass develops; it may be transilluminated.

Testicular torsion

○ A urologic emergency — scrotal swelling; sudden, severe pain; and, possibly, elevation of the affected testicle within the scrotum.
○ Most common before puberty.
○ Possible nausea and vomiting.

Testicular tumor

○ Scrotum swells and produces a sensation of excessive weight.
○ Typically, these tumors are painless, smooth, and firm.
○ With ureteral obstruction, urinary complaints are common.

Other causes

Surgery

○ Blood effusion from surgery can produce a hematocele, leading to scrotal swelling.

Nursing considerations

○ Place the patient on bedrest.
○ Give an antibiotic.
○ Provide fluids, fiber, and stool softeners.
○ Place a rolled towel under the scrotum to help reduce swelling.

○ For moderate swelling, suggest a loose-fitting athletic supporter.
○ Apply heat or ice packs to decrease inflammation.
○ Administer an analgesic, as needed.

Pediatric pointers

○ In children up to age 1, a hernia or hydrocele of the spermatic cord may cause scrotal swelling.
○ In infants, scrotal swelling may stem from ammonia-related dermatitis if diapers aren't changed often enough.
○ In prepubescent boys, scrotal swelling usually results from torsion of spermatic cord.

Patient teaching

○ Explain the importance of performing testicular self-examination, and teach the technique, if needed.

Seizures, complex partial

Overview

○ Complex partial seizures occur when focal seizures begin in the temporal lobe and cause partial alterations of consciousness.

○ Typically an aura — usually a complex hallucination, illusion, or sensation — precedes a psychomotor seizure.

○ Hallucination may be audiovisual, auditory, or olfactory.

○ Other types of auras include sensations of déjà vu, unfamiliarity with surroundings, or depersonalization.

○ After the seizure, the patient is confused, drowsy, and doesn't remember the seizure. (See *Seizures types*.)

Assessment

History

○ Ask about the occurrence of an aura.

○ Ask witnesses for a description of the seizure.

○ Ask about previous seizures or therapies.

Physical assessment

○ Examine the patient for injury after the seizure.

○ Ensure a patent airway.

○ Perform a complete neurologic assessment.

Seizure types

The various types of seizures — partial, generalized, status epilepticus, and unclassified — have distinct signs and symptoms.

Partial seizures

Arising from a localized area of the brain, partial seizures cause focal symptoms. These seizures are classified by their effect on consciousness and whether they spread throughout the motor pathway, causing a generalized seizure.

● A *simple partial seizure* begins locally and generally doesn't cause an alteration in consciousness. It may present with sensory symptoms (lights flashing, smells, and auditory hallucinations), autonomic symptoms (sweating, flushing, and pupil dilation), and psychic symptoms (dream states, anger, and fear). The seizure lasts for a few seconds and occurs without preceding or provoking events. This type can be motor or sensory.

● A *complex partial seizure* alters consciousness. Amnesia for events that occur during and immediately after the seizure is a differentiating characteristic. During the seizure, the patient may follow simple commands. This type of seizure usually lasts for 1 to 3 minutes.

Generalized seizures

As the term suggests, generalized seizures cause a generalized electrical abnormality within the brain. They can be convulsive or nonconvulsive and include several types:

● *Absence seizures* occur most commonly in children, although they may affect adults. They usually begin with a brief change in level of consciousness, indicated by a blinking or rolling of the eyes, a blank stare, and slight mouth movements. The patient retains his posture and continues preseizure activity without difficulty. Typically, each seizure lasts from 1 to 10 seconds. If not properly treated, seizures can recur as frequently as 100 times per day. An absence seizure is a nonconvulsive seizure, but it may progress to a generalized tonic-clonic seizure.

● *Myoclonic seizures* are brief, involuntary muscular jerks of the body or extremities, commonly occurring in the early morning.

● *Clonic* seizures are characterized by rhythmic movements.

● *Tonic* seizures are characterized by a sudden stiffening of muscle tone, usually of the arms, but possibly including the legs.

● *Generalized tonic-clonic seizures* typically begin with a loud cry, precipitated by air rushing from the lungs through the vocal cords. The patient then loses consciousness and falls to the ground. The body stiffens (tonic phase) and then alternates between episodes of muscle spasm and relaxation (clonic phase). Tongue biting, incontinence, labored breathing, apnea, and subsequent cyanosis may occur. The seizure stops in 2 to 5 minutes, when abnormal electrical conduction ceases. When the patient regains consciousness, he's confused and may have difficulty talking. If he can talk, he may complain of drowsiness, fatigue, headache, muscle soreness, and arm or leg weakness. He may fall into a deep sleep after the seizure.

● *Atonic seizures* are characterized by a general loss of postural tone and a temporary loss of consciousness. They occur in young children and are sometimes called *drop attacks* because they cause the child to fall.

Status epilepticus

Status epilepticus is a continuous seizure state that can occur in all seizure types. The most life-threatening example is generalized tonic-clonic status epilepticus, a continuous generalized tonic-clonic seizure. Status epilepticus is accompanied by respiratory distress leading to hypoxia or anoxia and can result from abrupt withdrawal of anticonvulsants, hypoxic encephalopathy, acute head trauma, metabolic encephalopathy, or septicemia caused by encephalitis or meningitis.

Unclassified seizures

The unclassified seizures category is reserved for seizures that don't fit the characteristics of partial or generalized seizures or status epilepticus. Events that lack the data necessary for making a definitive diagnosis are included in the category of unclassified seizures.

Medical causes

Brain abscess

○ If the temporal lobe is affected, complex partial seizures commonly occur after the abscess resolves.
○ Related findings include headache, nausea, vomiting, generalized seizures, and a decreased level of consciousness (LOC).
○ Central facial weakness, auditory receptive aphasia, hemiparesis, and ocular disturbances may also occur.

Head trauma

○ Trauma to the temporal lobe can produce complex partial seizures months or years later.
○ Seizures may decrease in frequency and eventually stop.
○ Generalized seizures and behavior and personality changes may also occur.

Temporal lobe tumor

○ Complex partial seizures may be the first sign.
○ Other findings include headache, pupillary changes, and mental dullness.
○ Increases intracranial pressure may cause a decreased LOC, vomiting, and papilledema.

Nursing considerations

○ After the seizure, reorient the patient to his surroundings and protect him from injury.
○ Keep the patient in bed until he's fully alert.
○ Remove harmful objects from the area.
○ Provide emotional support to the patient and family.
○ Monitor for therapeutic drug levels.

Pediatric pointers

○ Complex partial seizures in children may resemble absence seizures.
○ Complex partial seizures in children can result from birth injury, abuse, infection, or cancer.
○ Repeated complex partial seizures commonly lead to generalized seizures.

Patient teaching

○ Discuss methods for coping with seizures.
○ Instruct the patient and family in safety measures to take during a seizure.
○ Emphasize compliance with drug therapy.
○ Tell the patient to carry medical identification.

Seizures, generalized tonic-clonic

Overview

○ Are caused by paroxysmal, uncontrolled discharge of central nervous system neurons, leading to neurologic dysfunction (see *Recognizing a generalized tonic-clonic seizure*)
○ Extend to the entire brain

Assessment

History

○ Obtain a description of the seizure, including onset, duration, part of body affected, characteristics, and progression. (See *How to respond to a seizure*.)
○ Ask about unusual sensations before the seizure.
○ Find out about a personal and family history of seizures.
○ Take a drug history and determine compliance.
○ Ask about sleep deprivation or emotional or physical stress at time of seizure.

Physical assessment

○ If the patient may have sustained a head injury, observe him closely for loss of consciousness, unequal or nonreactive pupils, and focal neurologic signs.
○ Examine the arms, legs, and face (including tongue) for injury, residual paralysis, or limb weakness.
○ Take vital signs.
○ Complete a neurologic assessment.
○ Observe for adequate oxygenation.

Medical causes

Alcohol withdrawal syndrome

○ Seizures as well as status epilepticus may occur 7 to 48 hours after sudden withdrawal.
○ Other findings include restlessness, hallucinations, profuse diaphoresis, and tachycardia.

Arsenic poisoning

○ Generalized seizures may occur with a garlicky breath odor, increased salivation, generalized pruritus, diarrhea, nausea, vomiting, and abdominal pain.
○ Related findings include diffuse hyperpigmentation; sharply defined edema of the eyelids, face, and ankles; paresthesia of the extremities; alopecia; irritated mucous membranes; weakness; muscle aches; and peripheral neuropathy.

Assessment tip
Recognizing a generalized tonic-clonic seizure

Before the seizure
Prodromal signs and symptoms, such as myoclonic jerks, throbbing headache, and mood changes, may occur over several hours or days. The patient may have premonitions of the seizure. For example, he may report an aura, such as seeing a flashing light or smelling a characteristic odor.

During the seizure
If a generalized seizure begins with an aura, this indicates that irritability in a specific area of the brain quickly became widespread. Common auras include palpitations, epigastric distress rapidly rising to the throat, head or eye turning, and sensory hallucinations.

Next, *loss of consciousness* occurs as a sudden discharge of intense electrical activity overwhelms the brain's subcortical center. The patient falls and experiences brief, bilateral myoclonic contractures. Air forced through spasmodic vocal cords may produce a birdlike, piercing cry.

During the *tonic phase*, skeletal muscles contract for 10 to 20 seconds. The patient's eyelids are drawn up, his arms are flexed, and his legs are extended. His mouth opens wide, then snaps shut; he may bite his tongue. His respirations cease because of respiratory muscle spasm, and initial pallor of the skin and mucous membranes (the result of impaired venous return) changes to cyanosis caused by apnea. The patient arches his back and slowly lowers his arms. Other effects include dilated, nonreactive pupils; greatly increased heart rate and blood pressure; increased salivation and tracheobronchial secretions; and profuse diaphoresis.

During the *clonic phase*, lasting about 60 seconds, mild trembling progresses to violent contractures or jerks. Other motor activity includes facial grimaces (with possible tongue biting) and violent expiration of bloody, foamy saliva from clonic contractures of thoracic cage muscles. Clonic jerks slowly decrease in intensity and frequency. The patient is still apneic.

After the seizure
The patient's movements gradually cease, and he becomes unresponsive to external stimuli. Other postseizure features include stertorous respirations from increased tracheobronchial secretions, equal or unequal pupils (but becoming reactive), and urinary incontinence due to brief muscle relaxation. After about 5 minutes, the patient's level of consciousness increases, and he appears confused and disoriented. His muscle tone, heart rate, and blood pressure return to normal.

After several hours' sleep, the patient awakens exhausted and may have a headache, sore muscles, and amnesia about the seizure.

Brain abscess

○ Generalized seizures may occur in the acute stage of abscess formation or after the abscess disappears.
○ Constant headache, nausea, vomiting, and focal seizures are early signs and symptoms.
○ Other findings include decreased level of consciousness (LOC), ocular disturbances, aphasia, hemiparesis, abnormal behavior, and personality changes.

Brain tumor

○ Generalized seizures may occur, depending on the tumor's location and type.
○ Other findings include a slowly decreasing LOC, morning headache, dizziness, confusion, focal seizures, vision loss, motor and sensory disturbances, aphasia, and ataxia.
○ Later findings include papilledema, vomiting, increased systolic blood pressure, widening pulse pressure and, eventually, decorticate posture.

Cerebral aneurysm

○ Generalized seizures may occur.
○ Onset is typically abrupt with severe headache, nausea, vomiting, and decreased LOC.
○ Related findings vary with the site and amount of bleeding, but may include nuchal rigidity, irritability, hemiparesis, hemisensory defects, dysphagia, photophobia, diplopia, ptosis, and unilateral pupil dilation.

Eclampsia

○ Generalized seizures are a hallmark.
○ Related findings include severe frontal headache, nausea, vomiting, vision disturbances, increased blood pressure, fever, peripheral edema, oliguria, irritability, hyperactive deep tendon reflexes (DTRs), decreased LOC, and sudden weight gain.

Encephalitis

○ Seizures are an early sign, indicating a poor prognosis.
○ Seizures may also occur after recovery as a result of residual damage.
○ Other findings include fever, headache, photophobia, nuchal rigidity, neck pain, vomiting, aphasia, ataxia, hemiparesis, nystagmus, irritability, cranial nerve palsies, and myoclonic jerks.

Head trauma

○ Generalized seizures may occur at the time of injury; focal seizures may occur months later.
○ Related findings include decreased LOC; soft-tissue injury of the face, head, or neck; clear or bloody drainage from the mouth, nose, or ears; facial edema; bony deformity of the face, head, or neck; Battle's sign; and lack of response to oculocephalic and oculovestibular stimulation.

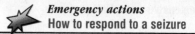

Emergency actions
How to respond to a seizure

If you witness the beginning of the seizure, first check the patient's airway, breathing, and circulation, and ensure that the cause isn't asystole or a blocked airway. Stay with the patient and ensure a patent airway. Focus your care on observing the seizure and protecting the patient. Place a towel under his head to prevent injury, loosen his clothing, and move any sharp or hard objects out of his way. Never try to restrain the patient or force a hard object into his mouth; you might chip his teeth or fracture his jaw. Only at the start of the ictal phase can you safely insert a soft object into his mouth.

If possible, turn the patient to one side *during* the seizure to allow secretions to drain and to prevent aspiration. Otherwise, do this at the end of the clonic phase when respirations return. (If they fail to return, check for airway obstruction and suction the patient, if needed. Cardiopulmonary resuscitation, intubation, and mechanical ventilation may be needed.)

Protect the patient after the seizure by providing a safe area in which he can rest. As he awakens, reassure and reorient him. Check his vital signs and neurologic status. Carefully record these data as well as your observations of the seizure.

If the seizure lasts longer than 4 minutes or if a second seizure occurs before full recovery from the first, suspect status epilepticus. Establish an airway, start an I.V. line, give supplemental oxygen, and begin cardiac monitoring. Draw blood for appropriate studies. Turn the patient on his side, with his head in a semi-dependent position, to drain secretions and prevent aspiration. Periodically turn him to the opposite side, check his arterial blood gas levels for hypoxemia, and administer oxygen by mask, increasing the flow rate if necessary. Administer diazepam or lorazepam by slow I.V. push, repeated two or three times at 10- to 20-minute intervals, to stop the seizures. If the patient isn't known to have epilepsy, an I.V. bolus of dextrose 50% (50 ml) with thiamine (100 mg) may be given. If the patient has hypoglycemia, extrose may stop the seizures. If his thiamine level is low, also give thiamine to guard against further damage.

If the patient is intubated, expect to insert a nasogastric (NG) tube to prevent vomiting and aspiration. If the patient hasn't been intubated, the NG tube itself can trigger the gag reflex and cause vomiting. Record your observations and the intervals between seizures.

○ Other findings include motor and sensory deficits, altered respirations, and signs of increasing ICP.

Hepatic encephalopathy

○ Generalized seizures may occur late.
○ Other findings include fetor hepaticus, asterixis, hyperactive DTRs, and a positive Babinski's sign.

Hypertensive encephalopathy

○ A life-threatening disorder — seizures with increased blood pressure, decreased LOC, intense headache, vomiting, transient blindness, paralysis, and Cheyne-Stokes respirations

Hypoglycemia

○ Generalized seizures usually occur in severe cases.
○ Other findings include blurred or double vision, motor weakness, hemiplegia, trembling, excessive diaphoresis, tachycardia, myoclonic twitching, and decreased LOC.

Hyponatremia

○ Seizure develops when sodium level falls below 125 mEq/L, especially if the decrease is rapid.
○ Other findings include orthostatic hypotension, headache, muscle twitching and weakness, fatigue, oliguria or anuria, cold and clammy skin, decreased skin turgor, irritability, lethargy, confusion, and stupor or coma.
○ Excessive thirst, tachycardia, nausea, vomiting, and abdominal cramps may also occur.

Hypoparathyroidism

○ Generalized seizures occur as a result of worsening tetany.
○ Chronic condition produces neuromuscular irritability, Chvostek's sign, dysphagia, tetany, and hyperactive DTRs.

Hypoxic encephalopathy

○ Generalized seizures, myoclonic jerks, and coma result.
○ Later, dementia, visual agnosia, choreoathetosis, and ataxia may occur.

Neurofibromatosis

○ Focal and generalized seizures occur.
○ Other findings include café-au-lait spots, multiple skin tumors, scoliosis, kyphoscoliosis, dizziness, ataxia, monocular blindness, and nystagmus.

Porphyria

○ Generalized seizures are a late sign of this disorder and indicate severe central nervous system involvement.
○ Other related findings include severe abdominal pain, tachycardia, muscle weakness, and psychotic behavior.

Renal failure (chronic)

○ Onset of twitching, trembling, myoclonic jerks, and generalized seizures is rapid.
○ Related signs and symptoms include anuria or oliguria, fatigue, malaise, irritability, decreased mental acuity, muscle cramps, peripheral neuropathies, pruritus, uremic frost, anorexia, and constipation or diarrhea.
○ Other findings include ammonia breath odor, nausea and vomiting, ecchymoses, petechiae, GI bleeding, mouth and gum ulcers, hypertension, and Kussmaul's respirations.

Sarcoidosis

○ Lesions may affect the brain, causing focal or generalized seizures.
○ Other related findings include nonproductive cough with dyspnea, substernal pain, malaise, fatigue, myalgia, weight loss, tachypnea, dysphagia, skin lesions, and impaired vision.

Stroke

○ Seizures (focal more often than generalized) may occur within 6 months of an ischemic stroke.
○ Other findings vary but may include decreased LOC, contralateral hemiplegia, dysarthria, dysphagia, ataxia, sensory loss on one side, apraxia, agnosia, aphasia, visual deficits, memory loss, personality changes, emotional lability, and incontinence.

Other causes

Barbiturate withdrawal

○ In chronically intoxicated patients, barbiturate withdrawal may produce generalized seizures 2 to 4 days after the last dose.

Diagnostic tests

○ Contrast agents used in radiologic tests may cause generalized seizures.

Drugs

○ Phenothiazines, tricyclic antidepressants, amphetamines, isoniazid, and vincristine may cause seizures in patients with preexisting epilepsy.
○ Toxic levels of some drugs, such as theophylline, lidocaine, meperidine, penicillins, and cimetidine may cause generalized seizures.

Nursing considerations

○ Monitor the patient after the seizure for recurring seizure activity.
○ Monitor for therapeutic drug levels.

Pediatric pointers

○ Common in children, generalized seizures may stem from fever, epilepsy, inborn errors of metabolism, perinatal injury, brain infection, Reye's syndrome,

Sturge-Weber syndrome, arteriovenous malformation, lead poisoning, hypoglycemia, and idiopathic causes.

Patient teaching

○ Teach the family how to observe and record seizure activity and explain the reasons for doing so.
○ Emphasize the importance of compliance with drug regimen and follow-up appointments.
○ Explain the possible adverse reactions of prescribed drugs.
○ Tell the patient to carry medical identification.

Seizures, simple partial

Overview

- Simple partial seizures result from an irritable focus in the cerebral cortex.
- They last about 30 seconds and don't alter level of consciousness (LOC).
- Type and pattern reflect the location of the irritable focus.
- They are classified as motor (including jacksonian seizures and *epilepsia partialis continua*) or somatosensory (including visual, olfactory, and auditory seizures). (See *Identifying body functions affected by focal seizures*.)

Assessment

History

- Obtain a description of the seizure activity.
- Ask about events before the seizure.
- Ask if the patient can describe an aura or recognize its onset.
- Inquire about loss of consciousness, tonicity and clonicity, cyanosis, tongue biting, and urinary incontinence.
- Explore any history of head trauma, stroke, or infection with fever, headache, or stiff neck.

Physical assessment

- Perform a complete physical assessment, focusing on the neurologic assessment.
- Check LOC.
- Test for residual deficits and sensory disturbances.

Medical causes

Brain abscess

- Seizures can occur in the acute stage of abscess formation or after resolution of the abscess.
- Decreased LOC varies from drowsiness to deep stupor.
- Early findings reflect increased intracranial pressure, such as a constant, intractable headache, nausea, and vomiting.
- Later findings include ocular disturbances, such as nystagmus, decreased visual acuity, and unequal pupils.

Assessment tip
Identifying body functions affected by focal seizures

The site of the irritable focus determines which body functions are affected by a focal seizure, as shown in this illustration.

Foot movement

Hand movement

Head turning

Facial movement

Hearing

Sight

Smell

○ Other findings vary with the abscess site and may include aphasia, hemiparesis, and personality changes.

Brain tumor

○ Focal seizures are commonly the earliest indicators.
○ Morning headache, dizziness, confusion, vision loss, and motor and sensory disturbances may occur.
○ Other findings include aphasia, generalized seizures, ataxia, decreased LOC, papilledema, vomiting, increased systolic blood pressure, widening pulse pressure and, eventually, decorticate posture.

Head trauma

○ Penetrating wounds are associated with focal seizures.
○ Seizures usually begin 3 to 15 months after injury, decrease in frequency after several years, and eventually stop.
○ Generalized seizures and a decreased LOC may progress to coma.

Multiple sclerosis

○ Focal or generalized seizures may occur in the late stages.
○ Other findings include visual deficits, paresthesia, constipation, muscle weakness, spasticity, paralysis, hyperreflexia, intention tremor, gait ataxia, dysphagia, dysarthria, emotional lability, impotence, and urinary frequency, urgency, and incontinence.

Neurofibromatosis

○ Multiple brain lesions cause focal seizures and, at times, generalized seizures.
○ Other findings include café-au-lait spots, multiple skin tumors, scoliosis, kyphoscoliosis, dizziness, ataxia, progressive monocular blindness, nystagmus, and endocrine abnormalities.

Stroke

○ Focal seizures may occur up to 6 months after a stroke's onset; generalized seizures may also occur.
○ Accompanying effects vary and may include decreased LOC, contralateral hemiplegia, dysarthria, dysphagia, ataxia, unilateral sensory loss, apraxia, agnosia, and aphasia.
○ Other findings include vision deficits, memory loss, poor judgment, personality changes, emotional lability, headache, urinary incontinence or retention, and vomiting.

Pediatric pointers

○ Focal seizures affect more children than adults and are likely to spread and become generalized; they typically cause the child's eyes, or his head and eyes, to turn to the side; in neonates, they cause mouth twitching, staring, or both.
○ Focal seizures in children can result from hemiplegic cerebral palsy, head trauma, child abuse, arteriovenous malformation, or Sturge-Weber syndrome.

Patient teaching

○ Teach family how to record seizures.
○ Emphasize the importance of complying with the prescribed drug regimen.
○ Provide information on maintaining a safe environment.
○ Tell patient to carry medical identification.

Nursing considerations

○ Remain with the patient during the seizure and reassure him.
○ Give anticonvulsants.
○ Provide emotional support.
○ Monitor for therapeutic drug levels.

Skin, bronze

Overview

- Results from excessive circulating melanin (see *Evaluating skin color variations*)
- Tends to appear at pressure points and in creases on the palms and soles
- May extend to the buccal mucosa and gums before covering the entire body

Assessment

History

- Ask about the onset of bronze skin.
- Determine whether the hue has changed.
- Inquire about the last exposure to sun or tanning source.
- Find out about a history of infection, illness, surgery, or trauma.
- Ask about abdominal pain, weakness, fatigue, diarrhea, constipation, or weight loss.
- Ask about patient's current maintenance therapy for adrenal insufficiency.
- Take a nutritional history.

Physical assessment

- Examine mucosa, gums, and scars for hyperpigmentation.

- Check pressure points — such as the knuckles, elbows, toes, and knees — for color changes.
- Check for signs of dehydration.
- Observe the abdomen for distention.
- Examine the entire body for loss of body hair and tissue and muscle wasting.
- Palpate for hepatosplenomegaly.

Medical causes

Adrenal hyperplasia

- A dark bronze tone develops within a few months.
- Other findings include visual field deficits; headache; signs of masculinization in females, such as clitoral enlargement and male distribution of hair, fat, and muscle mass.

Biliary cirrhosis

- Bronze skin develops on exposed areas of jaundiced skin, including the eyelids, palms, neck, and chest or back.
- Other findings include pruritus, weakness, fatigue, jaundice, dark urine, pale stools with steatorrhea, decreased appetite with weight loss, and hepatomegaly.

Hemochromatosis

- Progressive, generalized bronzing accentuated by metallic gray-bronze skin on sun-exposed areas, genitalia, and scars is an early sign.

Assessment tip
Evaluating skin color variations

To interpret your findings faster, refer to this chart.

Color	Distribution	Possible cause
Absent	• Small circumscribed areas • Generalized	• Vitiligo • Albinism
Blue	• Around lips or generalized	• Cyanosis (*Note:* In blacks, blue gingivae are normal.)
Deep red	• Generalized	• Polycythemia vera (increased red blood cell count)
Pink	• Local or generalized	• Erythema (superficial capillary dilation and congestion)
Tan to brown	• Facial patches	• Chloasma of pregnancy; butterfly rash of lupus erythematosus
Tan to brown bronze	• Generalized (not related to sun exposure)	• Addison's disease
Yellow to yellowish brown	• Sclera or generalized	• Jaundice from liver dysfunction (*Note:* In blacks, yellowish brown pigmentation of sclera is normal.)
Yellowish orange	• Palms, soles, and face; not sclera	• Carotenemia (carotene in the blood)

○ Other early associated effects include weakness, lethargy, weight loss, abdominal pain, loss of libido, polydipsia, and polyuria.

Malnutrition

○ Bronzing, apathy, lethargy, anorexia, weakness, and slow pulse and respiratory rates occur.
○ Other findings include paresthesia in the extremities; dull, sparse, dry hair; brittle nails; dark, swollen cheeks; dry, flaky skin; red, swollen lips; muscle wasting; and gonadal atrophy in males.

Primary adrenal insufficiency

○ Bronze skin is a classic sign.
○ Other findings include axillary and pubic hair loss, vitiligo, progressive fatigue, weakness, anorexia, nausea, vomiting, weight loss, orthostatic hypotension, weak and irregular pulse, abdominal pain, irritability, diarrhea or constipation, amenorrhea, and syncope.

Renal failure (chronic)

○ The skin becomes pallid, yellowish bronze, dry, and scaly.
○ Other findings include ammonia breath odor, oliguria, fatigue, decreased mental acuity, seizures, muscle cramps, peripheral neuropathy, bleeding tendencies, pruritus and, occasionally, uremic frost and hypertension.

Other causes

Drugs

○ Prolonged therapy with high doses of phenothiazines may cause a gradual bronzing of the skin.

Nursing considerations

○ Prepare the patient for diagnostic tests.
○ Encourage the patient to discuss concerns about changes in body image.
○ If fatigue is a problem, encourage frequent rest periods.

Pediatric pointers

○ Celiac disease can cause bronze skin in young children, beginning with the introduction of cereals and usually subsiding later in childhood.

Patient teaching

○ Emphasize the importance of rest periods.
○ Provide referral to nutritional counseling, if appropriate.

Skin, clammy

Overview

- Moist, cool, and usually pale skin
- A sympathetic response involving the release of epinephrine and norepinephrine, which causes cutaneous vasoconstriction and secretion of cold sweat from eccrine glands
- Usually on the palms, forehead, and soles
- Possibly with shock, acute hypoglycemia, anxiety reactions, arrhythmias, and heat exhaustion (see *Clammy skin: A key finding*)

Assessment

History

- Ask about a history of type 1 diabetes or cardiac disorder.
- Take a drug history, noting use of an antiarrhythmic.
- Find out about pain, chest pressure, nausea, epigastric distress, weakness, diarrhea, increased urination, or dry mouth.

Physical assessment

- Take vital signs.
- Perform cardiovascular assessment; then complete the physical assessment.
- Examine the pupils for dilation.
- Check for abdominal distention.
- Check blood glucose level.
- Test for increased muscle tension.

Medical causes

Anxiety

- Present on the forehead, palms, and soles.
- Pallor, dry mouth, tachycardia or bradycardia, palpitations, and hypertension or hypotension also occur.
- Other findings include possible tremors, breathlessness, headache, muscle tension, nausea, vomiting, abdominal distention, diarrhea, increased urination, and sharp chest pain.

Cardiac arrhythmias

- Generalized clammy skin occurs with mental status changes, dizziness, and hypotension.
- Pulse rate may be rapid, slow, or irregular.
- Other findings include palpitations, chest pain, diaphoresis, light-headedness, and weakness.

Cardiogenic shock

- Generalized clammy skin accompanies confusion, restlessness, hypotension, tachycardia, tachypnea, narrowing pulse pressure, cyanosis, and oliguria.
- Other signs and symptoms include anginal pain, dyspnea, jugular vein distention, ventricular gallop, and a bounding (early) or weak (late) pulse.

Heat exhaustion

- Generalized clammy skin, an ashen appearance, headache, confusion, syncope, giddiness and, possibly, a subnormal temperature develop with mild heat exhaustion.
- Other findings include a rapid and thready pulse, nausea, vomiting, tachypnea, oliguria, thirst, muscle cramps, and hypotension.

Hypoglycemia (acute)

- Generalized cool, clammy skin or diaphoresis may accompany irritability, tremors, palpitations, hunger, headache, tachycardia, and anxiety.
- Central nervous system findings include blurred vision, diplopia, confusion, motor weakness, hemiplegia, and coma.

Hypovolemic shock

- Generalized pale, cold, clammy skin accompanies subnormal body temperature, hypotension with narrowing pulse pressure, tachycardia, tachypnea, and rapid, thready pulse.
- Other findings are flat neck veins, increased capillary refill time, decreased urine output, poor skin turgor, confusion, and decreased level of consciousness.

Septic shock

- The cold shock stage causes generalized cold, clammy skin.
- Other findings include rapid and thready pulse, severe hypotension, persistent oliguria or anuria, and respiratory failure.

Nursing considerations

- Take vital signs frequently.
- Monitor urine output.
- Provide measures to correct the underlying cause.
- Provide emotional support to the patient and family.

Pediatric pointers

- Infants in shock don't have clammy skin because of immature sweat glands.

Geriatric pointers

- Elderly patients develop clammy skin easily because of decreased tissue perfusion.

Be alert for clammy skin. Why? Because it commonly accompanies emergency conditions, such as shock, acute hypoglycemia, and arrhythmias. To know what to do, review these typical clinical situations.

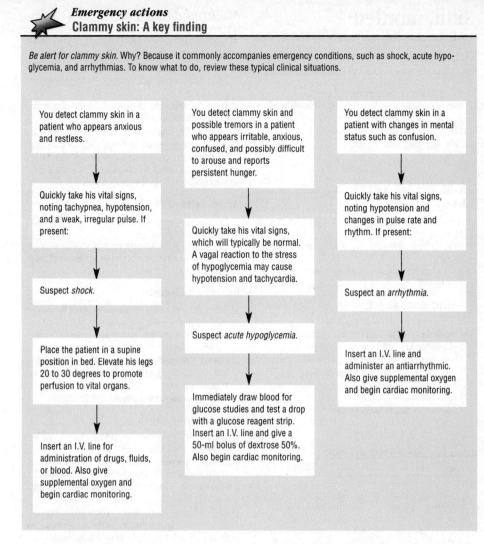

You detect clammy skin in a patient who appears anxious and restless.

↓

Quickly take his vital signs, noting tachypnea, hypotension, and a weak, irregular pulse. If present:

↓

Suspect *shock.*

↓

Place the patient in a supine position in bed. Elevate his legs 20 to 30 degrees to promote perfusion to vital organs.

↓

Insert an I.V. line for administration of drugs, fluids, or blood. Also give supplemental oxygen and begin cardiac monitoring.

You detect clammy skin and possible tremors in a patient who appears irritable, anxious, confused, and possibly difficult to arouse and reports persistent hunger.

↓

Quickly take his vital signs, which will typically be normal. A vagal reaction to the stress of hypoglycemia may cause hypotension and tachycardia.

↓

Suspect *acute hypoglycemia.*

↓

Immediately draw blood for glucose studies and test a drop with a glucose reagent strip. Insert an I.V. line and give a 50-ml bolus of dextrose 50%. Also begin cardiac monitoring.

You detect clammy skin in a patient with changes in mental status such as confusion.

↓

Quickly take his vital signs, noting hypotension and changes in pulse rate and rhythm. If present:

↓

Suspect an *arrhythmia.*

↓

Insert an I.V. line and administer an antiarrhythmic. Also give supplemental oxygen and begin cardiac monitoring.

○ Consider bowel ischemia in the differential diagnosis of older patients with cool, clammy skin, especially if abdominal pain or bloody stools occur.

Patient teaching
○ Explain the underlying illness.
○ Provide orientation to the intensive care unit, if applicable

Skin, mottled

Overview

○ Refers to patchy discoloration of the skin
○ Indicates changes of deep, middle, or superficial dermal blood vessels
○ May indicate an emergency condition (see *Mottled skin: Knowing what to do*)

Assessment

History

○ Ask about the onset of mottled skin (sudden or gradual).
○ Determine precipitating, aggravating, and alleviating factors.
○ Inquire about associated pain, numbness, or tingling in extremity.

Physical assessment

○ Observe the patient's skin color.
○ Palpate the arms and legs for skin texture, swelling, and temperature differences.
○ Check capillary refill time.
○ Palpate for pulses and note their quality.
○ Note breaks in the skin, muscle appearance, and hair distribution.
○ Assess motor and sensory function.

> **Emergency actions**
> ### Mottled skin: Knowing what to do
>
> If your patient's skin is pale, cool, clammy, and mottled at the elbows and knees or all over, he may be developing *hypovolemic shock*. Quickly take his vital signs and be sure to note tachycardia or a weak, thready pulse. Observe the neck for flattened veins. Does the patient appear anxious? If you detect these signs and symptoms, place the patient in a supine position in bed with his legs elevated 20 to 30 degrees. Administer oxygen by nasal cannula or face mask and begin cardiac monitoring. Insert a large-bore I.V. line for rapid fluid or blood product administration and prepare to insert a central line or a pulmonary artery catheter. Also prepare to insert a catheter to monitor urine output.
> Localized mottling in a pale, cool extremity that the patient says feels painful, numb, and tingling may signal acute arterial occlusion. Immediately check the patient's distal pulses. If they're absent or diminished, you'll need to insert an I.V. line in an unaffected extremity and prepare the patient for arteriography or immediate surgery.

Medical causes

Arterial occlusion (acute)

○ Temperature and color changes that develop at the level of obstruction are initial signs.
○ Pallor may change to blotchy cyanosis and livedo reticularis.
○ Color and temperature demarcation develop at the level of obstruction.
○ Other findings include sudden onset of pain in the extremity, diminished or absent pulses, cool extremity, increased capillary refill time, pallor, diminished reflexes and, possibly, paresthesia, paresis, and a sensation of cold in the affected area.

Arteriosclerosis obliterans

○ Leg pallor, cyanosis, blotchy erythema, and livedo reticularis develop.
○ Other findings include intermittent claudication, diminished or absent pedal pulses, paresthesia, and leg coolness.

Buerger's disease

○ Color changes and mottling, particularly livedo networking in the lower extremities, occur.
○ Also intermittent claudication and erythema along extremity blood vessels.
○ During cold exposure, feet become cold, cyanotic, and numb; later, they become hot, red, and tingling.
○ Possible findings include impaired peripheral pulses and peripheral neuropathy.

Hypovolemic shock

○ Vasoconstriction commonly produces skin mottling, initially in the knees and elbows.
○ As shock worsens, mottling becomes generalized.
○ Early signs include sudden onset of pallor, cool skin, restlessness, thirst, tachypnea, and slight tachycardia.
○ As shock progresses, other findings include cool, clammy skin; rapid, thready pulse; hypotension; narrowed pulse pressure; decreased urine output; subnormal temperature; confusion; and decreased level of consciousness.

Livedo reticularis (idiopathic or primary)

○ Symmetrical, diffuse mottling can involve the hands, feet, arms, legs, buttocks, and trunk.
○ Initially, networking is intermittent and most pronounced on exposure to cold or stress; eventually, mottling persists even with warming.

Polycythemia vera

○ Livedo reticularis, hemangiomas, purpura, rubor, ulcerative nodules, and scleroderma-like lesions are produced.
○ Other symptoms include headache, a vague feeling of fullness in the head, dizziness, vertigo, vision disturbances, dyspnea, and aquagenic pruritus.

Rheumatoid arthritis

○ Skin mottling may occur.
○ Early findings include joint pain and stiffness with subcutaneous nodules on the elbows.

Systemic lupus erythematosus

○ Livedo reticularis (mottling) occurs most commonly on outer arms.
○ Other findings include a butterfly rash, nondeforming joint pain and stiffness, photosensitivity, Raynaud's phenomenon, patchy alopecia, seizures, fever, anorexia, weight loss, lymphadenopathy, and emotional lability.

Other causes

Immobility

○ Prolonged immobility may cause bluish mottling, most noticeably in dependent extremities.

Thermal exposure

○ Prolonged thermal exposure, such as from a heating pad or hot water bottle, may cause a localized, reticulated, brown-to-red mottling.

Nursing considerations

○ Provide care to treat the underlying condition.

Pediatric pointers

○ A common cause of mottled skin in children is systemic vasoconstriction from shock.

Geriatric pointers

○ Decreased tissue perfusion can easily cause mottled skin.
○ Conditions producing mottled skin in older patients include arterial occlusion, polycythemia vera, and bowel ischemia.

Patient teaching

○ Encourage the avoidance of tight clothing and overexposure to cold or heating devices.
○ Teach the patient to recognize flare-up of underlying condition.

Skin, scaly

Overview

- Results when cells of the uppermost skin layer desiccate and shed
- Causes accumulation of loosely adherent flakes of keratin
- Appearance of scale indicates increased cell proliferation caused by altered keratinization
- Skin varies in texture from fine and delicate to branlike, coarse, or stratified
- Skin may be dry, brittle, and shiny or dull and greasy
- Color ranges from whitish gray, yellow, or brown to a silvery sheen

Assessment

History

- Ask about the onset, duration, and location of scaly skin.
- Find out if there was a preceding lesion or skin eruption.
- Find out about the use of topical skin products or prescribed drugs and the types of soap, cosmetics, skin lotion, and hair preparations used.
- Determine the frequency of bathing.
- Ask about recent joint pain, illness, or malaise.
- Note exposure to chemicals.
- Ask about a family history of skin disorders.

Physical assessment

- Examine the entire skin surface.
- Observe and record the pattern, location, and characteristics of skin lesions.
- Inspect the mucous membranes of the mouth, lips, and nose.
- Inspect the ears, hair, and nails.

Medical causes

Bowen's disease

- Painless, erythematous plaques are raised and indurated, with a thick, hyperkeratotic scale and, possibly, ulcerated centers.
- These occur most commonly on the head and neck.

Dermatitis

- In exfoliative dermatitis, desquamation, with fine scales or thick sheets, of all or most of the skin surface may cause life-threatening hypothermia; other findings include cardiac output failure, septicemia, fever, chills, malaise, lymphadenopathy, and gynecomastia.
- In nummular dermatitis, round, pustular lesions on the extensor surfaces of the limbs, posterior trunk, and buttocks, ooze purulent exudate, itch severely, and rapidly becomes encrusted and scaly.
- In seborrheic dermatitis, pruritic, erythematous, scaly papules progress to larger, dry or moist, greasy scales with yellowish crusts on the face, chest, and scalp.

Dermatophytosis

- Tinea capitis produces lesions with reddened, slightly elevated borders and a central area of dense scaling that become inflamed and pus-filled.
- Tinea pedis causes scaling and blisters between the toes.
- Tinea corporis produces crusty lesions; as they enlarge, their centers heal, causing the classic ringworm shape.

Discoid lupus erythematosus

- Separate or coalescing lesions, ranging from pink to purple, are covered with a yellow or brown crust.
- Enlarged hair follicles are filled with scales, and telangiectasia may be present.
- Commonly involves the face or sun-exposed areas of the neck, ears, scalp, lips, and oral mucosa.

Lichen planus

- Small, flat, violet lesions, with a fine scale and grey lines on the surface usually affect the lumbar region, genitalia, wrists, ankles, and anterior lower legs.

Lymphoma

- Hodgkin's disease may cause pruritic, scaling dermatitis that begins in the legs and spreads to the entire body.
- Non-Hodgkin's lymphoma produces erythematous patches with some scaling that become interspersed with nodules.

Pityriasis rosea

- Yellow-tan or erythematous patches with scaly edges erupt on the trunk and limbs a few days or weeks after onset.

Psoriasis

- Silvery white, micaceous scales cover erythematous plaques that have sharply defined borders.
- Usually appears on the scalp, chest, elbows, knees, back, buttocks, and genitalia.
- Other findings include nail pitting, pruritus, arthritis and, sometimes, pain from dry, cracked, encrusted lesion

Syphilis (secondary)

- Papulosquamous, slightly scaly eruptions are characteristic.
- A ring-shaped pattern of copper-red papules forms on the face, arms, palms, soles, chest, back, and abdomen.

- ○ Systemic findings include lymphadenopathy, malaise, weight loss, anorexia, nausea, vomiting, headache, sore throat, and fever.

Systemic lupus erythematosus

- ○ A bright-red maculopapular eruption that sometimes has scaling develops.
- ○ Patches are sharply defined and involve the nose and malar regions of the face in a butterfly pattern.
- ○ Other findings include photosensitivity, joint pain and stiffness, vasculitis, Raynaud's phenomenon, patchy alopecia, and mucous membrane ulcers.

Tinea versicolor

- ○ Slightly scaly, macular hypopigmented, fawn-colored, or brown patches commonly affect the upper trunk, arms, and lower abdomen.

Other causes

Drugs

- ○ Drugs, such as penicillins, sulfonamides, barbiturates, quinidine, diazepam, phenytoin, and isoniazid, can produce scaling patches.

Nursing considerations

- ○ If scaling results from corticosteroid therapy, withhold the drug.

Pediatric pointers

- ○ Scaly skin may stem from infantile eczema, pityriasis rosea, epidermolytic hyperkeratosis, psoriasis, various forms of ichthyosis, atopic dermatitis, a viral infection, seborrhea capitis, or an acute transient dermatitis.

Patient teaching

- ○ Instruct the patient or caregiver in proper skin care.
- ○ Explain the treatment of the underlying disorder.

Skin turgor, decreased

Overview

○ Pinched skin holds for up to 30 seconds, then slowly returns to its normal contour.
○ It's commonly assessed over the hand, arm, or sternum. (See *Evaluating skin turgor.*)
○ Decreased skin turgor results from dehydration or volume depletion, which moves interstitial fluid into the vascular bed to maintain circulating blood volume, leading to slackness in the skin's dermal layer.

Assessment

History

○ Ask about food and fluid intake and fluid loss.
○ Find out about recent vomiting, diarrhea, draining wounds, fever with sweating, or increased urination.
○ Take a drug history, noting use of diuretics.
○ Ask about use of alcohol.

Physical assessment

○ Take vital signs, noting orthostatic hypotension and tachycardia.
○ Evaluate level of consciousness.
○ Inspect the oral mucosa, the furrows of the tongue, and axillae for dryness.
○ Check jugular vein distention.
○ Check capillary refill.

Medical causes

Cholera

○ Cholera is characterized by abrupt watery diarrhea and vomiting, leading to severe water and electrolyte loss.
○ Other findings include intense thirst, weakness, muscle cramps, cyanosis, oliguria, tachycardia, falling blood pressure, fever, and hypoactive bowel sounds.

Dehydration

○ Decreased skin turgor occurs with moderate to severe dehydration.
○ Other findings include dry oral mucosa, decreased perspiration, resting tachycardia, orthostatic hypotension, dry and furrowed tongue, increased thirst, weight loss, oliguria, fever, and fatigue.
○ As dehydration worsens, findings include enophthalmos, lethargy, weakness, confusion, delirium or obtundation, anuria and shock.

Nursing considerations

○ Monitor intake and output.
○ Assess vital signs.
○ Turn the patient every 2 hours to prevent skin breakdown.
○ Administer I.V. fluid replacement, and frequently offer oral fluids.
○ Weight the patient daily.
○ Monitor electrolyte levels.

Pediatric pointers

○ Diarrhea from gastroenteritis is the most common cause of dehydration in children, especially up to age 2.

Assessment tip
Evaluating skin turgor

To evaluate skin turgor in an adult, pick up a fold of skin over the sternum or the arm, as shown at top. (In an infant, roll a fold of loosely adherent skin on the abdomen between your thumb and forefinger.) Then release it. Normal skin will immediately return to its previous contour. In decreased skin turgor, the skin fold will "hold," or "tent," as shown at bottom, for up to 30 seconds.

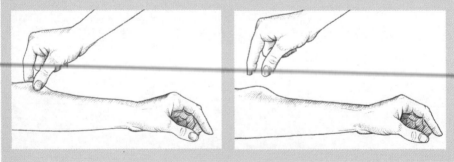

Geriatric pointers

○ Decreased skin turgor is a normal finding in elderly patients, making it an unreliable indicator of dehydration.

Patient teaching

○ Explain fluid replacement and its importance.
○ Explain the signs and symptoms the patient or caregiver needs to report.

Splenomegaly

Overview

- Splenomegaly refers to enlargement of the spleen.
- Enlargement may be detected by light palpation under the left costal margin. (See *Palpating for splenomegaly.*)
- Spleen functions as the body's largest lymph node.

⭐ ***Emergency actions***

If the patient has a history of abdominal or thoracic trauma, don't palpate the abdomen because this may aggravate internal bleeding. Instead, examine for left-upper-quadrant pain and signs of shock. If you detect these signs, suspect splenic rupture. Insert an I.V. line for emergency fluid and blood replacement, and administer oxygen. Catheterize the patient to evaluate urine output and begin cardiac monitoring. Prepare the patient for possible surgery.

Assessment

History

- Inquire about fatigue; frequent colds, sore throats, or other infections; bruising; left-upper-quadrant pain; abdominal fullness; and early satiety.

Physical assessment

- Complete an abdominal assessment.
- Examine the skin for pallor and ecchymoses.
- Palpate the axillae, groin, and neck for lymphadenopathy.

Medical causes

Cirrhosis

- Moderate to severe splenomegaly occurs with advanced cirrhosis.
- Late findings also include jaundice, hepatomegaly, leg edema, hematemesis, and ascites.
- Signs of hepatic encephalopathy may also occur, such as asterixis, fetor hepaticus, slurred speech, and decreased level of consciousness that may progress to coma.
- Other findings include jaundice, pruritus, bleeding tendencies, menstrual irregularities or testicular atrophy, gynecomastia, and right-upper abdominal pain.

Endocarditis (subacute infective)

- Spleen is enlarged but nontender.
- A suddenly changing murmur or the discovery of a new murmur in the presence of a fever is a classic sign.

- Other findings include anorexia, pallor, weakness, fever, night sweats, fatigue, tachycardia, weight loss, arthralgia, petechiae, hematuria, Osler's nodes, and Janeway lesions.

Hepatitis

- Splenomegaly may occur.
- Characteristic findings include dark urine, clay-colored stools, anorexia, malaise, pruritus, hepatomegaly, vomiting, jaundice, and fatigue.

Histoplasmosis

- Splenomegaly and hepatomegaly occur.
- Other findings include lymphadenopathy, jaundice, fever, anorexia, and signs and symptoms of anemia.

Hypersplenism (primary)

- Splenomegaly accompanies anemia, neutropenia, or thrombocytopenia.
- Left-sided abdominal pain may occur.
- With anemia, findings include weakness, fatigue, malaise, and pallor.
- With severe neutropenia, findings include frequent infections.
- With thrombocytopenia, easy bruising or spontaneous, widespread hemorrhage may occur.

Leukemia

- Moderate to severe splenomegaly is early sign.
- With chronic granulocytic leukemia, findings include hepatomegaly, lymphadenopathy, fatigue, malaise, pallor, fever, gum swelling, bleeding tendencies, weight loss, anorexia, and abdominal, bone, and joint pain.
- Acute leukemia may produce dyspnea, tachycardia, and palpitations.

Lymphoma

- Moderate to massive splenomegaly is late sign.
- Other late findings include hepatomegaly, painless lymphadenopathy, night sweats, fever, fatigue, weight loss, malaise, and scaly dermatitis with pruritus.

Mononucleosis (infectious)

- Splenomegaly, a common sign, is most pronounced during second and third weeks of illness.
- Triad includes sore throat, cervical lymphadenopathy, and fluctuating temperature with an evening peak.
- Hepatomegaly, jaundice, and a maculopapular rash may develop.

Pancreatic cancer

- Moderate to severe splenomegaly may occur if a tumor compresses the splenic vein.
- Other characteristic findings include abdominal or back pain, anorexia, nausea, vomiting, weight loss, GI bleeding, jaundice, pruritus, skin lesions, emotional lability, weakness, and fatigue.

Detecting splenomegaly requires skillful and gentle palpation to avoid rupturing the enlarged spleen. Follow these steps carefully:

- Place the patient in the supine position and stand at his right side. Place your left hand under the left costovertebral angle and push lightly to move the spleen forward. Then press your right hand gently under the left front costal margin.
- Have the patient take a deep breath and then exhale. As he exhales, move your right hand along the tissue contours under the border of the ribs, feeling for the

spleen's edge. The enlarged spleen should feel like a firm mass that bumps against your fingers. Remember to begin palpation low enough in the abdomen to catch the edge of a massive spleen.

- Grade the splenomegaly as slight (½″ to 1½″ [1 to 4 cm] below the costal margin), moderate (1½″ to 3″ [4 to 8 cm] below the costal margin), or great (greater than or equal to 3″ below the costal margin).
- Reposition the patient on his right side with his hips and knees flexed slightly to move the spleen forward. Then repeat the palpation procedure.

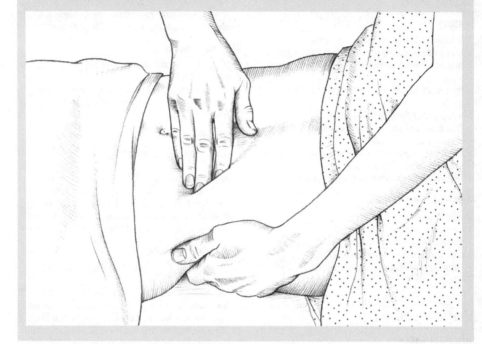

Polycythemia vera

○ Enlarged spleen resulting in easy satiety, abdominal fullness, and left-upper-quadrant abdominal pain or pleuritic chest pain late in the disease
○ Also finger and toe paresthesia, impaired mentation, tinnitus, blurred or double vision, scotoma, increased blood pressure, pruritus, epigastric distress, weight loss, hepatomegaly, bleeding tendencies, and intermittent claudication
○ Possible deep purplish red oral mucous membranes, headache, dyspnea, dizziness, vertigo, weakness, and fatigue

Splenic rupture

○ Splenomegaly may result from massive hemorrhage.
○ Other findings include left-upper-quadrant pain, abdominal rigidity, Kehr's sign, and signs of shock.

Nursing considerations

○ Prepare the patient for diagnostic tests.
○ Provide measures to treat the underlying disorder.

Pediatric pointers

○ Children may develop splenomegaly in congenital hemolytic anemia, Gaucher's disease, or sickle cell disease.
○ Splenic abscess is the most common cause of splenomegaly in immunocompromised children.

Patient teaching

○ Instruct the patient in avoiding infection.
○ Emphasize the importance of complying with drug therapy.

Stools, clay-colored

Overview

○ A result of hepatocellular degeneration or biliary obstruction that interferes with the formation or release of bile pigments
○ Commonly associated with jaundice and dark "cola-colored" urine

Assessment

History

○ Ask about the onset of clay-colored stools.
○ Explore associated abdominal pain, nausea and vomiting, fatigue, anorexia, weight loss, and dark urine.
○ Inquire about difficulty digesting fatty foods or heavy meals.
○ Note whether the patient bruises easily.
○ Take a medical history, noting gallbladder, hepatic, or pancreatic disorders.
○ Ask about recent barium studies or use of antacids.
○ Note a history of alcoholism.
○ Find out about exposure to toxic substances.

Physical assessment

○ Take vital signs.
○ Check for jaundice.
○ Inspect the abdomen for distention and ascites.
○ Auscultate for hypoactive bowel sounds.
○ Percuss and palpate for masses and rebound tenderness.

Medical causes

Bile duct cancer

○ Clay-colored stools may be accompanied by jaundice, pruritus, anorexia, weight loss, bleeding tendencies, and palpable mass.
○ Pain may develop in the epigastrium or right upper quadrant.

Biliary cirrhosis

○ Clay-colored stools typically follow unexplained pruritus that worsens at bedtime, weakness, fatigue, weight loss, and vague abdominal pain.
○ Other findings include jaundice; hyperpigmentation; signs of malabsorption; bone and back pain, hematemesis; ascites; edema; firm, nontender hepatomegaly; and xanthomas on the palms, soles, and elbows.

Cholangitis (sclerosing)

○ Clay-colored stools, chronic or intermittent jaundice, pruritus, right-upper-quadrant pain, weakness, fatigue, chills, and fever occur.

Cholelithiasis

○ Obstruction of the common bile duct may result in clay-colored stools.
○ Associated symptoms include dyspepsia and biliary colic.
○ Right-upper-quadrant pain intensifies over several hours, may radiate to the epigastrium or shoulder blades, and is relieved by antacids.
○ Pain is accompanied by tachycardia, restlessness, nausea, intolerance to certain foods, vomiting, upper abdominal tenderness, fever, chills, and jaundice.

Hepatic cancer

○ Weight loss, weakness, and anorexia precede clay-colored stools.
○ Later, nodular, firm hepatomegaly; jaundice; right-upper-quadrant pain; ascites; dependent edema; and fever develop.

Hepatitis

○ Clay-colored stools signal the start of the icteric phase.
○ Associated signs include mild weight loss, dark urine, anorexia, jaundice, and tender hepatomegaly.
○ Findings during the icteric phase include irritability, right-upper-quadrant pain, splenomegaly, enlarged cervical lymph nodes, and severe pruritus.

Pancreatic cancer

○ Common bile duct obstruction may cause clay-colored stools.
○ Classic associated findings include abdominal or back pain, jaundice, pruritus, nausea and vomiting, anorexia, weight loss, fatigue, weakness, and fever.
○ Other findings include diarrhea, skin lesions, emotional lability, splenomegaly, and signs of GI bleeding.

Pancreatitis (acute)

○ Clay-colored stools, dark urine, jaundice, and severe epigastric pain that's aggravated by lying down occur.
○ Other findings include nausea, vomiting, fever, abdominal rigidity and tenderness, hypoactive bowel sounds, and crackles at the lung bases.

Other causes

Biliary surgery

○ Biliary surgery may cause bile duct stricture, resulting in clay-colored stools.

Nursing considerations

○ Prepare the patient for diagnostic tests.
○ Encourage rest periods.
○ Give vaccines for hepatitis A and B.

Pediatric pointers

○ Clay-colored stools may occur in infants with biliary atresia.

Geriatric pointers

○ Because elderly patients with cholelithiasis have a greater risk of developing its complications, surgery should be considered.

Patient teaching

○ Explain ways to reduce abdominal pain.
○ Explain the dietary modifications the patient needs.
○ Explain the need for a restful environment.
○ Emphasize the importance of avoiding alcohol.

Stridor

Overview

- A loud, harsh, musical respiratory sound
- Results from an obstruction in the trachea or larynx
- Usually heard during inspiration, but it may also occur during expiration in severe upper airway obstruction
- May begin as a low-pitched croaking and progress to high-pitched crowing as respirations become more vigorous

Emergency actions

Check vital signs, including oxygen saturation, and examine the patient for signs of partial airway obstruction. Abrupt end of stridor signals complete airway obstruction. If you detect airway obstruction, clear the airway with back blows or abdominal thrusts. Give oxygen or prepare for emergency endotracheal intubation or tracheostomy and mechanical ventilation. (See Emergency endotracheal intubation.*) Suction any aspirated vomitus or blood. Connect the patient to a cardiac monitor and position the patient upright.*

Assessment

History

- Ask about the onset of stridor.
- Inquire about any previous instances of stridor.
- Note any current respiratory tract infection.
- Ask about a history of allergies, tumors, or respiratory and vascular disorders.
- Note recent exposure to smoke or noxious fumes or gases.
- Inquire about associated pain or cough.

Physical assessment

- Examine the mouth for excessive secretions, foreign matter, inflammation, and swelling.
- Assess neck for swelling, masses, subcutaneous crepitation, and scars.
- Observe chest for decreased or asymmetrical expansion.
- Auscultate for wheezes, rhonchi, crackles, rubs, and other abnormal breath sounds.
- Percuss for dullness, tympany, or flatness.
- Note burns or signs of trauma.

Medical causes

Airway trauma

- Acute obstruction is common and results in the sudden onset of stridor.

Emergency actions
Emergency endotracheal intubation

For a patient with stridor, you may have to perform emergency endotracheal (ET) intubation to establish a patent airway and administer mechanical ventilation. Just follow these essential steps:

- Gather the necessary equipment.
- Explain the procedure to the patient.
- Place the patient flat on his back with a small blanket or pillow under his head. This position aligns the axis of the oropharynx, posterior pharynx, and trachea.
- Check the cuff on the ET tube for leaks.
- After intubation, inflate the cuff, using the minimal leak technique.
- Check tube placement by auscultating for bilateral breath sounds or using a capnometer; observe the patient for chest expansion and feel for warm exhalations at the ET tube's opening.
- Insert an oral airway or bite block.
- Secure the tube and airway with tape applied to skin treated with compound benzoin tincture.
- Suction secretions from the patient's mouth and the ET tube as needed.
- Administer oxygen or initiate mechanical ventilation (or both).

After the patient has been intubated, suction secretions as needed and check cuff pressure once every shift (correcting any air leaks with the minimal leak technique). Provide mouth care every 2 to 3 hours and as needed. Prepare the patient for chest X-rays to check tube placement, and restrain and reassure him as needed.

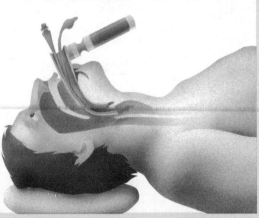

- Other findings include dysphonia, dysphagia, hemoptysis, cyanosis, accessory muscle use, intercostal retractions, nasal flaring, tachypnea, progressive dyspnea, and shallow respirations.

Anaphylaxis

- Upper airway edema and laryngospasm cause stridor and other signs of respiratory distress.
- Typically, these respiratory effects are preceded by a feeling of impending doom or fear, weakness, diaphoresis, sneezing, nasal pruritus, urticaria, erythema, and angioedema.
- Other common findings include chest or throat tightness, dysphagia and, possibly, signs of shock.

Anthrax (inhalation)

- The second stage develops abruptly with rapid deterioration marked by stridor, fever, dyspnea, and hypotension generally leading to death within 24 hours.
- Initial findings include fever, chills, weakness, cough, and chest pain.

Aspiration of foreign body

- A life-threatening situation — sudden stridor is characteristic.
- Other findings include abrupt onset of dry, paroxysmal coughing, gagging, or choking; hoarseness; tachycardia; wheezing; dyspnea; tachypnea; intercostal muscle retractions; diminished breath sounds; cyanosis; anxiety; and shallow respirations.

Epiglottiditis

- A life-threatening situation — stridor, caused by an erythematous, edematous epiglottis that obstructs the upper airway, occurs along with fever, sore throat, and a croupy cough.
- Cough may progress to severe respiratory distress with sternal and intercostal retractions, nasal flaring, cyanosis, and tachycardia.

Hypocalcemia

- Laryngospasm can cause stridor.
- Other findings include paresthesia, carpopedal spasm, hyperactive deep tendon reflexes, muscle twitching and cramping, and positive Chvostek's and Trousseau's signs.

Inhalation injury

- Laryngeal edema and bronchospasms, resulting in stridor, may develop within 48 hours after inhalation of smoke or noxious fumes.
- Other findings include singed nasal hairs, orofacial burns, coughing, hoarseness, sooty sputum, crackles, rhonchi, wheezes, dyspnea, accessory muscle use, intercostal retractions, and nasal flaring.

Laryngeal tumor

- A late sign, possible with dysphagia, dyspnea, enlarged cervical nodes, and pain that radiates to the ear.

- Preceded by hoarseness, minor throat pain, and a mild, dry cough.

Laryngitis (acute)

- Severe laryngeal edema, resulting in stridor and dyspnea, may occur.
- Mild to severe hoarseness is the chief sign.
- Other findings include sore throat, dysphagia, dry cough, malaise, and fever.

Mediastinal tumor

- Compression of the trachea and bronchi results in stridor.
- Other findings include hoarseness, brassy cough, tracheal shift or tug, dilated neck veins, swelling of the face and neck, stertorous respirations, dyspnea, dysphagia, suprasternal retractions on inspiration, and pain in the chest, shoulder, or arm.

Thoracic aortic aneurysm

- If the trachea is compressed, stridor, dyspnea, wheezing, and a brassy cough may result.
- Other findings include hoarseness or complete voice loss, dysphagia, jugular vein distention, prominent chest veins, tracheal tug, paresthesia or neuralgia, and edema of the face, neck, and arms.

Other causes

Diagnostic tests

- Bronchoscopy or laryngoscopy may precipitate laryngospasm and stridor.

Treatments

- Neck surgery, such as thyroidectomy, may cause laryngeal paralysis and stridor.
- After prolonged intubation, the patient may exhibit laryngeal edema and stridor when the tube is removed.

Nursing considerations

- Continue to monitor vital signs and oxygen saturation.
- Prepare the patient for diagnostic tests.
- Offer reassurance and calm the patient.

Pediatric pointers

- Causes of stridor in children include foreign-body aspiration, croup syndrome, laryngeal diphtheria, pertussis, retropharyngeal abscess, and congenital abnormalities of the larynx.

Patient teaching

- Explain all procedures and treatments.

Syncope

Overview

- Transient loss of consciousness
- Associated with impaired cerebral blood supply or cerebral hypoxia
- Abrupt and lasting for seconds to minutes

⭐ Emergency actions

If you see a patient faint, ensure a patent airway and patient safety. Take vital signs. Place the patient in supine position, elevate his legs, and loosen any tight clothing. Be alert for tachycardia, bradycardia, or an irregular pulse. Place the patient on a cardiac monitor to detect arrhythmias. If an arrhythmia appears, give oxygen and insert an I.V. line for drugs or fluids. Be ready to begin cardiopulmonary resuscitation. Cardioversion, defibrillation, or insertion of a temporary pacemaker may be required.

Assessment

History

- Obtain a description of the fainting episode and its duration.
- Inquire about precipitating factors.
- Ask about preceding symptoms, including weakness, light-headedness, nausea, or diaphoresis.
- Ask about associated headache.
- Obtain a history of previous fainting.

Physical assessment

- Take vital signs.
- Examine the patient for any injuries from falling during syncope.
- Perform a complete cardiac and neurologic assessment.

Medical causes

Aortic arch syndrome

- Syncope may be accompanied by weak or abruptly absent carotid pulses and unequal or absent radial pulses.
- Early findings include night sweats, pallor, nausea, anorexia, weight loss, arthralgia, and Raynaud's phenomenon.
- Other findings include hypotension in the arms; neck, shoulder, and chest pain; paresthesia; intermittent claudication; bruits; vision disturbances; and dizziness.

Aortic stenosis

- A classic late sign, syncope is accompanied by exertional dyspnea and angina.
- Fatigue, orthopnea, paroxysmal nocturnal dyspnea, palpitations, atrial and ventricular gallops, and diminished carotid pulses occur.
- A harsh, crescendo-decrescendo systolic ejection murmur that's loudest at the right sternal border of the second intercostal space may be heard.

Cardiac arrhythmias

- Decreased cardiac output and impaired cerebral circulation may cause syncope.

Carotid sinus hypersensitivity

- Syncope is triggered by compression of the carotid sinus.
- Preceding findings include palpitations, pallor, confusion, diaphoresis, dyspnea, and hypotension.
- Syncope may develop without warning in Stokes-Adams syndrome; asystole during syncope may precipitate spasm and myoclonic jerks if prolonged.

Hypoxemia

- Syncope, confusion, tachycardia, restlessness, tachypnea, dyspnea, cyanosis, and incoordination may occur.

Orthostatic hypotension

- Syncope occurs when the patient rises quickly from a recumbent position.
- Other findings include tachycardia, pallor, dizziness, blurred vision, nausea, and diaphoresis.

Transient ischemic attack

- Syncope and decreased level of consciousness may result.
- Other findings vary with the affected artery but may include vision loss, nystagmus, aphasia, dysarthria, unilateral numbness, hemiparesis or hemiplegia, tinnitus, facial weakness, dysphagia, and staggering or uncoordinated gait.

Vagal glossopharyngeal neuralgia

- Localized pressure may trigger pain in the base of the tongue, pharynx, larynx, tonsils, and ear, resulting in syncope.

Other causes

Drugs

- Occasionally, griseofulvin, indomethacin, and levodopa can produce syncope.
- Prazosin may cause severe orthostatic hypotension and syncope, usually after the first dose.
- Quinidine may cause syncope — and possibly death — associated with ventricular fibrillation.

Nursing considerations

○ Continue to monitor vital signs.
○ Prepare the patient for diagnostic studies.

Pediatric pointers

○ Syncope in children may result from a cardiac or neurologic disorder, allergies, or emotional stress.

Patient teaching

○ Encourage the patient to pace his activities.
○ Explain that he should avoid standing for prolonged periods of time.
○ Tell him what measures to take if feeling faint.

Tachycardia

Overview

○ Refers to a heart rate greater than 100 beats/minute
○ Detected by counting the apical, carotid, or radial pulse

Emergency actions

If the patient has tachycardia, increased or decreased blood pressure, drowsiness, and confusion, do an electrocardiograph (ECG). Give oxygen, and begin cardiac monitoring. Insert an I.V. line for fluid, blood product, and drug administration, and gather resuscitation equipment.

Assessment

History

○ Explore palpitations, dizziness, shortness of breath, weakness, fatigue, syncope, and chest pain.
○ Ask about a history of trauma, diabetes, and cardiac, pulmonary, or thyroid disorders.
○ Obtain an alcohol and drug history.

Physical assessment

○ Inspect for pallor or cyanosis.
○ Assess pulses and blood pressure and note peripheral edema.
○ Auscultate the heart and lungs for abnormal sounds and rhythms.

Medical causes

Acute respiratory distress syndrome

○ Tachycardia, crackles, rhonchi, dyspnea, tachypnea, nasal flaring, and grunting respirations
○ Cyanosis, anxiety, and decreased level of consciousness (LOC)

Adrenocortical insufficiency

○ A rapid, weak pulse with progressive weakness and fatigue
○ Abdominal pain, nausea, vomiting, altered bowel habits, weight loss, orthostatic hypotension, irritability, bronze skin, decreased libido, and syncope

Anemia

○ Tachycardia and bounding pulse
○ Fatigue, pallor, dyspnea, bleeding tendencies, atrial gallop, crackles, and a systolic bruit over the carotid arteries

Anxiety

○ Tachycardia, tachypnea, chest pain, cold and clammy skin, dry mouth, nausea, and light-headedness

Aortic insufficiency

○ Tachycardia with a bounding Corrigan's pulse that sounds like a water hammer and a large, diffuse apical heave
○ A high-pitched, blowing diastolic murmur starting with the second heart sound
○ Angina, dyspnea, palpitations, strong and abrupt carotid pulsations, pallor, and signs of heart failure

Aortic stenosis

○ Tachycardia, a weak and thready pulse, and an atrial gallop
○ Chiefly, dyspnea, angina, dizziness, and syncope
○ Palpitations, crackles, fatigue, and a harsh systolic ejection murmur

Cardiac arrhythmias

○ Tachycardia with hypotension, dizziness, palpitations, weakness, and fatigue
○ Tachypnea; decreased LOC; and pale, cool, clammy skin

Cardiac contusion

○ Tachycardia, substernal pain, dyspnea, hypotension, palpitations, sternal ecchymoses, and a pericardial rub or tamponade

Cardiac tamponade

○ A life-threatening disorder; tachycardia commonly with paradoxical pulse, dyspnea, and tachypnea
○ Anxiety, cyanosis, clammy skin, hypotension, jugular vein distention, narrowed pulse pressure, pericardial rub, muffled heart sounds, chest pain, and hepatomegaly

Chronic obstructive pulmonary disease

○ Tachycardia with cough, tachypnea, pursed-lip breathing, accessory muscle use, cyanosis, diminished breath sounds, rhonchi, crackles, wheezing and, in the late stages, barrel chest and clubbing

Diabetic ketoacidosis

○ Decreased LOC, dehydration, oliguria with ketosis, and a rapid, thready pulse with Kussmaul's respirations, its cardinal sign

Febrile illness

○ Tachycardia, chills, diaphoresis, headache, and weakness

Heart failure

○ Tachycardia with a ventricular gallop, fatigue, dyspnea, orthopnea, and leg edema

Hyperosmolar hyperglycemic nonketotic syndrome

○ A rapidly deteriorating LOC with tachycardia, hypotension, tachypnea, seizures, oliguria without ketosis, and severe dehydration

Hypertensive crisis

○ A life-threatening disorder; tachycardia with diastolic blood pressure over 120 mm Hg, systolic blood pressure that may exceed 200 mm Hg
○ Tachypnea, signs of pulmonary edema, chest pain, severe headache, confusion, anxiety, tinnitus, epistaxis, muscle twitching, seizures, nausea, and vomiting

Hypoglycemia

○ Tachycardia with nervousness, weakness, headache, hunger, nausea, diaphoresis, and moist, clammy skin

Hypovolemia

○ Tachycardia with hypotension, decreased urine output, fatigue, muscle weakness, decreased skin turgor, sunken eyeballs, thirst, syncope, and dry skin and tongue

Hypoxemia

○ Tachycardia with dyspnea, tachypnea, and cyanosis
○ Confusion, restlessness, and disorientation, progressing to coma

Myocardial infarction

○ A life-threatening disorder; tachycardia or bradycardia with crushing substernal chest pain that may radiate to the left arm, jaw, neck, or shoulder
○ Pallor, clammy skin, dyspnea, diaphoresis, atrial gallop, a new murmur, crackles, nausea, vomiting, anxiety, restlessness, and increased or decreased blood pressure

Orthostatic hypotension

○ Tachycardia with dizziness, syncope, pallor, blurred vision, diaphoresis, and nausea
○ Dim vision, spots before the eyes, and signs of dehydration

Pneumothorax

○ A life-threatening disorder; tachycardia and other signs and symptoms of distress, such as severe dyspnea and chest pain, tachypnea, and cyanosis
○ Dry cough, subcutaneous crepitation, absent or decreased breath sounds, reduced or absent chest movement on the affected side, and decreased vocal fremitus

Pulmonary embolism

○ Tachycardia preceded by sudden dyspnea, angina, or pleuritic chest pain
○ Weak peripheral pulse, tachypnea, low-grade fever, restlessness, diaphoresis, and a dry cough or a cough with blood-tinged sputum

Shock

○ Tachycardia, tachypnea, skin temperature changes, hypotension, apprehension, and decreaesed LOC before cardiac collapse

○ A life-threatening disorder whether source is cardiac, hypovolemic, neurologic, or septic

Thyrotoxicosis

○ Tachycardia, an enlarged thyroid, nervousness, heat intolerance, weight loss despite increased appetite, diaphoresis, tremors, palpitations and, possibly, exophthalmos are classic findings.

Other causes

Diagnostic tests

○ Cardiac catheterization and electrophysiologic studies may induce transient tachycardia.

Drugs and alcohol

○ Various drugs cause tachycardia, including acetylcholinesterase inhibitors, alpha blockers, anticholinergics, beta-adrenergic bronchodilators, nitrates, phenothiazines, sympathomimetics, and vasodilators.
○ Excessive caffeine intake and alcohol intoxication may also cause tachycardia.

Surgery and pacemakers

○ Cardiac surgery and pacemaker malfunction or wire irritation may cause tachycardia.

Nursing considerations

○ Continue to monitor the patient.
○ Explain ordered diagnostic tests.
○ Obtain a resting 12-lead ECG.

Pediatric pointers

○ Normal heart rates for children are higher than those for adults: 130 beats/minute for a neonate, 100 beats/minute for a child age 4, 90 beats/minute for a child age 8, and 75 to 80 beats/minute for an adolescent age 16.

Patient teaching

○ Explain the possibility of tachyarrhythmia recurring.
○ Explain the use of antiarrhythmics, internal defibrillator, or ablation therapy.

Tachypnea

Overview

○ Refers to an abnormally fast respiratory rate — 20 or more breaths/minute

Emergency actions

Evaluate cardiopulmonary status. Obtain vital signs, including oxygen saturation; check for cyanosis, chest pain, dyspnea, tachycardia, and hypotension. If the patient has paradoxical chest movement, suspect flail chest and immediately splint the chest with your hands or with sandbags. Administer supplemental oxygen, and, if possible, place the patient in semi-Fowler's position. If respiratory failure occurs, intubation and mechanical ventilation may be needed. Insert an I.V. line for fluid and drugs and begin cardiac monitoring.

Assessment

History

○ Ask about the onset, precipitating factors, and description of tachypnea.
○ Inquire about a history of pulmonary or cardiac conditions or anxiety attacks.
○ Find out about other signs and symptoms, such as diaphoresis, chest pain, or recent weight loss.
○ Take a drug history.

Physical assessment

○ Take vital signs, including oxygen saturation.
○ Auscultate the chest for abnormal heart and breath sounds.
○ Record the color, amount, and consistency of any sputum.
○ Check for jugular vein distention.
○ Examine the skin for pallor, cyanosis, edema, and warmth or coolness.

Medical causes

Acute respiratory distress syndrome

○ Tachypnea, an early finding, gradually worsens as fluid accumulates in the lungs.
○ Other findings include accessory muscle use, grunting expirations, suprasternal and intercostal retractions, crackles, and rhonchi.

Anemia

○ Tachypnea may occur, depending on the disorder.
○ Other findings include fatigue, pallor, dyspnea, tachycardia, postural hypotension, bounding pulse, atrial gallop, and a systolic bruit over the carotid arteries.

Anxiety

○ Tachypnea may occur with tachycardia, restlessness, chest pain, nausea, and light-headedness.

Aspiration of a foreign body

○ With partial obstruction, a dry, paroxysmal cough with rapid, shallow respirations develops abruptly.
○ Other findings include dyspnea, gagging or choking, intercostal retraction, nasal flaring, cyanosis, decreased or absent breath sounds, hoarseness, and stridor or coarse wheezing.

Asthma

○ Tachypnea is common along with mild wheezing and a dry cough progressing to mucous expectorating. in initial stages.
○ If left untreated, progresses to prolonged expirations, intercostal and supraclavicular retractions on inspiration, severe wheezing, rhonchi, flaring nostrils, tachycardia, diaphoresis, and flushing or cyanosis

Bronchitis (chronic)

○ Mild tachypnea may occur, accompanied by a dry, hacking cough, which later produces copious amounts of sputum.
○ Other findings include dyspnea, prolonged expirations, wheezing, scattered rhonchi, accessory muscle use, cyanosis, and late-stage clubbing and barrel chest.

Cardiac arrhythmias

○ Tachypnea may occur along with hypotension, dizziness, palpitations, weakness, fatigue and, possibly, decreased level of consciousness (LOC).

Cardiac tamponade

○ A life-threatening disorder; tachypnea may accompany tachycardia, dyspnea, and paradoxical pulse.
○ Related findings include muffled heart sounds, pericardial rub, chest pain, hypotension, narrowed pulse pressure, hepatomegaly, anxiety, cyanosis, clammy skin, and neck vein distention.

Emphysema

○ Tachypnea is accompanied by exertional dyspnea.
○ Accompanying findings include anorexia, malaise, peripheral cyanosis, pursed-lip breathing, accessory muscle use, chronic productive cough, and late-stage clubbing and barrel chest.

Febrile illness

○ Fever can cause tachypnea, tachycardia, chills, diaphoresis, headache, and weakness.

Flail chest

○ A life-threatening disorder; tachypnea usually appears early.
○ Other findings include paradoxical chest wall movement, rib bruises and palpable fractures, localized

chest pain, hypotension, diminished breath sounds, dyspnea, and accessory muscle use.

Head trauma

○ When trauma affects the brain stem, central neurogenic hyperventilation may produce a form of tachypnea marked by rapid, even, and deep respirations.
○ Other signs of life-threatening neurogenic dysfunction include coma, unequal and nonreactive pupils, seizures, hemiplegia, flaccidity, and hypoactive or absent deep tendon reflexes.

Hyperosmolar hyperglycemic nonketotic syndrome

○ Rapidly deteriorating LOC occurs with tachypnea, tachycardia, hypotension, seizures, oliguria, and signs of dehydration.

Hypoxia

○ Tachypnea occurs, possibly with restlessness, impaired judgment, tachycardia, dyspnea, and cyanosis.

Interstitial fibrosis

○ Tachypnea develops gradually and may become severe.
○ Other findings include exertional dyspnea; pleuritic chest pain; a paroxysmal, dry cough; crackles; late inspiratory wheezing; cyanosis; fatigue; weight loss; and late-stage clubbing.

Lung abscess

○ Tachypnea occurs with dyspnea and worsens with fever.
○ Chief sign is a productive cough with copious amounts of purulent, foul-smelling, usually bloody sputum.

Plague

○ Tachypnea, productive cough, chest pain, dyspnea, hemoptysis, and increasing respiratory distress and cardiopulmonary insufficiency

Pneumonia (bacterial)

○ Tachypnea is usually preceded by a painful, hacking, dry cough that rapidly becomes productive.
○ Other findings include high fever, shaking chills, headache, dyspnea, pleuritic chest pain, tachycardia, grunting respirations, nasal flaring, and cyanosis.

Pneumothorax

○ A life-threatening disorder; tachypnea is typically accompanied by severe, sharp, one-sided chest pain.
○ Other findings include dyspnea, tachycardia, accessory muscle use, asymmetrical chest expansion, dry cough, cyanosis, anxiety, and restlessness.
○ Deviated trachea occurs with tension pneumothorax.

Pulmonary edema

○ Tachypnea, an early sign, is accompanied by exertional dyspnea, paroxysmal nocturnal dyspnea and, later, orthopnea.
○ Other findings include productive cough with pink frothy sputum, crackles, tachycardia, and a ventricular gallop.

Pulmonary embolism (acute)

○ Sudden tachypnea with dyspnea
○ Angina or pleuritic pain, tachycardia, a dry or productive cough with blood-tinged sputum, fever, restlessness, and diaphoresis

Shock

○ Tachypnea, tachycardia. skin temperature changes, hypotension, apprehension, and decreased LOC before cardiac collapse

Tumor

○ A lung, pleural, or mediastinal tumor, causing tachypnea along with exertional dyspnea, cough, hemoptysis, and pleuritic chest pain
○ Tracheal shift, neck vein distention, weight loss, anorexia, and fatigue

Other causes

Drugs

○ Tachypnea may result from an overdose of salicylates.

Nursing considerations

○ Continue to monitor vital signs.
○ Keep suction and emergency equipment nearby.
○ Intubate the patient and provide mechanical ventilation if needed.

Pediatric pointers

○ Normal respiratory rate varies with the child's age.
○ Other causes include congenital heart defects, meningitis, metabolic acidosis, cystic fibrosis, hunger, and anxiety.

Geriatric pointers

○ Heart failure, chronic obstructive pulmonary disease, anxiety, or failure to take cardiac and respiratory drugs appropriately

Patient teaching

○ Explain that slight increases in respiratory rate may be normal.

Taste abnormalities

Overview

○ Include a loss of taste (ageusia), partial loss of taste (hypogeusia), a distorted sense of taste (dysgeusia), or an unpleasant sense of taste (cacogeusia)
○ Sensory receptors for taste (the taste buds): concentrated over the tongue's surface and scattered over the palate, pharynx, and larynx
○ Complex flavors perceived by taste and olfactory receptors

Assessment

History
○ Ask about the onset of taste abnormality.
○ Find out about a history of oral or other disorders.
○ Note recent flu, head trauma, or radiation treatments.
○ Ask about smoking habits.
○ Take a drug history.

Physical assessment
○ Evaluate taste: Withdraw the tongue with a gauze sponge, apply various flavors (such as salt or sugar) on the tongue, and ask the patient to identify the tastes.
○ Inspect the oral cavity for lesions, sores, and mucosal or taste bud abnormalities.
○ Evaluate sense of smell: Pinch one nostril and ask the patient to close his eyes and sniff through the open nostril to identify nonirritating odors such as coffee. Repeat test on the other nostril.

Medical causes

Basilar skull fracture
○ If the first cranial nerve is involved, the patient usually can't detect aromatic flavors.
○ Other findings include epistaxis, rhinorrhea, otorrhea, Battle's sign, raccoon eyes, headache, nausea, vomiting, hearing and vision loss, and a decreased level of consciousness.

Bell's palsy
○ Taste loss in the anterior two-thirds of the tongue is common along with hemifacial muscle weakness or paralysis.
○ Affected side of the face sags and is masklike.
○ Associated signs include drooling and tearing, diminished or absent corneal reflex, and difficulty blinking the affected eye.

Common cold
○ Impaired taste is usually from loss of smell.

○ Other common findings include rhinorrhea with nasal congestion, sore throat, headache, fatigue, myalgia, arthralgia, malaise, and a dry, hacking cough.

Geographic tongue
○ Taste abnormalities occur with areas of loss and regrowth of filiform papillae.
○ Affected areas are continually changing and produce a maplike appearance with denuded red patches surrounded by thick white borders.

Influenza
○ The patient may have hypogeusia, dysgeusia, or both as well as an impaired sense of smell.
○ Common complaints include sore throat, fever with chills, headache, weakness, malaise, muscle aches, cough and, occasionally, hoarseness and rhinorrhea.

Oral cancer
○ Tumors involving the tongue may destroy or damage taste buds.
○ Other findings include difficulty chewing and speaking, and halitosis.

Sjögren's syndrome
○ Impaired sense of taste occurs with ocular dryness, burning, and pain around the eyes and under the lids.
○ Other findings include photosensitivity; impaired vision; eye redness; mouth soreness; difficulty chewing, swallowing, and talking; a dry cough; hoarseness; epistaxis; dry, scaly skin; decreased sweating; abdominal distress; and polyuria.

Thalamic syndrome
○ A distorted sense of taste is preceded by contralateral sensory loss, transient hemiparesis, and homonymous hemianopia.
○ Later, sensation is gradually regained, and pain or hyperpathia may then be experienced.

Thrush
○ Cream-colored or bluish white patches of exudate on the tongue, mouth, or pharynx cause altered taste, pain, and burning.

Viral hepatitis (acute)
○ Hypogeusia commonly precedes jaundice by 1 to 2 weeks.
○ Associated preicteric findings include altered sense of smell, anorexia, nausea, vomiting, fatigue, malaise, headache, photophobia, muscle and joint aches, sore throat, and a cough.

Vitamin B$_{12}$ deficiency
○ Hypogeusia is accompanied by impaired sense of smell, anorexia, weight loss, abdominal discomfort, and glossitis.

- Yellow skin, peripheral neuropathy, dyspnea, ataxic gait, and dementia may also occur.

Zinc deficiency

- Idiopathic hypogeusia may occur with cacogeusia.
- Other findings include a distorted sense of smell, anorexia, soft and misshapen nails, hepatosplenomegaly, and sparse hair growth.

Other causes

Drugs

- Antithyroid drugs, captopril, griseofulvin, lithium, penicillamine, procarbazine, rifampin, vincristine, vinblastine, and antibiotics may distort the sense of taste.

Radiation therapy

- Irradiation of the head or neck may cause excessive dryness of the mouth, resulting in impaired taste sensation.

Nursing considerations

- Modify the patient's diet if needed.
- Encourage oral hygiene before and after meals.

Pediatric pointers

- Children may be unable to differentiate between abnormal taste sensation and taste dislike.

Geriatric pointers

- Aging reduces the number of taste buds, leading to impaired taste.

Patient teaching

- Emphasize proper oral hygiene.
- Discuss the use of spices to enhance flavors.
- Provide referral to a dietitian as needed.

Tearing, increased

Overview

- Refers to excessive lacrimation or tear production
- Also known as *epiphora*
- Usually results from inadequate tear drainage because of obstruction of the lacrimal drainage system or malposition of the lower lid
- May occur in response to emotional or physical stress (psychic lacrimation)
- May be neurogenic — lacrimation triggered by reflex stimulation associated with ocular trauma or inflammation or with exposure to environmental irritants
- *Decreased* tearing from aging, vitamin A deficiency, eye trauma, and certain drugs (see *Causes of decreased tearing*)

Assessment

History

- Ask about the onset and description of tearing.
- Find out about accompanying pain, irritation, or discharge.
- Inquire about a history of eye trauma or ocular and systemic disorders.
- Take a drug history.
- Discuss possible occupational hazards.

Physical assessment

- Examine the external structures of both eyes.

Causes of decreased tearing

Decreased tearing makes the patient's eyes uncomfortably dry. This symptom is usually associated with aging, but it may also result from the following:

- *Anticholinergics.* Decreased tearing commonly follows use of an anticholinergic (mydriatic), such as atropine, scopolamine, cyclopentolate, and tropicamide.
- *Keratoconjunctivitis sicca (dry eye syndrome).* With dry eye syndrome, atrophy of the lacrimal glands curtails tear production.
- *Ocular trauma.* Decreased tearing during healing and scar formation follows acute ocular trauma.
- *Sarcoidosis.* Decreased tearing results from inflammation of the lacrimal and salivary glands in this syndrome.
- *Stevens-Johnson syndrome.* With Stevens-Johnson syndrome, decreased tearing is accompanied by purulent conjunctivitis and severe eye pain.
- *Turner's syndrome.* Characterized by congenital absence of the lacrimal gland, Turner's syndrome causes decreased tearing.
- *Vitamin A deficiency.* Typically, vitamin A deficiency causes decreased tearing and poor night vision.

Nontraumatic decreased tearing is usually treated with artificial tears as either drops or ointment.

- Examine the eyelids for lesions and edema.
- Determine whether the eyeballs appear shrunken or swollen.
- Check for ptosis.
- Examine the conjunctiva for redness and abnormal drainage.
- Note the color of the sclera.
- Using a flashlight, examine the cornea and iris for scars, irregularities, and foreign bodies.
- Evaluate extraocular muscle function by testing the six cardinal fields of gaze.
- Test visual acuity.

Medical causes

Conjunctival foreign bodies and abrasions

- Increased tearing may occur with localized conjunctival injection, eye pain, and photophobia.
- A foreign-body sensation may be present.

Conjunctivitis

- Increased tearing, conjunctival injection, and itching
- With allergic conjunctivitis, a stringy discharge
- With bacterial conjunctivitis, copious, purulent discharge; burning; a foreign-body sensation; and eye pain if the cornea is involved
- With fungal conjunctivitis, lid edema; burning; photophobia; pain if the cornea is involved; and a copious, thick, purulent discharge that may form sticky crusts on the lids
- With viral conjunctivitis, a foreign-body sensation, slight exudate, and lid edema

Corneal abrasion

- Corneal pain with increased tearing and severe pain that's aggravated by itching and blinking.
- A foreign-body sensation, blurred vision, conjunctival injection, and photophobia

Corneal foreign body

- Increased tearing, blurred vision, a foreign-body sensation, photophobia, eye pain, miosis, and conjunctival injection occur.
- Dark specks may be visible in the cornea.

Corneal ulcers

- Increased tearing, severe photophobia, and eye pain aggravated by blinking
- Blurred vision, conjunctival injection, and a white, opaque cornea
- With bacterial ulcers, a copious, purulent discharge that may form sticky crusts on the lids.

Dacryocystitis

- Increased tearing and a purulent discharge are the chief complaints.

○ Other findings include pain and tenderness around the tear sac with marked eyelid edema and redness near the lacrimal punctum.
○ Pressing the tear sac produces a thick, purulent discharge or, in chronic cases, a mucoid discharge.

Dry eye syndrome

○ Excess tearing from excessive dryness of the cornea and conjunctiva
○ Eye pain, conjunctival injection, and itching

Episcleritis

○ Increased tearing and photophobia
○ If the sclera is inflamed, eye pain and tenderness on palpation
○ Conjunctival injection and edema, a purplish pink sclera, and episcleral edema

Herpes zoster

○ If the trigeminal nerve is affected, increased tearing.
○ Severe one-sided facial and eye pain that's followed by the eruption of vesicles within several days
○ Red and swollen eyelids, scanty serous discharge, conjunctival injection, and a white, cloudy cornea

Lid contractions

○ Increased tearing from stricture of the canaliculi

Psoriasis vulgaris

○ Lesions that affect the eyelids and extend into the conjunctiva may cause irritation, increased tearing, and a foreign-body sensation.
○ Early signs include chronic conjunctivitis and conjunctival injection.

Punctum misplacement

○ Increased tearing with keratitis

Thyrotoxicosis

○ Increased tearing in both eyes
○ In the eyes, ptosis, lid edema, photophobia, a foreign-body sensation, conjunctival injection, chemosis, diplopia and, at times, exophthalmos
○ Weight loss despite increased appetite, heat intolerance, nervousness, sweating, diarrhea, tremors, tachycardia, palpitations, and an enlarged thyroid

○ Follow standard precautions to prevent transmitting the infection.

Pediatric pointers

○ The most common causes of increased tearing in children are allergies, conjunctivitis, and the common cold.

Patient teaching

○ Explain the importance of avoiding cross-contamination.
○ Teach the patient good hand-washing techniques.

Other causes

Cholinergics

○ Miotics, such a pilocarpine

Nursing considerations

○ Obtain tear specimen for culture.
○ Prepare the patient for Schirmer's test and irrigation of lacrimal drainage system.

Throat pain

Overview

○ Refers to discomfort in pharynx
○ Ranges from sensation of scratchiness to severe pain
○ Typically accompanied by ear pain because cranial nerves IX and X innervate the pharynx as well as the middle and external ear

Assessment

History

○ Ask about the onset of throat pain.
○ Find out about fever, ear pain, or dysphagia.
○ Take a medical history, including throat problems and allergies.

Physical assessment

○ Examine the pharynx, oropharynx, and nasopharynx, noting redness, exudate, and swelling.
○ Observe the tonsils for redness, swelling, or exudate.
○ Obtain exudate specimen for culture.
○ Examine the nose, using a nasal speculum.
○ Check the ears using an otoscope.
○ Palpate neck and oropharynx for nodules or lymph node enlargement.

Medical causes

Agranulocytosis

○ Sore throat after progressive fatigue and weakness
○ Nausea, vomiting, anorexia, bleeding tendencies and, possibly, rough-edged ulcers with gray or black membranes on the gums, palate, or perianal area

Allergic rhinitis

○ Sore throat with nasal congestion with a thin nasal discharge, postnasal drip, paroxysmal sneezing, decreased sense of smell, frontal or temporal headache, and itchy eyes, nose, and throat

Bronchitis (acute)

○ Lower throat pain, fever, chills, productive cough, and muscle and back pain
○ Rhonchi, wheezing, and crackles on auscultation

Chronic fatigue syndrome

○ Incapacitating fatigue with sore throat, myalgia, lymphadenopathy, and cognitive dysfunction

Common cold

○ Sore throat with cough, sneezing, nasal congestion, mouth breathing, rhinorrhea, fatigue, headache, myalgia, and arthralgia
○ A transient loss of taste and smell

Contact ulcers

○ Ulcers appear symmetrically on the posterior vocal cords, resulting in sore throat.
○ Pain is aggravated by talking and may occur with referred ear pain and, occasionally, hemoptysis.

Foreign body

○ A foreign body lodged in the palatine or lingual tonsil and pyriform sinus may produce localized throat pain.

Gastroesophageal reflux disease

○ Chronic sore throat and hoarseness
○ Pyrosis is the most common symptom.

Glossopharyngeal neuralgia

○ Knifelike throat pain on one side in the tonsillar fossa, possibly radiating to the ear
○ From yawning, chewing, swallowing, or eating spicy foods

Herpes simplex virus

○ Sore throat may result from lesions on the oral mucosa.
○ After causing brief discomfort, lesions erupt into erythematous vesicles that eventually rupture and leave a painful ulcer, followed by a yellowish crust.

Influenza

○ Sore throat, fever, chills, headache, weakness, malaise, cough, muscle aches and, occasionally, hoarseness and rhinorrhea

Laryngeal cancer

○ With extrinsic laryngeal cancer, pain or burning in the throat when drinking citrus juice or hot liquids, or the patient feels a lump in the throat
○ With intrinsic laryngeal cancer, hoarseness for longer than 3 weeks
○ Later, during metastasis, dysphagia, dyspnea, a cough, enlarged cervical lymph nodes, and pain that radiates to the ear

Laryngitis (acute)

○ Sore throat with mild to severe hoarseness, its chief sign
○ Malaise, fever, dysphagia, dry cough, and tender, enlarged lymph nodes

Mononucleosis (infectious)

○ Sore throat, cervical lymphadenopathy, and fluctuating temperature
○ Possible hepatomegaly and splenomegaly

Necrotizing ulcerative gingivitis (acute)

○ Abrupt sore throat and gums that ulcerate and bleed
○ Gray exudate on the gums and pharyngeal tonsils
○ A foul taste in the mouth, halitosis, cervical lymphadenopathy, headache, malaise, and fever

Peritonsillar abscess

○ Severe throat pain, radiating to the ear
○ Dysphagia, drooling, dysarthria, halitosis, fever with chills, malaise, and nausea

Pharyngeal burns

○ Throat pain and dysphagia occur.
○ If the larynx is involved, laryngeal edema, bronchospasm, and stridor

Pharyngitis

○ With bacterial form, abrupt sore throat on one side
○ With fungal form, a diffuse, burning sore throat
○ With viral form, a diffuse sore throat, malaise, fever, and mild erythema and edema of the posterior oropharyngeal wall

Pharyngomaxillary space abscess

○ Mild throat pain with a bulge in the medial wall of the pharynx and swelling of the neck on the affected side
○ Fever, dysphagia, trismus and, possibly, signs of respiratory distress or toxemia

Sinusitis (acute)

○ Sore throat with purulent nasal discharge and postnasal drip
○ Halitosis, headache, malaise, cough, fever, and facial pain and swelling associated with nasal congestion

Tongue cancer

○ Localized throat pain around a white lesion or ulcer
○ Pain radiating to the ear with dysphagia

Tonsillar cancer

○ Throat pain that may radiate to the ear.
○ A superficial ulcer on the tonsil or one that extends to the base of the tongue.

Tonsillitis

○ With acute tonsillitis, mild to severe throat pain.
○ With chronic tonsillitis, mild sore throat
○ With lingual tonsillitis, throat pain on one or both sides, just above the hyoid bone

Uvulitis

○ Throat pain or a sensation of something in the throat
○ Swollen and red uvula; in allergic uvulitis, pale uvula

Other causes

Treatment

○ Endotracheal intubation and local surgery, such as tonsillectomy and adenoidectomy.

Nursing considerations

○ Provide analgesic sprays or lozenges to relieve throat pain.
○ Prepare the patient for throat culture, blood work, and a monospot test.

Pediatric pointers

○ Causes of sore throat include acute epiglottiditis, herpangina, scarlet fever, acute follicular tonsillitis, and retropharyngeal abscess.

Patient teaching

○ Explain the importance of completing full course of antibiotic treatment.
○ Discuss ways to soothe the throat.

Thyroid enlargement

Overview

○ Enlargement from inflammation, physiologic changes, iodine deficiency, and thyroid tumors or hormone imbalance
○ Hyperfunction or hypofunction, depending on the medical cause, with resulting excess or deficiency of the hormone thyroxine
○ *Goiter:* an enlarged thyroid that causes visible swelling in the front of the neck

Assessment

History

○ Ask about the onset of enlargement.
○ Inquire about the use of thyroid hormone replacement drugs.
○ Ask about previous irradiation of the thyroid gland or the neck and about recent infections.
○ Take a personal and family history, including thyroid disease.

Physical assessment

○ Inspect the trachea for midline deviation.
○ Palpate the enlarged gland; note the size, shape, consistency of gland, and the presence or absence of nodules. (See *Palpating the thyroid gland.*)
○ Using bell of stethoscope, listen over lobes of thyroid gland for a bruit.

Medical causes

Hypothyroidism

○ Enlarged thyroid; weight gain despite anorexia; fatigue; cold intolerance; constipation; menorrhagia; slowed intellectual and motor activity; dry, pale, cool skin; dry, sparse hair; and thick, brittle nails result
○ Eventually, the face assumes a dull expression with periorbital edema.

Thyroiditis

○ Autoimmune thyroiditis may not produce symptoms other than thyroid enlargement.
○ In subacute granulomatous thyroiditis, thyroid enlargement may follow an upper respiratory infection or a sore throat; other findings may include a painful and tender thyroid and dysphagia.

Assessment tip
Palpating the thyroid gland

To palpate the thyroid gland, you'll need to stand behind the patient. Give the patient a cup of water and have him extend his neck slightly. Place the fingers of both hands on the patient's neck, just below the cricoid cartilage and just alongside the trachea. Tell the patient to take a sip of water and swallow. The thyroid gland should rise as he swallows. Use your fingers to palpate on the sides and downward to feel the whole thyroid gland. Palpate over the midline to feel the isthmus of the thyroid.

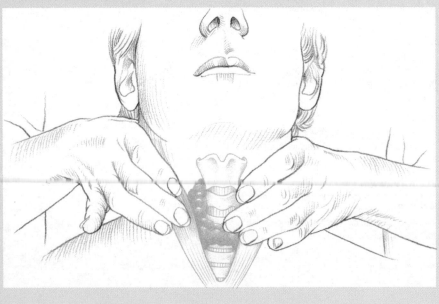

Thyrotoxicosis

○ An enlarged thyroid gland is a classic finding.
○ Other findings include nervousness; heat intolerance; fatigue; weight loss despite increased appetite; diarrhea; sweating; palpitations; tremors; smooth, warm, flushed skin; fine, soft hair; exophthalmos; nausea and vomiting; and oligomenorrhea or amenorrhea.

Tumors

○ An enlarged thyroid may be accompanied by hoarseness, loss of voice, and dysphagia.
○ A malignant tumor usually appears as a single nodule in the neck.
○ A nonmalignant tumor may appear as multiple nodules in the neck.

Other causes

Goitrogens

○ Certain drugs, including lithium, sulfonamides, phenylbutazone, and para-aminosalicylic acid, may decrease thyroxine production.
○ Foods containing goitrogens include peanuts, cabbage, soybeans, strawberries, spinach, rutabagas, and radishes.

Nursing considerations

○ Prepare the patient for diagnostic tests and surgery or radiation therapy, if needed.
○ Specific interventions depend on whether the patient is hypothyroid, has thyroiditis, or is recovering from a thyroidectomy.

Pediatric pointers

○ Congenital goiter, a syndrome of infantile myxedema or cretinism, is characterized by mental retardation, growth failure, and other signs and symptoms of hypothyroidism; early treatment can prevent mental retardation.

Patient teaching

○ Explain the signs and symptoms of hypothyroidism or hyperthyroidism to report.
○ Explain posttreatment precautions to a patient undergoing radioactive iodine therapy.
○ Explain thyroid hormone replacement therapy and signs of thyroid hormone overdose.

Tinnitus

Overview

- Refers to abnormal ringing, sizzling, buzzing, or humming occurring in the ear
- Can be classified as subjective or objective and as tinnitus aurium (the patient hears noise in his ears) or tinnitus cerebri (the patient hears noise in his head)

Assessment

History

- Ask about the onset, location, and description of the sound.
- Inquire about other symptoms, such as vertigo, headache, or hearing loss.
- Take a health and drug history.

Physical assessment

- Inspect the ears and examine the tympanic membrane, using an otoscope.
- Perform Weber's and Rinne tests to check for hearing loss.
- Auscultate for bruits in the neck.
- Compress the jugular or carotid artery to see if this affects the tinnitus.
- Examine the nasopharynx for masses that might cause eustachian tube dysfunction and tinnitus.

Medical causes

Acoustic neuroma

- Tinnitus in one ear precedes sensorineural hearing loss and vertigo in same ear.
- Facial paralysis, headache, nausea, vomiting, and papilledema may occur.

Anemia

- Mild tinnitus, if severe
- Pallor, weakness, fatigue, exertional dyspnea, tachycardia, bounding pulse, atrial gallop, and a systolic bruit over the carotid arteries

Atherosclerosis of the carotid artery

- Constant tinnitus can be stopped by applying pressure over the carotid artery.
- Auscultation over the upper part of the neck, on the auricle, or near the ear on the affected side may detect a bruit.
- Palpation may reveal a weak carotid pulse.

Cervical spondylosis

- Osteophytic growths may compress the vertebral arteries, resulting in tinnitus.

- A stiff neck and pain aggravated by activity accompany tinnitus.
- Other findings include brief vertigo, nystagmus, hearing loss, paresthesia, weakness, and pain that radiates down the arms.

Ear canal obstruction

- Tinnitus with conductive hearing loss, itching, blockage, and a feeling of fullness or pain in the ear

Eustachian tube patency

- Tinnitus, audible breath sounds, loud and distorted voice sounds, and a sense of fullness in the ear can occur.
- Use a pneumatic otoscope to see if the tympanic membrane moves with respiration.

Hypertension

- High-pitched tinnitus in both ears may occur with severe hypertension.
- Diastolic blood pressure over 120 mm Hg may also cause severe, throbbing headache; restlessness; nausea; vomiting; blurred vision; seizures; and decreased level of consciousness.

Intracranial arteriovenous malformation

- A large malformation may cause tinnitus accompanied by a bruit over the mastoid process.
- Other findings include severe headache, seizures, and progressive neurologic deficits.

Labyrinthitis (suppurative)

- Tinnitus with sudden, severe attacks of vertigo, sensorineural hearing loss in one or both ears, nystagmus, dizziness, nausea, and vomiting

Ménière's disease

- Attacks of tinnitus, vertigo, a feeling of fullness or blockage in the ear, and fluctuating sensorineural hearing loss for 10 minutes to several hours
- Severe nausea, vomiting, diaphoresis, and nystagmus

Ossicle dislocation

- Tinnitus and sensorineural hearing loss
- Possible bleeding from the middle ear

Otitis externa (acute)

- If debris in the external ear canal invades the tympanic membrane, tinnitus may result.
- More typical findings include pruritus, foul-smelling purulent discharge, and severe ear pain that are aggravated by manipulation of the tragus or auricle, teeth clenching, mouth opening, and chewing.
- External ear canal appears red and edematous and may be occluded by debris, causing partial hearing loss.

Otitis media

- Tinnitus and conductive hearing loss may occur.

○ More typical findings include ear pain, a red and bulging tympanic membrane, high fever, chills, and dizziness.

Otosclerosis

○ The patient may describe ringing, roaring, or whistling tinnitus or a combination of these sounds.
○ Progressive hearing loss and vertigo may occur.

Presbycusis

○ Tinnitus and a progressive, symmetrical, sensorineural hearing loss in both ears, usually of high-frequency tones.

Tympanic membrane perforation

○ Tinnitus is usually the chief complaint in a small perforation; hearing loss, in a larger perforation.
○ Other findings include pain, vertigo, and a feeling of fullness in the ear.

Other causes

Drugs and alcohol

○ Quinine, alcohol, and indomethacin may also cause reversible tinnitus.
○ Common drugs that may cause irreversible tinnitus include the aminoglycoside antibiotics and vancomycin.
○ Overdose of salicylates commonly causes reversible tinnitus.

Noise

○ Chronic exposure to noise, especially high-pitched sounds, can damage the ear's hair cells, causing temporary or permanent tinnitus and total hearing loss.

Nursing considerations

○ Educate the patient about strategies for adapting to the tinnitus.
○ A hearing aid may be used to amplify environmental sounds, thereby obscuring tinnitus.

Pediatric pointers

○ Maternal use of ototoxic drugs during the third trimester of pregnancy can cause labyrinthine damage in the fetus, resulting in tinnitus.

Patient teaching

○ Provide information about avoidance of excessive noise, ototoxic agents, and other things that may cause cochlear damage.

Tracheal deviation

Overview

- Signals an underlying condition that can compromise pulmonary function and possibly cause respiratory distress (see *Detecting slight tracheal deviation*)
- Occurs with disorders that produce mediastinal shift from asymmetrical thoracic volume or pressure
- A classic sign of life-threatening tension pneumothorax

⭐ Emergency actions

Look for signs and symptoms of respiratory distress. If possible, place the patient in semi-Fowler's position to aid chest expansion and improve oxygenation. Give supplemental oxygen, and intubate the patient if needed. Insert an I.V. line for fluid and drug administration. Palpate for subcutaneous crepitation in the neck and chest, a sign of tension pneumothorax. Chest tube insertion may be needed to release trapped air or fluid and to restore normal intrapleural and intrathoracic pressure gradients.

Assessment

History

- Take a history of pulmonary or cardiac disorders, surgery, trauma, or infection.
- Ask about smoking habits.
- Ask about other signs and symptoms, such as breathing difficulty, pain, and cough.

Physical assessment

- Take vital signs.
- Observe for respiratory distress.
- Perform a complete cardiopulmonary assessment.

Medical causes

Atelectasis

- Extensive lung collapse can produce tracheal deviation toward the affected side.
- Respiratory findings include dyspnea, tachypnea, pleuritic chest pain, dry cough, dullness on percussion, decreased vocal fremitus and breath sounds, inspiratory lag, and substernal or intercostal retractions.

Hiatal hernia

- Intrusion of abdominal viscera into the pleural space causes tracheal deviation toward the unaffected side.
- Other findings include pyrosis, regurgitation or vomiting, chest or abdominal pain, and respiratory distress.

Kyphoscoliosis

- Rib cage distortion and mediastinal shift produces tracheal deviation toward the compressed lung.
- Respiratory findings include dry cough, dyspnea, asymmetrical chest expansion and, possibly, asymmetrical breath sounds.
- Backache and fatigue are common.

Mediastinal tumor

- If large, a mediastinal tumor can press against the trachea and nearby structures, causing tracheal deviation and dysphagia.
- Other late findings include stridor, dyspnea, brassy cough, hoarseness, and stertorous respirations with suprasternal retraction.
- Shoulder, arm, or chest pain, and edema of the neck, face, or arm may develop.
- Neck and chest wall veins may be dilated.

Pleural effusion

- If the effusion is large, the mediastinum can shift to the contralateral side, producing tracheal deviation.
- Related findings include dry cough, dyspnea, pleuritic pain, pleural friction rub, tachypnea, decreased chest motion, decreased or absent breath sounds, egophony, flatness on percussion, decreased tactile fremitus, fever, and weight loss.

Pulmonary fibrosis

- Tracheal deviation as the mediastinum shifts toward the affected side
- Possible dyspnea, cough, clubbing, malaise, and fever

Pulmonary tuberculosis

- Tracheal deviation toward the affected side with asymmetrical chest excursion, and inspiratory crackles
- Insidious early findings, such as anorexia, weight loss, fever, chills, and night sweats
- Productive cough, hemoptysis, pleuritic chest pain, and dyspnea as the disease progresses

Tension pneumothorax

- A life-threatening disorder; tracheal deviation toward the unaffected side
- Sudden onset of respiratory distress, sharp chest pain, dry cough, severe dyspnea, tachycardia, wheezing, cyanosis, accessory muscle use, nasal flaring, air hunger, and asymmetrical chest movement
- Restlessness, anxiety, subcutaneous crepitation in the neck and upper chest, decreased or absent breath sounds on the affected side, jugular vein distention, and hypotension

Thoracic aortic aneurysm

- The trachea usually deviates to the right.
- Findings may include stridor; dyspnea; wheezing; brassy cough; hoarseness; dysphagia; edema of the

Although gross tracheal deviation is visible, detection of slight deviation requires palpation and perhaps even an X-ray. Try palpation first.

With the tip of your index finger, locate the patient's trachea by palpating between the sternocleidomastoid muscles. Then compare the trachea's position to an imaginary line drawn vertically through the suprasternal notch. Any deviation from midline is usually considered abnormal.

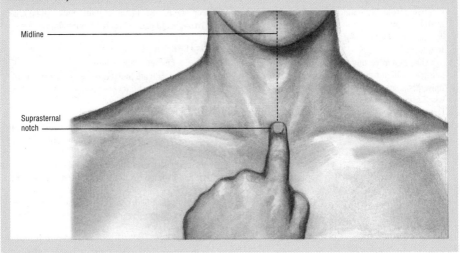

Midline

Suprasternal notch

face, neck, or arm; jugular vein distention; and substernal, neck, shoulder, or lower back pain.

Nursing considerations

○ Monitor respiratory and cardiac condition constantly.
○ Make sure that emergency equipment is readily available.
○ Give analgesics for comfort if needed.
○ Insert a large-bore needle into the pleural space or insert a thoracostomy tube for tension pneumothorax.
○ Give emotional support.

Pediatric pointers
○ Respiratory distress typically develops more rapidly in children than in adults.

Geriatric pointers
○ Tracheal deviation to the right commonly stems from an elongated, atherosclerotic aortic arch, but this deviation isn't considered abnormal.

Patient teaching
○ Teach the patient how to perform coughing and deep-breathing exercises.
○ Explain signs and symptoms of respiratory difficulty to report.

Tremors

Overview

- Refer to rhythmic, involuntary, oscillatory trembling that result from alternating contraction of opposing muscle groups
- Are characterized by their location, amplitude, and frequency
- Are classified as resting (occurs in extremity at rest, subsides with movement), intention (occurs with movement, subsides at rest) or postural (occurs when extremity or trunk is actively held in a particular position)

Assessment

History

- Ask about the onset, duration, and progression of tremor.
- Determine what aggravates or alleviates tremors.
- Find out about other symptoms, such as behavioral changes or memory loss.
- Explore personal and family history of neurologic, endocrine, or metabolic disorders.
- Obtain a drug history, especially use of phenothiazines.
- Ask about alcohol use.

Physical assessment

- Assess overall appearance and demeanor, noting mental condition.
- Test range of motion and strength in all major muscle groups while observing for chorea, athetosis, dystonia, and other involuntary movements.
- Check deep tendon reflexes (DTRs).
- Observe the patient's gait.

Medical causes

Alcohol withdrawal syndrome

- Resting and intention tremors as soon as 7 hours after the last drink and progressively worsen
- Early, diaphoresis, tachycardia, elevated blood pressure, anxiety, restlessness, irritability, insomnia, headache, nausea, and vomiting
- In severe withdrawal, profound tremors, agitation, confusion, hallucinations, and seizures

Alkalosis

- A severe intention tremor with twitching, carpopedal spasms, agitation, diaphoresis, and hyperventilation
- Dizziness, tinnitus, palpitations, and peripheral and circumoral cyanosis

Cerebellar tumor

- An intention tremor is a classic sign.
- Related findings include ataxia, nystagmus, incoordination, muscle weakness and atrophy, and hypoactive or absent DTRs.

Graves' disease

- Fine hand tremors, nervousness, weight loss, fatigue, palpitations, dyspnea, heat intolerance, an enlarged thyroid gland and, possibly, exophthalmos

Hypercapnia

- A rapid, fine intention tremor
- Headache, fatigue, blurred vision, weakness, lethargy, and decreased level of consciousness (LOC)

Hypoglycemia

- A rapid, fine intention tremor with confusion, weakness, tachycardia, diaphoresis, and cold, clammy skin
- Possible disappearing tremor as hypoglycemia worsens and hypotonia and decreased LOC become evident
- Early, headache, profound hunger, nervousness, and blurred or double vision

Kwashiorkor

- In the advanced stages, coarse intention and resting tremors
- Myoclonus, rigidity of all extremities, hyperreflexia, hepatomegaly, and pitting edema in the hands, feet, and sacral areas
- Flat affect, pronounced hair loss, and dry, peeling skin

Multiple sclerosis

- An intention tremor that waxes and wanes may be an early sign along with visual and sensory impairments.
- Other findings may include nystagmus, muscle weakness, paralysis, spasticity, hyperreflexia, ataxic gait, dysphagia, dysarthria, constipation, urinary frequency and urgency, incontinence, impotence, and emotional lability.

Parkinson's disease

- Tremors, a classic early sign, usually begin in the fingers and may eventually affect the foot, eyelids, jaw, lips, and tongue.
- Other characteristic findings include cogwheel rigidity, bradykinesia, propulsive gait with forward-leaning posture, monotone voice, masklike facies, drooling, dysphagia, dysarthria, and occasionally oculogyric crisis or blepharospasm.

Porphyria

- Resting tremor and rigidity with chorea and athetosis
- As the disease progresses, generalized seizures with aphasia and hemiplegia

Thalamic syndrome

○ Contralateral ataxic tremors and other abnormal movements occur along with Weber's syndrome, paralysis of vertical gaze, and stupor or coma occur with central midbrain syndromes.

○ Tremor, deep sensory loss, hemiataxia, and extrapyramidal dysfunction may occur with anteromedial-inferior syndrome.

Thyrotoxicosis

○ A rapid, fine intention tremor of the hands and tongue with clonus, and hyperreflexia

○ Tachycardia, cardiac arrhythmias, palpitations, anxiety, dyspnea, diaphoresis, heat intolerance, weight loss despite increased appetite, diarrhea, an enlarged thyroid and, possibly, exophthalmos

Wernicke's disease

○ An intention tremor is an early sign.

○ Other findings include ocular abnormalities, ataxia, apathy, confusion, orthostatic hypotension, and tachycardia.

West Nile encephalitis

○ In severe infections, headache, high fever, neck stiffness, stupor, disorientation, coma, tremors, occasional seizures, and paralysis

Other causes

Drugs

○ Phenothiazines and other antipsychotics may cause resting and pill-rolling tremors.

○ Infrequently, metoclopramide and metyrosine cause these tremors.

○ Amphetamines, lithium toxicity, phenytoin, and sympathomimetics can cause tremors that disappear with dose reduction.

Manganese toxicity

○ Early signs of manganese toxicity include resting tremor, chorea, propulsive gait, cogwheel rigidity, personality changes, amnesia, and masklike facies.

Mercury poisoning

○ Mercury poisoning is characterized by irritability, copious amounts of saliva, loose teeth, gum disease, slurred speech, and tremors.

Nursing considerations

○ Assist the patient with activities as needed.

○ Take precautions against possible injury during activities.

○ Encourage the patient to talk about changes in body image.

Pediatric pointers

○ Causes of pathologic tremors in children include cerebral palsy, fetal alcohol syndrome, and maternal drug addiction.

○ A normal neonate may display coarse tremors with stiffening — an exaggerated hypocalcemic startle reflex — in response to noises and chills.

Patient teaching

○ Reinforce the patient's independence.

○ Instruct the patient in the use of assistive devices as needed.

Tunnel vision

Overview

○ Also known as *tubular vision* (see *Comparing tunnel vision with normal vision*)
○ Reflects severe constriction of the visual field
○ Leaves only a small central area of sight
○ May be in one or both eyes

Assessment

History

○ Ask about the onset, progression, and description of loss of peripheral vision.
○ Explore personal and family history of ocular problems, especially progressive blindness that began at an early age.

Physical assessment

○ Test close visual acuity.
○ If your assessment findings suggest tunnel vision, refer the patient to an ophthalmologist for further evaluation, including visual field testing.

Assessment tip
Comparing tunnel vision with normal vision

The patient with tunnel vision experiences drastic constricting of his peripheral visual field. The illustrations here show how severe this constriction can be, comparing test findings for normal and tunnel vision.

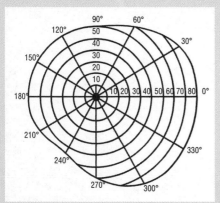

Normal field of vision in the right eye, as seen during visual field testing.

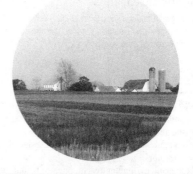

Normal field of vision in the right eye, as seen during visual field testing.

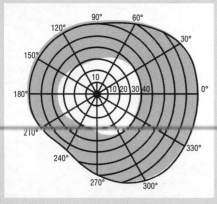

Tunnel vision in the right eye, as shown on a visual field chart.

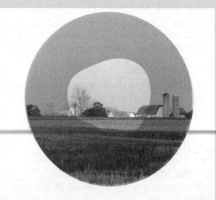

Tunnel vision in the right eye, as seen in advanced glaucoma during visual field testing.

Medical causes

Chronic open-angle glaucoma

○ Tunnel vision in both eyes occurs late and slowly progresses to complete blindness.
○ Other late findings include mild eye pain, halo vision, and reduced visual acuity, especially at night, that isn't correctable with glasses.

Retinal pigmentary degeneration

○ An annular scotoma progresses concentrically, causing tunnel vision and eventually resulting in complete blindness, usually by age 50.
○ Impaired night vision, the earliest symptom, typically appears during the first or second decade of life.
○ An ophthalmoscopic examination may reveal narrowed retinal blood vessels and a pale optic disk.

Nursing considerations

○ Remove all potentially dangerous objects and orient the patient to his surroundings.
○ Clearly explain diagnostic procedures.
○ Reassure the patient.

Pediatric pointers

○ In children with retinitis pigmentosa, night blindness foreshadows tunnel vision, which usually doesn't develop until later in the disease process.

Patient teaching

○ Teach the patient how to compensate for tunnel vision and avoid bumping into objects.

Urethral discharge

Overview

- Purulent, mucoid or thin, sanguineous discharge from the urinary meatus

Assessment

History

- Ask about the onset and description of discharge.
- Inquire about other pain or burning on urination, difficulty starting a urine stream, urinary frequency, fever, chills, and perineal fullness.
- Obtain a medical history, including prostate problems, sexually transmitted disease, or urinary tract infection.
- Find out about recent sexual contacts or a new sex partner.

Physical assessment

- Inspect the urethral meatus for inflammation and swelling.

Collecting a urethral discharge specimen

To obtain a urethral specimen from a man, follow these steps:

> Instruct the patient not to void for 1 hour before specimen collection to prevent flushing secretions from the urethra.

↓

> Provide privacy for the patient. Help him onto an examination table and into a supine position, and expose his penis. Have him grasp and raise his penis to allow you to see the urethra.

↓

> Wash your hands and put on sterile gloves. Then insert a thin, sterile urogenital alginate swab no more than ¾″ (2 cm) into the urethra. Rotate the swab, and leave it in place for 10 to 30 seconds to absorb organisms.

↓

> Remove the swab, allow it to dry, and then send it to the laboratory. Help the patient off the examination table, and tell him to dress.

- Obtain a culture specimen. (See *Collecting a urethral discharge specimen*.)
- Obtain a urine specimen for urinalysis and culture and a three-glass urine test. (See *Performing a three-glass urine test*.)

Medical causes

Prostatitis

- In the acute form, purulent urethral discharge, sudden fever, chills, lower back pain, myalgia, perineal fullness, arthralgia, frequent and urgent urination, dysuria, nocturia, and a tense, boggy, tender, and warm prostate
- In the chronic form, a persistent urethral discharge that's thin, milky, or clear at the meatus after not voiding for a long time, dull aching in the prostate or rectum, sexual dysfunction such as ejaculatory pain, and urinary disturbances, such as frequency, urgency, and dysuria

Reiter's syndrome

- Urethral discharge and other signs of acute urethritis 1 or 2 weeks after sexual contact
- Asymmetrical arthritis, conjunctivitis, and ulcerations on the oral mucosa, glans penis, palms, and soles

Urethritis

- Scant or profuse urethral discharge that's thin and clear, mucoid, or thick and purulent
- Urinary hesitancy, urgency, and frequency and itching and burning around the meatus.

Nursing considerations

- To relieve symptoms, suggest that the patient take hot sitz baths several times daily, increase his fluid intake, void frequently, and avoid caffeine, tea, and alcohol.
- Monitor for urine retention.

Pediatric pointers

- Evaluate a child with urethral discharge for evidence of sexual and physical abuse.

Geriatric pointers

- Urethral discharge in elderly patients isn't usually related to a sexually transmitted disease.

Patient teaching

- Advise the patient of the importance of avoiding sexual activity until acute symptoms subside.
- Explain that chronic symptoms can be relieved by engaging in regular sexual activity.

Performing the three-glass urine test

If a man complains of urinary frequency and urgency, dysuria, flank or lower back pain, or other signs or symptoms of urethritis, and if his urine specimen is cloudy, perform the three-glass urine test.

First, ask him to void into three conical glasses labeled with numbers 1, 2, and 3. First-voided urine goes into glass #1, midstream urine into glass #2, and the remainder into glass #3. Tell the patient to avoid interrupting the stream of urine when shifting glasses, if possible.

Next, observe each glass for pus and mucous shreds. Also note urine color and odor. Glass #1 will contain matter from the anterior urethra, glass #2 matter from the bladder, and glass #3 sediment from the prostate and seminal vesicles.

Some common findings are shown here. However, confirming diagnosis requires microscopic examination and a bacteriology report.

	Specimen 1	*Specimen 2*	*Specimen 3*
Acute or subacute urethritis	Cloudy	Clear	Clear
Acute posterior urethritis	Cloudy	Clear or cloudy	Cloudy
Chronic anterior urethritis	Small shreds	Clear	Clear
Chronic posterior urethritis	Large shreds	Clear	Clear
Chronic urethritis (anterior and posterior)	Small and large shreds	Clear	Clear
Prostatitis	Clear or large shreds	Clear	Cloudy or large shreds
Cystitis and pyelonephritis	Cloudy	Cloudy	Cloudy

Urinary frequency

Overview

○ Refers to increased incidence of the urge to void without an increase in the total volume of urine produced
○ A classic sign of urinary tract infection (UTI)

Assessment

History

○ Ask about current and previous voiding patterns.
○ Determine the onset and duration of urinary frequency.
○ Find out about dysuria, urgency, incontinence, hematuria, discharge, or lower abdominal pain with urination.
○ Obtain a medical history, especially of UTI, other urologic problems or recent urologic procedures, and neurologic disorders.
○ Inquire about a history of prostatic enlargement in men.
○ Inquire about the possibility of pregnancy in women.

Physical assessment

○ Obtain a clean-catch midstream specimen.
○ Palpate the suprapubic area, abdomen, and flanks, noting any tenderness.
○ Examine the urethral meatus for redness, discharge, or swelling.
○ Palpate the prostate gland.
○ Perform a neurologic assessment if the history reveals symptoms or a history of neurologic diseases.

Medical causes

Benign prostatic hyperplasia

○ Urinary frequency with nocturia and, possibly, incontinence and hematuria
○ Initially, reduced caliber and force of the urine stream, urinary hesitancy, tenesmus, inability to stop the stream of urine, a feeling of incomplete voiding, and occasionally urine retention

Bladder calculus

○ Urinary frequency and urgency, dysuria, hematuria at the end of micturition, and suprapubic pain from bladder spasms
○ If the calculus lodges in the bladder neck, overflow incontinence with greatest discomfort at the end of micturition

Bladder cancer

○ Urinary frequency, urgency, dribbling, and nocturia may develop.

○ The first sign commonly is gross, painless, intermittent hematuria (with clots).
○ Suprapubic or pelvic pain commonly occurs with invasive lesions.

Multiple sclerosis

○ Urinary frequency, urgency, and incontinence are common.
○ Vision problems (such as diplopia and blurred vision) and sensory impairment (such as paresthesia) are the earliest symptoms.
○ Other findings include constipation, muscle weakness, paralysis, spasticity, hyperreflexia, intention tremor, ataxic gait, dysarthria, impotence, and emotional lability.

Prostate cancer

○ In advanced stages, urinary frequency along with hesitancy, dribbling, nocturia, dysuria, bladder distention, perineal pain, constipation, and a hard, irregularly shaped prostate

Prostatitis

○ In the acute form, urinary frequency, urgency, dysuria, nocturia, and purulent urethral discharge are produced.
○ Other acute findings include fever, chills, lower back pain, myalgia, arthralgia, perineal fullness and, possibly, a tense, boggy, tender, and warm prostate.
○ In the chronic form, pain on ejaculation may occur as well as the same findings as in the acute form, but to a lesser degree.

Rectal tumor

○ Pressure from the tumor on the bladder may cause urinary frequency.
○ Early findings include changed bowel habits, commonly starting with an urgent need to defecate on arising or obstipation alternating with diarrhea; blood or mucus in the stool; and a sense of incomplete evacuation.

Reiter's syndrome

○ Urinary frequency 1 or 2 weeks after sexual contact
○ Asymmetrical arthritis of knees, ankles, and metatarsophalangeal joints; conjunctivitis; and small, painless ulcers on the mouth, tongue, glans penis, palms, and soles

Reproductive tract tumor

○ A tumor may compress the bladder, causing urinary frequency.
○ Other findings may include abdominal distention, menstrual disturbances, vaginal bleeding, weight loss, pelvic pain, and fatigue.

Spinal cord lesion

○ Urinary frequency, continuous overflow, dribbling, urgency, urinary hesitancy, and bladder distention from incomplete spinal cord transection

- Other findings below the level of the lesion, such as weakness, paralysis, sensory disturbances, hyperreflexia, and impotence

Urethral stricture

- Bladder decompensation produces urinary frequency, along with urgency and nocturia.
- Early signs include hesitancy, tenesmus, and reduced caliber and force of the urine stream.
- Overflow incontinence, urinoma, and urosepsis may also develop.

Urinary tract infection

- Urinary frequency, urgency, dysuria, hematuria, cloudy urine, and discharge
- Fever, bladder spasms, and a feeling of warmth during urination

Uterine prolapse

- Urinary frequency, hesitancy, infection, leakage, and retention
- Abdominal, vaginal, or lower back pain; painful intercourse
- Often gradual as pelvic muscles and ligaments weaken from age, childbirth, or abdominal surgery

Other causes

Diuretics

- Diuretics, including caffeine, reduce the body's total volume of water and salt by increasing urine excretion.

Treatments

- Radiation therapy may cause bladder inflammation, leading to urinary frequency.

Nursing considerations

- If mobility is impaired, keep a bedpan or commode by the bed.
- Document the patient's daily intake and output amounts.

Pediatric pointers

- UTI is a common cause of urinary frequency in children.

Geriatric pointers

- Men older than age 50 are prone to nonsexual UTIs.
- In postmenopausal women, decreased estrogen levels cause urinary frequency.

Patient teaching

- Emphasize safer sex practices.
- Instruct the patient in the proper way to clean genital area.

- Explain increasing fluid intake and frequency of voiding.
- Teach patient how to do Kegel exercises.

Urinary incontinence

Overview

- Refers to the uncontrollable passage of urine
- May be transient or permanent
- May involve large volumes of urine or scant dribbling
- Classified as stress, overflow, urge, or total

Assessment

History

- Ask about the onset and description of incontinence.
- Obtain a description of normal urinary pattern and fluid intake.
- Inquire about other urinary problems, such as hesitancy, frequency, urgency, nocturia, and decreased force or interruption of the urine stream.
- Ask about a history of urinary tract infection (UTI), prostate conditions, spinal injury or tumor, stroke, or surgery involving the bladder, prostate, or pelvic floor.
- Ask a woman about the number of pregnancies and childbirths she has had.

Physical assessment

- Have the patient empty his bladder.
- Inspect the urethral meatus for inflammation or defect.
- Have women bear down; note any urine leakage.
- Gently palpate the abdomen for bladder distention.
- Perform a complete neurologic assessment, noting motor and sensory function and obvious muscle atrophy.
- Assess post-void residual urine volume with a straight catheter.

Medical causes

Benign prostatic hyperplasia

- Overflow incontinence results from urethral obstruction and urine retention.
- Reduced caliber and force of the urine stream, urinary hesitancy, and a feeling of incomplete voiding constitute prostatism and are early findings.
- Urination becomes more frequent, with nocturia and, possibly, hematuria as the obstruction increases.
- Bladder distention and an enlarged prostate are revealed by examination.

Bladder calculus

- Overflow incontinence may occur if the calculus lodges in the bladder neck.

- Other findings may include those of an irritable bladder, such as urinary frequency and urgency, dysuria, hematuria, and suprapubic pain from bladder spasms.
- Pelvic pain and pain referred to the tip of the penis, vulva, lower back, or heel pain may occur.

Bladder cancer

- Urge incontinence and hematuria are early signs.
- Obstruction by a tumor may produce overflow incontinence.
- Other findings include frequency, dysuria, nocturia, dribbling, and suprapubic pain from bladder spasms after voiding.
- A mass may be palpable on bimanual examination.

Diabetic neuropathy

- Bladder distention with overflow incontinence may occur.
- Related findings include episodic constipation or diarrhea (which is commonly nocturnal), impotence and retrograde ejaculation, orthostatic hypotension, syncope, and dysphagia.

Guillain-Barré syndrome

- Urinary incontinence may occur early.
- Profound muscle weakness, which typically starts in the legs and extends to the arms and facial nerves within 24 to 72 hours, is the most prominent sign.
- Other findings include paresthesia, dysarthria, nasal speech, dysphagia, orthostatic hypotension, fecal incontinence, diaphoresis, drooling, tachycardia, and pain in the shoulders, thighs, or lumbar region.

Multiple sclerosis

- Urinary incontinence, urgency, and frequency are common urologic findings.
- Early findings include vision problems and sensory impairment.
- Other findings include constipation, muscle weakness, paralysis, spasticity, hyperreflexia, intention tremor, ataxic gait, dysarthria, impotence, and emotional lability.

Prostate cancer

- Urinary incontinence usually appears only in advanced stages.
- Other late findings include urinary frequency and hesitancy, nocturia, dysuria, bladder distention, perineal pain, constipation, and a hard, irregularly shaped, nodular prostate.

Prostatitis (chronic)

- Urinary incontinence may occur as well as urinary frequency and urgency, dysuria, hematuria, bladder distention, persistent urethral discharge, dull perineal pain that may radiate, ejaculatory pain, and decreased libido.

Spinal cord injury

○ Overflow incontinence follows rapid bladder distention.
○ Other findings include paraplegia, sexual dysfunction, sensory loss, muscle atrophy, anhidrosis, and
loss of reflexes far from the injury.

Stroke

○ Transient or permanent urinary incontinence
○ Impaired mentation, emotional lability, behavioral
changes, altered level of consciousness, and seizures
○ Headache, vomiting, vision deficits, and decreased
visual acuity
○ Sensorimotor findings, such as contralateral hemiplegia, dysarthria, dysphagia, ataxia, apraxia, agnosia, aphasia, and unilateral sensory loss

Urethral stricture

○ Eventually, overflow incontinence
○ Urinomas and urosepsis as obstruction increases

Urinary tract infection

○ Incontinence, urinary urgency, dysuria, hematuria,
and cloudy urine
○ Possible bladder spasms or a feeling of warmth during urination

Other causes

Surgery

○ Urinary incontinence after prostatectomy as a result
of urethral sphincter damage

Nursing considerations

○ Obtain a urine specimen.
○ Start bladder retraining.
○ If incontinence is neurologic, monitor the patient for
urine retention.

Pediatric pointers

○ Causes of incontinence in children include infrequent or incomplete voiding and an ectopic ureteral
orifice.

Geriatric pointers

○ Elderly patients with UTIs may present only with urinary incontinence or changes in mental status,
anorexia, or malaise.

Patient teaching

○ Instruct the patient in performing Kegel exercises.
○ Teach the patient self-catheterization techniques.
(See *Teaching self-catheterization.*)
○ Review with the patient which drugs he is taking.

Teaching self-catheterization

Teach a woman to hold the catheter in her dominant
hand as if it were a pencil or a dart, about ½" (1.3 cm)
from its tip. Keeping the vaginal folds separated, she
should slowly insert the lubricated catheter about 3"
(7.6 cm) into the urethra. Tell her to press down with
her abdominal muscles to empty the bladder, allowing
all urine to drain through the catheter and into the toilet or drainage container.

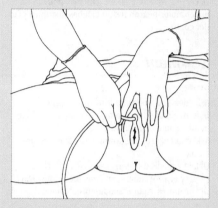

Teach a man to hold his penis in his nondominant
hand, at a right angle to his body. He should hold the
catheter in his dominant hand as if it were a pencil or a
dart and slowly insert it 7" to 10" (17.5 to 25 cm) into
the urethra until urine begins flowing. Then he should
gently advance the catheter about 1" (2.5 cm) farther,
allowing all urine to drain into the toilet or drainage
container.

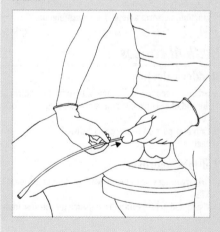

Urinary urgency

Overview

- Refers to a sudden, compelling urge to urinate
- Occurring with bladder pain is a classic symptom of urinary tract infection (UTI)
- Occurring without bladder pain may point to an upper-motor-neuron lesion that has disrupted bladder control

Assessment

History

- Ask about the onset and history of urgency.
- Inquire about other urologic symptoms, such as dysuria and cloudy urine.
- Ask about neurologic symptoms, such as paresthesia.
- Obtain a medical history, especially of UTIs and surgery or procedures involving the urinary tract.
- Obtain a prescription and nonprescription drug history.

Physical assessment

- Obtain a clean-catch specimen for urinalysis and culture.
- Note urine character, color, and odor; use a reagent strip to test for pH, glucose, and blood.
- Palpate the suprapubic area and both flanks for distention and tenderness.
- If the history or symptoms suggest neurologic dysfunction, perform a neurologic examination.

Medical causes

Bladder calculus

- Urinary urgency and frequency, dysuria, hematuria at the end of micturition, and suprapubic pain may occur.
- Pain may pass on to the penis, vulva, lower back, or heel.

Multiple sclerosis

- Urinary urgency can occur with or without frequent UTIs.
- Vision and sensory impairments are the earliest findings.
- Other findings include urinary frequency, incontinence, constipation, muscle weakness, paralysis, spasticity, intention tremor, hyperreflexia, ataxic gait, dysphagia, dysarthria, impotence, and emotional lability.

Reiter's syndrome

- Urgency occurs with other symptoms of acute urethritis 1 or 2 weeks after sexual contact primarily in men.
- Asymmetrical arthritis of knees, ankles, or metatarsal phalangeal joints; conjunctivitis; and ulcers on the penis, or skin, or in the mouth usually develop within several weeks after sexual contact.

Spinal cord lesion

- Urinary urgency can occur along with urinary frequency and difficulty initiating and inhibiting a urine stream; bladder distention and discomfort may also occur.
- Neuromuscular findings far from the lesion include weakness, paralysis, hyperreflexia, sensory disturbances, and impotence.

Urethral stricture

- Bladder decompensation produces urinary urgency, frequency, and nocturia.

Urinary tract infection

- Urinary urgency, frequency, and hesitancy; hematuria; dysuria; nocturia; and cloudy urine
- Bladder spasms; costovertebral angle tenderness; suprapubic, lower back, or flank pain; urethral discharge in males; fever; chills; malaise; nausea; and vomiting

Other causes

Treatments

- Radiation therapy may irritate and inflame the bladder, causing urinary urgency.

Nursing considerations

- Increase the patient's fluid intake.
- Give an antibiotic and a urinary anesthetic.

Pediatric pointers

- In young children, urinary urgency may appear as a change in toilet habits.
- Urgency may also result from urethral irritation by bubble bath salts.

Teaching Kegel exercises

These isometric exercises will strengthen the pubococ-cygeus (PC) muscle to increase voluntary control over urination. Teach your patient these techniques.

- Begin by sitting on the toilet with your legs spread. Then, without moving your legs, start and stop the flow of urine. The PC muscle is the one that contracts to help control urine flow.
- Now that you've identified the PC muscle, you can exercise it regularly. Kegel exercises can be performed almost anywhere — sitting at your desk, lying in bed, standing in line, and especially while urinating. Remember to breathe naturally — don't hold your breath.
- Contract the PC muscle as you did to stop the urine flow. Count slowly to three, then relax the muscle.

- Next, contract and relax the PC muscle as quickly as possible, without using your stomach or buttock muscles.
- Finally, slowly contract the entire vaginal area. Then bear down, using your abdominal muscles and your PC muscle.
- For the first week, repeat each exercise 10 times (1 set) for 5 sets daily. Then each week, add 5 repetitions of each exercise (15, 20, and so forth). Keep doing 5 sets daily.

    After about 2 weeks of practice, you'll notice improvement.

Patient teaching

○ Instruct the patient in safer sex practices.
○ Explain proper genital hygiene to women and girls.
○ Explain adequate fluid intake and frequent daily voiding.
○ Instuct the patient with a noninfective cause of urgency how to do Kegel exercises. (See *Teaching Kegel exercises.*)

Urticaria

Overview

- A vascular skin reaction
- Also known as *hives*
- Characterized by the eruption of transient pruritic wheals—smooth, slightly elevated patches with well-defined erythematous margins and pale centers of various shapes and sizes

Urticaria or angioedema?

The illustration below shows typical urticarial lesions: red, raised plaques that are surrounded by a white halo and can appear on any skin surface.

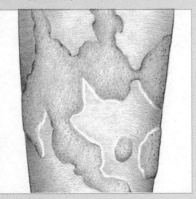

Angioedema is an urticarial swelling that occurs in the subcutaneous tissue. The skin over the angioedema may appear to be normal or may be reddened. Although it occurs frequently on the face and mucous membranes, angioedema can occur on other areas of the body, as shown below.

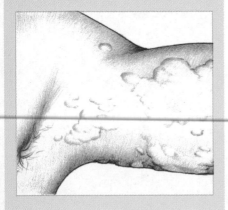

- Produced in response to the local release of histamine or other vasoactive substances as part of a hypersensitivity reaction
- Acute urticaria evolves rapidly and usually has a detectable cause.
- *Angioedema*, or giant urticaria, is characterized by the acute eruption of wheals involving the mucous membranes and, occasionally, the arms, legs, or genitals. (See *Urticaria or angioedema?*)

⭐ Emergency actions

In acute urticaria, quickly evaluate respiratory status and take vital signs. Ensure patent I.V. access if respiratory difficulty or signs of impending anaphylactic shock are present. As needed, give local epinephrine or apply ice to the affected site to decrease absorption through vasoconstriction. Maintain a patent airway, give oxygen as needed, and institute cardiac monitoring. Have resuscitation equipment at hand, and begin cardiopulmonary resuscitation if needed. Intubation or a tracheostomy may be required.

Assessment

History

- Ask about any known allergies.
- Inquire about a pattern of urticaria and what aggravates it.
- Find out about exposure to chemicals on the job or at home.
- Obtain a detailed drug history.
- Note any history of chronic or parasitic infection, skin disease, or a GI disorder.

Physical assessment

- Obtain vital signs.
- Perform a complete cardiopulmonary assessment, noting signs and symptoms of shock or respiratory distress.
- Assess for urticaria in other areas because new crops may continue to appear.

Medical causes

Anaphylaxis

- Rapid eruption of diffuse urticaria and angioedema develops; wheals range from pinpoint to palm-size or larger in this potentially life-threatening disorder.
- Lesions are usually pruritic and stinging; paresthesia commonly precedes their eruption.
- Other acute findings include profound anxiety; weakness; diaphoresis; sneezing; shortness of breath; profuse rhinorrhea; nasal congestion; dysphagia; and warm, moist skin.

Hereditary angioedema

○ Patches of nonpitting, nonpruritic edema develop on the arms, legs, or face.
○ Respiratory mucosal involvement can produce life-threatening acute laryngeal edema.

Lyme disease

○ Urticaria may result from erythema chronicum migrans.
○ Later findings include constant malaise and fatigue, intermittent headache, fever, chills, lymphadenopathy, neurologic and cardiac abnormalities, and arthritis.

Other causes

Drugs

○ Various drugs (most commonly aspirin, atropine, codeine, dextrans, immune serums, insulin, morphine, penicillin, quinine, sulfonamides, and vaccines) can produce urticaria.
○ Radiographic contrast medium commonly produces urticaria, especially when given I.V.

Nursing considerations

○ Apply a bland skin emollient or one containing menthol and phenol to help relieve discomfort.
○ Give an antihistamine, a systemic corticosteroid, or a tranquilizer.
○ Tepid baths and cool compresses may decrease pruritus.

Pediatric pointers

○ Acute papular urticaria (especially after insect bites) and urticaria pigmentosa (rare)

Patient teaching

○ Emphasize the importance of wearing medical identification for allergies.
○ Explain the risks of delayed symptoms.
○ Explain the signs and symptoms to report.
○ Stress ways to prevent anaphylaxis.
○ Teach the patient the proper use of an anaphylaxis kit.

Vaginal bleeding, postmenopausal

Overview

○ Refers to bleeding that occurs 6 or more months after menopause
○ Presents as slight, brown or red spotting, as oozing of fresh blood, or as bright red hemorrhage
○ An important indicator of gynecologic cancer; may also result from other causes such as infection, local pelvic disorder, atrophy of endometrium, and physiologic thinning and drying of vaginal mucosa

Assessment

History

○ Determine the patient's current age and age at menopause.
○ Ask about the onset of bleeding.
○ Obtain a thorough obstetric, gynecologic, and sexual history.
○ Find out all drugs used presently or within the time symptoms began, including douches and estrogen products.
○ Obtain a history of sexually transmitted disease, as needed.

Physical assessment

○ Observe the external genitalia, noting the character of any vaginal discharge and the appearance of the labia, vaginal rugae, and clitoris.
○ Palpate the breasts and lymph nodes for nodules or enlargement.
○ The patient will need pelvic and rectal examinations.

Medical causes

Atrophic vaginitis

○ Bloody staining may normally follow coitus or douching, but must be evaluated to rule out cancer.
○ Characteristic white, watery discharge may be accompanied by pruritus, dyspareunia, and a burning sensation in the vagina and labia.
○ Sparse pubic hair, a pale vagina with decreased rugae and small hemorrhagic spots, clitoral atrophy, and shrinking of the labia minora may also occur.

Cervical cancer

○ Spotting or heavier bleeding occurs early in invasive cervical cancer; bleeding may also normally follow coitus or douching.

○ Related findings include persistent, pink-tinged, and foul-smelling discharge, and postcoital pain occurs.
○ As the cancer spreads, back and sciatic pain, leg swelling, anorexia, weight loss, hematuria, dysuria, rectal bleeding, and weakness may occur.

Cervical or endometrial polyps

○ Spotting (possibly mucopurulent and pink) may occur after coitus, douching, or straining at stool.

Endometrial hyperplasia or cancer

○ Bleeding occurs early and is brownish and scant or red and profuse and usually follows coitus or douching.
○ Later, bleeding becomes heavier and more frequent, leading to clotting and anemia.
○ Pelvic, rectal, lower back, and leg pain may accompany bleeding.
○ Uterus may be enlarged.

Ovarian tumor (feminizing)

○ Endometrial shedding may occur and cause heavy bleeding.
○ A palpable pelvic mass, increased cervical mucus, breast enlargement, and spider angiomas may be present.

Vaginal cancer

○ Characteristic spotting or bleeding may be preceded by thin, watery discharge.
○ Bleeding may be spontaneous but usually follows coitus or douching.
○ A firm, ulcerated vaginal lesion may be present.
○ Dyspareunia, urinary frequency, bladder and pelvic pain, rectal bleeding, and vulvar lesions may develop later.

Vulval cancer

○ Bleeding, itching, groin pain, unusual lumps or sores, and abnormal urination and defecation

Other causes

Drugs

○ Unopposed estrogen replacement therapy may cause abnormal vaginal bleeding, but cancer must always be ruled out.
○ Antibiotics may change the normal vaginal pH and flora.

Nursing considerations

○ Until a diagnosis is made, stop estrogen.
○ Prepare the patient for diagnostic tests.

Geriatric pointers

○ Endometrial atrophy may cause postmenopausal bleeding, but malignancy should be ruled out.

Patient teaching

○ Reassure the patient that postmenopausal vaginal bleeding may be benign, but careful assessment is still needed.

Vaginal discharge

Overview

- Normal discharge is mucoid, clear or white, non-bloody, and odorless.
- A marked increase or change in discharge color, odor, or consistency can signal disease.

Assessment

History

- Ask about the onset and description of the discharge.
- Find out about other symptoms, such as dysuria and perineal pruritus and burning.
- Determine recent changes in sexual habits or hygiene practices.
- Ask about previous discharge or infection and treatment used.
- Take a drug history, including use of antibiotics, oral estrogens, and contraceptives.
- Ask about the possibility of pregnancy.

Physical assessment

- Examine the external genitalia and note the character of the discharge. (See *Identifying causes of vaginal discharge.*)
- Observe vulvar and vaginal tissues for redness, edema, and excoriation.
- Palpate the inguinal nodes for tenderness or enlargement.
- Palpate the abdomen for tenderness.
- A pelvic examination may be needed.
- Obtain vaginal discharge specimens for testing.

Medical causes

Atrophic vaginitis

- A thin, scant, watery white vaginal discharge may be accompanied by pruritus, burning, and tenderness.
- Sparse pubic hair, a pale vagina with decreased rugae and small hemorrhagic spots, clitoral atrophy, and shrinking of the labia minora may also occur.

Bacterial vaginosis

- Thin, foul-smelling, green or gray-white discharge adheres to the vaginal walls and can be easily wiped away.
- Pruritus, redness, and other signs of vaginal irritation may occur.

Candidiasis

- A profuse, white, curdlike discharge with a yeasty, sweet odor is produced.
- Onset of discharge is abrupt, usually just before menses or during a course of antibiotics.

- Exudate may be lightly attached to the labia and vaginal walls and is commonly accompanied by vulvar redness and edema.
- The inner thighs may be covered with a fine, red dermatitis and weeping erosions.
- Intense labial itching and burning and external dysuria may also occur.

Chlamydial infection

- A yellow, mucopurulent, odorless, or acrid vaginal discharge is produced.
- Other findings include dysuria, dyspareunia, and vaginal bleeding after douching or coitus, especially following menses.

Endometritis

- A scant, serosanguineous discharge with a foul odor can result.
- Other findings include fever, lower back and abdominal pain, abdominal muscle spasm, malaise, dysmenorrhea, and an enlarged uterus.

Genital warts

- A profuse, mucopurulent vaginal discharge, which may be foul-smelling if the warts are infected, may be produced.
- Mosaic, papular vulvar lesions occur, frequently with burning or paresthesia around the vaginal opening.

Gonorrhea

- Occasionally, yellow or green, foul-smelling discharge can be expressed from Bartholin's or Skene's ducts, but 80% of women have no symptoms.
- Other findings include dysuria, urinary frequency and incontinence, bleeding, vaginal redness and swelling, fever, and severe pelvic and abdominal pain.

Gynecologic cancer

- Chronic, watery, bloody or purulent vaginal discharge may be foul-smelling.
- Other findings include abnormal vaginal bleeding and, later, weight loss; pelvic, back, and leg pain; fatigue; urinary frequency; and abdominal distention.

Herpes simplex (genital)

- Copious mucoid discharge results, but the initial complaint is painful, indurated vesicles and ulcerations on the labia, vagina, cervix, anus, thighs, or mouth.
- Erythema, marked edema, and tender inguinal lymph nodes may occur with fever, malaise, and dysuria.

Trichomoniasis

- A foul-smelling discharge, which may be frothy, green-yellow, and profuse or thin, white, and scant, may be produced, although about 70% of patients are asymptomatic.

The color, consistency, amount, and odor of your patient's vaginal discharge provide important clues about the underlying disorder. For quick reference, use this chart to match common characteristics of vaginal discharge and their possible causes.

Characteristics	Possible causes
Thin, scant, watery white discharge	Atrophic vaginitis
Thin, green or gray-white, foul-smelling discharge	Bacterial vaginosis
White, curdlike, profuse discharge with yeasty, sweet odor	Candidiasis
Mucopurulent, foul-smelling discharge	Chancroid
Yellow, mucopurulent, odorless, or acrid discharge	Chlamydial infection
Scant, serosanguineous, or purulent discharge with foul odor	Endometritis
Copious mucoid discharge	Genital herpes
Profuse, mucopurulent discharge, possibly foul-smelling	Genital warts
Yellow or green, foul-smelling discharge from the cervix or occasionally from Bartholin's or Skene's ducts	Gonorrhea
Chronic, watery, bloody, or purulent discharge, possibly foul-smelling	Gynecologic cancer
Frothy, green-yellow, and profuse (or thin, white, and scant) foul-smelling discharge	Trichomoniasis

○ Other findings include pruritus; a red, inflamed vagina with tiny petechiae; dysuria and urinary frequency; and dyspareunia, postcoital spotting, menorrhagia, or dysmenorrhea.

Other causes

Contraceptive creams and jellies

○ Contraceptive creams and jellies can increase vaginal secretions.

Drugs

○ Drugs that contain estrogen can cause increased mucoid vaginal discharge.
○ Antibiotics may increase the risk of candidal vagina infection and discharge.

Radiation therapy

○ Irradiation of reproductive tract can cause a watery, odorless, vaginal discharge.

Nursing considerations

○ Obtain cultures of the discharge.
○ Give antibiotics, antivirals, or other drugs, if needed.

○ Observe standard precautions to prevent the spread of infection.

Pediatric pointers

○ Newborn girls who have been exposed to their mother's estrogens in utero may have a white, mucous, vaginal discharge for the first month after birth; a yellow mucous discharge indicates disease.
○ In an older child, purulent, foul-smelling, and possibly bloody vaginal discharge commonly results from a foreign object placed in the vagina. Consider the possibility of sexual abuse.

Geriatric pointers

○ Incidence of vaginitis increases in elderly patients.

Patient teaching

○ Explain the importance of keeping the perineum clean and dry and avoiding tight-fitting clothing.
○ Suggest douching with vinegar and water to relieve discomfort.
○ Stress compliance with prescribed drugs.
○ Instruct the patient to avoid intercourse until symptoms of infection clear.
○ Provide information on safer sex practices.

Venous hum

Overview

- A functional or innocent murmur heard above the clavicles throughout the cardiac cycle (see *Detecting a venous hum*)
- Loudest during diastole
- May be low-pitched, rough, or noisy
- Commonly accompanies a thrill or, possibly, a high-pitched whine
- Results from increased blood flow through the internal jugular veins
- Occurs in hyperdynamic states such as thyrotoxicosis
- A common normal finding in children and pregnant women
- May be mistaken for a heart murmur or thyroid bruit
- Disappears with jugular vein compression and waxes and wanes with head turning; murmurs and thyroid bruit persists despite jugular vein compression and head turning.

Assessment

History

- Ask about a history of anemia or thyroid disorders.
- Note associated palpitations, dyspnea, nervousness, tremors, heat intolerance, weight loss, fatigue, or malaise.
- Take a drug history.

Physical assessment

- Take vital signs, noting especially tachycardia, hypertension, a bounding pulse, and widened pulse pressure.
- Auscultate the heart for gallops or murmurs.
- Examine the skin and mucous membranes for pallor.

Medical causes

Anemia

- In severe cases, a venous hum occurs with pale skin and mucous membranes, dyspnea, crackles, tachycardia, bounding pulse, atrial gallop, systolic bruits over the carotid arteries, bleeding tendencies, weakness, fatigue, and malaise.

Thyrotoxicosis

- A loud venous hum may be audible whether the patient is sitting or in a supine position.
- An atrial or ventricular gallop may be present.
- Additional findings include tachycardia, palpitations, weight loss despite increased appetite, diarrhea, an enlarged thyroid, dyspnea, nervousness, difficulty

---

Assessment tip
Detecting a venous hum

To detect a venous hum, have your patient sit upright; place the bell of the stethoscope over his right supraclavicular area. Gently lift his chin and turn his head toward the left, which increases the loudness of the hum.

If you still can't hear the hum, press his jugular vein with your thumb. The hum will disappear with pressure but will suddenly return, temporarily louder than before, when you release your thumb—a result of the turbulence created by pressure changes.

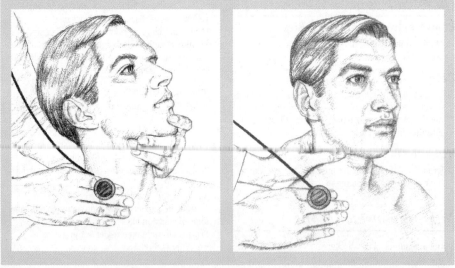

concentrating, tremors, diaphoresis, heat intolerance, decreased libido and, possibly, exophthalmos.
○ Women may have oligomenorrhea or amenorrhea; men may have gynecomastia.

Nursing considerations

○ Prepare the patient for diagnostic tests, such as a complete blood count or thyroid study.

Pediatric pointers
○ A cervical venous hum occurs normally in more than two-thirds of children ages 5 to 15.

Patient teaching
○ Explain ways to manage the underlying disorder.
○ Stress the importance of rest periods.

Vertigo

Overview

- Refers to an illusion of movement in which the patient feels that he's revolving in space (subjective) or the feeling of the surroundings revolving around the individual (objective)
- May be temporary or permanent, mild or severe
- Commonly occurs with nausea, vomiting, nystagmus, and tinnitus or hearing loss
- May worsen with movement and subside when lying down

Assessment

History

- Ask about the onset and description of vertigo.
- Note what aggravates and alleviates vertigo.
- Ask about motion sickness.
- Obtain a recent drug history.
- Ask about alcohol use.

Physical assessment

- Perform a neurologic assessment, focusing particularly on eighth cranial nerve function.
- Observe gait and posture.

Medical causes

Acoustic neuroma

- Mild, intermittent vertigo occurs with sensorineural hearing loss in one ear.
- Other findings include tinnitus, postauricular or sub-occipital pain, and — with cranial nerve compression — facial paralysis.

Benign positional vertigo

- Debris in a semicircular canal produces vertigo on head position change, lasting a few minutes.

Brain stem ischemia

- Sudden, severe vertigo may become episodic and later persistent.
- Other findings include ataxia, nausea, vomiting, increased blood pressure, tachycardia, nystagmus, and lateral deviation of the eyes toward the side of the lesion.
- Hemiparesis and paresthesia may also occur.

Head trauma

- Persistent vertigo occurs soon after injury along with spontaneous or positional nystagmus and, if the temporal bone is fractured, hearing loss.
- Other findings include headache, nausea, vomiting, and decreased level of consciousness (LOC).

- Behavioral changes, diplopia or visual blurring, seizures, motor or sensory deficits, and signs of increased intracranial pressure may also develop.

Herpes zoster

- Infection of the eighth cranial nerve produces sudden onset of vertigo, facial paralysis, hearing loss in the affected ear, and herpetic vesicular lesions in the auditory canal.

Labyrinthitis

- Severe vertigo begins abruptly and may occur in a single episode or recur over months or years.
- Associated findings include nausea, vomiting, progressive sensorineural hearing loss, and nystagmus.

Ménière's disease

- Labyrinthine dysfunction causes abrupt onset of vertigo, lasting minutes, hours, or days.
- Unpredictable episodes of severe vertigo and unsteady gait may cause the patient to fall.
- During an attack, any sudden motion of the head or eyes can precipitate nausea or vomiting.

Motion sickness

- Vertigo, nausea, vomiting, and headache occur in response to rhythmic or erratic motions.
- Headache, dizziness, fatigue, diaphoresis, hypersalivation, and dyspnea may also occur.

Multiple sclerosis

- Episodic vertigo may occur early and become persistent.
- Other early findings include diplopia, visual blurring, and paresthesia.
- Nystagmus, constipation, muscle weakness, paralysis, spasticity, hyperreflexia, intention tremor, and ataxia may also occur.

Posterior fossa tumor

- Positional vertigo occurs and lasts a few seconds.
- Other findings include papilledema, headache, memory loss, nausea, vomiting, nystagmus, apneustic respirations, and elevated blood pressure.

Seizures

- Temporal lobe seizures may produce vertigo, usually associated with other symptoms of partial complex seizures.
- Seizures may be heralded by an aura and followed by several minutes of mental confusion.

Vestibular neuritis

- Severe vertigo usually begins abruptly and lasts several days, without tinnitus or hearing loss.
- Other findings include nausea, vomiting, and nystagmus.

Other causes

Diagnostic tests

○ Caloric testing (irrigating the ears with warm or cold water) can induce vertigo.

Drugs and alcohol

○ High or toxic doses of certain drugs (such as salicylates, aminoglycosides, antibiotics, quinine, and hormonal contraceptives) or alcohol may produce vertigo.

Surgery and other procedures

○ Use of overly warm or cold eardrops or irrigating solutions can cause vertigo.
○ Ear surgery may cause vertigo that lasts for several days.

Nursing considerations

○ Place the patient in a comfortable position.
○ Monitor vital signs and LOC.
○ Keep the bed's side rails up; if the patient is standing, help him to a chair.
○ Darken the room and keep the patient calm.
○ Give drugs to control nausea and vomiting and decrease labyrinthine irritability.

Pediatric pointers

○ Ear infection and vestibular neuritis may cause vertigo.

Patient teaching

○ Explain the need for moving around with assistance.
○ Explain the need to avoid sudden position changes and dangerous tasks.

Vesicular rash

Overview

- Appears as a scattered or linear distribution of sharply circumscribed, blisterlike lesions that are usually less than 0.5 cm in diameter
- May be filled with clear, cloudy, or bloody fluid
- May be mild or severe and temporary or permanent

Assessment

History

- Ask about the onset and characteristics of rash.
- Take a drug history.
- Ask about other signs and symptoms.
- Find out about a family history of skin disorders.
- Ask about a history of allergies.
- Inquire about recent infections, insect bites, or exposure to allergens.

Physical assessment

- Note if skin is dry, oily, or moist.
- Observe the distribution of the lesions; record their location.
- Note the color, shape, and size of the lesions.
- Check for crusts, scales, scars, macules, papules, or wheals.
- Palpate the vesicles or bullae to determine if they're flaccid or tense.

Medical causes

Burns (second-degree)

- Vesicles and bullae, erythema, swelling, pain, and moistness

Dermatitis

- With contact dermatitis, small vesicles are surrounded by redness and marked edema; vesicles may ooze, scale, and cause severe pruritus.
- With dermatitis herpetiformis, vesicular, papular, bullous, pustular, or erythematous lesions form; severe pruritus, burning, and stinging may also occur.
- With nummular dermatitis, groups of pinpoint vesicles and papules appear on erythematous or pustular lesions, pustular lesions may ooze a purulent exudate, itch severely, and rapidly become crusted and scaly.

Dermatophytid

- Pruritic and tender vesicular lesions develop on the hands.
- Other findings include fever, anorexia, generalized adenopathy, and splenomegaly.

Erythema multiform

- Heralded by a sudden eruption of erythematous macules, papules, and occasionally vesicles and bullae
- Vesiculobullous lesions usually appear on the mucous membranes, especially the lips and buccal mucosa—where they may rupture and ulcerate producing thick, yellow or white exudate.
- A characteristic rash appears symmetrically over the hands, arms, feet, legs, face and neck.

Herpes simplex

- Vesicles that are 2 to 3 mm in size and on an inflamed base most commonly appear on the lips and lower face.
- Vesicles are preceded by itching, tingling, burning, or pain.
- Eventually, vesicle rupture, forming a painful ulcer followed by a yellowish crust.

Herpes zoster

- A vesicular rash is preceded by erythema and, occasionally, by a nodular skin eruption and sharp pain along a dermatome.
- About 5 days later, lesions erupt and the pain becomes burning; vesicles dry and scab about 10 days after eruption.
- Other findings include fever, malaise, pruritus, and paresthesia or hyperesthesia of the involved area.
- If the cranial nerves are involved, facial palsy, hearing loss, dizziness, loss of taste, eye pain, and impaired vision occur.

Insect bites

- Vesicles appear on red papules and may become hemorrhagic.
- Other findings include fever, myalgia, headache, lymphadenopathy, nausea, and vomiting.

Pemphigus

- Groups of tiny vesicles erupt on normal skin or mucous membranes.
- Vesicles are thin-walled, flaccid, and easily broken, producing small denuded areas that eventually form crusts; itching and burning of the skin may also occur.

Pompholyx (dyshidrosis or dyshidrosis eczema)

- Symmetrical vesicular lesions that can become pustular appear on the palms and soles.
- Pruritic lesions are more common on the palms than on the soles with possible minimal erythema.

Scabies

- Small vesicles erupt on an erythematous base and may be at the end of a threadlike burrow.
- Pustules and excoriations may occur.
- Pruritus occurs and may worsen with inactivity, warmth, and nightfall.

Smallpox

○ A maculopapular rash on the mucosa of the mouth, pharynx, face and forearms spreads to the trunk and legs, then turns vesicular within 2 days and later pustular.
○ Initial findings include high fever, malaise, prostration, severe headache, backache, and abdominal pain.
○ After 8 to 9 days, the pustules form a crust; later, the scab separates from the skin, leaving a pitted scar.

Tinea pedis

○ Vesicles and scaling develop between the toes.
○ Inflammation, pruritus, and difficulty walking occur with severe infection.

Nursing considerations

○ If skin eruptions cover a large skin surface, start an I.V. line to replace fluid and electrolytes.
○ Keep the environment warm and free from drafts.
○ Obtain cultures to determine the standard causative organism.
○ Look for signs of secondary infection.
○ Give the patient an antibiotic and apply corticosteroid or antimicrobial ointment to the lesions.

Pediatric pointers

○ May be caused by staphylococcal infections, varicella, hand-foot-and-mouth disease, contact dermatitis, and prickly heat.

Patient teaching

○ Explain importance of frequent hand-washing.
○ Instruct the patient to avoiding touching the lesions.
○ Explain the use of tepid baths or cold compresses to relieve itching.

Vision loss

Overview

- An inability to perceive visual stimuli that ranges from slight impairment to total blindness
- Can be sudden or gradual, temporary or permanent
- If sudden, can be an ocular emergency (see *Managing sudden vision loss*)

Assessment

History

- Ask about the characteristics of vision loss.
- Find out about associated photosensitivity or eye pain.
- Obtain an ocular history and family history of eye problems or systemic diseases that may lead to eye problems, such as hypertension; diabetes mellitus; thyroid, rheumatic, or vascular disease; infections; and cancer.
- Determine current drug profile, especially eye drops.

Physical assessment

- If the patient has perforating or penetrating ocular trauma, don't touch his eye.
- Assess visual acuity, with best available correction in each eye. (See *Testing visual acuity*.)
- Inspect the eyes, noting edema, foreign bodies, drainage, or conjunctival or scleral redness.
- Observe whether lid closure is complete or incomplete and check for ptosis.

> ### Emergency actions
> ### Managing sudden vision loss
>
> Sudden vision loss can signal central retinal artery occlusion or acute angle-closure glaucoma — ocular emergencies that require immediate intervention. If your patient reports sudden vision loss, immediately notify an ophthalmologist for an emergency examination, and perform these interventions:
>
> *For a patient with suspected central retinal artery occlusion,* perform light massage over his closed eyelid. Increase his carbon dioxide level by administering a set flow of oxygen and carbon dioxide through a Venturi mask, or have the patient rebreathe in a paper bag to retain exhaled carbon dioxide. These steps will dilate the artery and, possibly, restore blood flow to the retina.
>
> *For a patient with suspected acute angle-closure glaucoma,* measure intraocular pressure (IOP) with a tonometer. (You can also estimate IOP without a tonometer by placing your fingers over the patient's closed eyelid. A rock-hard eyeball usually indicates increased IOP.) Instill timolol drops and administer I.V. acetazolamide to help decrease IOP.

- Using a flashlight, examine the cornea and iris for scars, irregularities, and foreign bodies.
- Observe the size, shape, and color of the pupils.
- Test the direct and consensual light reflex and the effect of accommodation.

Medical causes

Amaurosis fugax

- Recurrent attacks of vision loss in one eye may last from a few seconds to a few minutes.
- Vision is normal at other times.
- Transient one-sided weakness, hypertension, and elevated intraocular pressure (IOP) in the affected eye may also develop.

Cataract

- Painless and gradual blurring of vision precedes vision loss.
- As the disease progresses, the pupil turns milky white.
- Night blindness and halo vision may be early signs.

Concussion

- Vision may be temporarily blurred, doubled, or lost.
- Other findings include headache, anterograde and retrograde amnesia, transient loss of consciousness, nausea, vomiting, dizziness, irritability, confusion, lethargy, and aphasia.

Diabetic retinopathy

- Retinal edema and hemorrhage lead to blurred vision, which may progress to blindness.
- Loss of central vision and color vision may also occur.
- Usually a sign of poorly controlled, brittle or advanced diabetes.

Endophthalmitis

- Permanent unilateral vision loss may result as well as headache, photophobia, and ocular discharge.

Glaucoma

- Gradual blurring of vision may progress to total blindness.
- Acute angle-closure glaucoma, an ocular emergency, may produce blindness within 3 to 5 days, inflammation, and pain in one eye; eye pressure; moderate pupil dilation; nonreactive pupillary response; a cloudy cornea; reduced visual acuity, photophobia; nausea; vomiting; and perception of blue or red halos around lights.
- Chronic open-angle glaucoma typically causes a slowly progressive peripheral vision loss, peripheral vision loss, aching eyes, halo vision, and reduced visual acuity.

Use a Snellen letter chart to test visual acuity in the literate patient older than age 6. Have the patient sit or stand 20′ (6 m) from the chart. Tell him to cover his left eye and read aloud the smallest line of letters that he can see. Record the fraction assigned to that line on the chart (the numerator indicates distance from the chart; the denominator indicates the distance at which a normal eye can read the chart). Normal vision is 20/20. Repeat the test with the patient's right eye covered.

If your patient can't read the largest letter from a distance of 20′, have him approach the chart until he can read it. Record the distance between him and the chart as the numerator of the fraction. For example, if he can see the top line of the chart at a distance of 3′ (1 m), record the test result as 3/20.

Use a Snellen symbol chart to test children ages 3 to 6 and illiterate patients. Follow the same procedure as for the Snellen letter chart, but ask the patient to indicate the direction of the E's fingers as you point to each symbol.

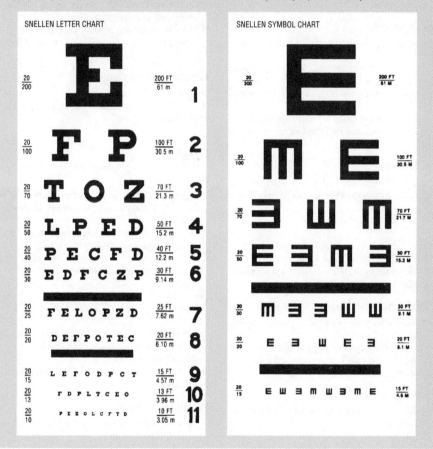

Herpes zoster

○ When the nasociliary nerve is affected, vision loss with eyelid lesions, conjunctivitis, skin lesions, and ocular muscle palsies.

Hyphema

○ Blood in the anterior chamber can reduce vision to light perception only.
○ Other findings include moderate pain, conjunctival injection, and eyelid edema.

Keratitis

○ Complete vision loss in one eye with an opaque cornea, increased tearing, irritation, and photophobia.

Ocular trauma

○ Vision loss is sudden, total or partial, permanent or temporary, and in one or both eyes.
○ Eyelids may be reddened, edematous, and lacerated; intraocular contents may be extruded.

Optic atrophy

○ Irreversible loss of the visual field and changes in color vision result.
○ Pupillary reactions are sluggish, and optic disk pallor is evident.

Optic neuritis

○ Vision loss in one eye is temporary but severe.
○ Pain around the eye occurs, especially with movement of the globe.
○ Visual field defects and a sluggish pupillary response may also occur.

Paget's disease

○ Vision loss may develop because of bony impingements on the cranial nerves.
○ Hearing loss, tinnitus, vertigo, and severe, persistent bone pain also occur. Cranial enlargement may be noticeable frontally and occipitally, and headaches may occur.
○ Sites of bone involvement are warm and tender, and impaired mobility and pathologic fractures are common.

Papilledema

○ Acute papilledema may lead to momentary blurring or transiently obscured vision; chimeric papilledema may cause vision loss.

Pituitary tumor

○ Blurred vision progresses to hemianopsia and, possibly, unilateral blindness as tumor grows.
○ Double vision, nystagmus, ptosis, limited eye movement, and headaches may also occur.

Retinal artery occlusion (central)

○ An ocular emergency—partial or complete vision loss in one eye is sudden.
○ Permanent blindness may occur within hours.
○ A sluggish direct pupillary response and a normal consensual response occur.

Retinal detachment

○ Painless vision loss may be gradual or sudden and total or partial.
○ With partial vision loss, visual field defects or a shadow or curtain over the visual fields, and visual floaters may be reported.
○ Total blindness occurs with macular involvement.

Retinal vein occlusion (central)

○ Decrease in visual acuity in one eye may occur with variable vision loss.
○ IOP may be elevated in both eyes.

Senile macular degeneration

○ Painless blurring or loss of central vision occurs.
○ Vision loss may proceed slowly or rapidly, may eventually affect both eyes, and may be worse at night.

Temporal arteritis

○ Vision blurring and loss with a throbbing headache are characteristic.
○ Other findings include malaise, anorexia, weight loss, weakness, low-grade fever, generalized muscle aches, and confusion.

Uveitis

○ Inflammation of the uveal tract may cause unilateral vision loss.
○ Anterior uveitis produces moderate to severe eye pain, severe conjunctival injection, photophobia, and a small, nonreactive pupil.
○ Posterior uveitis may produce insidious onset of blurred vision, conjunctival injection, visual floaters, pain, and photophobia.

Vitreous hemorrhage

○ Vision loss in one eye is sudden.
○ Visual floaters and partial vision with a reddish haze may occur.

Other causes

Drugs

○ Digoxin derivatives, indomethacin, ethambutol, quinine sulfate, and methanol toxicity may also cause vision loss.
○ Chloroquine therapy may cause patchy retinal pigmentation that typically leads to blindness.
○ Phenylbutazone may cause vision loss and increased susceptibility to retinal detachment.

Nursing considerations

○ If the patient has photophobia, darken the room and suggest wearing sunglasses during the day.
○ Obtain cultures of eye drainage.
○ Get the patient a referral to an ophthalmologist for evaluation.

Pediatric pointers

○ Optic nerve gliomas and retinoblastomas may cause vision loss in children.
○ Congenital rubella and syphilis may cause vision loss in infants.

Geriatric pointers

○ Reduced visual acuity may be caused by morphologic changes in the choroid, pigment epithelium, and retina or by decreased function of the rods, cones, and other neural elements.

Patient teaching

○ Give the patient orientation to his environment.
○ Explain safety measures to prevent injury.

○ Emphasize importance of frequent hand washing and avoiding rubbing the eyes.
○ If loss is progressive or permanent, refer patient to appropraite social service agencies for assistance with adaptation and equipment.

Visual blurring

Overview

○ The loss of visual acuity with indistinct visual details

Assessment

History

○ Ask about eye pain, trauma, sudden vision loss, or discharge.
○ Find out about the onset of visual blurring.
○ Ask about recent accidents or injuries.
○ Obtain a medical and drug history.

Physical assessment

○ Inspect the eye; note lid edema, drainage, conjunctival or scleral redness, an irregularly shaped iris, and excessive blinking.
○ Assess for pupillary changes.
○ Test visual acuity in both eyes.

Medical causes

Brain tumor

○ Visual blurring with decreased level of consciousness (LOC), headache, apathy, behavioral changes, memory loss, decreased attention span, dizziness, and confusion
○ Aphasia, seizures, ataxia, and signs of hormonal imbalance
○ Later, vomiting, increased systolic blood pressure, widened pulse pressure, and decorticate posture

Cataract

○ Gradual blurring with halo vision (an early sign), visual glare in bright light, progressive vision loss, and a gray pupil that turns milky white

Concussion

○ Blurred, double, or temporarily lost vision.
○ Changes in LOC and behavior

Conjunctivitis

○ Visual blurring with photophobia, pain, burning, tearing, itching, and a feeling of fullness around the eyes
○ Redness near the fornices (brilliant red suggests a bacterial cause; milky red, an allergic cause) and drainage (copious, mucopurulent, and flaky in bacterial conjunctivitis; stringy in allergic conjunctivitis)
○ With viral conjunctivitis, copious tearing, minimal exudate, and an enlarged preauricular lymph node

Corneal abrasions

○ Visual blurring with severe eye pain
○ Photophobia, redness, and excessive tearing

Diabetic retinopathy

○ Retinal edema and hemorrhage produce gradual blurring, which may progress to blindness.
○ Loss of central vision and color vision may occur.

Eye tumor

○ If the macula is involved, blurring may be the first symptom.
○ Other findings include varying visual field losses.

Glaucoma

○ With acute angle-closure glaucoma, an ocular emergency, visual blurring and severe pain begin suddenly in one eye.
○ Other acute findings include halo vision; a moderately dilated, nonreactive pupil; conjunctival injection; a cloudy cornea; and decreased visual acuity.
○ With chronic angle-closure glaucoma, transient visual blurring and halo vision may precede pain and blindness.

Hypertension

○ Visual blurring and a constant morning headache
○ With a diastolic blood pressure over 120 mm Hg, a severe throbbing headache
○ Restlessness, confusion, nausea, vomiting, seizures, and decreased LOC

Hyphema

○ Visual blurring from blunt eye trauma with hemorrhage into the anterior chamber causes moderate pain, diffuse conjunctival injection, visible blood in the anterior chamber, ecchymoses, eyelid edema, and a hard eye.

Iritis

○ Sudden blurring, moderate to severe eye pain, photophobia, conjunctival injection, and a constricted pupil

Migraine headache

○ Blurring and paroxysmal attacks of severe, throbbing, headache
○ Nausea, vomiting, sensitivity to light and noise, and sensory or visual auras

Multiple sclerosis

○ In the early stage, blurred vision, diplopia, and paresthesia
○ In later stages, nystagmus, muscle weakness, paralysis, spasticity, hyperreflexia, intention tremor, and ataxic gait
○ Urinary frequency, urgency, and incontinence

Optic neuritis

- An acute attack of blurring and vision loss from inflammation, degeneration, or demyelinization of the optic nerve
- Scotomas and eye pain
- Hyperemia of the optic disk, large vein distention, blurred disk margins, and filling of the physiologic cup revealed upon ophthalmoscopic examination

Retinal detachment

- Sudden visual blurring may be the first symptom, followed by visual floaters and recurring light flashes.
- Progressive detachment increases vision loss.

Retinal vein occlusion (central)

- Gradual visual blurring and varying degrees of vision loss in one eye

Senile macular degeneration

- Initially, painless visual blurring worsens at night.
- Other findings include loss of central vision and progressive vision loss.

Serous retinopathy (central)

- Blurring with darkened vision in the affected eye
- A blind spot in the visual field with distorted straight lines

Stroke

- Brief attacks of visual blurring before or with a stroke
- Decreased LOC, contralateral hemiplegia, dysarthria, dysphagia, ataxia, unilateral sensory loss, agnosia, aphasia, homonymous hemianopsia, diplopia, disorientation, and apraxia
- Urine retention or incontinence, constipation, personality changes, emotional lability, and seizures

Temporal arteritis

- Sudden blurred vision with vision loss and a throbbing headache
- First, malaise, anorexia, weight loss, weakness, low-grade fever, and generalized muscle aches
- Confusion; disorientation; swollen, nodular, tender temporal arteries; and erythema of overlying skin

Uveitis (posterior)

- Blurred vision, conjunctival injection, visual floaters, pain, and photophobia

Vitreous hemorrhage

- Sudden visual blurring and varying vision loss in one eye
- Visual floaters or dark streaks and partial vision with a reddish haze

Other causes

Drugs

- Cycloplegics, guanethidine, reserpine, clomiphene, phenylbutazone, thiazide diuretics, antihistamines, anticholinergics, or phenothiazines

Nursing considerations

- Prepare the patient for diagnostic tests.
- Initiate safety measures to prevent injury.
- Provide emotional support as needed.

Pediatric pointers

- Blurring may stem from congenital syphilis or cataracts, refractive errors, eye injuries or infections, and increased intracranial pressure.

Patient teaching

- Teach the patient to instill eyedrops properly.
- Explain the need for orientation to his environment.
- Instruct the patient in safety measures.

Vomiting

Overview

- The forceful expulsion of gastric contents through the mouth
- A coordinated sequence of abdominal muscle contractions and reverse esophageal peristalsis
- Characteristically preceded by nausea

Assessment

History

- Ask about the onset, duration, and intensity of vomiting. (See *Identifying causes of vomiting*.)
- Determine aggravating or alleviating factors.
- Ask about nausea, abdominal pain, anorexia, weight loss, changes in bowel habits, excessive belching or flatus, and bloating or fullness.
- Obtain a medical history, including GI, endocrine, and metabolic disorders; infections; and cancer, including chemotherapy and radiation therapy.
- Ask about current drug use and alcohol consumption.
- Find out if pregnancy is possible.

Physical assessment

- Inspect the abdomen for distention.
- Auscultate for bowel sounds and bruits.
- Palpate for rigidity and tenderness, and test for rebound tenderness.
- Palpate and percuss the liver for enlargement.
- Assess buccal mucosa and skin turgor for sufficient hydration.

Medical causes

Adrenal insufficiency

- Commonly, vomiting, nausea, anorexia, and diarrhea
- Weakness; fatigue; weight loss; bronze skin; orthostatic hypotension, and weak, irregular pulse

Anthrax (GI)

- Vomiting, loss of appetite, nausea, and fever after eating contaminated food
- May progress to abdominal pain, severe bloody diarrhea, and hematemesis

Appendicitis

- Vomiting and nausea after or with abdominal pain
- Vague epigastric or periumbilical discomfort, rapidly progressing to severe, stabbing pain the right-lower-quadrant

- A positive McBurney's sign — severe pain and tenderness on palpation about 2" (5 cm) from the right anterior superior spine of the ilium, on a line between that spine and the umbilicus
- Abdominal rigidity and tenderness, anorexia, constipation or diarrhea, cutaneous hyperalgesia, fever, tachycardia, and malaise

Bulimia

- Polyphagia that alternates with self-induced vomiting, fasting, or diarrhea
- Anorexia, a morbid fear of obesity, and calloused knuckles (from self-induced vomiting)

Cholecystitis (acute)

- Nausea and mild vomiting after severe right-upper-quadrant pain that may radiate to the back or shoulders
- Abdominal tenderness and, possibly, rigidity and distention, fever, and diaphoresis

Cholelithiasis

- Nausea and vomiting with severe unlocalized right-upper-quadrant or epigastric pain after ingestion of fatty foods
- Abdominal tenderness and guarding, flatulence, belching, epigastric burning, pyrosis, tachycardia, and restlessness

Cirrhosis

- In the early stage, nausea and vomiting, anorexia, aching abdominal pain, and constipation or diarrhea
- In later stages, jaundice, hepatomegaly, and abdominal distention

Cholera

- Vomiting with abrupt watery diarrhea
- Thirst, weakness, muscle cramps, decreased skin turgor, oliguria, tachycardia, and hypotension from severe water and electrolyte loss

Escherichia coli 0157:H7

- Vomiting, watery or bloody diarrhea, nausea, fever, and abdominal cramps
- Acute renal failure in children younger than 5 and elderly patients

Ectopic pregnancy

- A life-threatening disorder; vomiting, nausea, vaginal bleeding, and lower abdominal pain
- A tender abdominal mass and a 1- to 2-month history of amenorrhea

Electrolyte imbalances

- Nausea and vomiting frequently occur along with arrhythmias, tremors, seizures, anorexia, malaise, and weakness.

When you collect a sample of the patient's vomitus, observe it carefully for clues to the underlying disorder. Here's what vomitus may indicate:

Bile-stained (greenish) vomitus
Obstruction below the pylorus, as from a duodenal lesion

Bloody vomitus
Upper GI bleeding (if bright red may result from gastritis or a peptic ulcer; if dark red, from esophageal or gastric varices)

Brown vomitus with a fecal odor
Intestinal obstruction or infarction

Burning, bitter-tasting vomitus
Excessive hydrochloric acid in gastric contents

Coffee-ground vomitus
Digested blood from slowly bleeding gastric or duodenal lesion

Undigested food
Gastric outlet obstruction, as from gastric tumor or ulcer

Food poisoning
○ Commonly, vomiting, diarrhea, severe and cramping abdominal pain, prostration, and fever

Gastritis
○ Commonly, nausea and vomiting of mucus or blood
○ Epigastric pain, belching, and fever

Gastroenteritis
○ Nausea, vomiting (often of undigested food), diarrhea, and abdominal cramping
○ Fever, malaise, hyperactive bowel sounds, and abdominal pain and tenderness

Heart failure
○ Nausea and vomiting, especially with right-sided heart failure
○ Tachycardia, ventricular gallop, fatigue, dyspnea, crackles, peripheral edema, and neck vein distention

Hepatitis
○ In the early stage, nausea and vomiting, fatigue, myalgia, arthralgia, headache, photophobia, anorexia, pharyngitis, cough, and fever

Hyperemesis gravidarum
○ Unremitting nausea and vomiting are that last beyond the first trimester
○ Undigested food, mucus, and small amounts of bile in the vomitus early in the disorder; later, a coffee-ground appearance
○ Weight loss, headache, and delirium

Increased intracranial pressure
○ Projectile vomiting not preceded by nausea
○ Decreased level of consciousness (LOC), and Cushing's triad (bradycardia, hypertension, and respiratory pattern changes)
○ Headache, widened pulse pressure, impaired motor movement, vision disturbances, pupillary changes, and papilledema

Intestinal obstruction
○ Commonly, nausea and vomiting (bilious or fecal)
○ Usually episodic and colicky abdominal pain, possibly becoming severe and steady
○ Constipation early in large intestinal obstruction and late in small intestinal obstruction)
○ Obstipation in complete obstruction
○ High pitched and hyperactive bowel sounds in partial obstruction and hypoactive or absent in complete obstruction

Labyrinthitis
○ Nausea, vomiting, severe vertigo, progressive hearing loss, nystagmus and, possibly, otorrhea

Listeriosis
○ After ingesting food contaminated with *Listeria monocytogenes*, vomiting, fever, abdominal pain, myalgias, nausea, and diarrhea

Ménière's disease
○ Sudden, brief, recurrent attacks of nausea and vomiting, dizziness, vertigo, hearing loss, tinnitus, and nystagmus

Mesenteric artery ischemia
○ A life-threatening disorder; nausea and vomiting and severe, cramping abdominal pain, especially after meals
○ Diarrhea or constipation, abdominal tenderness and bloating, anorexia, weight loss, and abdominal bruits

Mesenteric venous thrombosis
○ Nausea, vomiting, and abdominal pain with diarrhea or constipation, abdominal distention, hematemesis, and melena

Metabolic acidosis
○ Nausea, vomiting, anorexia, diarrhea, Kussmaul's respirations, and decreased LOC

Migraine headache

○ Premonitory nausea and vomiting
○ Fatigue, photophobia, light flashes, increased noise sensitivity and, possibly, partial vision loss and paresthesia

Motion sickness

○ Nausea and vomiting with headache, vertigo, dizziness, fatigue, diaphoresis, and dyspnea

Myocardial infarction

○ Nausea and vomiting may occur, but the main symptom is severe substernal chest pain, which may radiate to the left arm, jaw, or neck.
○ Dyspnea, pallor, clammy skin, diaphoresis, and restlessness may occur.

Pancreatitis (acute)

○ In the early stage, vomiting, usually preceded by nausea
○ Steady and severe epigastric or left-upper-quadrant pain that may radiate to the back, abdominal tenderness and rigidity, hypoactive bowel sounds, anorexia, and fever
○ In severe cases, tachycardia, restlessness, hypotension, skin mottling, and cold, sweaty extremities

Peptic ulcer

○ Nausea and vomiting may follow sharp, burning or gnawing epigastric pain.
○ Pain occurs especially when the stomach is empty or after ingestion of alcohol, caffeine, or aspirin.
○ Hematemesis or melena may also occur.

Peritonitis

○ Nausea and vomiting usually with acute abdominal pain
○ High fever with chills; tachycardia; hypoactive or absent bowel sounds; abdominal distention, rigidity, and tenderness; weakness; pale, cold skin; diaphoresis; hypotension; signs of dehydration; and shallow respirations

Preeclampsia

○ Nausea and vomiting with rapid weight gain, epigastric pain, edema, elevated blood pressure, oliguria, severe frontal headache, and blurred or double vision

Q fever

○ In this rickettsial infection, vomiting with fever, chills, severe headache, malaise, chest pain, nausea, and diarrhea

Rhabdomyolysis

○ Vomiting along with muscle weakness or pain, fever, nausea, malaise, and dark urine

Thyrotoxicosis

○ Nausea and vomiting with the classic findings of severe anxiety, heat intolerance, weight loss despite increased appetite, diaphoresis, diarrhea, tremors, tachycardia, and palpitations
○ Exophthalmos, ventricular or atrial gallop, and an enlarged thyroid

Ulcerative colitis

○ Vomiting, nausea, and anorexia with the common sign of recurrent diarrhea with blood, pus, and mucus
○ Fever, chills, and weight loss

Volvulus

○ Vomiting with rapid, marked abdominal distention and sudden, severe abdominal pain
○ Twisting of intestine at least 180 degress in its mesentery, leading to blood vessel compression and ischemia
○ In adults, common in sigmoid bowel; in children, small bowel
○ Can also be in the stomach or cecum

Other causes

Drugs

○ Anesthetics, antibiotics, antineoplastics, chloride replacements, estrogens, ferrous sulfate, levodopa, opiates, oral potassium, quinidine, and sulfasalazine
○ Overdoses of cardiac glycosides and theophylline
○ Syrup of ipecac (used for overdoses by inducing vomiting)

Radiation and surgery

○ Radiation therapy if it disrupts the gastric mucosa.
○ Commonly, postoperative nausea and vomiting, especially after abdominal surgery

Nursing considerations

○ Draw blood to determine electrolyte and acid-base balance.
○ Position the patient to prevent aspiration of vomitus.
○ Monitor vital signs and intake and output.
○ Maintain hydration with sips of water or ice chips if tolerated or by I.V. fluids if hospitalized. (See *Managing a dehydration emergency.*)

○ Give drugs for pain promptly. If possible, give these by injection or suppository.

○ If an opioid is used, monitor bowel sounds, flatus, and bowel movements.

Pediatric pointers

○ In a neonate, pyloric obstruction may cause projectile vomiting; Hirschsprung's disease may cause fecal vomiting.

○ Intussusception may lead to vomiting of bile and fecal matter.

○ Infants and young children are susceptible to dehydration—a medical emergency—if vomiting persists for 2 days without the ability to retain fluids.

Geriatric pointers

○ Rule out intestinal ischemia first because it's especially common in elderly patients.

○ Debilitated and undernourished patients are more susceptible to dehydration.

Patient teaching

○ Explain deep-breathing techniques.

○ Explain how to replace fluid losses.

○ Teach the patient to adjust his diet by starting with clear liquids and advancing to a bland diet.

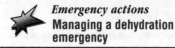

Emergency actions
Managing a dehydration emergency

Signs and symptoms:
- Increased thirst
- Decreased urination
- Weakness or light-headedness
- Dry mouth and mucous membranes
- Dry eyes and few tears when crying
- Decreased skin turgor
- Sunken cheeks, eyes, possibly abdomen, fontanelle in infants
- Irritability
- Listlessness, low energy level

Actions:
- Notify physician.
- Institute I.V. fluid replacement therapy.
- Draw blood for electrolytes, renal studies, liver function tests, and complete blood count.
- Assess vital signs frequently until stable.
- Administer antiemetic (such as prochlorperazine, metoclopramide, droperidol, ondansetron, granisetron, or lorazepam depending on source of vomiting and effectiveness).
- Offer supportive care while patient is vomiting.
- Provide careful mouthcare after episodes.

Vulvar lesions

Overview

- Cutaneous lumps, nodules, papules, vesicles, or ulcers that appear on the vulva

Assessment

History

- Ask about the onset of vulvar lesions.
- Inquire about associated findings, such as swelling, pain, or discharge.
- Question the patient about sexual activity and the potential for sexually transmitted disease (STD) exposure.

Physical assessment

- Examine the lesion and obtain cultures. (See *Recognizing common vulvar lesions*.)
- Examine the rest of the skin for rashes and lesions.

Medical causes

Basal cell carcinoma

- Tumor is nodular and has a central ulcer and a raised, poorly rolled border.
- Pruritus, bleeding, discharge, and a burning sensation may occur.

Benign cysts

- Epidermal inclusion cysts (usually round) appear on labia majora.
- Bartholin's duct cysts are usually tense, and nontender and on one side of the posterior labia minora.
- Bartholin's abscess causes gradual pain and tenderness.

Genital warts

- Painless red and pink swellings on vulva, vagina, and cervix
- Pruritus, erythema, and a profuse, mucopurulent, vaginal discharge

Gonorrhea

- Vulvar lesions, usually confined to Bartholin's glands, with pruritus, a burning sensation, pain, and a green-yellow vaginal discharge, but most patients are asymptomatic
- Dysuria, urinary incontinence, severe pelvic and lower abdominal pain, and vaginal redness, swelling, bleeding, and engorgement

Herpes simplex (genital)

- Fluid-filled vesicles appear on cervix and, possibly, on vulva, labia, perianal skin, or vagina.

- Initially painless, vesicles may rupture and develop into extensive, shallow, painful ulcers, with redness and edema, and tender inguinal lymph nodes.
- Other findings include fever, malaise, and dysuria.

Molluscum contagiosum

- Raised vulvar papules are 1 to 2 mm in diameter and pearly or flesh-colored with umbilicated centers and white cores.

Pediculosis pubis

- Erythematous vulvar papules occur with pruritus and irritation.
- Adult pubic lice and nits are visible on pubic hair.

Squamous cell carcinoma

- Invasive carcinoma may produce vulvar pruritus, pain, and a lump.
- Carcinoma in situ produces a vulvar lesion that may be white or red, raised, well defined, moist, crusted, and isolated.

Squamous cell hyperplasia

- Vulvar lesions may be well delineated or poorly defined; localized or extensive; and red, brown, white, or both red and white.
- Intense pruritus, possibly with vulvar pain, intense burning, and dyspareunia, is the cardinal symptom.

Syphilis

- Papules with indurated, raised edges and clear bases on the vulva, vagina, or cervix 10 to 90 days after initial contact
- A maculopapular, pustular, or nodular rash; headache; malaise; anorexia; weight loss; fever; nausea; vomiting; lymphadenopathy; and a sore throat

Viral disease (systemic)

- Varicella, measles, and other systemic viral diseases may produce vulvar lesions.

Nursing considerations

- Give a systemic antibiotic, an antiviral, a topical corticosteroid, a topical testosterone, or an antipruritic.

Pediatric pointers

- Vulvar lesions in children may result from congenital syphilis or gonorrhea; assess for sexual abuse.

Geriatric pointers

- Vulvar dystrophies and neoplasia occur more frequently with advancing age.

Patient teaching

- Explain that sitz baths may make the patient more comfortable.
- Provide instruction in safer sex practices.

Various disorders can cause vulvar lesions. For example, sexually transmitted diseases account for most vulvar lesions in premenopausal women, whereas vulvar tumors and cysts account for most lesions in women ages 50 to 70. The illustrations below will help you recognize some of the most common lesions.

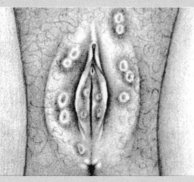

Primary genital herpes produces multiple ulcerated lesions surrounded by red halos.

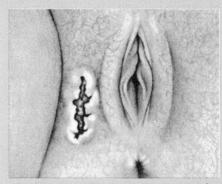

Basal cell carcinoma can produce an ulcerated lesion with raised, poorly rolled edges.

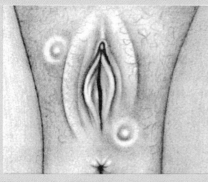

Primary syphilis produces chancres that appear as ulcerated lesions with raised borders.

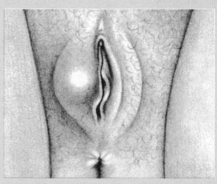

Epidermal inclusion cysts produce a round lump that usually appears on the labia majora.

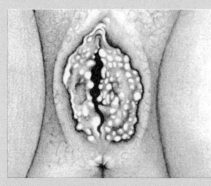

Squamous cell carcinoma can produce a large, granulomatous-appearing ulcer.

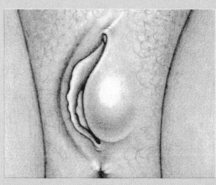

Bartholin's duct cysts produce a tense, nontender, palpable lump that usually appears on the labia minora.

Weight gain, excessive

Overview

- When ingested calories exceed body requirements for energy, resulting in increased adipose tissue storage
- May also occur when fluid retention causes edema

Assessment

History

- Ask about previous pattern of weight gain and loss.
- Find out about a family history of obesity, thyroid disease, or diabetes mellitus.
- Note eating and activity patterns.
- Determine exercise habits.
- Ask about vision disturbances, hoarseness, paresthesia, or increased urination and thirst, impotence, or menstrual irregularities.
- Take a drug history.

Physical assessment

- Note mental status, memory, and response time.
- Measure skin-fold thickness.
- Note fat distribution and the presence of edema.
- Note overall nutritional status.
- Inspect for other abnormalities, such as abnormal body hair distribution or hair loss and dry skin.
- Take vital signs.
- Determine body mass index.

Medical causes

Acromegaly

- Moderate weight gain occurs with coarsened facial features, prognathism, enlarged hands and feet, increased sweating, oily skin, deep voice, back and joint pain, lethargy, sleepiness, and heat intolerance.
- Hirsutism may occur occasionally.

Diabetes mellitus

- Increased appetite may lead to weight gain, although weight loss may also occur.
- Other findings include fatigue, polydipsia, polyuria, polyphagia, nocturia, weakness, and somnolence.

Heart failure

- Weight gain from edema
- Paroxysmal nocturnal dyspnea, tachypnea, nausea, orthopnea, and fatigue

Hypercortisolism

- Excessive weight gain, usually over the trunk and the back of the neck (buffalo hump)

- Slender extremities, moon face, weakness, purple striae, emotional lability, and increased susceptibility to infection.
- In men, gynecomastia occurs.
- In women, hirsutism, acne, and menstrual irregularities occur.

Hyperinsulinism

- Increased appetite leads to weight gain.
- Emotional lability, indigestion, weakness, diaphoresis, tachycardia, vision disturbances, and syncope also occur.

Hypogonadism

- Weight gain is common.
- Prepubertal hypogonadism cause eunuchoid body proportions with relatively sparse facial and body hair and a high-pitched voice.
- Postpubertal hypogonadism causes loss of libido, impotence, and infertility.

Hypothyroidism

- Weight gain despite anorexia
- Fatigue; cold intolerance; constipation; menorrhagia; slowed intellectual and motor activity; dry, pale, cool skin; dry, sparse hair; and thick, brittle nails
- Possible myalgia, hoarseness, hypoactive deep tendon reflexes, bradycardia, and abdominal distention.
- Eventually, a dull facial expression with periorbital edema

Nephrotic syndrome

- Weight gain results from edema.
- In severe cases, anasarca develops — increasing body weight as much as 50%.
- Related findings include abdominal distention, orthostatic hypotension, and lethargy.

Pancreatic islet cell tumor

- Excessive hunger leads to weight gain.
- Other findings include emotional lability, weakness, malaise, fatigue, restlessness, diaphoresis, palpitations, tachycardia, vision disturbances, and syncope.

Preeclampsia

- Rapid weight gain with nausea and vomiting, epigastric pain, elevated blood pressure, and blurred or double vision

Other causes

Drugs

- Corticosteroids, phenothiazines, and tricyclic antidepressants (from fluid retention and increased appetite)
- Hormonal contraceptives (from fluid retention), cyproheptadine (from increased appetite), and lithium (from hypothyroidism)

Nursing considerations

○ Psychological counseling may be necessary.
○ If the patient is obese or has a cardiopulmonary disorder, exercises should be monitored closely.
○ Perform studies to rule out possible secondary causes should include serum thyroid-stimulating hormone determination and dexamethasone suppression testing.
○ Perform laboratory tests for thyroid function and serum cholesterol, triglyceride, and glucose levels should be performed.

Pediatric pointers

○ Weight gain can result from an endocrine disorder or from inactivity caused by Prader-Willi syndrome, Down syndrome, Werdnig-Hoffmann disease, muscular dystrophy, and cerebral palsy.
○ Other causes include poor eating habits, sedentary recreation, and emotional problems.

Geriatric pointers

○ Normal weight increases with age, but shouldn't exceed 15% over normal body weight.
○ Aerobic and muscle-building exercise is beneficial for longevity as well as weight control.

Patient teaching

○ Discuss the importance of weight control.
○ Explain the importance of behavior modification and dietary compliance.
○ Provide guidance in appropriate exercise.

Weight loss, excessive

Overview

○ From decreased food intake, decreased food absorption, increased metabolic requirements, or a combination of these

Assessment

History

○ Take a diet history.
○ Question the patient about why he isn't eating properly, if applicable.
○ Ask about previous weight and if weight loss is intentional.
○ Take a diet history, noting use of diet pills and laxatives.
○ Note sources of anxiety or depression.
○ Ask about changes in bowel habits, nausea, vomiting, abdominal pain, excessive thirst, excessive urination, or heat intolerance.

Physical assessment

○ Check height and weight.
○ Take vital signs and note general appearance.
○ Examine the skin for turgor and abnormal pigmentation.
○ Look for signs of infection or irritation on the roof of the mouth; note hyperpigmentation of the buccal mucosa.
○ Check the eyes for exophthalmos and the neck for swelling.
○ Evaluate breath sounds.
○ Inspect the abdomen for wasting; palpate for masses, tenderness, and an enlarged liver.

Medical causes

Adrenal insufficiency

○ Weight loss, anorexia, weakness, fatigue, irritability, syncope, nausea, vomiting, abdominal pain, and diarrhea or constipation
○ Hyperpigmentation at the joints, belt line, palmar creases, lips, gums, tongue, and buccal mucosa

Anorexia nervosa

○ Self-imposed weight loss of 10% to 50% of premorbid weight
○ A morbid fear of becoming fat, skeletal muscle atrophy, loss of fatty tissue, hypotension, constipation, dental caries, susceptibility to infection, blotchy or sallow skin, cold intolerance, hairiness on the face and body, dryness or loss of scalp hair, and amenorrhea

○ Dehydration or metabolic acidosis or alkalosis from self-induced vomiting or use of laxatives and diuretics

Cancer

○ Weight loss occurs with findings specific to the tumor, including fatigue, pain, nausea, vomiting, anorexia, abnormal bleeding, or a palpable mass.

Crohn's disease

○ Weight loss, chronic cramping, abdominal pain, and anorexia
○ Diarrhea, nausea, fever, tachycardia, abdominal tenderness and guarding, hyperactive bowel sounds, abdominal distention, and pain

Cryptosporidiosis

○ Weight loss with profuse watery diarrhea, abdominal cramping, flatulence, anorexia, malaise, fever, nausea, vomiting, and myalgia

Depression

○ Excessive weight loss or gain with insomnia or hypersomnia, anorexia, apathy, fatigue, suicidal thoughts, and feelings of worthlessness

Diabetes mellitus

○ Weight loss despite increased appetite
○ Polydipsia, polyuria, weakness, fatigue, and blurred vision

Esophagitis

○ Avoidance of eating and weight loss from painful inflammation of the esophagus
○ Intense pain in the mouth and anterior chest with hypersalivation, dysphagia, tachypnea, and hematemesis

Gastroenteritis

○ Malabsorption and dehydration cause sudden weight loss in acute viral infections or gradual weight loss in parasitic infections.
○ Other findings include poor skin turgor, dry mucous membranes, tachycardia, hypotension, diarrhea, abdominal pain and tenderness, hyperactive bowel sounds, nausea, vomiting, fever, and malaise.

Herpes simplex 1

○ Painful fluid-filled blisters in and around mouth make eating painful, causing decreased food intake and weight loss.
○ Fever and pharyngitis may also occur.

Leukemia

○ Acute form causes progressive weight loss; severe prostration; high fever; swollen, bleeding gums; and bleeding tendencies.
○ Chronic form causes progressive weight loss, malaise, fatigue, pallor, enlarged spleen, bleeding

tendencies, anemia, skin eruptions, anorexia, and fever.

Lymphoma
○ Gradual weight loss
○ Fever, fatigue, night sweats, malaise, hepatosplenomegaly, and lymphadenopathy

Pulmonary tuberculosis
○ Weight loss, fatigue, weakness, anorexia, night sweats, and low-grade fever
○ A cough with bloody or mucopurulent sputum, dyspnea, and pleuritic chest pain

Stomatitis
○ Weight loss from inability to eat caused by inflammation of the oral mucosa (usually red, swollen, and ulcerated)
○ Fever, increased salivation, malaise, mouth pain, anorexia, and swollen, bleeding gums

Thyrotoxicosis
○ Increased metabolism causes weight loss.
○ Other characteristic findings include nervousness, heat intolerance, diarrhea, increased appetite, palpitations, tachycardia, diaphoresis, fine tremor, an enlarged thyroid, and exophthalmos.

Ulcerative colitis
○ Weight loss is a late sign.
○ Bloody diarrhea with pus or mucus is an initial characteristic sign.
○ Weakness, crampy lower abdominal pain, tenesmus, anorexia, low-grade fever, and nausea and vomiting may also occur.

Other causes

Drugs
○ Amphetamines and inappropriate dosage of thyroid preparations commonly lead to weight loss.
○ Chemotherapeutics cause stomatitis, which, when severe, causes weight loss.
○ Laxative abuse may cause a malabsorptive state that leads to weight loss.

Nursing considerations

○ Take daily calorie counts and weigh the patient weekly.
○ Consult a nutritionist to determine an appropriate diet with adequate calories.
○ Administer hyperalimentation or tube feedings to maintain nutrition.

Pediatric pointers
○ In infants, weight loss may be from failure-to-thrive syndrome.

○ In children, severe weight loss may be the first indication of diabetes mellitus.

Geriatric pointers
○ Some elderly patients experience mild, gradual weight loss from changes in body composition.
○ Rapid, unintentional weight loss is highly predictive of morbidity and mortality in elderly patients.
○ Other causes include tooth loss, difficulty chewing, social isolation, and alcoholism.

Patient teaching
○ Provide guidance in proper diet and keeping a food diary.`
○ Instruct the patient in good oral hygiene.
○ Provide a referral to psychological counseling, if appropriate.

Wheezing

steroids, bronchodilators, and sedatives. Perform the abdominal thrust maneuver for airway obstruction.

Overview

- Adventitious breath sounds with a high-pitched, musical, squealing, creaking, or groaning quality
- Caused by air flowing at a high velocity through a narrowed airway
- Also known as *sibilant rhonchi*
- Can't be cleared by coughing

⚡ Emergency actions

Examine the degree of respiratory distress. (See Evaluating breath sounds.) Take other vital signs, and note hypotension or hypertension, decreased oxygen saturation, and an irregular, weak, rapid, or slow pulse. Help the patient relax, give humidified oxygen, and encourage slow, deep breathing. Have emergency resuscitation equipment readily available. Supply intermittent positive-pressure breathing and nebulization treatments with bronchodilators. Insert an I.V. line for administration for drugs, such as diuretics,

Assessment

History

- Ask what triggers wheezing.
- Ask about smoking habits.
- Find out about the onset, productivity, and frequency of coughing; obtain a description of any sputum.
- Inquire about a history of asthma, allergies, cancer, or pulmonary or cardiac disorders.
- Find out about recent surgery, illness, or trauma, or changes in appetite, weight, exercise tolerance, or sleep patterns.
- Take a drug history.
- Ask about exposure to irritants and toxic fumes.
- Ask about onset, quality, duration, intensity, aggravating or alleviating factors, and radiation of chest pain.

Physical assessment

- Examine the nose and mouth for congestion, drainage, or signs of infection.

🖐 Assessment tip
Evaluating breath sounds

Diminished or absent breath sounds indicate some interference with airflow. If pus, fluid, or air fills the pleural space, breath sounds will be quieter than normal. If a foreign body or secretions obstruct a bronchus, breath sounds will be diminished or absent over distal lung tissue. Increased thickness of the chest wall, such as with a patient who's obese or extremely muscular, may cause breath sounds to be decreased, distant, or inaudible. Absent breath sounds typically indicate loss of ventilation power.

When air passes through narrowed airways or through moisture, or when the membranes lining the chest cavity become inflamed, adventitious breath sounds will be heard. These include crackles, rhonchi, wheezes, and pleural friction rubs. Usually, these sounds indicate pulmonary disease.

Follow the auscultation sequences shown to assess the patient's breath sounds. Have the patient take full, deep breaths, and compare sound variations from one side to the other. Note the location, timing, and character of any abnormal breath sounds.

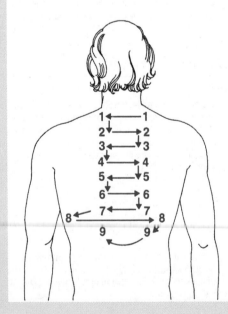

POSTERIOR

- If coughing produces sputum, obtain a sample for examination.
- Check for cyanosis, pallor, clamminess, masses, tenderness, swelling, distended neck veins, and enlarged lymph nodes.
- Inspect the chest for abnormal configuration and asymmetrical motion.
- Determine if the trachea is midline.
- Auscultate for crackles, rhonchi, or pleural friction rubs. *(See* Evaluating breath sounds.*)*
- Percuss for dullness or hyperresonance.
- Auscultate for heart and breath sounds.

Medical causes

Anaphylaxis

- Tracheal edema or bronchospasm can result in severe wheezing and stridor.
- Initial findings include fright, weakness, sneezing, dyspnea, nasal pruritus, urticaria, erythema, angioedema, and signs of respiratory distress.
- Other findings include nasal edema and congestion; profuse, watery rhinorrhea; chest or throat tightness; and dysphagia.

- Arrhythmias and hypotension may also result.

Aspiration of a foreign body

- Partial obstruction produces sudden onset of wheezing and possibly stridor; a dry, paroxysmal cough; gagging; and hoarseness.
- Other findings include tachycardia, dyspnea, decreased breath sounds, and possibly cyanosis.
- Fever, pain, and swelling may be produced by a retained foreign body.

Aspiration pneumonitis

- Wheezing with tachypnea, marked dyspnea, cyanosis, tachycardia, fever, productive (eventually purulent) cough, and pink, frothy sputum

Asthma

- Wheezing heard at the mouth during expiration is an initial and classic sign.
- An initially dry cough later becomes productive with thick mucus.
- Other findings include apprehension, prolonged expiration, intercostal and supraclavicular retractions, rhonchi, accessory muscle use, nasal flaring, and tachypnea.

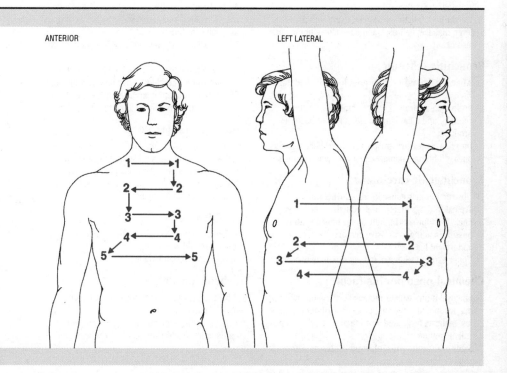

When wheezing stops

If you no longer hear wheezing in a patient having an acute asthma attack, the attack may be far from over. When bronchospasm and mucosal swelling become severe, little air can move through the airways. As a result, wheezing stops.

If all the assessment criteria — labored breathing, prolonged expiratory time, and accessory muscle use — point to acute bronchial obstruction (a medical emergency), maintain the patient's airway and give oxygen and medications as ordered to relieve the obstruction. The patient may begin to wheeze again when the airways open more.

○ Tachycardia, diaphoresis, and flushing or cyanosis also occur. (See *When wheezing stops.*)

Bronchial adenoma

○ Severe wheezing with chronic cough and recurring hemoptysis
○ In later stages, symptoms of airway obstruction

Bronchiectasis

○ Excessive mucus causes intermittent and localized or diffuse wheezing.
○ A copious, foul-smelling, mucopurulent cough is classic and is accompanied by hemoptysis, rhonchi, and coarse crackles.
○ Weight loss, fatigue, weakness, exertional dyspnea, fever, malaise, halitosis, and late-stage clubbing may also occur.

Bronchitis (chronic)

○ Wheezing that varies in severity, location, and intensity
○ Prolonged expiration, coarse crackles, scattered rhonchi, and a hacking cough that later becomes productive
○ Dyspnea, accessory muscle use, barrel chest, tachypnea, clubbing, edema, weight gain, and cyanosis

Bronchogenic carcinoma

○ Obstruction may cause localized wheezing.
○ Typical findings include a productive cough, dyspnea, hemoptysis (initially blood-tinged sputum, possibly leading to massive hemorrhage), anorexia, and weight loss.
○ Upper extremity edema and chest pain may occur.

Chemical pneumonitis (acute)

○ Mucosal injury causes increased secretions and edema, leading to wheezing, dyspnea, orthopnea, crackles, malaise, fever, and a productive cough with purulent sputum.
○ Signs of conjunctivitis, pharyngitis, laryngitis, and rhinitis may also occur.

Emphysema

○ Mild to moderate wheezing
○ Dyspnea, malaise, tachypnea, diminished breath sounds, peripheral cyanosis, pursed-lip breathing, accessory muscle use, barrel chest, a chronic productive cough, clubbing, anorexia, and malaise

Inhalation injury

○ Wheezing after initial findings of hoarseness and coughing, singed nasal hairs, orofacial burns, and soot-stained sputum
○ In later stages, crackles, rhonchi, and respiratory distress

Pneumothorax (tension)

○ A life-threatening disorder — wheezing, dyspnea, tachycardia, tachypnea, and sudden, severe, sharp chest pain (often one-sided)
○ A dry cough, cyanosis, accessory muscle use, asymmetrical chest wall movement, anxiety, and restlessness

Pulmonary coccidioidomycosis

○ Wheezing and rhonchi with cough, fever, chills, pleuritic chest pain, headache, weakness, fatigue, sore throat, backache, malaise, anorexia, and an itchy, macular rash

Pulmonary edema

○ A life-threatening disorder — wheezing with coughing, exertional and paroxysmal nocturnal dyspnea and, later, orthopnea
○ Tachycardia, tachypnea, crackles, and a diastolic gallop
○ In severe pulmonary edema, rapid, labored respirations; diffuse crackles; a productive cough and frothy, bloody sputum; arrhythmias; cold, clammy, cyanotic skin; hypotension; and thready pulse

Pulmonary tuberculosis

○ Fibrosis causes wheezing in the late stages.
○ Common findings include a mild to severe productive cough with pleuritic chest pain and fine crackles, night sweats, anorexia, weight loss, fever, malaise, dyspnea, and fatigue.

Thyroid goiter

○ Wheezing, dysphagia, and respiratory difficulty from a compressed airway
○ Swollen and distended neck

Tracheobronchitis

○ Wheezing, rhonchi, and moist or coarse crackles may be auscultated.
○ Related findings include a cough, fever, sudden chills, muscle and back pain, and substernal tightness.

Nursing considerations

○ Place the patient in semi-Fowler's position to ease breathing.
○ Perform pulmonary physiotherapy as necessary.
○ Give an antibiotic to treat infection, a bronchodilator to relieve bronchospasm and maintain patent airways, a steroid to reduce inflammation, and a mucolytic or expectorant to increase the flow of secretions.
○ Provide humidification to thin secretions.

Pediatric pointers

○ Primary causes of wheezing in children include bronchospasm, mucosal edema, and accumulation of secretions, which may occur with such disorders as cystic fibrosis, aspiration of a foreign body, acute bronchiolitis, and pulmonary hemosiderosis.
○ Children are especially susceptible to wheezing because their small airways allow rapid obstruction.

Patient teaching

○ Tell the patient how to promote drainage and prevent pooling of secretions, if needed.
○ Explain deep-breathing and coughing techniques.
○ Explain the importance of increasing fluid intake.
○ Provide information about taking prescribed drugs.

Additional signs and symptoms

Alternating pulse

○ A beat-to-beat change in the size and intensity of a peripheral pulse, but pulse rhythm remains regular; strong and weak pulsations alternate.

○ A sign of severe left-sided heart failure.

○ Have the patient hold his breath during palpation because the small changes in arterial pressure that occur during normal respirations may obscure this abnormal pulse.

○ Apply light pressure to avoid obliterating the weaker pulse.

Amnesia

○ Amnesia is a disturbance in, or loss of, memory.

○ *Anterograde amnesia* means memory loss for events that occurred after the onset of the causing trauma or disease.

○ *Retrograde amnesia* involves memory loss for events that occurred before the onset.

○ *Organic (true) amnesia* results from temporal lobe dysfunction; it characteristically spares patches of memory. A common symptom in patients with seizures or head trauma and an early indicator of Alzheimer's disease.

○ *Hysterical amnesia* has a psychogenic origin and characteristically causes complete memory loss.

○ *Treatment-induced amnesia* is usually transient.

Analgesia

○ The absence of sensitivity to pain that commonly indicates a specific type and location of spinal cord lesion.

○ Occurs with loss of temperature sensation (thermanesthesia).

○ Can also occur with such sensory deficits as paresthesia, loss of proprioception and vibratory sense, and tactile anesthesia in disorders involving the peripheral nerves, spinal cord, and brain. Analgesia is tested for by lightly touching different skin points with a pin.

Apnea

○ Breathing has stopped.

○ Common causes include trauma, cardiac arrest, neurologic disease, aspiration of foreign objects, bronchospasm, and drug overdose — life-threatening emergencies that require immediate intervention.

Apneustic respirations

○ Prolonged, gasping inspirations, with a pause at full inspiration.

○ An important localizing sign of severe brain stem damage.

Asterixis

○ A coarse movement, characterized by sudden relaxation of muscle groups holding a sustained posture.

○ Also known as a *liver flap* or *flapping tremor*.

○ Commonly observed in the wrists and fingers but may also appear during any sustained voluntary action.

○ Typically signals hepatic, renal, or pulmonary disease and may signal serious metabolic deterioration.

Biot's respirations

○ An irregular and unpredictable respiratory rate, rhythm, and depth.

○ A late and ominous sign of neurologic deterioration and may reflect increased pressure on the medulla coinciding with brain stem compression.

Breast dimpling

○ Puckering or retraction of skin on the breast from abnormal attachment of the skin to underlying tissue.

○ Suggests an inflammatory or malignant mass beneath the skin surface and usually represents a late sign of breast cancer.

○ Usually affects women older than age 40 but occasionally affects men.

Breast ulcer

○ The destruction of the skin and subcutaneous tissue on the nipple, areola, or the breast itself.

○ Usually a late sign of cancer, appearing well after the confirming diagnosis.

○ May be the first sign of breast cancer in men, who are more apt to dismiss earlier breast changes.

○ Can also result from trauma, infection, or radiation.

Buffalo hump

○ An accumulation of cervicodorsal fat.

○ May indicate hypercortisolism, resulting from long-term glucocorticoid therapy, adrenal carcinoma, adrenal adenoma, ectopic corticotropin production, or Cushing's disease.

Café-au-lait spots

○ Flat, light brown, uniformly hyperpigmented macules or patches on the skin surface.
○ Usually appear during the first 3 years of life but may develop at any age.
○ Can be differentiated from freckles and other benign birthmarks by their larger size (a few millimeters to ⅝" [1.5 cm] or larger) and irregular shape.
○ Usually have no significance; however, six or more café-au-lait spots may signal an underlying neurologic disorder such as neurofibromatosis.

Cat's cry

○ Mewing, kittenlike sound occurs during infancy.
○ The primary indicator of cat's cry (also known as *cri du chat*) syndrome and thought to result from abnormal laryngeal development.

Cold intolerance

○ Increased sensitivity to cold temperatures.
○ Reflects damage to the body's temperature-regulating mechanism, based on interactions between the hypothalamus and the thyroid gland.
○ In elderly patients, cold intolerance reflects normal age-related changes.

Corneal reflex, absent

○ The corneal reflex is tested by drawing a fine-pointed wisp of sterile cotton from a corner of each eye to the cornea. If both eyes blink, the reflex is present.
○ When the reflex is absent, neither eyelid closes when the cornea of one is touched.
○ Absence of the corneal reflex in one or both eyes may result from damage to the trigeminal or facial nerves (cranial nerves V and VII).

Cry, high-pitched

○ Characterized by a brief, sharp, piercing vocal sound produced by a neonate or infant.
○ Also called a *cephalic cry.*
○ A late sign of increased intracranial pressure (ICP).
○ The acute onset of a high-pitched cry demands emergency treatment to prevent permanent brain damage or death.

Depression

○ A mood disturbance that's characterized by feelings of sadness, despair, and loss of interest or pleasure in activities.
○ With changes in appetite, sleep disturbances, restlessness or lethargy, decreased concentration, and thoughts of injuring one's self, death, or suicide.

Drooling

○ The flow of saliva from the mouth.
○ May stem from facial muscle paralysis or weakness that prevents mouth closure, from neuromuscular disorders or local pain that causes dysphagia or, less commonly, from the effects of drugs or toxins that induce salivation.

○ Because it signals an inability to handle secretions, drooling warns of potential aspiration.

Dysmenorrhea

○ Painful menstruation.
○ May involve sharp, intermittent pain or dull, aching pain.
○ Usually characterized by mild to severe cramping or colicky pain in the pelvis or lower abdomen that may radiate to the thighs and lower sacrum.
○ The pain may precede menstruation by several days or may accompany it. The pain gradually subsides as bleeding tapers off.

Dyspareunia

○ Painful or difficult coitus.
○ May occur with attempted penetration or during or after coitus.
○ May stem from friction of the penis against perineal tissue or from jarring of deeper adnexal structures.
○ Common with pelvic disorders, but may also result from diminished vaginal lubrication from with aging, the effects of drugs, and psychological factors — most notably, fear of pain or injury.

Dystonia

○ Slow, involuntary movements of large-muscle groups in the limbs, trunk, and neck.
○ May involve flexion of the foot, hyperextension of the legs, extension and pronation of the arms, arching of the back, and extension and rotation of the neck (spasmodic torticollis).
○ Typically aggravated by walking and emotional stress and relieved by sleep.
○ May last just a few minutes or be continuous and painful. Occasionally, it causes permanent contractures, resulting in a grotesque posture.
○ May be hereditary or idiopathic, but usually results from extrapyramidal disorders or drugs.

Enophthalmos

○ The sinking of the eye into the orbit.
○ Usually from trauma, but may come from severe dehydration and eye disorders.
○ In elderly patients, senile atrophy of orbital fat may produce physiologic enophthalmos.
○ Because enophthalmos allows the upper lid to droop over the sunken eye, this sign is commonly mistaken for ptosis.

Enuresis

○ Night time urinary incontinence in girls age 5 and older and boys age 6 and older.
○ This sign rarely continues into adulthood but may occur in some adults with sleep apnea.
○ Primary enuresis describes a child who has never achieved bladder control.
○ Secondary enuresis describes a child who achieved bladder control for at least 3 months but has lost it.

- Delayed development of detrusor muscle control, unusually deep or sound sleep, organic disorders (such as urinary tract infection or obstruction), and psychological stress.
- Psychological stress — probably the most important factor — commonly results from the birth of a sibling, the death of a parent or loved one, divorce, or premature, rigorous toilet training.

Fasciculations

- Local muscle contractions, which represent the spontaneous discharge of a muscle fiber bundle innervated by a single motor nerve filament.
- Cause visible dimpling or wavelike twitching of the skin, but they aren't strong enough to cause a joint to move.
- Occur irregularly at frequencies ranging from once every several seconds to two or three times per second; infrequently, myokymia — continuous, rapid fasciculations that cause a rippling effect — may occur.
- Benign fasciculations are common and normal and occur in tense, anxious, or overtired people and typically affect the eyelid, thumb, or calf.
- May indicate a severe neurologic disorder, most notably a diffuse motor neuron disorder that causes loss of control over muscle fiber discharge or an early sign of pesticide poisoning.

Fetor hepaticus

- A distinctive musty, sweet breath odor.
- Characterizes hepatic encephalopathy, a life-threatening complication of severe liver disease.

Fontanel bulging

- Widened, tense, and pulsating fontanel in infants.
- A main sign of meningitis associated with increased intracranial pressure — a medical emergency.
- Can be an indication of encephalitis or fluid overload.
- Because prolonged coughing, crying, or lying down can cause normal, transient bulging, the infant's head should be observed and palpated while the infant is upright and relaxed to detect abnormal bulging.

Fontanel depression

- Depression of the anterior fontanel below the surrounding bony ridges of the skull.
- May be a sign of dehydration, possibly from insufficient fluid intake, but typically reflects excessive fluid loss from severe vomiting or diarrhea.
- May also reflect insensible water loss, pyloric stenosis, or tracheoesophageal fistula.
- To detect fontanel depression, it's best to assess the fontanel when the infant is in an upright position and isn't crying.

Gag reflex abnormalities

- Normal gag reflex, or pharyngeal reflex, is a protective mechanism that prevents aspiration of food, fluid, and vomitus.
- Elicited by touching the posterior wall of the oropharynx with a tongue depressor or by suctioning the throat.
- Prompt elevation of the palate, constriction of the pharyngeal musculature, and a sensation of gagging indicate a normal gag reflex.
- An abnormal gag reflex — either decreased or absent — interferes with the ability to swallow and, more important, increases susceptibility to life-threatening aspiration.
- An impaired gag reflex can result from any lesion that affects its mediators — cranial nerves IX (glossopharyngeal) and X (vagus) or the pons or medulla.
- Can also occur during a coma, in muscle diseases such as severe myasthenia gravis, or as a temporary result of anesthesia.

Gait, bizarre

- Also called a *hysterical gait*.
- Has no consistent pattern and no obvious organic basis but is produced unconsciously by a person with a somatoform disorder (hysterical neurosis) or consciously by a malingerer.
- May mimic an organic impairment but characteristically has a more theatrical or bizarre quality with key elements missing, such as a spastic gait without hip circumduction, or leg "paralysis" with normal reflexes and motor strength.
- May include wild gyrations, exaggerated stepping, leg dragging, or mimicking unusual walks, such as that of a tightrope walker.

Gait, propulsive

- Also called a *festinating gait*.
- The patient's head and neck are bent forward; his flexed, stiffened arms are held away from the body; his fingers are extended; and his knees and hips are stiffly bent. While walking, the body's center of gravity is shifted forward, impairing balance and causing increasingly rapid, short, shuffling steps with involuntary acceleration (festination) and lack of control over forward motion (propulsion) or backward motion (retropulsion).
- A classic sign of advanced Parkinson's disease.

Gait, scissors

- A stiff, short gait in which the thighs overlap with each step.
- The patient's legs flex slightly at the hips and knees, so he looks as if he's crouching.
- With each step, his thighs adduct and his knees hit or cross in a scissorslike movement. His steps are short, regular, and laborious, as if he were wading through waist-deep water. His feet may be plantar-flexed and turned inward, with a shortened Achilles

tendon; as a result, he walks on his toes or on the balls of his feet and may scrape his toes on the ground.
○ Results from bilateral spastic paresis (diplegia).

Gait, spastic

○ Sometimes referred to as paretic, hemiplegic, or weak gait.
○ A stiff, foot-dragging walk.
○ The affected leg becomes rigid, with a marked decrease in flexion at the hip and knee and possibly plantar flexion and equinovarus deformity of the foot.
○ Because the patient's leg doesn't swing normally at the hip or knee, his foot tends to drag or shuffle, scraping his toes on the ground.
○ To compensate, the pelvis of the affected side tilts upward in an attempt to lift the toes, causing the patient's leg to abduct and circumduct.
○ Also, arm swing is hindered on the same side as the affected leg.
○ Caused by one leg muscle's hypertonicity and indicates focal damage to the corticospinal tract.
○ Usually develops after a period of flaccidity (hypotonicity) in the affected leg.

Gait, steppage

○ Also called *equine, paretic, prancing,* or *weak steppage gait.*
○ The foot hangs with the toes pointing down while taking a step.
○ Typically results from footdrop caused by weakness or paralysis of pretibial and peroneal muscles, usually from lower motor neuron lesions, causing the foot to scrape on the ground.
○ To compensate, the hip rotates outward and the hip and knee flex in an exaggerated fashion to lift the advancing leg off the ground. The foot is thrown forward and the toes hit the ground first, producing an audible slap.
○ The rhythm of the gait is usually regular, with even steps and normal upper body posture and arm swing.

Gait, waddling

○ A ducklike walk.
○ An important sign of muscular dystrophy, spinal muscle atrophy or, rarely, congenital hip displacement.
○ Results from deterioration of the pelvic girdle muscles — primarily the gluteus medius, hip flexors, and hip extensors. Weakness in these muscles hinders stabilization of the weight-bearing hip during walking, causing the opposite hip to drop and the trunk to lean toward that side in an attempt to maintain balance.
○ Typically, the legs assume a wide stance and the trunk is thrown back to further improve stability, exaggerating lordosis and abdominal protrusion.

○ In severe cases, leg and foot muscle contractures may cause equinovarus deformity of the foot combined with circumduction or bowing of the legs.

Gum swelling

○ An increase in the size of existing gum cells (hypertrophy) or an increase in their number (hyperplasia).
○ May involve one or many papillae — the triangular bits of gum between adjacent teeth.
○ Usually results from the effects of phenytoin; less commonly, from nutritional deficiency and certain systemic disorders.
○ Happens normally during the first and second trimesters of pregnancy when hormonal changes make the gums highly vascular; even slight irritation causes swelling and gives the papillae a characteristic raspberry hue (pregnancy epulis).
○ Irritating dentures may also cause swelling associated with red, soft, movable masses on the gums.

Heat intolerance

○ The inability to withstand high temperatures or to maintain a comfortable body temperature.
○ Produces a continuous feeling of being overheated and, at times, profuse diaphoresis.
○ Mainly results from thyrotoxicosis.
○ Although rare, hypothalamic disease may also cause intolerance to heat and cold.

Hiccups

○ Also called a *singultus.*
○ An involuntary, spasmodic contraction of the diaphragm followed by sudden closure of the glottis. The characteristic sound reflects the vibration of closed vocal cords as air suddenly rushes into the lungs.
○ In a patient with a neurologic disorder, may indicate increasing intracranial pressure or extension of a brain stem lesion.
○ May also occur after ingestion of hot or cold liquids or other irritants, after exposure to cold, or with irritation from a drainage tube.
○ Persistent hiccups cause considerable distress and may lead to vomiting.
○ Increased level of carbon dioxide may inhibit hiccups; decreased level may accentuate them.

Hyperpigmentation

○ Also called *hypermelanosis.*
○ Excessive skin coloring that usually reflects overproduction, abnormal location, or maldistribution of the pigment melanin.
○ Can also reflect abnormalities of other skin pigments: carotenoids (yellow), oxyhemoglobin (red), and hemoglobin (blue).
○ Most commonly results from exposure to sunlight.
○ Can also result from metabolic, endocrine, neoplastic, and inflammatory disorders; chemical poisoning; drugs; genetic defects; thermal burns; ionizing radia-

tion; and localized activation by sunlight of certain photosensitizing chemicals on the skin.
- Many types of benign hyperpigmented lesions occur normally.
- Some, such as acanthosis nigricans and carotenemia, may also accompany certain disorders.
- Chronic nutritional insufficiency may lead to dyspigmentation—increased pigmentation in some areas and decreased pigmentation in others.

Hypopigmentation

- Also called *hypomelanosis*
- A decrease in normal skin, hair, mucous membrane, or nail color from deficiency, absence, or abnormal degradation of the pigment melanin.
- Caused by genetic disorders, nutritional deficiency, chemicals and drugs, inflammation, infection, and physical trauma.

Janeway lesions

- Small erythematous lesions on the palms and soles that are slightly raised but usually flat, irregular, and nontender and disappear spontaneously.
- Blanch with pressure or elevation of the affected extremity and occasionally, form a diffuse rash over the trunk and extremities.
- Were once a common finding in those with infective endocarditis, possibly reflecting an immunologic reaction to the infecting organisms (usually bacteria), but are rarely seen today because the disease is now detected and managed at an earlier stage.

Kehr's sign

- Referred to as left shoulder pain.
- Elicited when the patient assumes the supine position or lowers his head, increasing the contact of free blood or clots with the left diaphragm and involving the phrenic nerve.
- A classic sign of hemorrhage within the peritoneal cavity or a ruptured spleen, but also occurs in ruptured ectopic pregnancy.

Lid lag

- Also called *Graefe's sign.*
- The inability of the upper eyelid to follow the eye's downward movements.
- To test for the sign, hold a finger, penlight, or other target above the patient's eye level and then move it downward, observing eyelid movement as his eyes follow the target.
- The sign is positive when a rim of sclera appears between the upper lid margin and the iris when the patient lowers his eyes, when one lid closes more slowly than the other, or when both lids close slowly and incompletely with jerky movements.
- A classic sign of thyrotoxicosis.

Low birth weight

- Neonates born weighing less than the normal minimum birth weight of 2,500 g.

- A premature neonate born before the 37th week of gestation weighs an appropriate amount for his gestational age and probably would have matured normally if carried to term, but the small-for-gestational-age (SGA) neonate weighs less than the normal amount for his age except his organs are mature.
- Can signal a life-threatening emergency.
- Usually results from a disorder that prevents the uterus from retaining the fetus, interferes with the normal course of pregnancy, causes premature separation of the placenta, or stimulates uterine contractions before term.
- In the SGA neonate, intrauterine growth may be retarded by a disorder that interferes with placental circulation, fetal development, or associated with higher neonate morbidity and mortality.

Masklike facies

- A total loss of facial expression.
- Results from bradykinesia usually from extrapyramidal damage.
- The rate of eye blinking is reduced to 1 to 4 blinks per minute, producing a characteristic reptilian stare.
- The sign often develops insidiously, at first mistaken by the observer for depression or apathy.
- A neurologic disorder is the most common cause.
- Can result from certain systemic diseases and the effects of drugs and toxins.

Menorrhagia

- Abnormally heavy or long menstrual bleeding.
- Can result from endocrine and hematologic disorders, stress, and certain drugs and procedures.

Metrorrhagia

- Uterine bleeding that occurs irregularly between menstrual periods.
- Usually light bleeding, although it can range from staining to hemorrhage.
- Reflects slight bleeding from the endometrium during ovulation.
- May be the only indication of an underlying gynecologic disorder.
- Can result from stress, drugs, treatments, and intrauterine devices.

Miosis

- Pupillary constriction.
- Occurs normally as a response to fatigue, increased light, or administration of a miotic; as part of the eye's accommodation reflex; and as part of the aging process.
- Can stem from an ocular or neurologic disorder, trauma, use of a systemic drug, or contact lens overuse.
- A rare form of miosis—Argyll Robertson pupils—can stem from tabes dorsalis and neurologic disorders; miotic (often pinpoint), unequal, and irregularly shaped pupils don't dilate properly with mydri-

atic use and fail to react to light, although they do constrict on accommodation.

Moon face

○ A distinctive facial adiposity.
○ Marked facial roundness and puffiness, a double chin, a prominent upper lip, and full supraclavicular fossae.
○ Usually indicates hypercortisolism resulting from ectopic or excessive pituitary production of corticotropin, adrenal adenoma or carcinoma, or long-term glucocorticoid therapy.

Muscle flaccidity

○ Profoundly weak and soft muscles that have decreased resistance to movement, increased mobility, and greater than normal range of motion.
○ Results from disrupted muscle innervation and can be localized to a limb or muscle group or generalized over the entire body.
○ Onset may be acute, as in trauma, or chronic, as in neurologic disease.

Nasal flaring

○ The abnormal dilation of the nostrils.
○ Usually during inspiration, but occasionally during expiration or throughout the respiratory cycle.
○ Indicates respiratory dysfunction, ranging from mild difficulty to potentially life-threatening respiratory distress.

Paroxysmal nocturnal dyspnea

○ An attack of dyspnea that abruptly awakens the patient.
○ A sign of left-sided heart failure.
○ May result from decreased respiratory drive, impaired left ventricular function, enhanced reabsorption of interstitial fluid, or increased thoracic blood volume.
○ Diaphoresis, coughing, wheezing, and chest discomfort.
○ Attack subsides after the patient sits up or stands for several minutes, but may recur every 2 to 3 hours.

Pica

○ Craving and ingestion of normally inedible substances, such as plaster, charcoal, clay, wool, ashes, paint, or dirt.
○ Typically from nutritional deficiencies with children are most commonly affected.
○ Commonly seen in pregnant patients and may be associated with iron deficiency anemia.
○ May reflect a psychological disturbance.
○ Can lead to poisoning and GI disorders.

Postnasal drip

○ Nasal discharge, frequent throat clearing, and mucoid or mucopurulent secretions in the posterior pharynx suggest postnasal drip, typically from infection or allergies.

○ A thick, tenacious, and purulent discharge suggests infection, whereas a watery discharge usually suggests an allergy.
○ Can be from environmental irritants.

Priapism

○ A urologic emergency characterized by a persistent, painful erection that's unrelated to sexual excitation.
○ This relatively rare sign may begin during sleep and appear to be a normal erection, but it may last for several hours or days.
○ With a severe, constant, dull aching in the penis.
○ Despite the pain, the patient may be too embarrassed to seek medical help. He may try to achieve detumescence through continued sexual activity.
○ Without prompt treatment, penile ischemia and thrombosis occur.
○ In about half of all cases, priapism is idiopathic and develops without apparent predisposing factors.
○ Secondary priapism can result from a blood disorder, neoplasm, trauma, or use of certain drugs.

Psoas sign

○ Evident if the patient experiences increased abdominal pain when he moves his leg against resistance.
○ A positive psoas sign indicates direct or reflexive irritation of the psoas muscles that can be elicited on the right or left side.
○ Usually indicates appendicitis but may also occur with localized abscesses.
○ Elicit in a patient with abdominal or lower back pain after completion of an abdominal examination to prevent spurious assessment findings.

Purple striae

○ Thin, purple streaks on the skin.
○ Characteristically occur in hypercortisolism along with other cushingoid signs, such as a buffalo hump and moon face.
○ Although hypercortisolism can be caused by adrenocortical carcinoma, adrenal adenoma, and pituitary adenoma, it usually results from excessive use of glucocorticoids.
○ Although purple striae are most common over the abdominal area, they may also occur over the breasts, hips, buttocks, thighs, and axillae.

Salt craving

○ A compensatory response to the body's failure to adequately conserve sodium.
○ From drenal insufficiency (primary) and adrenal crisis, a potentially fatal condition.

Seizures, absence

○ Benign, generalized seizures thought to originate subcortically of unknown cause.
○ Usually last 3 to 20 seconds and can occur 100 or more times a day and without warning.
○ Usually begin between ages 4 and 12, first noticed as deteriorating schoolwork and behavior.

- The patient suddenly stops all purposeful activity and stares blankly ahead, as if he were daydreaming.
- They may produce automatisms, such as repetitive lip smacking, or mild clonic or myoclonic movements, including mild jerking of the eyelids. The patient may drop an object that he's holding, and muscle relaxation may cause him to drop his head or arms or to slump. After the attack, the patient resumes activity, typically unaware of the episode.

Setting-sun sign

- Also known as *sunset eyes*.
- A late and ominous sign of increased intracranial pressure on cranial nerves III, IV, and VI in an infant or young child.
- Both eyes are rotated downward, typically revealing an area of sclera above the irises; occasionally, the irises appear to be forced outward.
- Pupils are sluggish, responding to light unequally.

Spider angioma

- Also known as an *arterial spider*, a s*pider nevus*, a *spider telangiectasia*, a *stellate angioma*, or a *vascular spider*.
- A fiery red vascular lesion with an elevated central body, branching spiderlike legs, and a surrounding flush.
- A form of telangiectasia, this characteristic lesion ranges from a few millimeters to several centimeters in diameter and may occur singly or in multiples.
- Usually appear on the face and neck; less commonly, they occur on the shoulders, thorax, arms, backs of the hands and fingers, and mucous membranes of the lips and nose.
- Typically associated with cirrhosis but can also be found in hyperestrogenism such in pregnant women or in those taking hormonal contraceptives.
- May erupt in the second or third month of pregnancy, enlarge and multiply, then disappear about 6 weeks after delivery.
- May also appear in elderly patients.

Tics

- An involuntary, repetitive movement of a specific group of muscles—usually those of the face, neck, shoulders, trunk, and hands.
- Typically occurs suddenly and intermittently.
- May involve a single isolated movement, such as lip smacking, grimacing, blinking, sniffing, tongue thrusting, throat clearing, hitching up one shoulder, or protruding the chin or it may involve a complex set of movements. Mild tics, such as twitching of an eyelid, are especially common.
- Usually psychogenic and may be aggravated by stress or anxiety.
- Commonly begin between ages 5 and 10 as voluntary, coordinated, and purposeful actions that the child feels compelled to perform to decrease anxiety.
- Also associated with Tourette syndrome.

Tracheal tugging

- Known as *Cardarelli's sign, Castellino's sign,* or *Oliver's sign.*
- A visible recession of the larynx and trachea that occurs in synchrony with cardiac systole.
- Commonly results from an aneurysm or a tumor near the aortic arch.
- May signal dangerous compression or obstruction of major airways. The tugging movement, best observed with the patient's neck hyperextended, reflects abnormal transmission of aortic pulsations because of compression and distortion of the heart, esophagus, great vessels, airways, and nerves.

Trismus

- Commonly known as *lockjaw.*
- The prolonged and painful tonic spasm of the masticatory jaw muscles.
- A characteristic early sign of tetanus produced by the neuromuscular effects of tetanospasmin, a potentially lethal exotoxin.
- Can also result from drug therapy; occasionally, a milder form may accompany neuromuscular involvement in other disorders or infection or disease of the jaw, teeth, parotid glands, or tonsils.

Uremic frost

- A fine white powder, believed to be urate crystals, that covers the skin.
- A characteristic sign of end-stage renal failure or uremia. The frost typically appears on the face, neck, axillae, groin, and genitalia.

Urine cloudiness

- Cloudy, murky, or turbid urine.
- Reflects the presence of bacteria, mucus, leukocytes or erythrocytes, epithelial cells, fat, or phosphates (in alkaline urine).
- Characteristic of urinary tract infection but can also result from prolonged storage of a urine specimen at room temperature.

Violent behavior

- The use of physical force to violate, injure, or abuse an object or person, sometimes self-directed.
- It may result from an organic or psychiatric disorder or from the use of certain drugs.

Wristdrop

- The flexed position of the hand from paresis of the extensor muscles of the hand, wrist, and fingers.
- May be slight or severe and temporary or permanent.
- May occur unilaterally and suddenly with a radial nerve injury or bilaterally and gradually with a neurologic disorder, such as myasthenia gravis, Guillain-Barré syndrome, or multiple sclerosis.

Evaluating a symptom

Your patient may be vague in describing his chief complaint. Using your interviewing skills, you may discover his problem is related to abdominal distention. Now what? This flowchart will help you decide what to do next, using abdominal distention as the patient's chief complaint.

Ask the patient to identify what's bothering him physically. He tells you, "My stomach gets bloated."

↓

Form a first impression. Does the patient's condition alert you to an emergency? For example, does he say the bloating developed suddenly? Does he mention that other signs or symptoms occur with it, such as sweating or light-headedness? (Both are indicators of hypovolemia.)

YES

Take a brief history to gather more clues. For example, ask the patient if he has severe abdominal pain or difficulty breathing or if he ever had an abdominal injury.

↓

Perform a focused physical examination to quickly determine the severity of the patient's condition. Check for bruising, lacerations, abnormal bowel sounds, or abdominal rigidity.

NO

Take a thorough history to get an overview of the patient's condition. Ask him about associated signs or symptoms. Note especially GI disorders that can lead to abdominal distention.

↓

Thoroughly examine the patient to evaluate the chief sign or symptom and to detect additional signs and symptoms.
Place the patient in a recumbent position, and observe him for abdominal asymmetry. Inspect the skin, auscultate for bowel sounds, percuss and palpate the abdomen, and measure his abdomina girth.

Evaluate your findings. Are emergency signs or symptoms present, such as abdominal rigidity or abnormal bowel sounds?

YES

Based on your findings, intervene appropriately to stabilize the patient's condition. Notify the doctor immediately, place the patient in a supine position, administer oxygen, and start an I.V. line. GI or nasogastric tube insertion and emergency surgery may be needed.

↓

After the patient's condition is stabilized, review your findings to consider possible causes, such as trauma, large-bowel obstruction, mesenteric artery occlusion, or peritonitis.

NO

Review your findings to consider possible causes, such as cancer, bladder distention, cirrhosis, heart failure, or gastric dilation.

↓

Evaluate your findings and devise an appropriate care plan. Position the patient comfortably, give analgesics, and prepare the patient for diagnostic tests.

Selected references

Andrews, M., and Boyle, J. *Transcultural Concepts in Nursing Care,* 4th ed. Philadelphia: Lippincott Williams & Wilkins, 2003.

Baranoski, S., and Ayello, E.A. *Wound Care Essentials: Practice Principles.* Philadelphia: Lippincott Williams & Wilkins, 2004.

Bender, K., and Thompson, F.E., Jr. "West Nile Virus: A Growing Challenge," *AJN* 103(6):32-39, June 2003.

Berry, B., and Pinard, A. "Assessing Tissue Oxygenation," *Critical Care Nurse* 22(3):22-40, June 2002.

Bickley, L.S. *Bates' Guide to Physical Examination and History Taking,* 8th ed. Philadelphia: Lippincott Williams & Wilkins, 2005.

Braunwald, E., et al. *Harrison's Manual of Medicine,* 15th ed. New York: McGraw-Hill Professional, 2003.

ECG Interpretation. Just the Facts series. Philadelphia: Lippincott Williams & Wilkins, 2005.

Eliopoulos, C. *Gerontological Nursing,* 6th ed. Philadelphia: Lippincott Williams & Wilkins, 2005.

Fetrow, C.W., and Avila, J.R. *Professional's Handbook of Complementary and Alternative Medicines,* 3rd ed. Philadelphia: Lippincott Williams & Wilkins, 2004.

Green-Hernandez, C., et al. *Primary Care Pediatrics.* Philadelphia: Lippincott Williams & Wilkins, 2001.

Habif, T.P. *Clinical Dermatology,* 4th ed. St. Louis: Mosby–Year Book, Inc., 2004.

Henderson, D., et al. *Bioterrorism: Guidelines for Medical and Public Health Management.* Chicago: American Medical Association, 2002.

Hickey, J. *The Clinical Practice of Neurological and Neurosurgical Nursing,* 5th ed. Philadelphia: Lippincott Williams & Wilkins, 2003.

Hockenberry, M.J., et al. *Wong's Nursing Care of Infants and Children,* 7th ed. St. Louis: Mosby–Year Book, Inc., 2003.

Ignatavicius, D.D., and Workman, M. L. *Medical-Surgical Nursing: Critical Thinking for Collaborative Care,* 4th ed. Philadelphia: W.B. Saunders Co., 2002.

Kemp, C. "Bioterrorism: Introduction and Major Agents," *Journal of the American Academy of Nurse Practitioners* 13(11):483-91, November 2001.

Kozier, B., et al. *Fundamentals of Nursing: Concepts, Process, and Practice,* 7th ed. Upper Saddle River, N.J.: Prentice Hall Health, 2004.

Pillitteri, A. *Maternal and Child Health Nursing,* 4th ed. Philadelphia: Lippincott Williams & Wilkins, 2003.

Porth, C.M. *Pathophysiology,* 7th ed. Philadelphia: Lippincott Williams & Wilkins, 2005.

Professional Guide to Pathophysiology. Philadelphia: Lippincott Williams & Wilkins, 2003.

Rakel, R., and Bope, E. *Conn's Current Therapy 2004.* Philadelphia: W.B. Saunders Co., 2003.

Shives, L. *Basic Concepts of Psychiatric-Mental Health Nursing,* 6th ed. Philadelphia: Lippincott Williams & Wilkins, 2005.

Tierney, L., et al. *Current Medical Diagnosis and Treatment 2004,* 43rd ed. New York: McGraw-Hill/Appleton & Lange, 2004.

Woods, S., et al. *Cardiac Nursing,* 5th ed. Philadelphia: Lippincott Williams & Wilkins, 2005.

Index

i refers to an illustration; t refers to a table.

i refers to an illustration; t refers to a table.

Arteriosclerotic occlusive disease,
    cyanosis in, 118
Arteriovenous malformation,
    intracranial, tinnitus in, 418
Arthritis. *See also specific type.*
    jaw pain in, 228
    paresthesia in, 302
Asbestosis, pleural rub in, 312
Aspiration pneumonitis
    productive cough in, 112
    wheezing in, 463
Asterixis, 468
Asthma
    accessory muscle use in, 12
    anxiety in, 28
    barrel chest in, 45
    chest pain in, 84, 85
    crackles in, 114
    dyspnea in, 144
    grunting respirations in, 356
    nonproductive cough in, 108
    productive cough in, 112
    rhonchi in, 368
    shallow respirations in, 358
    tachypnea in, 408
    wheezing in, 463-464
Asthma attack, costal and sternal
    retractions in, 364
Ataxia, 36-37
Atelectasis
    nonproductive cough in, 108
    shallow respirations in, 358
    tracheal deviation in, 420
Atherosclerosis
    blood pressure increase in, 52
    bruits in, 75
    of the carotid artery, tinnitus in,
        418
Athetosis, 38-39
    distinguishing, from chorea, 38i
Atonic seizures, 380
Atopic dermatitis. *See also* Dermatitis.
    erythema in, 162
    pruritus in, 320
Atrial fibrillation, pulse rhythm in,
    337t
Atrial gallop, 184-185
Atrioventricular block, atrial gallop
    in, 185
Atrophic vaginitis
    postmenopausal vaginal bleeding
        in, 436
    vaginal discharge in, 438
Aural polyps, otorrhea in, 288
Autonomic hyperreflexia
    anxiety in, 28
    diaphoresis in, 128

B
Babinski's reflex, 40-41
    testing for, 41i

Back pain, 42-43
    severe, managing, 42
Bacteremia, chills and, 90
Balanitis, genital lesions in male in,
    188
Balanoposthitis, genital lesions in
    male in, 188
Barbiturate withdrawal, generalized
    tonic-clonic seizures in, 384
Barotrauma, earache in, 148
Barrel chest, 44-45, 44i
Basal cell carcinoma, vulvar lesions
    in, 456, 457i
Basal ganglia, calcification of,
    athetosis in, 38
Basilar artery insufficiency, dysarthria
    in, 138
Basilar skull fracture
    Battle's sign in, 46
    nasal obstruction in, 266
    otorrhea in, 288
    raccoon eyes in, 350-351
    rhinorrhea in, 366
    taste abnormalities in, 410
Battle's sign, 46-47
Bell's palsy
    increased salivation in, 374
    paralysis in, 300
    taste abnormalities in, 410
Benign cysts, vulvar lesions in, 456,
    457i
Benign positional vertigo, 442
Benign prostatic hyperplasia
    bladder distention in, 48
    nocturia in, 274
    urinary frequency in, 428
    urinary incontinence in, 430
Bile duct cancer, clay-colored stools
    in, 400
Biliary cirrhosis
    bronze skin in, 388
    clay-colored stools in, 400
Biliary obstruction, epistaxis in, 158
Biliary surgery, clay-colored stools
    and, 400
Biot's respirations, 468
Bizarre language, 322
Bladder calculi
    hematuria in, 206
    urinary frequency in, 428
    urinary incontinence in, 430
    urinary urgency in, 432
Bladder cancer
    bladder distention in, 48
    dysuria in, 146
    flank pain in, 178
    hematuria in, 206
    nocturia in, 274
    urinary frequency in, 428
    urinary incontinence in, 430

Bladder distention, 48-49
    abdominal distention in, 2
    abdominal mass in, 4
Bladder trauma, hematuria in, 206
Blastomycosis, pustular rash in, 346
Blepharitis
    conjunctival injection in, 100
    eye pain in, 168
Blood pressure
    decrease in, 50-51
    increase in, 52-53
Blumberg's sign. *See* Rebound
    tenderness.
Bone cancer, leg pain in, 234
Botulism
    dysarthria in, 138
    dysphagia in, 142
    hypoactive deep tendon reflexes in,
        126
    nonreactive pupils in, 340
    ptosis in, 324
Bowel obstruction, halitosis in, 194
Bowel sounds
    absent, 54-55
    characteristics of, 56
    hyperactive, 56-57
    hypoactive, 58-59
    silent, 54-55
Bowen's disease
    genital lesions in male in, 188
    scaly skin in, 394
Bradycardia, 60-61
    life-threatening, 60
Bradypnea, 62-63
Brain abscess
    aphasia in, 30
    apraxia in, 32
    complex partial seizures in, 381
    decorticate posture in, 122
    decreased level of consciousness
        in, 236
    generalized tonic-clonic seizures
        in, 383
    headache in, 196
    simple partial seizures in, 386-387
Brain stem infarction
    absent doll's eye reflex in, 136
    decerebrate posture in, 120
Brain stem ischemia, vertigo in, 442
Brain stem tumor
    absent doll's eye reflex in, 136
    decerebrate posture in, 120
Brain tumor
    anosmia and, 24
    aphasia in, 30
    apraxia in, 32-33
    athetosis in, 38
    Babinski's reflex in, 40
    confusion in, 98
    decorticate posture in, 122-123
    decreased level of consciousness
        in, 236

i refers to an illustration; t refers to a table.

i refers to an illustration; t refers to a table.

Cerebral aneurysm *(continued)*
ptosis in, 324
Cerebral contusion, decreased level
of consciousness in, 236
Cerebral infarction
athetosis in, 38
chorea in, 92
Cerebral lesion, decerebrate posture
in, 120
Cerebral perfusion, decreased,
confusion in, 98
Cerumen impaction, earache in, 148
Cervical cancer, postmenopausal
vaginal bleeding in, 436
Cervical extension injury, neck pain
in, 270
Cervical nerve root compression, arm
pain in, 34
Cervical polyps, postmenopausal
vaginal bleeding in, 436
Cervical spinal injury, bradycardia in,
60
Cervical spine fracture, neck pain in,
270
Cervical spine tumor, neck pain in,
270
Cervical spondylosis
neck pain in, 270
tinnitus in, 418
Cervical stenosis, neck pain in, 270
Chalazion
eye pain in, 168
facial edema in, 154
Chancroid, genital lesions in male in,
188, 189i
Chemical burns, conjunctival
injection in, 100
Chemical irritants
dysuria and, 147
epistaxis and, 159
gum bleeding and, 191
Chemical pneumonitis
crackles in, 114
productive cough in, 112
wheezing in, 464
Chest expansion, asymmetrical, 82-83
recognizing life-threatening causes
of, 83i
Chest pain, 84-87
severe, managing, 85
Chest physiotherapy, positioning
infant for, 357i
Cheyne-Stokes respirations, 88-89
respiratory pattern of, 88i
Chills, 90-91
Chinese restaurant syndrome, chest
pain in, 87
Chlamydial infection, vaginal
discharge in, 438
Cholangitis
chills in, 90
clay-colored stools in, 400

Cholangitis *(continued)*
jaundice in, 226
Cholecystitis
abdominal mass in, 4
abdominal pain in, 6-7
chest pain in, 85
jaundice in, 226
nausea in, 268
vomiting in, 452
Cholelithiasis
abdominal mass in, 4
abdominal pain in, 7
clay-colored stools in, 400
dyspepsia in, 140
jaundice in, 226
nausea in, 268
vomiting in, 452
Cholera
blood pressure decrease in, 50
decreased skin turgor in, 396
muscle spasms in, 254
vomiting in, 452
Cholestasis, jaundice in, 226
Cholesteatoma, hearing loss in, 200
Cholesterol emboli, purpura in, 344
Cholinergics, increased tearing and,
413
Chondrodermatitis nodularis
chronica, earache in, 148
Chorea, 92-93
distinguishing, from athetosis, 38i
Choriocarcinoma, nipple discharge
in, 272
Chorioretinitis, scotoma in, 376-377
Chronic bronchitis
accessory muscle use in, 12
barrel chest in, 45
crackles in, 114
hemoptysis in, 210
nonproductive cough in, 108
productive cough in, 112
tachypnea in, 408
wheezing in, 464
Chronic fatigue syndrome
fatigue in, 172
lymphadenopathy in, 240
throat pain in, 414
Chronic obstructive pulmonary
disease
anxiety in, 28
cyanosis in, 118
fatigue in, 172
orthopnea in, 284
paradoxical pulse in, 298
tachycardia in, 406
Chronic renal failure. *See also* Acute
renal failure *and* Renal failure.
agitation in, 14
anorexia in, 22
bronze skin in, 389
generalized tonic-clonic seizures
in, 384

Chronic renal failure *(continued)*
gynecomastia in, 192
halitosis in, 194-195
nocturia in, 274-275
oliguria in, 282
pruritus in, 321
Chvostek's sign, 94-95
eliciting, 94i
Cirrhosis
abdominal distention in, 2
abdominal pain in, 7
anorexia in, 22
dyspepsia in, 140
epistaxis in, 158
flatulence in, 180
generalized edema in, 150
gum bleeding in, 190
gynecomastia in, 192
hepatomegaly in, 212
jaundice in, 226
nausea in, 268
splenomegaly in, 398
vomiting in, 452
Clonic seizures, 380
Clostridium difficile infection,
diarrhea in, 130
Clubbing, 96-97
checking for, 96i
Cluster headache, rhinorrhea in, 366
Coagulation disorders
epistaxis in, 158
hematemesis in, 202
hematochezia in, 204
hematuria in, 206
hemoptysis in, 210
Coarctation of the aorta, absent or
weak pulse in, 326
Cold intolerance, 469
Colitis, hematochezia in, 204
Colon cancer
abdominal mass in, 4
flatulence in, 180
hematochezia in, 204
melena in, 246
Colorectal polyps, hematochezia in,
204
Common cold
halitosis in, 194
nasal obstruction in, 266
nonproductive cough in, 109
productive cough in, 112
rhinorrhea in, 366
taste abnormalities in, 410
throat pain in, 414
Compartment syndrome
arm pain in, 34
leg pain in, 234
muscle atrophy in, 252
Complex partial seizures, 380-381
Concussion
vision loss in, 446
visual blurring in, 450

i refers to an illustration; t refers to a table.

i refers to an illustration; t refers to a table.

i refers to an illustration; t refers to a table.

i refers to an illustration; t refers to a table.

i refers to an illustration; t refers to a table.

i refers to an illustration; t refers to a table.

Hepatic encephalopathy
  agitation in, 14
  apraxia in, 33
  athetosis in, 38
  decerebrate posture in, 120
  generalized tonic-clonic seizures
    in, 383
  halitosis in, 194
  hyperactive deep tendon reflexes
    in, 124
  myoclonus in, 264
Hepatic porphyria, constipation in,
  102
Hepatitis
  abdominal pain in, 8
  anorexia in, 23
  clay-colored stools in, 400
  dyspepsia in, 140
  epistaxis in, 158
  hepatomegaly in, 212
  jaundice in, 227
  nausea in, 268
  splenomegaly in, 398
  taste abnormalities in, 410
  vomiting in, 453
Hepatobiliary disease, pruritus in,
  320
Hepatocerebral degeneration, ataxia
  in, 36
Hepatomegaly, 212-213
  abdominal mass in, 5
Herbal products, flatulence and, 180
Hereditary angioedema, urticaria in,
  435
Hernia, scrotal swelling in, 378
Herniated disk
  footdrop in, 182
  Kernig's sign in, 232
  muscle atrophy in, 252
  muscle weakness in, 258
  neck pain in, 270
  paresthesia in, 302
Herpes simplex
  excessive weight loss in, 460
  mouth lesions in, 248
  throat pain in, 414
  vaginal discharge in, 438
  vesicular rash in 444
  vulvar lesions in, 456, 457i
Herpes zoster
  abdominal pain in, 8
  chest pain in, 85
  increased tearing in, 413
  mouth lesions in, 248
  nipple discharge in, 272
  paresthesia in, 302
  pruritus in, 320
  sluggish pupils in, 342
  vertigo in, 442
  vesicular rash in, 444
  vision loss in, 447

Herpes zoster ophthalmicus
  eye discharge in, 166-167
  eye pain in, 169
  facial edema in, 154
Herpes zoster oticus
  earache in, 148
  facial pain in, 170
Hiatal hernia
  chest pain in, 85
  dyspepsia in, 140
  pyrosis in, 348
  tracheal deviation in, 420
Hiccups, 471
High cardiac output states, pulsus
  biferiens in, 339
Hirsutism, 214-215
Histoplasmosis, splenomegaly in, 398
Hives, 434-435, 434i
Hoarseness, 216-217
Hodgkin's disease
  alopecia in, 16
  chills in, 90
  diaphoresis in, 128
  lymphadenopathy in, 240
  muscle weakness in, 258
  neck pain in, 270
  nonproductive cough in, 109
  pruritus in, 320
Homans' sign, 218-219
  eliciting, 218i
Hordeolum
  eye pain in, 169
  facial edema in, 154
Human immunodeficiency virus
  infection, papular rash in, 296
Huntington's disease
  athetosis in, 38
  chorea in, 92
Hydrocele, scrotal swelling in, 378
Hydronephrosis, abdominal mass in,
  5
Hyperaldosteronism, orthostatic
  hypotension in, 286
Hypercalcemia
  constipation in, 102
  polydipsia in, 314
  polyuria in, 318
Hypercalcemic nephropathy, nocturia
  in, 274
Hypercapnia, tremors in, 422
Hypercortisolism
  excessive weight gain in, 458
  fatigue in, 172
  muscle atrophy in, 252
  muscle weakness in, 258
Hyperemesis gravidarum
  nausea in, 268
  vomiting in, 453
Hyperinsulinism, excessive weight
  gain in, 458
Hyperkalemia, muscle weakness in,
  259

Hypermelanosis, 471-472
Hypernatremia, decreased level of
  consciousness in, 238
Hyperosmolar hyperglycemic
  nonketotic syndrome
  decreased level of consciousness
    in, 238
  tachycardia in, 406
  tachypnea in, 409
Hyperpigmentation, 471-472
Hyperpnea, 220-221
  managing, 221
Hyperprolactinemia, hirsutism in,
  214
Hypersensitivity pneumonitis,
  nonproductive cough in, 109
Hypersensitivity reaction, agitation in,
  14
Hypersplenism, splenomegaly in, 398
Hypertension
  atrial gallop in, 185
  blood pressure increase in, 52
  dizziness in, 134
  epistaxis in, 158
  headache in, 196
  palpitations in, 292
  tinnitus in, 418
  visual blurring in, 450
Hypertensive crisis, tachycardia in,
  407
Hypertensive encephalopathy
  Cheyne-Stokes respirations and, 88
  generalized tonic-clonic seizures
    in, 384
Hyperthermia, ataxia in, 36
Hyperthyroidism, anxiety in, 28
Hypertrophic cardiomyopathy,
  murmurs in, 250
Hypertrophic obstructive
  cardiomyopathy, pulsus
  biferiens in, 339
Hyperventilation syndrome
  anxiety in, 28
  dizziness in, 134
  hyperpnea in, 220
  paresthesia in, 302
Hypervolemia, jugular vein distention
  in, 231
Hyphema
  conjunctival injection in, 101
  eye pain in, 169
  vision loss in, 447
  visual blurring in, 450
Hypocalcemia
  carpopedal spasm in, 80
  Chvostek's sign in, 94
  dysphagia in, 143
  hyperactive deep tendon reflexes
    in, 124
  muscle spasms in, 254
  palpitations in, 292
  paresthesia in, 302-303

i refers to an illustration; t refers to a table.

i refers to an illustration; t refers to a table.

Intracranial pressure, increased (continued)
signs of, 47t
vomiting in, 453
widened pulse pressure in, 334
Intraductal papilloma
breast nodule in, 64
breast pain in, 66
nipple discharge in, 272
Intraocular foreign bodies
conjunctival injection in, 101
eye pain in, 169
Involuntary guarding, 10-11
Involuntary rigidity, distinguishing, from voluntary rigidity, 10
Iridoplegia, traumatic, mydriasis in, 263
Iritis
conjunctival injection in, 101
photophobia in, 310
sluggish pupils in, 342
visual blurring in, 450
Iron deficiency anemia, pruritus in, 320
Irritable bowel syndrome
abdominal distention in, 3
abdominal pain in, 8
constipation in, 102-103
diarrhea in, 130
flatulence in, 180
nausea in, 269
Ischemic bowel disease, diarrhea in, 130
I.V. therapy, chills in, 91

J

Janeway lesions, 472
Jaundice, 226-227
Jaw pain, 228-229
Jock itch, 189, 189i
Jugular vein distention, 230-231
evaluating, 230i

K

Kaposi's sarcoma, papular rash in, 296
Kegel exercises, 433
Kehr's sign, 472
Keratitis
interstitial, photophobia in, 310
vision loss in, 447
Keratoconjunctivitis
conjunctival injection in, 101
eye discharge in, 167
eye pain in, 169
Kernig's sign, 232-233
eliciting, 232i
as sign of central nervous system crisis, 233

Ketoacidosis. *See also specific type.*
fruity breath odor and, 70
hyperpnea in, 220
Kidneys, palpating, 147i
Kinetic apraxia, 32t
Klinefelter's syndrome, gynecomastia in, 192
Kussmaul's respirations, 220, 221
Kwashiorkor, tremors in, 422
Kyphoscoliosis
asymmetrical chest expansion in, 82
shallow respirations in, 359-360
tracheal deviation in, 420

L

Labyrinthitis
nausea in, 269
nystagmus in, 276
tinnitus in, 418
vertigo in, 442
vomiting in, 453
Lacrimal gland tumor
exophthalmos in, 164
eye pain in, 169
Lactose intolerance
diarrhea in, 130
flatulence in, 180
nausea in, 269
Language centers in brain, 30i
Large-bowel cancer, diarrhea in, 130
Large-bowel obstruction. *See also Intestinal obstruction and Small-bowel obstruction.*
abdominal distention in, 3
fecal breath odor in, 68
visible peristaltic waves in, 308
Laryngeal cancer
dysphagia in, 143
hemoptysis in, 210
hoarseness in, 216
neck pain in, 270
throat pain in, 414
Laryngeal leukoplakia, hoarseness in, 216
Laryngeal tumor
nonproductive cough in, 110
stridor in, 403
Laryngitis
hoarseness in, 216
nonproductive cough in, 110
stridor in, 403
throat pain in, 414
Laryngotracheobronchitis
barking cough in, 106
costal and sternal retractions in, 364
Lead poisoning
anosmia in, 24
chorea in, 92
diarrhea in, 130

Lead poisoning (continued)
dysphagia in, 143
ptosis in, 324-325
Legionnaires' disease
chest pain in, 85
chills in, 90
crackles in, 114-115
nonproductive cough in, 110
productive cough in, 112
Leg muscles, testing strength of, 261i
Leg pain, 234-235
Leg trauma, leg edema in, 156
Leriche's syndrome, intermittent claudication in, 224
Leukemia
epistaxis in, 158
excessive weight loss in, 460-461
gum bleeding in, 190
hepatomegaly in, 213
lymphadenopathy in, 240
purpura in, 344
splenomegaly in, 398
Leukoplakia, mouth lesions in, 248
Levator muscle maldevelopment, ptosis in, 324
Level of consciousness, decreased, 236-239
Lichen amyloidosis, papular rash in, 296
Lichen planus
genital lesions in male in, 188
mouth lesions in, 248-249, 249i
papular rash in, 296
scaly skin in, 394
Lichen simplex chronicus, pruritus in, 320
Lid contractions, increased tearing in, 413
Lid lag, 472
Lifestyle, pyrosis and, 348
Listeriosis
abdominal pain in, 8
diarrhea in, 130-131
vomiting in, 453
Livedo reticularis, mottled skin in, 392
Liver abscess, diaphoresis and, 128
liver cancer, hepatomegaly in, 213
Liver disease
erythema in, 163
purpura in, 344
Liver, percussing, 212i
Lockjaw, 474
Low birth weight, 472
Lower esophageal ring, dysphagia in, 143
Ludwig's angina, jaw pain in, 228
Lumbosacral sprain, back pain in, 43
Lung abscess
clubbing in, 96-97
crackles in, 115
diaphoresis in, 129

i refers to an illustration; t refers to a table.

i refers to an illustration; t refers to a table.

i refers to an illustration; t refers to a table.

i refers to an illustration; t refers to a table.

i refers to an illustration; t refers to a table.

i refers to an illustration; t refers to a table.

i refers to an illustration; t refers to a table.

Rheumatoid arthritis *(continued)*
  muscle atrophy in, 253
  muscle weakness in, 259
  neck pain in, 271
  pleural rub in, 312
Rhinitis
  anosmia in, 24
  facial edema in, 155
  nasal obstruction in, 266
  rhinorrhea in, 366
Rhinorrhea, 366-367
Rhonchi, 368-369
  characteristics of, 369t
Rib fracture, chest pain and, 87
Rift Valley fever, dizziness in, 135
Right ventricular infarction,
      paradoxical pulse in, 298
Rinne test, 199i
Rocky Mountain spotted fever
  chills in, 91
  purpura in, 345
Romberg's sign, 370-371
  assessing, 370i
Rosacea
  butterfly rash in, 76-77
  erythema in, 163
  papular rash in, 296
  pustular rash in, 346
Rubella, erythema in, 163

S

Sacroiliac strain, back pain in, 43
Salivary duct obstruction, decreased
      salivation in, 373
Salivary glands, examining, 372i
Salivation
  decreased, 372-373
  increased, 374-375
Salt craving, 473
Sarcoidosis
  alopecia in, 17
  crackles in, 115
  epistaxis in, 159
  generalized tonic-clonic seizures
      in, 384
  lymphadenopathy in, 240-241
  nonproductive cough in, 110
  papular rash in, 296
Scabies
  genital lesions in male in, 188
  pruritus in, 321
  pustular rash in, 346
  vesicular rash in, 444
Sciatica, leg pain in, 234
Scleritis
  exophthalmos in, 164
  photophobia in, 311
Scleroderma, pyrosis in, 348
Scotoma, 376-377
  locating, 376i
Scrotal swelling, 378-379

Scrotal trauma, scrotal swelling in,
      378
Sebaceous cyst, breast pain in, 66
Seborrheic dermatitis. *See also*
      Dermatitis.
  alopecia in, 17
  butterfly rash in, 77
  erythema in, 162
  genital lesions in male in, 188
  otorrhea in, 288
  scaly skin in, 394
Seborrheic keratosis, papular rash in,
      296
Second-degree atrioventricular heart
      block, pulse rhythm in, 337t
Seizures. *See also specific type.*
  aphasia in, 31
  confusion in, 99
  decreased level of consciousness
      in, 238
  generalized, 380
  muscle weakness in, 259
  paralysis in, 301
  paresthesia in, 303
  partial, 380
  responding to, 383
  vertigo in, 442
Self-catheterization, patient teaching
      for, 431i
Sepsis
  hyperpnea in, 220
  oliguria in, 283
Septal fracture, anosmia in, 25
Septal hematoma, anosmia in, 25
Septicemia, purpura in, 345
Septic shock
  absent or weak pulse in, 327
  blood pressure decrease in, 51
  chills in, 91
  clammy skin in, 390
  generalized edema in, 150
  narrowed pulse pressure in, 333
Setting-sun sign, 474
Severe acute respiratory syndrome
  dyspnea in, 145
  fever in, 176
  headache in, 197
  nonproductive cough in, 110
S_3 heart sound, 186-187
S_4 heart sound, 184-185
Shingles. *See* Herpes zoster.
Shock. *See also specific type.*
  absent or weak pulse in, 327
  cyanosis in, 119
  decreased level of consciousness
      in, 238
  dyspnea in, 145
  hyperpnea in, 220
  increased capillary refill time in, 78
  narrowed pulse pressure in, 333
  pallor in, 291
  tachycardia in, 407

Shock. *(continued)*
  tachypnea in, 409
Shortness of breath, 144-145
Shy-Drager syndrome, anhidrosis in,
      20
Sibilant rhonchi, 462-463
Sickle cell anemia
  hematuria in, 207
  jaundice in, 227
  polydipsia in, 314
  polyuria in, 318
Sickle cell crisis
  abdominal pain in, 9
  chest pain in, 87
Silicosis
  crackles in, 115
  hemoptysis in, 211
  productive cough in, 113
Simple partial seizure, 380, 386-387
  body functions affected by, 386i
Singultus, 471
Sinus arrhythmia, pulse rhythm in,
      337t
Sinusitis
  anosmia in, 25
  epistaxis in, 159
  facial edema in, 155
  facial pain in, 170
  halitosis in, 195
  headache in, 197
  jaw pain in, 228-229
  nasal obstruction in, 266
  nonproductive cough in, 110
  rhinorrhea in, 366
  throat pain in, 415
Sinus tumor
  anosmia in, 24
  rhinorrhea in, 366
Sjögren's syndrome
  decreased salivation in, 373
  taste abnormalities in, 410
Skin
  bronze, 388-389
  clammy, 390-391, 391i
  evaluating color variations in, 388t
  mottled, 392-393
  scaly, 394-395
Skin cancer, alopecia and, 17
Skin lesions, 294-295i
Skin turgor
  decreased, 396-397
  evaluating, 396i
Skull fracture. *See also* Basilar skull
      fracture.
  epistaxis in, 159
  hearing loss in, 200
Sleep apnea
  insomnia in, 222
  stertorous respirations in, 362
Small-bowel obstruction. *See also*
      Intestinal obstruction *and*
      Large-bowel obstruction.

i refers to an illustration; t refers to a table.

Small-bowel obstruction *(continued)*
  abdominal distention in, 3
  fecal breath odor and, 68
  visible peristaltic waves in, 308
Small-bowel tumors, melena in, 246
Small-intestine cancer, hematochezia in, 205
Smallpox
  abdominal pain in, 9
  fever in, 176
  headache in, 197
  papular rash in, 297
  pustular rash in, 347
  vesicular rash in, 445
Smell, absent sense of, 24-25
Solvent poisoning, paresthesia in, 302
Somatoform disorder, anxiety in, 29
Spermatocele, scrotal swelling in, 378
Sphenopalatine neuralgia, facial pain in, 170
Spider angioma, 474
Spider nevus, 474
Spider telangiectasia, 474
Spinal accessory nerve, functions of, 46
Spinal cerebellar degeneration, Romberg's sign in, 371
Spinal cord disease, Romberg's sign in, 371
Spinal cord injury
  accessory muscle use in, 13
  Babinski's reflex in, 40-41
  footdrop in, 182
  muscle atrophy in, 253
  muscle spasticity in, 257
  paralysis in, 301
  paresthesia in, 303
  shallow respirations in, 360
  urinary incontinence in, 431
Spinal cord lesions
  anhidrosis in, 20
  constipation in, 103
  erectile dysfunction in, 160
  fecal incontinence in, 174
  hyperactive deep tendon reflexes in, 124
  hypoactive deep tendon reflexes in, 126-127
  urinary frequency in, 428-429
  urinary urgency in, 432
Spinal cord tumor
  Babinski's reflex in, 41
  Kernig's sign in, 232
  paralysis in, 301
  paresthesia in, 303
Spinal injury or disease, muscle spasms in, 254
Spinal neoplasms, bladder distention in, 48
Spinal stenosis, back pain in, 43
Spinal trauma and disease, muscle weakness in, 259

Spinocerebellar ataxia, 37
Spinous process fracture, neck pain in, 271
Splenic infarction, abdominal pain in, 9
Splenic rupture, splenomegaly in, 399
Splenomegaly, 398-399
  abdominal mass in, 5
  palpating for, 399i
Sprain, leg pain in, 234
Squamous cell carcinoma
  mouth lesions in, 249, 249i
  otorrhea in, 289
  vulvar lesions in, 456, 457i
Squamous cell hyperplasia, vulvar lesions in, 456
Staphylococcal scalded skin syndrome, erythema in, 163
Starvation ketoacidosis
  fruity breath odor in, 70
  hyperpnea in, 220
Status epilepticus, 380
Stellate angioma, 474
Stomatitis
  excessive weight loss in, 461
  increased salivation in, 374
  mouth lesions in, 249, 249i
Stools, clay-colored, 400-401
Strain, leg pain in, 234
Stridor, 402-403
Stroke
  aphasia in, 31
  apraxia in, 33
  ataxia in, 37
  Babinski's reflex in, 41
  decorticate posture in, 123
  decreased level of consciousness in, 238
  diplopia in, 132
  dysarthria in, 139
  fecal incontinence in, 174
  footdrop in, 182
  generalized tonic-clonic seizures in, 384
  hemianopsia in, 208
  hyperactive deep tendon reflexes in, 125
  muscle atrophy in, 253
  muscle spasticity in, 257
  muscle weakness in, 259
  nystagmus in, 276
  ocular deviation in, 279
  paralysis in, 301
  paresthesia in, 303
  simple partial seizures in, 387
  urinary incontinence in, 431
  visual blurring in, 451
Subarachnoid hemorrhage
  Brudzinski's sign in, 73
  headache in, 197
  Kernig's sign in, 232, 233
  neck pain in, 271

Subarachnoid hemorrhage *(continued)*
  paralysis in, 301
Subclavian steal syndrome, bruits in, 75
Subdural hematoma
  decreased level of consciousness in, 239
  headache in, 197
  ptosis in, 324
Sunset eyes, 474
Superior vena cava obstruction, jugular vein distention in, 231
Superior vena cava syndrome
  arm edema in, 153
  facial edema in, 155
Suppurative parotitis, jaw pain in, 229
Surgery
  amenorrhea and, 19
  anosmia and, 25
  carpopedal spasm and, 80
  constipation and, 103
  dyspepsia in, 141
  erectile dysfunction and, 160
  facial edema and, 155
  fecal incontinence and, 174
  hearing loss and, 201
  hypoactive bowel sounds and, 58
  mydriasis and, 263
  nasal obstruction and, 267
  nausea and, 269
  nipple discharge and, 273
  raccoon eyes and, 351
  rhinorrhea and, 367
  scrotal swelling and, 378
  shallow respirations and, 360
  tachycardia and, 407
  urinary incontinence and, 431
  vertigo and, 443
  vomiting and, 454
Swallowing difficulty, 142-143
Sweat, deficiency of, 20-21
Sweating, profuse, 128-129
Sympathectomy, orthostatic hypotension and, 286
Symptom, evaluating, 475i
Syncope, 404-405
Syphilis
  genital lesions in male in, 188
  increased salivation in, 374
  lymphadenopathy in, 241
  mouth lesions in, 249, 249i
  papular rash in, 297
  scaly skin in, 394-395
  sluggish pupils in, 342
  vulvar lesions in, 456, 457i
Systemic lupus erythematosus
  alopecia in, 16-17
  butterfly rash in, 77
  epistaxis in, 159
  fatigue in, 173
  hematuria in, 207

i refers to an illustration; t refers to a table.

i refers to an illustration; t refers to a table.

i refers to an illustration; t refers to a table.

Vitamin B$_6$ deficiency, agitation in, 14
Vitamin B$_{12}$ deficiency, taste
    abnormalities in, 410-411
Vitamin K deficiency, gum bleeding in,
    191
Vitreous hemorrhage
  vision loss in, 448
  visual blurring in, 451
Vocal cord paralysis, hoarseness in,
    216
Vocal cord polyps or nodules,
    hoarseness in, 216
Volkmann's ischemic contracture,
    muscle atrophy in, 252
Voluntary rigidity, distinguishing, from
    involuntary rigidity, 10
Volvulus, vomiting in, 454
Vomiting, 452-455
Vomitus, characteristics of, 453
Vulval cancer, postmenopausal
    vaginal bleeding in, 436
Vulvar lesions, 456-457, 457i

W

Weber's test, 199i
Wegener's granulomatosis
  nasal obstruction in, 266-267
  rhinorrhea in, 366
Weight gain, excessive, 458-459
Weight loss, excessive, 460-461
Wernicke's aphasia, 30i, 31t
Wernicke's disease
  ataxia in, 37
  nonreactive pupils in, 341
  sluggish pupils in, 342
  tremors in, 423
West Nile encephalitis
  decreased level of consciousness
      in, 239
  fever in, 177
  paralysis in, 301
  tremors in, 423
Wheal, 295i
Wheezes, characteristics of, 369t
Wheezing, 462-465
Wilson's disease
  athetosis in, 38
  chorea in, 92
Wristdrop, 474

XY

Xerostomia, 372-373

Z

Zinc deficiency, taste abnormalities in,
    411

i refers to an illustration; t refers to a table.